USING OLD SOLUTIONS TO NEW PROBLEMS - NATURAL DRUG DISCOVERY IN THE 21ST CENTURY

Edited by **Marianna Kulka**

Using Old Solutions to New Problems - Natural Drug Discovery in the 21st Century
http://dx.doi.org/10.5772/46069
Edited by Marianna Kulka

Contributors

Ray Syvitski, Nadine Merkley, Ian Burton, Tobias Karakach, Marianna Kulka, Susan Douglas, Gailene Tobin, Ruwani Kalupahana, Bourlaye Fofana, Kaushik Ghose, Bob Chapman, Kevin Sanderson, Robert Hurta, Priyanka Pundir, Xiaofeng Wang, Kathryn Vanya Ewart, Juergen Krause, Yanwen Wang, H.P. Vasantha Rupasinghe, Wasundara Fernando

Published by InTech

Janeza Trdine 9, 51000 Rijeka, Croatia

Publishing Process Manager Oliver Kurelic
Technical Editor InTech DTP team
Cover InTech Design team

Additional hard copies can be obtained from orders@intechopen.com

Using Old Solutions to New Problems - Natural Drug Discovery in the 21st Century, Edited by Marianna Kulka
p. cm.
ISBN 978-953-51-1158-0

For EU product safety concerns:
IN TECH d.o.o., Prolaz Marije Krucifikse Kozulić 3, 51000 Rijeka, Croatia,
info@intechopen.com or visit our website at intechopen.com.

Meet the editor

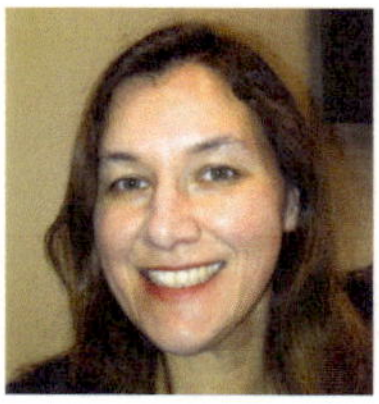

Dr. Marianna Kulka obtained her PhD from the University of Alberta in Edmonton, Alberta, Canada where she studied the role of ion channels in mast cell activation. Dr. Kulka completed her research fellowship at the National Institutes of Health in Bethesda, Maryland, USA where she became interested in human mast cell differentiation and expression of pathogen recognition receptors. Dr. Kulka was a Research Assistant Professor at Northwestern University and investigated mast cells and their role in allergic inflammation until she accepted a research position at the National Research Council (NRC) Canada in 2007. At the NRC, Dr. Kulka has established an immunology research group that is interested in skin microenvironments, human mast cell biology and the use of nanotechnology to improve human health.

Contents

Preface

Modern medicine has been, and will continue to be, extremely dependent upon the discovery of new drugs. As our modern civilization continues to develop, we will be challenged with new and more difficult-to-treat diseases. In large part, these diseases will be the consequence of our rapidly changing lifestyles to which we have not had time to evolve appropriate biological coping mechanisms – obesity and our sedentary lifestyle being just one obvious example. The rise in obesity-related disease, allergic inflammation and certain types of cancers has challenged us to create a new arsenal of drugs that are capable of treating or even preventing these complex diseases. If our search for new medicines is to be successful, we must consider naturally-sourced bioactives as a good starting point. After all, many of our modern drugs are derivatives of natural products and this historical pharmacopeia probably contains a great deal more compounds that have beneficial biologic activity.

The word "drug" is not always associated with herbs and naturally-derived medicine. In fact, herbal and naturopathic remedies have been dissociated from one another in our modern medical lexicon. In essence, however, herbal and folk medicines were the first drugs in the truest sense of the term. The word "drug" is etymologically derived from the Middle Dutch or German word droog or droge meaning "dry barrels" or droge waere, meaning "dry wares" but specifically drugs and spices. The word drogue was later used in Old French in the 14th century meaning "supply, stock or provision" again probably referring to the supply of dried herbs and plants used for medicinal purposes. The word drug was associated with poisons in the 16th century and was later applied to narcotics and opiates in the late 19th century.

Today, the word drug can be generally defined as any chemical or biological agent that affects biologic processes. Drugs can have medicinal, enhancing or intoxicating effects on any living organism, including humans. Drugs can be chemical compounds used in the diagnosis, treatment or prevention of disease but drugs can also be biological products (such as blood products or hormones) used to enhance an athlete's performance in a sport, for example.

Drugs are defined according to their specific ability to affect or modify an abnormal biological condition such as disease or illness. However, medicine has always incorporated a variety of strategies to achieve health – not just drugs – and our modern understanding of healthy diets and enriched foods has given rise to a number of new terms that represent these various approaches to modern health. Therefore, it is useful to define some of these terms like "functional foods" and "nutraceuticals" in the context of what constitutes a drug. "Natural Health Products" or NPH are defined in the US as .....

Nutritional foods consumed for healthy and normal biological functions are not considered drugs, but if the same foods are consumed, often in a more pure form, with the specific purpose of treating a pathological condition, they may be classified as a drug. Foods that have been infused with biological compounds that give them more healthful characteristics (vitamin-enriched water, for example) have been classified as "functional foods" because they function to either prevent disease or alleviate symptoms associated with a particular illness. Still yet are nutraceuticals which refers to products that range from isolated nutrients, dietary supplements and herbal products and is a term that was first coined by Dr. Stephen L. DeFelice, founder and chairman of the Foundation of Innovation Medicine in Crawford, New Jersey. In the US, the term nutraceutical has no legal meaning and most "nutraceutical" products are regulated as drugs, dietary supplements, food ingredients or food. In Canada, the term is defined by Health Canada as "a product isolated or purified from foods that is generally sold in medicinal forms not usually associated with food. A nutraceutical is demonstrated to have a physiological benefit or provide protection against chronic disease." The term nutriceutical is new, but the idea is not. Hippocrates, considered by many to be the father of modern medicine, wrote in his corpus wrote "let food by thy medicine" and health practitioners have promoted certain foods and drinks as fundamentally "healthy" for centuries. It is from these origins that drug discovery undoubtedly began.

The ancient Egyptians, Indians and Chinese all had extensive treatises of herbs or mixtures to alleviate and treat disease. The Ebers Papyrus, dating back to 1550 BC, for example, lists about 800 ancient Egyptian prescriptions for over 700 remedies. Most of the Egyptian drugs have been identified with drugs and active compounds that have been described in current formulations and recipes. The Indian Ayurveda, dating back to 900BC, has been used in India for thousands of years and describes the use of plants for ailments such as hypertension and mental disease. Greek and Latin medicine was heavily influenced by Egyptian medicine and reached a peak during Dioscorides in the first century AD. Claudius Galen was a physician and pharmacist and his approach to therapy often involved complex mixtures called "galenicals" from which he believed the body would select the appropriate medicinal ingredient that it needed.

With the fall of the Roman Empire, the use of medicinal plants came to be associated with witchcraft and sorcery and ancient science was, for the most part, neglected by western society. However, some scholars preserved and transmitted some of this vast information and Islamic schools and monastic abbeys played an important part in this process. By the Renaissance, some of this ancient information was re-discovered and revised. Valerius Cordus was a German botanist who in 1542 wrote a botanic treatise in which he introduced "laudanum," a formulation that contained opium extract and was used widely by European and North American doctors until the mid-19th century.

Modern drug discovery began with the breakthroughs in chemical and biological sciences in the 19th century wherein the isolation, chemical characterization and analytical determination of bioactive molecules could be done. It was at this point that the chemical identity of these bioactive compounds could finally be defined and this knowledge was used to create more effective, potent and targeted drugs that were also more stable and had fewer side-effects. This new field of drug discovery is beautifully examined in the first chapter of this book.

As drug discovery progressed, we made new leaps in our understanding of molecular structures and how they can be manipulated to make bioactive compounds much more potent or more specific. This allowed us to not only create "designer" drugs but gave us the opportunity to go back to the ancient pharmacopeia to find similar compounds.

As our population ages, our need for new and more dynamic medications will increase. The diverse set of professionals that are now involved in drug discover must all work together to achieve this goal.

Marianna Kulka
National Research Council Canada ,
Canada

Section 1

Agronomy and Molecular Characterization

Chapter 1

Discovery, Development, and Regulation of Natural Products

Juergen Krause and Gailene Tobin

Additional information is available at the end of the chapter

http://dx.doi.org/10.5772/56424

1. Introduction

Natural products have historically been an extremely productive source for new medicines in all cultures and continue to deliver a great variety of structural templates for drug discovery and development. Although products derived from natural sources may not necessarily represent active ingredients in their final form, the majority of all drugs in the market have their origin in nature [1, 2]. Therefore, the foremost emphasis in this chapter is given to aspects concerning the identification, properties, and development of potential drug candidates from natural products. It is the intention to give a high-level overview of the current status and developments in the field. Many important aspects in the arena of natural therapeutics including natural product sources, discovery, characterization, development and uses have been addressed and covered in depth in excellent recent reviews by extremely competent authors referenced in this contribution.

1.1. Definition of a natural product

The extent to which the term natural product has been characterized is both limited and debatable. Therefore, a common definition that is accepted by all involved disciplines will remain a moving target, but likely will evolve as researchers unveil the vast amount of compounds projected to be discovered in this field [3]. In the simplest of terms, a natural product is a small molecule that is produced by a biological source [3]. As a central theme of exploration bordering chemistry and biology, natural products research focuses on the chemical properties, biosynthesis and biological functions of secondary metabolites [3]. In this context, the task of defining "natural" is more straight forward and encompasses isolation from a native organism, synthesis in a laboratory, biosynthesis *in vitro*, or isolation from a metabolically engineered organism whereby the chemical structure has been determined and the resultant compound is chemically equivalent to the original natural product [3]. Thus, in summary, and for the purposes of this chapter, one can still agree with the refuted definition that a natural product is a pharmacologically or biologically active chemical compound or substance, which is found in nature and produced by a living organism and can even be considered as such if it can be prepared by a totally synthetic approach [4]. Albeit, we realize this definition can be challenged as many biosynthetic enzymes are nonspecific and may result in the production of multiple analogs combined with the fact that identifying the entirety of natural products is in the infant stage [5].

Generally the term "natural product" is regarded as being synonymous with "secondary metabolite" [6]. Secondary metabolites are organic compounds in the correct chiral configuration to exert biological activity, but have no "primary" function directly involved in the normal growth, development or reproduction of an organism [7]. Natural products are usually relatively small molecules with a molecular weight below 3,000 Daltons and exhibit considerable structural diversity [6]. The product categories in which natural compounds can be found as active ingredients include prescription and non-prescription drugs (pharmaceuticals), cosmetic ingredients (cosmeceuticals) and dietary supplements and natural health product ingredients (nutriceuticals) [8].

The respective studies leading to the identification, isolation, and characterization of natural products constitute an important part of the scientific field of pharmacognosy. The American Society of Pharmacognosy defines pharmacognosy as "*the study of natural product molecules (typically secondary metabolites) that are useful for their medicinal, ecological, gustatory, or other functional properties. The natural species that are the source of the compounds under study span all biological kingdoms, most notably marine invertebrates, plants, fungi, and bacteria*" [9]. Amongst the various assortments and exciting capacities that are being explored within the arena of pharmacognosy, this chapter will mostly address the study of health relevant medicinal properties of natural compounds for drug discovery and development.

1.2. History

Natural substances have evolved over a very long selection process to form optimal interactions with biological macromolecules [10] which have activity on a biological system that is relevant to the target disease. They have historically been the most productive source of active compounds and chemical lead structures for the discovery and development of new medicines [11]. Since ancient times, civilizations used plants and plant extracts to ameliorate diseases and foster healing. Early historic examples for medical treatments from natural sources include the discovery of the beneficial effects of *cardiotonic digitalis* extracts from foxglove for treating some manifestations of heart disease in the 18th century, the use of the bark of the willow and cinchona trees in treating fever and the effectiveness of poppy extracts in the treatment of dysenteries [12]. Morphine, largely reproducing the analgesic and sedative effect of opium, was isolated from opium obtained from the seed pots of the poppy plant in 1804 [12]. Throughout the century, purified bioactive natural products were extracted from the Peruvian bark cinchoa (quinine), from cocoa (cocaine), and from many other plants [12]. By 1829, scientists discovered that the compound salicin, in willow trees, was responsible for pain relief and in 1838 salicylic acid was isolated [13]. The problem was that salicylic acid was harsh on the stomach and in the second half of the 19th century acetylsalicylic acid was synthesized which served as a less-irritating replacement for standard common salicylate medicines [13]. A number of additional plants served as sources of natural product derived agents that are still used in current routine medical practice [14].

The discovery of valuable therapeutic agents from natural sources continued into the 20th century. Inspired by the discovery and benefits of penicillin, pharmaceutical research expanded after the Second World War into intensive screening of microorganisms for new antibiotics [12]. The study of new bacterial and fungal strains resulted in the expansion of the antibacterial arsenal with additional agents such as cephalosporins, tetracyclines, aminoglycosides, rifamycins, chloramphenicol, and lipopeptides [15, 16]. In the 1950's, two nucleosides isolated from Caribbean marine sponges paved the way for the synthesis of vidarabine, and the related compound cytarabine, which eventually received approval as therapeutics for clinical use in viral diseases and cancer, respectively [17]. A more recent example is the cancer therapeutic paclitaxel (Taxol®) derived from the Yew tree, which was discovered in the 1970s, but due to difficulties in obtaining commercial compound quantities only reached the market in late 1992 [18-20]. Overall, only 244 prototypic chemical structures (over 80% came from animal, plant, microbial or mineral origin) have been used as templates to produce medicines up to 1995, and relatively few new scaffolds have appeared since [21,22]. About half of the marketed agents in today's arsenal of drugs are derived from biological sources with the large majority being based on terrestrial natural product scaffolds [23]. Approximately 50% of the new drugs introduced since 1994 were either natural products or derivatives thereof [21, 23, 24].

2. Discovery and development

2.1. Discovery

Drug discovery involves the identification of new chemical entities (NCEs) of potential therapeutic value, which can be obtained through isolation from natural sources, through chemical synthesis or a combination of both. The field of natural products drug discovery, despite the success stories of penicillin, paclitaxel, etc., also had aspects that made it less attractive. In the traditional approach, drug targets were exposed to crude extracts, and in case of evidence of pharmacological activity the extract was fractionated and the active compound isolated and identified. This method was slow, labor intensive, inefficient, and provided no guarantee that a lead from the screening process would be chemically workable or even patentable [25, 26]. As natural products usually are molecules with more complex structures, it was more difficult to extract, purify or synthesize sufficient quantities of a NCE of interest for discovery and development activities [25]. Enriched or pure material is needed for the initial characterization of the chemical and biological properties as well as the elucidation of structure-activity relationships in drug discovery studies; furthermore, even larger quantities need to be supplied for potential later development activities and ultimately, the market [24, 27].

The pharmaceutical industry's interest in natural products diminished with the advent of such promising new technologies like combinatorial chemistry (CC) and high throughput screening (HTS) [28]. The prospect of such disciplines, aimed at accelerating drug discovery efforts for NCEs, led some companies to dismiss their natural product programs [28]. Combinatorial chemistry employs parallel synthesis techniques allowing the creation of libraries containing hundreds of thousands of compounds, whereas HTS allows rapid testing of large numbers of compounds [28]. High-throughput screening grew out of automated clinical analyzer technologies and miniaturization in the late 1980's, as drug companies focused on methods aiming to increase the pace of testing and lower the cost per sample [12]. As a result, large libraries of synthetic molecules could be exploited very quickly. These new synthetic libraries were also given preference because of the lack of compatibility of traditional natural product extract libraries with HTS assays [28-30]. Compounds obtained from commercial libraries, in-house collections of pharmaceutical companies containing hundreds of thousands of compounds and new libraries generated through CC could be now screened rapidly [21]. Although the initial hopes for such advances were high, they were not fulfilled by either of the improved technologies. To be successful, HTS needed appropriate therapeutic targets matched to collections of NCEs that are highly diverse in their structural and physicochemical properties. The approach to exclusively bank on synthetic compounds did not meet the initial expectations, as the newly created compound libraries had limited structural diversity and did not provide enough quality hits to be of value. For CC, the most valuable role of parallel synthesis therefore appears to be in expanding on an existing lead, rather than creating new screening libraries [12]. Consequently, the interest in natural sources experienced some renaissance; however, even if natural product extracts were tested first, the pace of their isolation made it difficult to keep up with the demand for testing candidates in high-throughput models [25, 26, 29]. Therefore, natural products, and derivatives thereof, are still under-represented in the typical screening decks of the pharmaceutical and biopharmaceutical industry [31]. Specifically, it has been noted that major pharmaceutical companies in the United States continue to favor approaches that do not enable the integration of natural products of marine origin into their screening libraries [32]. More risk friendly institutions like academic laboratories, research institutes and small biotech companies venturing in the natural products arena have now a greater role in drug discovery and feed candidates into the development pipelines of big pharmaceutical companies[32].

Overall, there are limited systematic approaches to exploring traditionally used natural products for compounds that could serve as drug leads. Additionally, the pharmaceutical industry has decreased their emphasis on natural product discovery from sources in various countries. Both of these facts may be based on possible uncertainties and concerns over expectations about benefits sharing resulting from the United Nations Convention on Biological Diversity (CBD) [21, 33, 34]. Countries are increasingly protective of their natural assets in flora and fauna and may not authorize the collection of sample species without prior approval [35]. In this context, potential handicaps may arise for companies as they develop and market new products from natural sources in the form of very difficult to negotiate agreements as well as significant intellectual property and royalty issues [25, 26, 28, 35].

Nonetheless, natural products continue to provide a valuable and rich pool for the discovery of templates and drug candidates and are suitable for further optimization by synthetic means because the chemical novelty associated with natural products is higher than that of structures from any other source [10]. This fact is of particular importance when seeking out lead molecules against newly discovered targets where no small molecule lead exists or in mechanistic and pathway studies when searching for chemical probes [24]. It is assumed that. in many cases, structures devised by nature and evolution are far superior to even the best synthetic moieties in terms of diversity, specificity, binding efficiency, and propensity to interact with biological targets [24]. In comparing a large number of natural products to compounds from CC and synthetic drugs derived from natural substances, it has become evident that drugs and products obtained from natural sources exhibited more diverse and chemically complex structures [36]. In fact, only a moderate structural overlap was found when comparing natural product scaffolds to drug collections with the natural product database containing a significantly larger number of scaffolds and exhibiting higher structural novelty [37]. The structural diversity of these naturally sourced compounds supports the belief that the assortment of natural products represents a greater variety and better exemplifies the 'chemical space' of drug-like scaffolds than those of synthetic origin [30, 38, 39]. As Newman and Cragg (2012) have stated, and demonstrated in their reviews for the 30-year period of 1981 to 2010, natural products do play a dominant role in the discovery of lead structures for the development of drugs for the treatment of human diseases [1]. We agree with these authors in their assumption that it is highly probable that in the near future totally synthetic variations of even complex natural products will be part of the arsenal of physicians [1].

In general, there is growing awareness of the limited structural diversity in existing compound collections. The historic focus of the pharmaceutical industry on a relatively small set of 'druggable' targets has resulted in the exploration of a very narrow chemical space appropriate for these targets [40]. The 207 human targets described for small-molecule drugs correspond to only about 1% of the human genome and half of all drugs target only four protein classes [41]. So called 'undruggable' targets, such as protein-protein interactions and phosphatases, still await the identification of lead structures with the required qualities for lead or development candidates [40]. Although the expectations in natural products for the future are still high, an analysis of the distinct biological network between the targets of natural products and disease genes revealed that natural products, as a group, may still not contain enough versatility to yield suitable treatments for all heritable human diseases [42]. Nevertheless, the importance of natural product related compound collections, as the most promising avenue to explore new bioactive chemical space for drug discovery, continues to be emphasized; consequently, efforts have been made over the last decade to generate CC libraries inspired by natural product scaffolds [31, 43, 44]. Those scaffolds, which have presumably undergone evolutionary selection over time, might possess favorable properties in terms of bioactivity and selectivity and therefore provide biologically validated valuable starting points for the design and generation of new combinatorial libraries [25, 26, 45, 46]. Thomas and Johannes state that the production of relatively small natural product like libraries have revealed biologically active compounds, while modification of natural products identified activity that is entirely unrelated to the parent molecules [31].

Libraries of small molecules of natural origin have already served as templates for the majority of approved therapeutics including important compounds for the treatment of life-threatening conditions. Moreover, these small molecule libraries are constantly growing through products extracted from various natural sources. Harvey *et al.* reviewed the current approaches for expansion of natural product based compound libraries and CBD compliant collections exist at the U.S. National Cancer Institute, academic institutions and commercial companies [11]. However, large collections of pure natural products are rare and the quantities of individual compounds that are isolated are typically small. A more recent strategy has been to use natural product scaffolds as templates for creating libraries of semi-synthetic and synthetic analogues [21, 28, 47]. Rosen *et al.* identified several hundred unique natural products which could serve as starting points in the search for novel leads with particular properties [48]. Based on the continuous efforts of researchers in the field of marine drug discovery, more potent bioactive lead structures are expected with new or unknown mechanisms of action [23, 48]. The progress made in the areas of cellular biology, genomics, and molecular mechanisms increased the number of druggable targets, allowing screening for candidates of natural compound libraries against an ever increasing number of potential molecular sites for therapeutic intervention. This increase in defined molecular targets combined with more automatization, more sensitive detection instruments, and faster data processing allows for high throughput assays, which can rapidly screen large existing libraries of new and specific biological targets.

In the last decade there has also been a major shift to technologically advanced and more complex screening assays conducted in cells, including those in which biological function is directly measured. These more complex approaches provide higher stringency which can mean lower hit rates. However, the specificity of such hits results in an increase in the quality of leads with more desired biological properties [12]. In this context, bioassays based on zebrafish embryos are noteworthy, as they can be used in 96-well plates and allow for *in vivo* bioactivity screening of crude extracts and natural substances at the microgram scale [49-52]. A further improvement, potentially leading to new secondary metabolites of interest for drug discovery, is based on the development of refined analytical and spectroscopic methods. This involves rapid identification and structural elucidation (dereplication) of natural products in complex mixtures (such as crude or pre-fractionated extracts) in parallel with profiling their bioactivity in information-rich bioassays [53]. In addition, stress can be applied to stimulate the number and levels of bioactive compounds in organisms. Wolfender and Queiroz presented examples of dynamic responses resulting from stress, which induced chemical defenses in elicitation experiments in both plants and microorganisms [30]. A significantly increased number of hits, including antibacterial, antifungal and anticancer agents were described for extracts from elicited plants [30]. New groups of microorganisms obtained through small scale, high-through-put cultivation methods and employing nutrient deficient media, specific nutrients and long cultivation times constitute another approach potentially leading to new secondary metabolites of interest for drug discovery [54]. Genome mining, the analyses of plant and microbial genome sequences for genes and gene clusters encoding proteins, is a further recent approach which has allowed the discovery of numerous novel natural products and also revealed gene clusters and novel pathways for the biosynthesis of several known natural compounds [55, 56].

Although plants are still the major source for many natural products and remedies, microbes and marine organisms also constitute promising, abundant, and valuable sources for bioactive natural compounds [57]. Like it is true for plants, also for these, only a very small fraction of structures of potential therapeutic relevance have been chemically analyzed or examined in a broad panel of screening models or bioassays. But even if discovered and identified, active substances from natural sources may not be readily available for further investigations, development or introduction to the market. A number of biologically relevant natural products can only be isolated in small amounts, consequently adding to efforts, timelines and costs by forcing the development of an economically viable synthesis [31].

2.2. Development

The time required to develop a pharmaceutical can range from only a few to as many as 20 years. For natural products, an additional challenge can be the provision of sufficient quantities from natural sources for development and consequently commercial market supplies. Early *in vitro* tests may only require microgram to milligram amounts but the demand for compound quantities will increase quickly when *in vivo* animal models, safety and toxicology studies, formulation development and ultimately clinical trials are initiated. As mentioned earlier, one of the more recent respective examples is the cancer drug paclitaxel (Taxol®), which was discovered in 1967 as the cytotoxic active ingredient in extracts of *Taxus brevifolia* but only approved for the market in 1992 [20]. From 1967 to 1993, almost all paclitaxel produced was derived from bark from the Pacific yew tree [18]. Harvesting of the bark kills the tree in the process, however, this production method was replaced by a more sustainable approach using a precursor of Taxol® isolated from the leaves and needles of cultivated yew tree species [18, 20].

The compounds in development today target a variety of indications, mainly cancer and infectious diseases (bacterial, viral, fungal, and parasitic), but also address other therapeutic areas such as cardiovascular diseases, neurological illnesses and depression, metabolic diseases (like diabetes and cholesterol management), and inflammatory diseases (like arthritis) [1, 15, 16, 25, 26]. The cytotoxic properties of many secondary metabolites from marine organisms and bacteria are of particular interest for the development of new anticancer treatments [58]. For infectious diseases, natural products are effective because most of these compounds evolved from microbial warfare and show activity against other microorganisms at low concentrations [25, 26, 29]. The renewed interest in natural drugs is determined by the urgent need to find and develop effective means to fight infections caused by viruses, like HIV (Human Immunodeficiency Virus) and so called "superbugs" (bacteria with multiple resistance against antibiotics) currently in use [29]. Pathogens having only limited and rather expensive treatment options include penicillin-resistant *Streptococcus pneumonia*, methicillin-resistant *Staphylococcus aureus* (MRSA), vancomycin-resistant *Enterococcus* (VRE), *Clostridium difficile*, and *Mycobacterium tuberculosis* [29]. However, some new structures identified from marine fungi exhibited activity against bacteria like MRSA [59].

Before the advent of high throughput screening and the post-genomic era, more than 80% of drug substances or active ingredients were natural products, semisynthetic analogs thereof, or were obtained using structures of natural compounds as templates for synthetic modification [60, 61]. Chin reported 23 drugs from natural sources being approved between 2000 and 2005 [2]. Between 1998 and 2007 a total of 34 natural products and natural product-derived drugs were approved in different international markets [15, 62, 63].

According to Brahmachari (2011), 38 natural product-derived drugs were approved in the decade from 2000 to 2010 for various indications including 15 for infectious diseases, 7 each for oncology, neurological diseases and cardiovascular disorders, 4 for metabolic disorders and 1 for diabetes [22]. It is therefore not surprising that by 2008 more than a hundred new drug candidates from natural sources like plants, bacteria, fungi and animals or those obtained semi-synthetically were reported to be in clinical development with a similar number in preclinical development [60]. Of those in clinical development, 91 were described to be plant-derived [63]. Although this was a lower number than in the years before, the interest in natural sources to obtain pharmacologically active compounds has recently been rekindled with improved access to a broader base of sources including those from new microbial and marine origins [23, 64]. Brahmachari (2011) reported 49 plant-derived, 54 microorganism-derived, 14 marine organism derived (including 2 from fish and 1 from a cone snail), and 1 terrestrial animal-derived (bovine neutrophils) drug candidate(s) in various phases of clinical evaluation [22].

Natural products have been the biggest single source of anti-cancer drugs as evidenced by the historical data reviewed by Newman and Cragg [1]. Of the 175 anti-cancer agents developed and approved over the seven decades from 1940 until 2010 in Western countries and Japan, 85 compounds representing 48.6%, were natural products or directly derived from natural products [1]. The four major structural classes of plant derived cancer treatments include Vinca alkaloids, Epipodophyllotoxin lignans, Taxane diterpenoids and Camptotectin quinolone alkaloid derivatives. Approximately 30 plant derived anti-cancer compounds have been reported to be clinically active against various types of tumors and are currently used in clinical trials [65].

A potential development candidate is typically isolated from its natural source only in milligram quantities [6]. Testing *in vitro* occurs in assays such as the U.S National Cancer Institute 60-cell-line panel, followed by human tumor-derived cell lines in primary culture and *in vivo* animal models such as the above mentioned zebrafish embryos, the hollow-fiber human tumor cell assay or human tumor xenografts in rodents [6, 50, 52, 66]. Harvey and Cree have recently reviewed current screening systems for anti-cancer activity suitable for use with collections of natural products. These include quantification of cell growth or cell death in standard cancer cell, three-dimensional and primary cell culture, as well as cell-based reporter and molecular assays [50]. The quantification of cell growth or cell death in culture using signals like caspase-3 as a marker for apoptosis come with the handicap that the artificial culture environment may not be suitable to predict activity in *in vivo* animal models or cancer patients [50]. Another concern raised is the fact that compounds which kill readily proliferating cancer cells in culture may not eliminate the tumor because of the persistence of cancer stem cells for which suitable screening assays with significant throughput are still lacking [50]. Cancer stem cells are only present in low abundance and remain in a quiescent state until receiving environmental cues such as overexpression of growth factors, cytokines, or chemokines resulting in recurrence of cancer after initially successful treatment and loss of efficacy of the initial treatment agent in the relapsed disease [67].

Dietary sources of compounds assumed to have anti-cancer benefits include fruits, vegetables and spices yielding biologically active components such as curcumin, resveratrol, cucurbitacins, isoflavones, saponins, phytosterols, lycopene, and many others [68]. A number of these are gaining importance as adjuvant anti-cancer agents with curcumin, resveratrol and cucurbitacins having activity reported against cancer stem cells [67]. Bhanot *et al* list 39 natural compounds from marine species, mostly invertebrates, and 10 from microorganisms, mostly from bacteria of the *Streptomyces* genus, as potential new anti-cancer agents [68]. It is assumed that many prokaryotic and eukaryotic natural product sources may still reveal a number of valuable anti-cancer compounds in the future and even ancient animal species have been suggested as a particularly valuable source [69].

Anti-virals constitute another important class of needed therapeutics. The HIV type-1 (HIV-1) is the cause of the Acquired Immune Deficiency Syndrome (AIDS), a major human viral disease with over 34 million people infected worldwide in 2012 and approximately 1.7 million dying per year [70]. Failure of anti-HIV therapy is observed due to the emergence of drug resistance and the significant side effect profile of existing therapies [71]. Hence, the quest for novel prospective drug candidates with fewer side effects and increased efficacy against various HIV strains also relies on natural products. Naturally derived anti-HIV compounds found to be most promising for the treatment HIV infections, with the potential to overcome drug-resistance of mutated HIV strains, were described to be flavonoids, coumarins, terpenoids, tannins, alkaloids, polyphenols, polysaccharides or proteins [72, 73]. Despite the need for affordable, effective, and better tolerated treatments, the vast majority of the potential natural anti-HIV compounds described have so far only been tested as *in vitro, ex vivo* or *in silico* approaches to identify activity; the findings have not yet been confirmed in relevant *in vivo* systems. Only a few of the many natural products that have been reported to exhibit anti-HIV activities have reached clinical trials and none of them made it on the list of conventional antiretroviral drugs [71, 72].

Antiviral agents from marine sources which demonstrated activity against HIV were recently reviewed by Vo and Kim (2010). These include phlorotannins from brown algae, sulfated derivatives of chitin from the shells of crabs and shrimps including chitosan (produced commercially by deacetylation of chitin), sulfated polysaccharides from marine algae, lectins or carbohydrate-binding proteins from a variety of different species (ranging from prokaryotes to corals, algae, fungi, plants, invertebrates and vertebrates) as well as bioactive peptides isolated by enzymatic hydrolysis of marine organisms [73]. Until now, most of the anti-HIV activities of these marine-derived inhibitors were also only observed in *in vitro* assays or in mouse model systems and still await confirmation of their value in clinical trials [73].

3. Natural product sources

Historically, the most important sources for biologically active natural products have been terrestrial plants and microorganisms such as fungi and bacteria. Terrestrial and aquatic species of plants and microorganisms, especially those of marine origin, produce unique bioactive substances yielding a large variety of valuable therapeutics and lead structures for potential new drugs. Even though natural products may not have coevolved with human proteins, they have emerged in nature to interact with biomolecules [74]. Natural products interact with a wide variety of proteins and other biological targets, acting also as modulators of cellular processes when they inhibit the difficult to target protein-protein interactions [27, 40].

Since the middle of the last century, marine species and microorganisms have consistently and increasingly raised interest as sources for new agents and scaffolds [75]. In recent years, other less conventional sources like alcoholic and non-alcoholic beverages, spices, animal and human excreta, and many more have generated interest for natural product researchers [75]. The more conventional sources for secondary metabolites like plants, marine organisms and microorganisms will be described in more detail in the following sections.

3.1. Plants

A significant number of drugs have been derived from plants that were traditionally employed in ethnomedicine or ethnobotany (the use of plants by humans as medicine as in Ayurvedic or Traditional Chinese Medicine), while others were discovered initially (through random screening of plant extracts in animals) or later, by determining their *in vitro* activity against HIV or cancer cell lines [6, 50, 71-73]. An avenue that may have influenced ethnopharmacology suggests that some traditionally used remedies may have arisen from observations of self-medication by animals [76]. Studies have shown that wild animals often consumed plants and other material for medical rather than nutritional reasons, treating parasitic infections and possible viral and bacterial diseases [11, 60, 76, 77]. For drug discovery, the chemical and pharmacologic investigation of ethnobotanical information offers a viable alternative to high-throughput screening and the body of existing ethnomedical knowledge has led to great developments in health care. It would appear that selection of plants, based on long-term human use in conjunction with appropriate biologic assays that correlate with the ethnobotanical uses, should be most successful [78]. Nevertheless, therapeutic approaches based on active principles from single plant and polyherbal formulations from traditional medicines, like the ones mentioned in Ayurvedic texts, still require scientific validation and sufficient pharmacoepidemiological evidence supporting their safety and efficacy [79]. This is evidenced by the example of aristolochic acid, a constituent of *Aristolochia* vines, which are used in complementary and alternative therapies. Aristolochic acid is a powerful nephrotoxin and a human carcinogen associated with chronic kidney disease and upper urinary tract urothelial carcinomas (UUC) [80]. These dual toxicities and the target tissues were revealed when a group of otherwise healthy Belgian women developed renal failure and UUC after ingesting *Aristolochia* herbs in conjunction with a weight-loss regime; subsequently, more cases were reported in Taiwan and countries throughout the world [80]. Importantly, the traditional practice of Chinese herbal medicine in Taiwan mirrors that in China and other Asian countries making it likely that these toxicities are also prevalent in these and in other countries where *Aristolochia* herbs have long been used for treatment and prevention of disease, thereby creating an international public health problem of considerable magnitude [80, 81].

In the early 1900's, 80% of all medicines were obtained from roots, barks and leaves and it is estimated is that approximately 25% of all drugs prescribed today still originate from plants [14, 19, 78]. The plant kingdom, with 300,000 to 400,000 higher species (estimated levels reach from 215,000 up to 500,000 [78], was always a key source of new chemical entities (NCEs) for active pharmaceutical ingredients and lead compounds [12]. It is estimated that only 5% to 15% of these terrestrial plants have been chemically and pharmacologically investigated in a systemic fashion [19]. Approximately 10,000 to 15,000 of the world's plants have documented medicinal uses and roughly 150-200 have been incorporated in western medicine [19, 82]. Marine plants like microalgae, macroalgae (seaweeds) and flowering plants (such as mangroves) have been studied to a much lesser extent and are mostly reported in connection with nutritional, supplemental or ethnopharmacological uses [83]. For over 20 years the U.S. National Cancer Institute has collected higher plants for screening, with the current collection composed of ~ 30,000 species [84]. Only a small percentage of these have reportedly been screened for biological or phytochemical activity until a decade ago and large numbers are constantly being tested for their possible pharmacological value today [35, 78]. Based on their research, the authors justify their assumption that the plant kingdom still holds many species containing substances of medicinal value and for potential pharmaceutical applications, which have yet to be discovered. However, such assumptions may be diminished as the loss of valuable natural sources increases due to factors such as deforestation, environmental pollution, and global warming [85].

Saslis-Lagoudakis *et al.* provided evidence through phylogenetic cross-cultural comparisons that related plants from different geographic regions are used to treat medical conditions in the same therapeutic areas [86]. Accordingly, there has been a recent surge in interest in the components of traditional Chinese medicines and Ayurvedic remedies [11]. Limitations of this approach include the fact that both of these ancient traditions use polyherbal preparations (botanicals) for the majority of prescriptions and that plants as biological systems have an inherent potential variability in their chemistry and resulting biological activity [12, 35]. Fabricant and Farnsworth reported that 25% of all plants showing biological activity in their assay system failed to reproduce the activity on sub-sequent recollections [35]. This may be caused by factors coming into play after the collection of a specimen, however, for plants it is common to dry the collected plant parts thoroughly in the field before extraction to assure that the material does not compose before reaching the laboratory [12].

Rout *et al.* describe the approaches for using individual plants as therapeutic agents as follows: (i) to isolate bioactive compounds for direct use as drugs, (ii) to produce bioactive derivatives of known compounds as new structures, (iii) to use substances as pharmacologic agents or tools, and (iv) to use a whole or partial plant as herbal remedy and provide examples for each category [78]. Mixtures of plant-derived products are known as botanicals, and the term is defined by the United States (US) Food and Drug Administration (FDA) to describe finished, labeled products that contain vegetable matter as ingredients which can include plant materials, algae, macroscopic fungi, and combinations thereof [87]. They can fall under the classification of a food (including a dietary supplement), a drug (including a biological drug), a medical device, or a cosmetic [87]. The vast majority of plant-derived treatments are based on synthetic, semisynthetic, or otherwise highly purified or chemically modified drugs [87, 88]. According to the most recent report by BCC Research, the global plant-derived drug market was valued at US$ 22.1 billion in 2012 and sales are projected to grow to US$ 26.6 billion by 2017 at a compound annual growth rate (CAGR) of 3.8% [89]. The botanicals subgroup currently has only one approved drug, Veregen, with an expected revenue increase from US $ 2.8 million in 2010 to 599 million in 2017 [89].

3.2. Marine life

Given the fact that oceans cover nearly 70% of the earth's surface and that life originated in the oceans with the first marine organisms evolving more than 3.5 billion years ago, the enormous diversity of organisms in the marine environment is not surprising and largely unexplored [90]. On some coral reefs, their density can reach up to 1,000 species per square meter, which is believed to be a higher biodiversity than observed in tropical rainforests and inspired researchers for decades to search for novel compounds from marine sources [57, 91]. As the greatest biodiversity is found in the oceans, it is estimated that between 250,000 and one million marine species could provide an immense resource to discover NCEs serving as unprecedented novel bioactive structures and scaffolds that have the potential to serve as medical treatments or templates for new therapeutics [23, 92].

The interest in novel chemical structures from marine organisms started in the 1950s as marine animal taxonomy advanced significantly, but progressed at a slow pace for the first two decades before it started to burgeon in the 1970s [91-94]. Since then, approximately 30,000 structurally diverse natural products with a vast array of bioactivities have been discovered from marine organisms including microbes, algae and invertebrates [92, 95]. Invertebrates alone comprise approximately 60% of all marine animals and were described as the source of almost 10,000 new natural products since 1990 with a pronounced increase to about 1,000 compounds per year in more recent years [23, 32, 93].

By the turn of the 21st century larger percentages of bioactive NCEs were reported for marine organisms in comparison to terrestrial organisms, but nevertheless, marine chemical ecology is still several decades behind its terrestrial counterpart with respect to the total number of characterized and documented natural products [93, 96]. Kong *et al.* specifically compared natural products from terrestrial and marine sources. They found that compounds from marine organisms exhibited a higher chemical novelty and that over 2/3 of those scaffolds were exclusively used by marine species, but alerted readers to concerns of the suitability of the new scaffolds as drug templates because of their unsuitably high hydrophobicity [96]. As is the case for plant derived natural compounds, the U.S. National Cancer Institute also plays an important role for establishing marine organism collections since the 1980s and has a vast National repository of invertebrate derived compounds and extracts from specimens rigorously identified by taxonomic experts [92].

Many marine natural products appear to arise from multi-functional enzymes that are also present in terrestrial systems, exhibiting a cross phylum activity with terrestrial biota [94, 95]. However, a large number of marine derived compounds also possess a substantial amount of functional groups, which were not previously described from terrestrial metabolites [91, 94, 95]. They range from derivatives of amino acids and nucleosides to macrolides, porphyrins, terpenoids, aliphatic cyclic peroxides, and sterols [91]. These secondary metabolites resulted from evolutionary pressure threatening many marine organisms, especially those which are soft bodied and have a sedentary life style, forcing them to develop the ability to synthetize toxic compounds which serve to deter predators, manage competitors or immobilize prey [57, 91, 93, 94]. The search for new drug candidates from marine species has expanded into circumpolar regions for cold-adapted species as well as harsh environments like deep-sea hydrothermal vents; these approaches have been particularly successful with filter-feeders such as sponges, tunicates and bryozoans [23, 97].

The fact that marine invertebrates contain astounding levels of microbial diversity and form highly complex microbial communities led to the assumption, followed by confirmation in recent examples, that microbial symbionts like bacteria are important producers of natural products derived from marine species [58]. In particular, these include polyketides and non-ribosomally synthesized peptides as well as unique biosynthetic enzymes which emerged as potent biocatalysts in medicinal chemistry [58, 97].

By 2010, four drugs of marine origin had obtained approval for the treatment of human disorders [98]. Cytarabine (Cytosar-U®; Upjohn/Pfizer) for the treatment of white blood cell cancers, vidarabine (Vira-A®; discontinued by distributor Monarch Pharmaceuticals) an ophtalmic antiviral, and ziconotide (Prialt®; Elan) for pain management were FDA approved and trabectedin (Yondelis®; Pharmamar), an anticancer compound against soft tissue and ovarian cancer was approved in Europe [98]. Vidarabine and cytarabine originate from marine sponges, ziconotide is the synthetic equivalent of a conopeptide originating from a marine cone snail, and trabectedin, now produced synthetically, originates from a bacterial symbiont of a tunicate or sea squirt [32, 99]. At the same time, 13 marine organism-derived drug candidates were listed to be in clinical development (3 in Phase III, 7 in Phase II, and 3 in Phase I) and hundreds are in pre-clinical testing as ion channel blockers, enzyme inhibitors, DNA-interactive and microtubule-interfering agents, with the majority of the latter compounds being tested for anti-tumor and cytotoxic properties [91, 94, 98]. Natural products of marine origin with biological activity of interest include, but are not limited to, curacin A, eleutherobin, discodermolide, bryostatins, dolostatins, cephalostatins [16].

3.3. Microorganisms

Microorganisms were identified early on as sources of valuable natural products as evidenced by the discovery of penicillin by from the fungus *Penicillium rubens* by Alexander Fleming in 1928 [100]. Historically, microorganisms (amongst them mostly bacteria and fungi) have played an important role in providing new structures, like antibiotics for drug discovery and development. The terrestrial microbial populations are immensely diverse which is also reflected in the number of compounds and metabolites isolated from these microorganisms. As mentioned above, the similarity of many compounds from marine invertebrates like sponges, ascidians, soft corals and bryozoans to those isolated from terrestrial microbes led to the hypothesis that associated microorganisms might be responsible for their production. Over time it became more and more evident, that a significant number of marine natural products are actually not produced by the originally assumed invertebrate but rather by microbes living in symbioses with their invertebrate host [92, 101]. In some instances it could indeed be demonstrated early on that the isolated marine microbes are the original source of the new compounds or secondary metabolites discovered and in recent years marine bacteria have emerged more and more as a source of NCEs [58, 91, 94, 95]. Besides bacteria, marine fungi and deep-sea hydrothermal vent microorganisms are reported to produce bioactive compounds and metabolites [91, 94]. Deep-sea vent sites offer harsh conditions in depth below 200 meters with complete absence of light, pressures in excess of 20 atmospheres, temperatures of up to 400°Celius, pH extremes and high sulfide concentrations and are populated by highly dense and unique, biologically diverse communities [91, 94, 102].

Unique microorganisms are abundant on land, in freshwater and all areas of the ocean. However, the enormous biological diversity of free-living and symbiotic marine microbes has so far only been explored to a very limited extent. The estimates extrapolate the number of marine species to at least a million, but for marine microbial species, including fungi and bacteria, the estimated numbers reach as high as tens or even hundreds of millions [23]. Over 74,000 known species of fungi are reported including around 3,000 aquatic species of which only about 465 are described as marine species, but a vast geographical area has not yet been sampled and estimates for the potential total number of species reach from 0.5 to 9.9 million with about 1.5 million considered as most realistic [103, 104]. The overlap is assumed to be relatively high between species in terrestrial and freshwater habitats, but not between these two and the marine habitat [104]. Nevertheless, a large percentage of the over 270 secondary metabolites isolated from marine fungi resembles analogues of compounds previously discovered from terrestrial fungi but some of the new substances identified exhibited potent activities against tumor cells, microbes or bacteria like methicillin-resistant *Staphylococcus aureus* (MRSA) or even antifouling properties [59, 105]. In comparison to bacteria, fungi appear to be rare in marine environments and few marine fungi isolates exist in culture [106]. Marine bacteria are assumed to constitute approximately 10% of the living biomass carbon and inhabit mainly sediments but can also be found in open oceans and in association with marine organisms [90, 91, 94]. Many marine invertebrates are associated with large amounts of epibiotic and endobiotic microorganisms and for many sponges bacteria can make up to 40% of the animal biomass and even resemble new species [97]. In fact it is assumed that almost all marine organisms host bacteria on their surface and that the vast majority bare epibiotic films of variable density and composition, which can affect the basibiont's physiology and interactions with its environment in beneficial, detrimental, or ambiguous manners [107]. This constitutes a vast pool for the discovery of new structures and scaffolds if the source can be unanimously established.

To identify the source of a compound, the determination of its mere presence in a certain organism is not sufficient, as this could be the result of active or passive accumulation and does not necessarily reflect the true site of its biosynthetic production. As Gulder and Moore further explain: *"An unambiguous assignment of the biosynthetic origin of a natural product derived from a complex assemblage of marine organisms thus has to originate at the genomic level. This is particularly true for bacterial symbionts, which have to date eluded cultivation"* [58]. These microbes generally organize their biosynthetic genes for each secondary metabolite in compact clusters, which will, following identification and sequencing of the cluster responsible for the respective pathways, allow the transfer of the respective bacterial genes into effective heterologous producers, like *Escherichia coli (E. coli)* [55, 58, 97]. In terms of microbial sources, culturing of the respective microorganism may generally be a viable approach to increase quantities. A major difference between microorganisms from terrestrial and marine sources is the fact that marine pelagic bacteria are much more difficult to grow in culture than the soil borne actinomycetes; therefore determining the conditions for replication, growth of sufficient quantities and induction of metabolite production can be a tedious challenge [12, 17]. This again may necessitate the production in a heterologous system like that observed for *E. coli.*

4. Challenges

Natural products, although a valuable and precious resource, also come with their fair share of challenges in a variety of aspects. As mentioned before, one of the major issues concerning the use of natural products are the difficulties associated with obtaining sufficient amounts of material pure enough for discovery and development activities. If a compound is derived from a plant growing only in small quantities or remote locations or a marine organism residing in great depth or difficult to access regions, re-supply becomes a problem.

The threat of losing potentially valuable natural sources of pharmacologically active ingredients is constantly increasing due to the threat of extinction by deforestation of large landmasses and environmental pollution in remote areas as well as global warming [85]. It is estimated that about 70% of the supply of herbal raw material for Ayurveda and other homeopathic medicines in India comes from the wild [82, 85]. To meet the increasing demand for raw material, to conserve wild resources, and to reduce the potential variability in the active ingredient content in medicinal plants from different collection areas, it is important to implement more controlled cultivation programs to ensure quality and to protect resources [82, 85].

Tissues of marine invertebrates present unique problems for extraction, because of their high water and salt content, and the promising compounds may be present only in low amounts and/or can be very difficult to isolate. Sponges and their microbial fauna are mostly not suitable for culture, and the compounds of interest need to be extracted and purified from specimens collected in the wild [17, 93]. Marine organisms and microbes constitute a valuable potential source of NCEs and structural templates for drug discovery in the future, but may necessitate tons of raw material to isolate milligram to gram amounts of the compound of interest [97]. This difficulty combined with the challenges for synthetic approaches to obtain significant quantities of potential new drug candidates, based on their often highly complex structures, are obstacles that can hamper their use in discovery and development [58, 97]. In some cases, supply issues could be resolved by semi-synthesis or total synthesis of the compound, the development of synthetic analogs with more manageable properties, or by design of a pharmacophore of reduced complexity, which can then be synthesized [17, 92, 97]. Fragments or synthetic analogs with simplified structures may retain bioactivity or even show improved activity towards the target [12].

Furthermore, environmental aspects can constitute significant hurdles for supplying material for discovery and development as the product may stem from an endangered species or the wild collection of the producing species may be detrimental to its originating terrestrial or marine ecosystem. Additionally, as mentioned above, because of their low abundance many compounds of interest from natural sources need to be extracted and purified from large quantities of specimen collected in the wild, which in turn carries the risks of over-exploitation and habitat destruction [17, 93]. Radjasa *et al.* provide a positive outlook for marine ecosystems and state "*There is optimism for the future because the international marine bioorganic community clearly recognizes that invertebrates must be harvested and studied in an environmentally sustainable manner*" [92]. Although aquaculture of marine species or culture of bacteria seem like logical alternative sources to obtain product, they are not viable avenues in most cases because it proves difficult to impossible to culture the source organisms (especially invertebrates and/or their microbial symbionts like bacteria etc.) or they may not produce the compound of interest under the given culture conditions [12, 17, 95, 97]. Findings indicate, that the bacterial composition on invertebrates is largely independent from sponge taxonomy or locality of collection and the bacteria most likely are contaminants from the ocean water rather than specific symbionts, which further exacerbates the cultivation problem [97, 108].

Another challenge can result from redundant activity determination in assay systems and the mixed composition of natural product extracts. With over 150,000 known small molecules characterized from natural sources, previously known natural products are often re-isolated in the course of bioassay-guided fractionation [84]. While this may be acceptable if the biological activity is new, it is frustrating to waste resources on the *de novo* structure elucidation of known compounds. Furthermore, not all compounds contained in natural product extracts are drug leads and it is extremely desirable to remove "nuisance compounds" like tannins, phorbol esters, saponins, and anionic polysaccharides; the latter, for instance, being highly active in cellular HIV bioassays [35].

Last, but not least, intellectual property rights can pose a significant hurdle that is difficult to manage. In general, patent protection can be obtained if the active principles derived from natural sources have novel structures and relevant biological activity. However, as mentioned before, additional handicaps may arise in the context of developing and marketing products from natural sources in the form of potentially significant intellectual property issues as well as, possibly, very difficult and costly negotiations to obtain agreements to collect and develop natural products from species collected in foreign countries [25, 26, 35].

5. Regulatory requirements and risks

The regulatory requirements for different product categories containing natural substances like pharmaceuticals, nutraceuticals, and cosmeceuticals vary from rather stringent to generous to non-existent at an International level. To exemplify regulatory approaches for the three aforementioned categories, an overview of the current situation in North America (U.S. and Canada) and the European Union is summarized. In many areas we have presented exact wording from the respective governing websites, as the phrasing of such represents the official context and any deviation thereof could be misleading.

5.1. Natural product-derived pharmaceuticals

Natural products constitute a key source of pharmacologically active ingredients in a variety of novel agents with therapeutic potential in a wide range of diseases. Pharmaceuticals containing natural products or compounds derived from natural product scaffolds or templates have to undergo the same stringent approval process as drugs obtained from purely synthetic origin.

5.1.1. North America

5.1.1.1. United States of America (U.S.)

The U.S. Government Office for the Control of Food and Drug Administration (FDA) oversees the regulatory control of pharmaceuticals including new treatments based on natural products [109]. The FDA's Center for Drug Evaluation and Research (CDER) role is to evaluate and approve new drugs before they can be sold ensuring that drugs are safe and effective for intended use and that their health benefits outweigh their known risks [109].

5.1.1.2. Canada

In Canada, Health Canada fulfills the same role as the US FDA according to the mandate under the authority of the Food and Drugs Act and the Food and Drug Regulations [110].

5.1.2. European Union

The European Medicines Agency (EMA) with headquarters in London/England regulates drugs and medicinal products in the European Union (EU) [111]. On April 30th, 2011 the EU entered into force the directive on herbal medicine products called Traditional Herbal Medicinal Products Directive 2004/24/EC, THMPD [111]. The regulation came as a sub-directive for the act on Human Medicinal Products Directive 2001/83/EC claiming a unique set of information on a herbal substance or herbal preparation for all EU Member States. Such could be used when evaluating marketing applications for herbal medicinal products from companies and covers medicinal products containing herbal substances/preparations [111]. To reach the market, these must fall within one of the following three categories, as outlined on the EMA website [111]:

1. a product can be classified under traditional medicinal use provisions ('traditional use') accepted on the basis of sufficient safety data and plausible efficacy: the product is granted a traditional use registration (simplified registration procedure) by a Member State,

2. a product can be classified under well-established medicinal use provisions ('well-established use'). This is demonstrated with the provision of scientific literature establishing that the active substances of the medicinal products have been in well-established medicinal use within the Union for at least ten years, with recognized efficacy and an acceptable level of safety. As a result the product is granted a marketing authorization usually by a Member State or by the European Medicines Agency. While both classifications have specific requirements, both regulatory paths involve the assessment of mostly bibliographic safety and efficacy data.

3. a product can be authorized after evaluation of a marketing authorization application consisting of only safety and efficacy data from the company's own development ('stand alone') or a combination of own studies and bibliographic data ('mixed application'). As a result the product is granted a marketing authorization by a Member State or by the Agency via the centralized procedure if all requirements are met.

In summary, while safety needs to be shown for products, proof of efficacy is not always a requirement and only the traditional indications in specified conditions must be plausible. Nonetheless, and irrespective of the regulatory pathway to access the market, the quality of the herbal medicinal product must always be demonstrated [111].

The Directive provides definitions for herbal medicinal products, herbal preparations and herbal substances, as follows [111]:

- *Herbal medicinal product:* Any medicinal product, exclusively containing as active ingredients one or more herbal substances or one or more herbal preparations, or one or more such herbal substances in combination with one or more such herbal preparations.

- *Herbal substances:* All mainly whole, fragmented or cut plants, plant parts, algae, fungi, lichen in an unprocessed, usually dried, form, but sometimes fresh. Certain exudates that have not been subjected to a specific treatment are also considered to be herbal substances. Herbal

http://dx.doi.org/10.5772/56424

substances are precisely defined by the plant part used and the botanical name according to the binomial system (genus, species, variety and author).

- *Herbal preparations:* Preparations obtained by subjecting herbal substances to treatments such as extraction, distillation, expression, fractionation, purification, concentration or fermentation. These include comminuted or powdered herbal substances, tinctures, extracts, essential oils, expressed juices and processed exudates

Additionally, it has been noted that from a herbal substance (e.g. valerian root) different herbal preparations (e.g. a valerian root extract using 70% ethanol) can be made; in such cases, both can represent the active ingredient in an individual herbal medicinal product [111].

5.2. Nutraceuticals — Dietary supplements (U.S.)/Natural health products (Canada)

Even if natural health products (NHPs) or dietary supplements are considered as or expected to be safe, they may still carry potential risks in themselves or through interactions with prescription or Over The Counter (OTC) drugs. This is illustrated by the previously described example of *aristolochic acid*, a powerful nephrotoxin and a human carcinogen associated with chronic kidney disease and upper urinary tract urothelial carcinomas after ingesting *Aristolochia* herbs in conjunction with a weight-loss regime [80, 81]. Furthermore, interactions between NHPs and prescription medicines are of increasing concern and need to be considered by physicians and patients alike [112]. Mills *et al*, in their evaluation of 47 trials which examined drug interactions with 19 different herbal preparations, observed potentially clinically significant drug interactions with St. Johns Wort, garlic, and American ginseng [113].

5.2.1. North America

5.2.1.1. United States of America

In the U.S., biologically active food and dietary supplements are regulated by the FDA and are classified as food and nutrition, not drugs [88]. The FDA website provides a detailed overview of their regulatory approach concerning nutraceuticals. The following paragraphs reflect some core points as outlined on the FDA's respective website [88].

- The FDA regulates both finished dietary supplement products and dietary ingredients under a different set of regulations than those covering "conventional" foods and drug products (prescription and OTC). Under the Dietary Supplement Health and Education Act (DSHEA) of 1994, the dietary supplement or dietary ingredient manufacturer is responsible for ensuring that a dietary supplement or ingredient is safe before it is marketed. The FDA is responsible for taking action against any unsafe dietary supplement product after it reaches the market. Generally, manufacturers do not need to register their products with the FDA nor get FDA approval before producing or selling dietary supplements.

- The Federal Food, Drug, and Cosmetic Act requires that manufacturers and distributors who wish to market dietary supplements that contain "new dietary ingredients" notify the Food and Drug Administration about these ingredients, which must include information that is the basis on which manufacturers/distributors have concluded that a dietary supplement containing a new dietary ingredient will reasonably be expected to be safe under the conditions of use recommended or suggested in the labeling [87].

- The U.S. Congress defined the term "dietary supplement" and both of the terms "dietary ingredient" and "new dietary ingredient" as components of dietary supplements in the DSHEA. A dietary supplement is a product taken by mouth that contains a "dietary ingredient" intended to supplement the diet.
- In order to be a "dietary ingredient," it must be one or any combination of the following substances:
- A "new dietary ingredient" is one that meets the above definition for a "dietary ingredient" and was not sold in the U.S. in a dietary supplement before October 15, 1994.
- Dietary supplements can also be extracts or concentrates, and may be found in many forms such as tablets, capsules, softgels, gelcaps, liquids, or powders [88]. They can also be in other forms, such as a bar, but if they are, information on their label must not represent the product as a conventional food or a sole item of a meal or diet [88]. Whatever their form may be, the DSHEA places dietary supplements in a special category under the general umbrella of "foods," not drugs, and requires that every supplement be labeled a dietary supplement.

5.2.1.2. Canada

In Canada, the use and sale of natural health products (NHPs) is on the rise [8]. A 2010 Ipsos-Reid survey showed that 73% of Canadians regularly take natural health products (NHPs) like vitamins and minerals, herbal products, and homeopathic medicines [114]. Health Canada defines natural health products under the Natural Health Products Regulations as:

- Vitamins and minerals
- Herbal remedies
- Homeopathic medicines
- Traditional medicines such as traditional Chinese medicines
- Probiotics
- Other products like amino acids and essential fatty acids [115].

Natural Health Products must be safe to use as OTC products and not need a prescription to be sold [115]. Natural products, compounds and active ingredients derived from natural sources or totally synthesized and needing a prescription are regulated as drugs under the Food and Drug Regulations [115].

5.2.2. European Union

Herbal supplements and nutritional supplements are not regulated on a harmonized EU wide basis and remain under the control of the relevant medical institutions of the individual EU member states.

5.3. Cosmeceuticals

Although the term is not recognized by the US Food and Drug Administration (FDA) or by the European Medicines Agency (EMA), it has been widely adopted by the cosmetics industry, which is rapidly expanding in spite of global economic woes in recent years [116]. The global cosmeceuticals market references the seven most developed markets including the U.S. and the top five European countries, namely the UK, France, Germany, Italy and Spain; as well as Japan [116]. In 2011, the global cosmeceuticals market was estimated to be worth $30.9 billion (with the aforementioned European countries accounting for approximately 65% of overall revenues) and is expected to reach $42.4 billion by 2018 [116]. Three major categories have been noted in the cosmeceutical industry including skin care, hair care, and others, with the skin care segment accounting for the largest share of the market at 43% [117]. Dominated by anti-aging products, the skin-care market is expected to contribute significantly to future growth based on the aging populations in the top seven aforementioned markets [116].

Cosmeceuticals are topically applied and represent a hybrid of cosmetics and pharmaceuticals usually containing vitamins, herbs, various oils, and botanical extracts or a mixture thereof including antioxidants, growth factors, peptides, anti-inflammatories/botanicals, polysaccharides, and pigment-lightening agents [117, 118]. The combination of cosmetics and foods resulted in products termed nutricosmetics. Nutricosmetics are foods and supplements claiming cosmetic effects with major ingredients like soy isoflavone proteins, lutein, lycopene, vitamins (A, B_6, E), omega-3 fatty acids, beta-carotene probiotics, sterol esters, chondrotin and coenzyme Q10 [119, 120]. These compounds act as antioxidants and the respective nutricosmetics containing them are being promoted for their skin care properties as for instance in anti-aging by fighting free radicals generated as a by-product of biochemical reactions through skin exposure to the sun [119].

5.3.1. North America

5.3.1.1. United States of America

In the US, products that can be put in both the cosmetics and drugs category, such as cosmetic products with active ingredients which claim therapeutic use, require New Drug Application (NDA) approval or must comply with the appropriate monograph for an (OTC) drug. Moreover, the FDA also has specific guidelines for Good Manufacturing Practice (GMP) for cosmetics [116].

While the *Federal Food, Drug, and Cosmetic Act (FD&C Act)* does not recognize the term "cosmeceutical", the cosmetic industry uses this word to refer to cosmetic products that have medicinal or drug-like benefits [118]. The FD&C Act defines drugs as those products that cure, treat, mitigate or prevent disease or that affect the structure or function of the human body [121]. Under the FD&C Act, cosmetic products and ingredients, with the exception of color additives, do not require FDA approval before they go on the market [121]. Therefore, while drugs are subject to a review and approval process by the FDA, cosmetics are not approved by the FDA prior to sale. However, when a product makes a therapeutic claim (e.g. to prevent or treat disease), it is classified as a drug and therefore requires evaluation by the FDA's Center for Drug Evaluation and Research (CDER) and a drug identification number (DIN) before it can be sold.

5.3.1.2. Canada

In Canada, the term "cosmeceutical" (used to describe a cosmetic product with pharmaceutical-like benefits) is not employed by Health Canada [122]. Therefore cosmeceuticals fall under either cosmetics or drugs (depending on the claims made and/or the composition of the product) and are subject to the provisions of the Food and Drugs Act and its Cosmetic Regulations regarding composition, safety, labeling and advertising and they are subject to the provisions of the Consumer Packaging and Labeling Act and Regulations [122]. The three most significant features of the Canadian cosmetic regulatory system are mandatory notification of all cosmetic products, safety of ingredients and products, and product labeling [122]. According to Health Canada, a "cosmetic" is defined as *"any substance or mixture of substances, manufactured, sold or represented for use in cleansing, improving or altering the complexion, skin, hair or teeth and includes deodorants and perfumes"* [122].

5.3.2. European Union

In Europe, EMA guidelines place a clear demarcation between drugs and cosmetics, whereby a cosmetic is a product that is to be applied topically with an intended cosmetic function and products cannot fall under both categories, unlike in the US [116]. On November 30th (2009), the new Cosmetic Products Regulation, EU Regulation 1223/2009 was adopted, replacing the Cosmetics Directive [123]. With the new Cosmetics Regulation, Europe claims to have a robust, internationally recognized regime, which reinforces product safety taking into consideration the latest technological developments [123]. Most of the provisions of this new regulation will be applicable as of July 11th, 2013 [123].

6. Conclusion

A natural product or secondary metabolite is a pharmacologically or biologically active chemical compound or substance, which is found in nature and produced by a living organism. The lengthy process of natural products evolution has resulted in optimal interactions with biological macromolecules and targets. Historically, natural substances have been the most productive source of active compounds and chemical lead structures. Natural products have traditionally provided a large fraction of the drugs in use today and millions of terrestrial and marine plants, organisms and microorganisms provide an immense resource to discover unprecedented novel bioactive scaffolds. These have the potential to serve as medical treatments or templates for new therapeutics and may be suitable for production via a synthetic routes or in a heterologous system like *E. coli.* About half of the agents in today's arsenal of marketed drugs are derived from biological sources with the large majority being based on terrestrial natural product scaffolds. Approximately 50% of the new drugs introduced since 1994 were either natural products or derived from natural products. As of today, only a very small fraction of bioactive structures of potential therapeutic relevance from plants, microbes, and marine organisms have been chemically analyzed or examined in a broad panel of screening models or bioassays. The discovery of valuable therapeutic agents from natural sources continues in the 21th century by reaching into new and untapped terrestrial and marine source organisms as the chemical novelty associated with natural products is higher than that of structures from any other source.

There is growing awareness of the limited structural diversity in existing compound collections and the extreme chemical diversity, the high biological potency, and the potential to frequently discover drug-like characteristics in natural products. Therefore, they constitute a valuable platform for the development of new therapeutics for a variety of indications, although they may still not contain enough versatility to yield suitable treatments for all heritable human diseases.

As some major pharmaceutical companies terminated their natural product programs, the future role to discover and feed candidates into the development pipelines will reside increasingly with research institutes and small biotech companies. Over a hundred new drug candidates from natural sources like plants, bacteria, fungi and animals or obtained semi-synthetically are in clinical development with a similar number in preclinical development. They target a variety of indications, mainly cancer and infectious diseases (bacterial, viral, fungal, and parasitic) but also other therapeutic areas such as cardiovascular diseases, neurological illnesses and depression, metabolic diorders and inflammatory diseases.

Natural products, although a valuable and precious resource, also come with their fair share of challenges concerning the provision of sufficient amounts of pure enough material for discovery and development activities. As mentioned earlier, such apprehensions are based on the threat of losing potentially valuable natural sources through extinction resulting from deforestation of large landmasses, environmental pollution in remote areas as well as global warming. Countries are also increasingly protective of their natural assets in flora and fauna and may not authorize the collection of sample species without significant demands and very difficult negotiations. The regulatory requirements for different product categories containing natural substances like pharmaceuticals, nutraceuticals, and cosmeceuticals vary from rather stringent over generous to non-existent at an international level. Even if natural health products or dietary supplements are considered as or expected to be safe, they may still carry potential risks in themselves or through interactions with prescription or OTC drugs. Therefore, the discovery and development of natural products require cientific validation and sufficient pharmacoepidemiological evidence to support their safety and efficacy.

Acknowledgements

Funding for the publication of this chapter was provided by the School of Business Administration and the Centre for Health and Biotech Management Research, University of Prince Edward Island, Charlottetown, PE, Canada. We are grateful to BCC Research (Wellesley, MA,

USA) for providing us with applicable sections from their 2013 market report, namely "Botanical and Plant-derived Drugs: Global Markets".

Author details

Juergen Krause[1*] and Gailene Tobin[2]

*Address all correspondence to: jukrause@upei.ca

1 School of Business Administration and Centre for Health and Biotech Management Research, University of Prince Edward Island, Charlottetown, PE, Canada

2 Department of Biomedical Sciences, University of Prince Edward Island, Charlottetown, PE, Canada

References

[1] Newman DJ, Cragg GM. Natural products as sources of new drugs over the 30 years from 1981 to 2010. Journal of natural products. 2012 Mar 23;75(3):311-35. PubMed PMID: 22316239.

[2] Chin YW, Balunas MJ, Chai HB, Kinghorn AD. Drug discovery from natural sources. The AAPS journal. 2006;8(2):E239-53. PubMed PMID: 16796374. Pubmed Central PMCID: 3231566.

[3] All natural. Nat Chem Biol. 2007; 3:[351]. Available from: http://dx.doi.org/10.1038/nchembio0707-351.

[4] Natural Product. Feb 7, 2013. Available from: http://www.thefreedictionary.com/Natural+product.

[5] Fischbach MA, Clardy J. One pathway, many products. Nat Chem Biol. 2007 Jul;3(7):353-5. PubMed PMID: 17576415.

[6] Kinghorn AD, Chin YW, Swanson SM. Discovery of natural product anticancer agents from biodiverse organisms. Current opinion in drug discovery & development. 2009 Mar;12(2):189-96. PubMed PMID: 19333864. Pubmed Central PMCID: 2877274.

[7] Zähner H. What are secondary metabolites? Folia Microbiol. 1979 1979/10/01;24(5):435-43.

[8] Chernyak M. Canadian NHP Market: Headed In The Right Direction2012; (November). Available from: http://www.nutraceuticalsworld.com/issues/2012-11/view_features/canadian-nhp-market-headed-in-the-right-direction/.

[9] What-is-pharmacognosy? [Internet]. 2011. Available from: http://www.pharmacognosy.us/what-is-pharmacognosy/.

[10] Ertl P, Schuffenhauer A. Cheminformatics analysis of natural products: lessons from nature inspiring the design of new drugs. Progress in drug research Fortschritte der Arzneimittelforschung Progres des recherches pharmaceutiques. 2008;66:217, 9-35. PubMed PMID: 18416307.

[11] Harvey AL, Clark RL, Mackay SP, Johnston BF. Current strategies for drug discovery through natural products. Expert opinion on drug discovery. 2010 Jun;5(6):559-68. PubMed PMID: 22823167.

[12] Beutler JA. Natural Products as a Foundation for Drug Discovery. Current protocols in pharmacology / editorial board, SJ Enna. 2009 Sep 1;46:9 11 1-9 21. PubMed PMID: 20161632. Pubmed Central PMCID: 2813068.

[13] Jeffreys D. Aspirin: The Remarkable Story of a Wonderdrug: Bloomsbury Publishing PLC; 2004.

[14] Schwartsmann G. Marine organisms and other novel natural sources of new cancer drugs. Annals of oncology : official journal of the European Society for Medical Oncology / ESMO. 2000;11 Suppl 3:235-43. PubMed PMID: 11079147.

[15] Butler MS. Natural products to drugs: natural product derived compounds in clinical trials. Natural product reports. 2005 Apr;22(2):162-95. PubMed PMID: 15806196.

[16] Mishra BB, Tiwari VK. Natural Products in Drug Discovery; Clinical Evaluations and Investigations. Research Signpost. 2011:1-62.

[17] Molinski TF, Dalisay DS, Lievens SL, Saludes JP. Drug development from marine natural products. Nature reviews Drug discovery. 2009 Jan;8(1):69-85. PubMed PMID: 19096380.

[18] Goodman JW, V. The Story of Taxol: Nature and Politics in the Pursuit of an Anti-Cancer Drug. . British Medical Journal. 2001;323 (1704)(July 14):115. Pubmed Central PMCID: PMC1120731.

[19] McChesney JD, Venkataraman SK, Henri JT. Plant natural products: back to the future or into extinction? Phytochemistry. 2007 Jul;68(14):2015-22. PubMed PMID: 17574638.

[20] Wani MC, Taylor HL, Wall ME, Coggon P, McPhail AT. Plant antitumor agents. VI. The isolation and structure of taxol, a novel antileukemic and antitumor agent from Taxus brevifolia. Journal of the American Chemical Society. 1971 May 5;93(9):2325-7. PubMed PMID: 5553076.

[21] Harvey A. The role of natural products in drug discovery and development in the new millennium. IDrugs. 2010 Feb;13(2):70-2. PubMed PMID: 20127553.

[22] Brahmachari G. Bioactive Natural Products: World Scientific Publishing Co. ; 2011.

[23] Montaser R, Luesch H. Marine natural products: a new wave of drugs? Future medicinal chemistry. 2011 Sep;3(12):1475-89. PubMed PMID: 21882941. Pubmed Central PMCID: 3210699.

[24] Carlson EE. Natural products as chemical probes. ACS chemical biology. 2010 Jul 16;5(7):639-53. PubMed PMID: 20509672. Pubmed Central PMCID: 2926141.

[25] Rouhi AM. Rediscovering Natural Products. Chem. Eng. News. 2003 October 13, :pp. 104-7.

[26] Rouhi AM. Moving Beyond Natural Products. Chem. Eng. News. 2003 October 13, :pp. 77-91.

[27] Koehn FE, Carter GT. The evolving role of natural products in drug discovery. Nature reviews Drug discovery. 2005 Mar;4(3):206-20. PubMed PMID: 15729362.

[28] Ortholand JY, Ganesan A. Natural products and combinatorial chemistry: back to the future. Current opinion in chemical biology. 2004 Jun;8(3):271-80. PubMed PMID: 15183325.

[29] Molinari G. Natural products in drug discovery: present status and perspectives. Advances in experimental medicine and biology. 2009;655:13-27. PubMed PMID: 20047031.

[30] Wolfender JL, Queiroz EF. New approaches for studying the chemical diversity of natural resources and the bioactivity of their constituents. Chimia. 2012;66(5):324-9. PubMed PMID: 22867545.

[31] Thomas GL, Johannes CW. Natural product-like synthetic libraries. Current opinion in chemical biology. 2011 Aug;15(4):516-22. PubMed PMID: 21684804.

[32] Glaser KB, Mayer AM. A renaissance in marine pharmacology: from preclinical curiosity to clinical reality. Biochemical pharmacology. 2009 Sep 1;78(5):440-8. PubMed PMID: 19393227.

[33] Cragg GM, Katz F, Newman DJ, Rosenthal J. The impact of the United Nations Convention on Biological Diversity on natural products research. Natural product reports. 2012 Dec;29(12):1407-23. PubMed PMID: 23037777.

[34] Kirsop B. The convention on Biological Diversity: Some implications for microbiology and microbial culture collections. Journal of Industrial Microbiology and Biotechnology. 1996;17(5):505-11.

[35] Fabricant DS, Farnsworth NR. The value of plants used in traditional medicine for drug discovery. Environmental health perspectives. 2001 Mar;109 Suppl 1:69-75. PubMed PMID: 11250806. Pubmed Central PMCID: 1240543.

[36] Feher M, Schmidt JM. Property distributions: differences between drugs, natural products, and molecules from combinatorial chemistry. Journal of chemical information and computer sciences. 2003 Jan-Feb;43(1):218-27. PubMed PMID: 12546556.

[37] Lee ML, Schneider G. Scaffold architecture and pharmacophoric properties of natural products and trade drugs: application in the design of natural product-based combinatorial libraries. Journal of combinatorial chemistry. 2001 May-Jun;3(3):284-9. PubMed PMID: 11350252.

[38] Larsson J, Gottfries J, Muresan S, Backlund A. ChemGPS-NP: tuned for navigation in biologically relevant chemical space. Journal of natural products. 2007 May;70(5): 789-94. PubMed PMID: 17439280.

[39] Yongye AB, Waddell J, Medina-Franco JL. Molecular scaffold analysis of natural products databases in the public domain. Chemical biology & drug design. 2012 Nov;80(5):717-24. PubMed PMID: 22863071.

[40] Barker A, Kettle JG, Nowak T, Pease JE. Expanding medicinal chemistry space. Drug discovery today. 2012 Oct 29. PubMed PMID: 23117010.

[41] Pors K, Goldberg FW, Leamon CP, Rigby AC, Snyder SA, Falconer RA. The changing landscape of cancer drug discovery: a challenge to the medicinal chemist of tomorrow. Drug discovery today. 2009 Nov;14(21-22):1045-50. PubMed PMID: 19638319.

[42] Dancik V, Seiler KP, Young DW, Schreiber SL, Clemons PA. Distinct biological network properties between the targets of natural products and disease genes. Journal of the American Chemical Society. 2010 Jul 14;132(27):9259-61. PubMed PMID: 20565092. Pubmed Central PMCID: 2898216.

[43] Hong J. Role of natural product diversity in chemical biology. Current opinion in chemical biology. 2011 Jun;15(3):350-4. PubMed PMID: 21489856. Pubmed Central PMCID: 3110584.

[44] Lopez-Vallejo F, Giulianotti MA, Houghten RA, Medina-Franco JL. Expanding the medicinally relevant chemical space with compound libraries. Drug discovery today. 2012 Jul;17(13-14):718-26. PubMed PMID: 22515962.

[45] Shang S, Tan DS. Advancing chemistry and biology through diversity-oriented synthesis of natural product-like libraries. Current opinion in chemical biology. 2005 Jun;9(3):248-58. PubMed PMID: 15939326.

[46] Zhang HY, Chen LL, Li XJ, Zhang J. Evolutionary inspirations for drug discovery. Trends in pharmacological sciences. 2010 Oct;31(10):443-8. PubMed PMID: 20724009.

[47] Balamurugan R, Dekker FJ, Waldmann H. Design of compound libraries based on natural product scaffolds and protein structure similarity clustering (PSSC). Molecular bioSystems. 2005 May;1(1):36-45. PubMed PMID: 16880961.

[48] Rosen J, Gottfries J, Muresan S, Backlund A, Oprea TI. Novel chemical space exploration via natural products. Journal of medicinal chemistry. 2009 Apr 9;52(7):1953-62. PubMed PMID: 19265440. Pubmed Central PMCID: 2696019.

[49] Crawford AD, Liekens S, Kamuhabwa AR, Maes J, Munck S, Busson R, et al. Zebrafish bioassay-guided natural product discovery: isolation of angiogenesis inhibitors from East African medicinal plants. PloS one. 2011;6(2):e14694. PubMed PMID: 21379387. Pubmed Central PMCID: 3040759.

[50] Harvey AL, Cree IA. High-throughput screening of natural products for cancer therapy. Planta medica. 2010 Aug;76(11):1080-6. PubMed PMID: 20635309.

[51] Mandrekar N, Thakur NL. Significance of the zebrafish model in the discovery of bioactive molecules from nature. Biotechnology letters. 2009 Feb;31(2):171-9. PubMed PMID: 18931972.

[52] Mimeault M, Batra SK. Emergence of zebrafish models in oncology for validating novel anticancer drug targets and nanomaterials. Drug discovery today. 2013 Feb; 18(3-4):128-40. PubMed PMID: 22903142. Pubmed Central PMCID: 3562372.

[53] Koehn FE. High impact technologies for natural products screening. Progress in drug research Fortschritte der Arzneimittelforschung Progres des recherches pharmaceutiques. 2008;65:175, 7-210. PubMed PMID: 18084916.

[54] Leeds JA, Schmitt EK, Krastel P. Recent developments in antibacterial drug discovery: microbe-derived natural products--from collection to the clinic. Expert opinion on investigational drugs. 2006 Mar;15(3):211-26. PubMed PMID: 16503759.

[55] Corre C, Challis GL. New natural product biosynthetic chemistry discovered by genome mining. Natural product reports. 2009 Aug;26(8):977-86. PubMed PMID: 19636446.

[56] Zerikly M, Challis GL. Strategies for the discovery of new natural products by genome mining. Chembiochem : a European journal of chemical biology. 2009 Mar 2;10(4):625-33. PubMed PMID: 19165837.

[57] Haefner B. Drugs from the deep: marine natural products as drug candidates. Drug discovery today. 2003 Jun 15;8(12):536-44. PubMed PMID: 12821301.

[58] Gulder TA, Moore BS. Chasing the treasures of the sea - bacterial marine natural products. Current opinion in microbiology. 2009 Jun;12(3):252-60. PubMed PMID: 19481972. Pubmed Central PMCID: 2695832.

[59] Bhatnagar I, Kim SK. Immense essence of excellence: marine microbial bioactive compounds. Marine drugs. 2010;8(10):2673-701. PubMed PMID: 21116414. Pubmed Central PMCID: 2993000.

[60] Harvey AL. Natural products in drug discovery. Drug discovery today. 2008 Oct; 13(19-20):894-901. PubMed PMID: 18691670.

[61] Katiyar C, Gupta A, Kanjilal S, Katiyar S. Drug discovery from plant sources: An integrated approach. Ayu. 2012 Jan;33(1):10-9. PubMed PMID: 23049178. Pubmed Central PMCID: 3456845.

[62] Butler MS. Natural products to drugs: natural product-derived compounds in clinical trials. Natural product reports. 2008 Jun;25(3):475-516. PubMed PMID: 18497896.

[63] Saklani A, Kutty SK. Plant-derived compounds in clinical trials. Drug discovery today. 2008 Feb;13(3-4):161-71. PubMed PMID: 18275914.

[64] Galm U, Shen B. Natural product drug discovery: the times have never been better. Chemistry & biology. 2007 Oct;14(10):1098-104. PubMed PMID: 17961822.

[65] Nirmala M, Samundeeswari A. Sankar PD. . Natural plant resources in anti-cancer therapy-A review. Research in Plant Biology. 2011 1(13):1-14.

[66] Metzger KL, Shoemaker JM, Kahn JB, Maxwell CR, Liang Y, Tokarczyk J, et al. Pharmacokinetic and behavioral characterization of a long-term antipsychotic delivery system in rodents and rabbits. Psychopharmacology. 2007 Feb;190(2):201-11. PubMed PMID: 17119931.

[67] Vira D, Basak SK, Veena MS, Wang MB, Batra RK, Srivatsan ES. Cancer stem cells, microRNAs, and therapeutic strategies including natural products. Cancer metastasis reviews. 2012 Dec;31(3-4):733-51. PubMed PMID: 22752409.

[68] Bhanot A SR, Noolvi M. Natural sources as potential anti-cancer agents: A review. International Journal of Phytomedicine. 2011;3 (1).

[69] Ma X, Wang Z. Anticancer drug discovery in the future: an evolutionary perspective. Drug discovery today. 2009 Dec;14(23-24):1136-42. PubMed PMID: 19800414.

[70] The Foundation for Aids Research. Statistics Worldwide: The Regional Picture. 2012 (Nov). Available at: www.amfar.org.

[71] Hupfeld J, Efferth T. Review. Drug resistance of human immunodeficiency virus and overcoming it by natural products. In vivo. 2009 Jan-Feb;23(1):1-6. PubMed PMID: 19368117.

[72] Asres K, Seyoum A, Veeresham C, Bucar F, Gibbons S. Naturally derived anti-HIV agents. Phytotherapy research : PTR. 2005 Jul;19(7):557-81. PubMed PMID: 16161055.

[73] Vo TS, Kim SK. Potential anti-HIV agents from marine resources: an overview. Marine drugs. 2010;8(12):2871-92. PubMed PMID: 21339954. Pubmed Central PMCID: 3039460.

[74] Piggott AM, Karuso P. Quality, not quantity: the role of natural products and chemical proteomics in modern drug discovery. Combinatorial chemistry & high throughput screening. 2004 Nov;7(7):607-30. PubMed PMID: 15578924.

[75] Tulp M, Bohlin L. Unconventional natural sources for future drug discovery. Drug discovery today. 2004 May 15;9(10):450-8. PubMed PMID: 15109950.

[76] Health in the Wild. Animal Doctors. The Economist. 2002.

[77] Richards S. Natural-born Doctors. The Scientist. 2012.

[78] Rout SP. Choudary K, Kar, DM., Das, LM. Jain, A. Plants in Traditional Medicinal Ststem - Future Source of New Drugs. International Journal of Pharmacy and Pharmaceutical Sciences. 2009 July-Sep.;Vol. 1(Issue 1).

[79] Patwardhan B, Vaidya AD. Natural products drug discovery: accelerating the clinical candidate development using reverse pharmacology approaches. Indian journal of experimental biology. 2010 Mar;48(3):220-7. PubMed PMID: 21046974.

[80] Chen CH, Dickman KG, Moriya M, Zavadil J, Sidorenko VS, Edwards KL, et al. Aristolochic acid-associated urothelial cancer in Taiwan. Proceedings of the National Academy of Sciences of the United States of America. 2012 May 22;109(21):8241-6. PubMed PMID: 22493262. Pubmed Central PMCID: 3361449.

[81] Alternative Medicines. The Scientist. (2012). Available at: http://www.the-scientist.com/?articles.view/articleNo/32219/title/Alternative-Medicines/

[82] Birari RB, Bhutani KK. Pancreatic lipase inhibitors from natural sources: unexplored potential. Drug discovery today. 2007 Oct;12(19-20):879-89. PubMed PMID: 17933690.

[83] Boopathy Raja A, Elanchezhiyan C, Sethupathy S. Antihyperlipidemic activity of Helicteres isora fruit extract on streptozotocin induced diabetic male Wistar rats. European review for medical and pharmacological sciences. 2010 Mar;14(3):191-6. PubMed PMID: 20391957.

[84] Beutler JA. Natural products as a foundation for drug discovery. Current protocols in pharmacology / editorial board, SJ Enna. 2009 Sep;Chapter 9:Unit 9 11. PubMed PMID: 22294405.

[85] Bhutani KK, Gohil VM. Natural products drug discovery research in India: status and appraisal. Indian journal of experimental biology. 2010 Mar;48(3):199-207. PubMed PMID: 21046972.

[86] Saslis-Lagoudakis CH, Savolainen V, Williamson EM, Forest F, Wagstaff SJ, Baral SR, et al. Phylogenies reveal predictive power of traditional medicine in bioprospecting. Proceedings of the National Academy of Sciences of the United States of America.

2012 Sep 25;109(39):15835-40. PubMed PMID: 22984175. Pubmed Central PMCID: 3465383.

[87] Guidance for Industry; Botanical Drug Products U.S. Department of Health and Human Services. 2004 June. Available from: http://www.fda.gov/cder/guidance/index.htm.

[88] Dietary Supplements. U.S. Department of Health and Human Services. Available from: http://www.fda.gov/Food/DietarySupplements/default.htm.

[89] Lawson K. Botanical and Plant-derived Drugs: Global Markets. Wellesley, MA. USA: BCC Research; 2013.

[90] Parkes RJ CB, Bale SJ, Getlifff JM, Goodman K, Rochelle PA, Fry JC, Weightman AJ, Harvey SM. Deep bacterial biosphere in Pacific Ocean sediments. Nature. 1994;371(Sep):410-3.

[91] Thakur NL TA, Müller WE. Marine natural products in drug discovery. 471-477 [Internet]. 2005; 4 (6):[471-7 pp.].

[92] Radjasa OK, Vaske YM, Navarro G, Vervoort HC, Tenney K, Linington RG, et al. Highlights of marine invertebrate-derived biosynthetic products: their biomedical potential and possible production by microbial associants. Bioorganic & medicinal chemistry. 2011 Nov 15;19(22):6658-74. PubMed PMID: 21835627. Pubmed Central PMCID: 3205244.

[93] Leal MC, Puga J, Serodio J, Gomes NC, Calado R. Trends in the discovery of new marine natural products from invertebrates over the last two decades--where and what are we bioprospecting? 2012;7(1):e30580. PubMed PMID: 22276216. Pubmed Central PMCID: 3262841.

[94] Thakur GA, Duclos RI, Jr., Makriyannis A. Natural cannabinoids: templates for drug discovery. Life sciences. 2005 Dec 22;78(5):454-66. PubMed PMID: 16242157.

[95] Salomon CE, Magarvey NA, Sherman DH. Merging the potential of microbial genetics with biological and chemical diversity: an even brighter future for marine natural product drug discovery. Natural product reports. 2004 Feb;21(1):105-21. PubMed PMID: 15039838.

[96] Kong DX, Jiang YY, Zhang HY. Marine natural products as sources of novel scaffolds: achievement and concern. Drug discovery today. 2010 Nov;15(21-22):884-6. PubMed PMID: 20869461.

[97] Piel J. Bacterial symbionts: prospects for the sustainable production of invertebrate-derived pharmaceuticals. Current medicinal chemistry. 2006;13(1):39-50. PubMed PMID: 16457638.

[98] Mayer AM, Glaser KB, Cuevas C, Jacobs RS, Kem W, Little RD, et al. The odyssey of marine pharmaceuticals: a current pipeline perspective. Trends in pharmacological sciences. 2010 Jun;31(6):255-65. PubMed PMID: 20363514.

[99] Rath CM, Janto B, Earl J, Ahmed A, Hu FZ, Hiller L, et al. Meta-omic characterization of the marine invertebrate microbial consortium that produces the chemotherapeutic natural product ET-743. ACS chemical biology. 2011 Nov 18;6(11):1244-56. PubMed PMID: 21875091. Pubmed Central PMCID: 3220770.

[100] Houbraken J, Frisvad JC, Samson RA. Fleming's penicillin producing strain is not *Penicillium chrysogenum* but *P. rubens*. IMA fungus. 2011 Jun;2(1):87-95. PubMed PMID: 22679592. Pubmed Central PMCID: 3317369.

[101] Newman DJ, Cragg GM. Natural products as sources of new drugs over the last 25 years. Journal of natural products. 2007 Mar;70(3):461-77. PubMed PMID: 17309302.

[102] Thornburg CC, Zabriskie TM, McPhail KL. Deep-sea hydrothermal vents: potential hot spots for natural products discovery? Journal of natural products. 2010 Mar 26;73(3):489-99. PubMed PMID: 20099811.

[103] DL. H. The magnitude of fungal diversity: the 1 5 million species estimate revisited. Mycological research. 2001 Dec;105(12):1422-32.

[104] Shearer CA DE, Kohlmeyer B, Kohlmeyer J, Marvanova L, Padgett D, Porter D, Raja HA, Schmit JP,Thorton HA, Voglymayr H. . Fungal biodiversity in aquatic habitats. . Biodivers Conserv. 2006;16:49-67.

[105] Bhadury P, Mohammad BT, Wright PC. The current status of natural products from marine fungi and their potential as anti-infective agents. Journal of industrial microbiology & biotechnology. 2006 May;33(5):325-37. PubMed PMID: 16429315.

[106] Richards TA, Jones MD, Leonard G, Bass D. Marine fungi: their ecology and molecular diversity. Annual review of marine science. 2012;4:495-522. PubMed PMID: 22457985.

[107] Wahl M, Goecke F, Labes A, Dobretsov S, Weinberger F. The second skin: ecological role of epibiotic biofilms on marine organisms. Frontiers in microbiology. 2012;3:292. PubMed PMID: 22936927. Pubmed Central PMCID: 3425911.

[108] Hentschel U, Hopke J, Horn M, Friedrich AB, Wagner M, Hacker J, et al. Molecular evidence for a uniform microbial community in sponges from different oceans. Applied and environmental microbiology. 2002 Sep;68(9):4431-40. PubMed PMID: 12200297. Pubmed Central PMCID: 124103.

[109] How Drugs Are Developed and Approved. Available from: http://www.fda.gov/drugs/developmentapprovalprocess/howdrugsaredevelopedandapproved/default.htm.

[110] Drugs and Health Products 2012. U.S. Department of Health and Human Services. Available from: www.hc-sc.gc.ca/dph-mps/prodpharma/index-eng/php.

[111] Herbal Medicinal Products. European Medicines Agency. Available from: (http://www.ema.europa.eu/ema/index.jsp?curl=pages/regulation/general/general_content_000208.jsp).

[112] Gilmour J, Harrison C, Asadi L, Cohen MH, Vohra S. Natural health product-drug interactions: evolving responsibilities to take complementary and alternative medicine into account. Pediatrics. 2011 Nov;128 Suppl 4:S155-60. PubMed PMID: 22045857.

[113] Mills E, Wu P, Johnston BC, Gallicano K, Clarke M, Guyatt G. Natural health product-drug interactions: a systematic review of clinical trials. Therapeutic drug monitoring. 2005 Oct;27(5):549-57. PubMed PMID: 16175124.

[114] Reid I. Natural Health Product Tracking Survey – 2010; Final Report. Health Canada; 2011.

[115] What are Natural Health Products? 2012. U.S. Department of Health and Human Services. Available from: www.hc-sc.gc.ca/dhp/mps/prodnatur/index-eng.php.

[116] Global Cosmeceuticals Market Poised to Reach $42.4 Billion by 2018: Technological Advances and Consumer Awareness Boost Commercial Potential for Innovative and Premium-Priced Products.2013. Available from: http://www.giiresearch.com/press/7470.shtml.

[117] Dover J. Cosmeceuticals: A Practical Approach. Skin therapy letter. 2008;3(1):1-7.

[118] Choi CM, Berson DS. Cosmeceuticals. Seminars in cutaneous medicine and surgery. 2006 Sep;25(3):163-8. PubMed PMID: 17055397.

[119] Sullivan and Frost. Nutricosmetics - Health and Beauty Within and Without! (2007). May 25. Available at: http://www.frost.com/sublib/display-market-insight.do?id=99171683

[120] Anunciato TP, da Rocha Filho PA. Carotenoids and polyphenols in nutricosmetics, nutraceuticals, and cosmeceuticals. Journal of cosmetic dermatology. 2012 Mar;11(1):51-4. PubMed PMID: 22360335.

[121] Cosmetics: Guidance, Compliance and Regulatory Information. Available from: www.fda.gov/Cosmetics/GuidanceComplianceRegulatoryinformation/default.htm.

[122] General Requirements for Cosmetics2012. Available from: www.hc-sc.gc.ca/cps-spc/cosmet-person/indust/require-exige/index-eng.php

[123] Cosmetic Products Regulation EU Regulation 1223/2009. European Medicines Agency. Available from: ec.europa.eu/consumers/sectors/cosmetics/documents/revision/index_en.htm.

Chapter 2

Genetic, Agronomy, and Metabolomics of Prince Edwards Island Wild Rose Collection and Promise for Cultivar Development

Bourlaye Fofana, Kaushik Ghose, Bob Chapman and Kevin Sanderson

Additional information is available at the end of the chapter

http://dx.doi.org/10.5772/54688

1. Introduction

Agriculture – the control of plants for human consumption – is believed to have appeared and developed during the paleolitic/neolitic period, ~ 10,000 years ago [1]. The first agriculture had no single or simple origin since a wide variety of plants and animals have been independently domesticated at different times and different places [1-4]. The origin of agriculture and crops domestication is intertwined. Plant domestication involves changes in the plant's genetic makeup and morphological appearance following successive selections within wild plants and based upon on the variations that are best suitable for humans needs [5]. Domestication is therefore an artificial selection process conducted by humans for the production of plants showing fewer undesirable traits compared to its wild related plants, and making them more dependent on the new artificial environments for their continued survival and development. The concept of selection assumes the existence of a population or group of individuals from which choices can be made. Thus, the diversity of morphotypes or genetic diversity is considered as the backbone for plant domestication and crop improvement. Nonetheless, the way this genetic diversity was probed across time has constantly evolved while being a continuum from the first day. Moreover, while the selection criteria for the desired traits and purposes in the ancient domestication process were certainly exclusively based on morphology (size, color, shape of leaves and fruits, easiness for identification) and to satisfy man's energy supply needs (taste and flavour, satiety potential), today, the required traits and purposes for plant domestication (seen as continuum) have been refined and expanded. Indeed, new technologies have been developed for probing the genetic diversity whereas human needs have increased to include health and wellbeing. As a consequence more specific and defined traits such as a targeted and defined ingredient or metabolite are sought. To date, the pace of plant domestication has slowed down mainly due to the loss of biodiversity but also because of our ability to satisfy our current food needs. Nevertheless, few new crops species are still being introduced into farming system to fill the growing gaps in the need of humans and pets. Although domestication, as a concept, is not the main focus of this chapter (reader can refer to [3, 4, 6-9]), this review will look at some aspects of plant domestication in the 21st century as compared with ancient domestication process, the extent of genetic diversity within North American roses, the challenges associated with the domestication and agronomy of Atlantic Canada wild rose species taken as an example, and how the current biotechnology tools can contribute to an economic crop production.

2. Domestication as a science

2.1. Definition

Domestication was defined by De Wet [8] as "changes in adaptation that insure total fitness in habitats especially prepared by man for his cultigens". Van Raamsdonk [7] refined this definition by taking into account Simmond's [6] observations on plant domestication syndrome because a considerable number of crop plants are dependent on man for establishing new generations due to non-dehiscence, non-shattering, and absence of seed dormancy. Domestication was thus better defined by van Raamsdonk as a process leading to characteristics that are beneficial to humans but generally unprofitable for plants in natural habitats and in the decrease or total lack of capability to disseminate viable offspring [7]. As such defined, the goal for crop domestication appears obvious: setting plant for human's benefits. However, the paths and process followed, and the tools used towards developing a new crop from its wild related plant can greatly vary (Table 1).

2.2. Domestication process and goal

An artificial selection results in a phenotypic evolution [10]. In fact, agriculture started ~10,000 years ago by probing the diversity present within wild plant species and by planting the selected specimens, first in the garden and then in the field setting, a process known as domestication. Although all crops and plant varieties known to man today did not undergo through this classic process (case of known semi-domesticates) [3], the vast majority did go through, and thus being fully or super domesticated [3], depending on era, needs and advances in technology. Domestication is generally considered to be the end-point of a continuum that starts with exploring wild plants, continues through cultivation of plants selected from the wild but not yet genetically different from wild plants, and terminates in the fixation (at some extent), through human selection, of morphological and hence genetic differences distinguishing a domesticate from its wild progenitor. Wild and cultivated populations differ statistically in various characters targeted by human selection, although the cultivated plants may be morphologically indistinguishable from the wild plants [3]. Therefore, cultivated populations are not genetically fixed for any characters distinguishing them from wild populations, but the frequencies of alleles governing the characters subjected to human selection presumably differ [3]. Casas et al. [11] considered that changes in allele frequencies resulting from human selection constitute at least an incipient domestication, i.e. a nascent domestication. These authors analyzed the morphological variations in wild, managed *in situ*, and cultivated populations of the columnar cactus *Stenocereus stellatus* in central Mexico. They investigated whether morphological divergence has occurred between manipulated and wild populations by the domestication processes. Multivariate statistical analyses showed that individuals grouped according to management options and the fruit characteristics were the most relevant for grouping. Sweet fruits with non-red pulp colors were more frequent in cultivated populations. The fruits were also larger, contained more and bigger seeds, had thinner peel, and fewer spines in cultivated populations than fruits in wild individuals. Phenotypes common in managed *in situ* and cultivated populations generally occur also in the wild but at lower frequencies. However, Gepts [12] considered cultivation as a necessary but insufficient condition for domestication which, at least incipient or semi-domestication, may occur without cultivation by selective removal of undesirable phenotypes and/or enhancement of desirable phenotypes in wild populations [11]. How these different domestication processes and the available tools may apply to wild rosehip is one of the main topics developed in this review.

2.3. Domestication tools

2.3.1. Ancient tools

The oldest cultivated garden rose was *R x richardii* grown and depicted in art works by the Minoan civilization in Crete more than 3500 years ago. Roses were extensively cultivated during the Roman era (625 BC- 476 AD). After the demise of the Roman Empire, the less-appreciated wild-growing roses in Europe and Asia, belonging to *Rosa* section *Canina* and known today as Dogroses were maintained in monasteries for their reputed medicinal properties [13]. By the 18th century, five rose species (*R. gallica, R. alba, R. damascena, R. centrifolia, and R. centrifolia moscosa*) sharing a number of features such as double flower, flagrance, flower colour, frost hardiness, spring flowering, resistance to black spot and rust, and susceptibility to mildew had emerged [14]. These five species fall into 5 broad rose classes namely Gallica, Alba, Damask, Centrifolia, and Moss rose, respectively, and referred to as old European roses. These traditional European roses were crossed with roses from China (*R. chinensis*) leading to *Rosa x hybrid*, the modern rose selected for defined traits such as shape, colour and flagrance of the flower bud and flower qualities, stem length, and vase life. During these times, probing the genetic diversity within wild populations and selection of progenies from crosses were solely based on morphology.

2.3.1.1. Probing the genetic diversity

During ancient times, botanists such as Linnaeus [15] have played a crucial role in probing rose genetic diversity and defining boundaries between species. Linaeus [15] was one of the first botanists to acknowledge the complexity of the genus *Rosa*. In his book "*Species Planta-*

rum" Linaeus stated that "the species of the genus *Rosa* are difficult to distinguish and determine, I have the impression that nature combines just for fun a number of them and then forms a new one out of the lot, those who have seen only some distinguish them more easily than those who have examined many". The complexity of the genus has remained enigmatic to taxonomists of the twentieth century [13, 16-19] as the morphological characters are continuous and possibly polygenic making difficult in assigning genotypes that clearly define taxa. Nonetheless, similar to any other plant species, end-uses have been instrumental drivers for probing the genetic diversity and guiding in the selection process.

2.3.1.2. Process and goal for probing the genetic diversity (food and ornamentals)

During the Middle Ages, dogroses were cultivated at monasteries as a medicinal plant and, all parts including rosehips, seeds, petals, leaves and roots were virtually used. Later on in the 19th century, dogroses served as rootstocks to graft modern rose cultivars either as frost or soil born disease resistance sources [13]. They have also been used as a rustic and hardly living fence for fields and public spaces. In the twentieth century, roses have become important horticultural and cosmetic crops receiving much attention from geneticists, breeders, and general public. Hybrid Tea varieties of roses (*Rosa hybrida* L.) are among the most economically important cut-flower plants. The first Hybrid Tea rose was introduced in 1867, and since then more than 10,000 varieties have been released.

The Centre for Variety Research, the Netherlands, has submitted more than 2,800, predominantly Hybrid Tea varieties, for Plant Breeders Rights. This number is increasing annually with 80 applications on average each year. This registration and protection process is based on morphological and physiological characteristics as described by the UPOV (Union Internationale pour la Protection des Obtentions Végétales) guidelines [20]. Wild roses, semi-domesticated and commercial varieties, serve as breeding materials for creating new genetic stocks. These breeding materials generally selected as seed or pollen parents, for flowers that are often flagrant, commonly rose-colored flowers although white or more rarely yellow flowers can be observed in some species [21] are used in crosses. Hence, seedlings of interest with differences in flagrance, colour, shapes, disease resistance genes are selected through extensive field trials and advanced in the registration process [22]. Among the many wild rose species, the selection was obviously based on easy availability, attractiveness of characters, seed set potential, but also the plant morphology such as dwarfness and small size of flowers [22]. During these times less emphasis was made on the wild rose fruit characteristics.

2.3.2. Modern tools

In modern times, these classical methods become less and less efficient as the number of varieties to be tested increases and the genetic distances between varieties becomes smaller [20]. As well, because the needs, objectives, and challenges associated with the rose industry are now changing both in terms of flower and fruit production, combination of morphological, cytological, conventional breeding and biotechnological methods are being widely used for the determination of *Rosa* species as well as for the development of new rose cultivars [23-28].

2.3.2.1. *Probing the genetic diversity*

Domestication and crop improvement involve the selection of specific alleles at genes controlling key morphological and agronomic traits, resulting in reduced genetic diversity relative to unselected genes [10]. This artificial selection process that operates also in almost all agro-systems, including agroforestry, favours abundance of the preferred targeted phenotypes, and acts with more intensity in household gardens [29]. In the 20th century, probing for crops and their wild relative's genetic diversity has been the focus of extensive investigations. In roses in particular, morphometric [13, 30-34], cytological characters [25, 35] were the most used in the *Rosa sp* taxonomy and phylogeny. But these methods have been proven not to be sufficient in assigning individual genotypes that clearly defined taxa [13]. The 21st century is characterized by a remarkable explosion of molecular tools, highly polymorphic and with high discrimination power, for deciphering differences based on DNA nucleotide sequences. The development of these tools were achieved mostly with the event of polymerase chain reaction (PCR) in the mid 1980's [36], which has revolutionized the field of biology by inspiring the development of many PCR-based technologies, large DNA sequence databases, and increased computer power by bioinformatics. Despite the success of these powerful tools and its speed in advancing our current knowledge of the *Rosa* phylogeny [16, 17, 19, 37-43], there is still not exist at present a single method or tool for tracing a clear cut relative phylogenetic position between *Rosa* subgenera, sections and species within the genus [16], mainly due to low sequence divergence, natural hybridization between taxa, and polyploidy [44]. Rather, complementary methods (morpho-cytology, ploidy level, and DNA sequences from both chloroplast and nuclear genomes) using extensive data computing, with iterations and bootstrapping, are now the approach commonly sought [16, 17, 39, 40, 44, 45, 46, 47]. Nonetheless, for well-defined *Rosa* species, the DNA sequence analysis for single nucleotide polymorphism [47] and SSR polymorphism [48] are the preferred choice for distinguishing between genotypes and varieties [20]. The current *Rosa* phylogeny relies mainly on Rehder [49] who subdivided the genus into 4 subgeneras: *Hulthemia, Platyrhodon, hesperhodon,* each with 1 or 2 species, and *Rosa*. Likewise, the large *Rosa* subgenus was divided into 10 sections (*Pimpinellifoliae, Rosa, Caninae, Carolinae, Cinnamomae, Synstylae, Indicae, Banksianae, Laevigatae, Bracteatae*). However, recent molecular evidences do not support distinct subgenera status [16, 50] but did support the presence of 2 main clades. One clade includes subgenera *Rosa* species of sections *Carolinae, Cinnamomae,* and *Pimpinellifoliae* (clade 1) and the other clade (clade 2) includes all remaining subgenera *Rosa* sections, excluding the section *Banksianae* which comprises *R. Banksiae* (section *Banksianae*), *R. roxburhii* (subgenera *Platyrhodon*), and *R. persica* (subgenera *Hulthemia*), found to be sister to clade 2 [16]. The section *Caninae* DC forms a large and well-defined group of polyploid taxa and known as dogroses. In this section, pentaploids are the most common, but tetraploid and hexaploids also occur [18]. Bruneau et al. [16] also showed that sections *Cinnamomae* and *Carolinae* form a monophyletic group, and should be merged into one section, referred to as sect *Cinnamomae*. Indeed, section *Cinnamomae* comprises more than 40% of the species in the genus *Rosa*.

2.3.2.2. *Process and goal (life quality)*

One of the main current questions is whether the process and goal for probing rose genetic diversity has changed over time. Although crop domestication and improvement process is a continuum, it evolves constantly with the available technologies in order to meet and fulfill the societal needs. In the present global economy, the scale of demands for any good has increased and the trade has become multidirectional (selling in all part of globe) with multiple layers (one product could be found in many other products as additive or supplement) (Table 1). Thus, probing the genetic diversity of a plant species which end-product would satisfy these new needs both in terms of quality, quantity, sustainability and stability has become the new challenge for plant products developers. Hence, the need for well characterized germplasm with stable and preserved genetic identity is becoming the landmark for todays and tomorrow's natural product designers and developers. Therefore, sophisticated molecular tools [51, 52] as well as mass tissue culture and plant propagation tools are being employed to insure stability and sustainability.

	Ancient domestication	**Domestication in the 21st century**	**References**
Purposes	Food, medicine clothing, energy, sustainability	Food, clothing, energy, health, life quality, sustainability	[28, 53, 54]
Screening methods	Morphology, taste, flavour, energy	Morphology, genetic DNA markers, QTLs, taste, flavour, energy, metabolite profiles,	[20, 41, 51, 52]
Production paths	Gathering, yards and small farms sowing and harvesting, human and animal force	Experimental tubes, growth chambers, greenhouse and fields, large commercial fields, high throughput management, human and animal force and mechanization	[28, 53]
Purity	Composite	Composite, variety	
Ecosystem	Complex	Simple	[53]
Yield	Low	High	[28, 55, 56]
Value chain	Self, local consumption,	Global, processing, distribution and marketing networks	

Table 1. Comparative pathways of ancient and modern plant domestication processes: purposes, tools, and expectations

3. Plant domestication in the 21st century: A case study with PEI wild rosehips

One of the most recent and successful domestication of a wild species is that of the North American ginseng [57]. Similar to ginseng, interests in wild rosehip products are increasing worldwide due to its nutraceutical and natural health products properties [13]. With aging and changing eating lifestyles, the incidence of chronic diseases is increasing worldwide. Despite success achieved in fighting these diseases, prevention measures have become top priorities for citizens and public health systems. Recently, increasing interest has been expressed in plant natural products as preventative agents. Hence, plant product preparations such as those from rosehip have been used as food and medicine for centuries. The genus *Rosa* contains more than 150 species. They are widespread in North America within the *Cinnamomae* section and are renowned for the vitamin C content [58-61]. Although formulations from *Rosa canina* have been associated with the treatment and symptom reduction of inflammation and arthritis, the vast majority of wild rose species are fully unexplored for their heath potential. To date, most of the reported studies were focused mainly on *Rosa* species within the *Caninae* section which comprises 20 – 30 *Rosa* species known as dogroses [18, 42] and is currently the focus of major domestication research programs for the production and commercialisation of rosehips (fruits) around the world, particularly in Northern Europe, Germany, Turkey, Eastern Europe and Chile [13]. So far, less emphasis has been made on *Rosa* species belonging to *R. carolina* complex within the *Cinnamomae* section and the rosehips production from the eastern North American native wild roses is new and emerging [55, 56]. This section deals with the genetic diversity of PEI wild rosehips, the challenges associated with their domestication as well as the agronomic practices that could ensure an economic production.

3.1. Introduction to the genus *Rosa*

The genus *Rosa* (*Rosaceae*) originated in the temperate regions of the northern hemisphere, including North America, Europe, Asia, and the Middle East, with the greatest diversity of species found in western China, where it is endemic, and is now widespread all over the globe [18]. With this wide distribution range and the high number of species (more than 150 shrub species), the delimitation of the species bounbaries remained a challenge for taxonomists and molecular biologists [16, 21, 41, 44].

3.2. *Rosa* species phylogeny and biodiversity

3.2.1. Global Rosa species biodiversity and phylogeny

The taxonomy and breeding system of the genus *Rosa* has been recently reviewed by several authors [13, 16, 21, 38, 49, 62, 63] and the reader is invited to find more details in these treatments. Of particular interests are works reported by Werlemark and Nybom [13] and Macphail and Kevan [21] on one hands, and those by Bruneau et al. [16] and Joly and Bruneau [44] on the other hands, focusing on the European Dogroses from section *Caninae* and the North American *Rosa* species from section *Cinnamomae*, respectively. Wild rose species from these two sections are currently extensively investigated for domestication purposes and commercial rosehip production [13, 55, 64-67]. As our interest lies mainly in the domestication of North American wild roses, the next section of this review will put more emphasis on the biodiversity and phylogeny of wild rose species commonly encountered in this part of the globe and more specifically in Canada, a country as large as the whole Europe (West and East taken together, excluding the former USSR).

3.2.2. North American Rosa species biodiversity and phylogeny

Biodiversity of the North American wild roses has been investigated by botanists in the early 1900's. Watson [68], Crepin [69, 70], Erlanson MacFarlane [71, 72] have described and defined 13 - 22 *Rosa* species in North America. This important polymorphism in *Rosa* species, especially in eastern North America, together with hybridization and polyploidy have long been considered as the major causes of taxonomic confusion in the genus [17]. Alfred Rehder (1869-1949) established the first foundation of *Rosa* species taxonomic relationship in a book entitled "*The Manual of Cultivated Trees and Shrubs Hardy in North America Exclusive of the Subtropical and Warmer Temperate Regions*" published in 1940 [49]. Rehder provided concise physical description, time of flowering, region of native habitat, hardiness zone, distinguishing features and pertinent information on North American roses, and subdivided the genus *Rosa* into 4 subgenera and 10 sections, including the *Rosa carolina* L. complex of section *Cinnamomae*. East of the Rocky Mountain, the *Rosa Carolina* complex is composed of five diploid species (*R. blanda*, Ait., *R. foliolosa* Nutt., *R. nitida* Wild., *R. palustris* March., and *R. Woodsii* Lindl.), three tetraploid species (*R. carolina* L., *R. virginiana* Mill., and *R. arkansana* Porter) and one hexaploid/octaploid species (*R. acicularis* Lindl.) which is morphologically distinct from all other species [17]. The taxonomic problems are well known at the diploid level, where some species hybridize and are also morphologically difficult to distinguish (which is particular true for *R. blanda* and *R. woodsii*), but are even more acute at the polyploidy level. *Rosa carolina* which is widespread East of the Mississipi river hybridizes with *R. Arkansana* in the western part of its distribution [71] but also in the East with *R. virginiana*. Moreover, the morphological similarity cuts across ploidy levels and no single morphological character can be used to distinguish one species to another [17]. Thanks to molecular tools (AFLP, SNP), haplotype network analysis using statistical parsimony, genealogical approach, and multivariate analysis of 25 morphological characters including ploidy determination based on stomatal guard cell lengths, Joly et al. [17] and Joly and Bruneau [44] determined four species at the diploid level and that were separated into 2 groups in the east of the Rocky Mountains: one group consists of *R. blanda* - *R. woodsii* (which were indistinguishable and should be considered as a single species), and the other group is consisted of *R. foliolosa*, *R. nitida*, and *R. palustris*. The authors also determined 3 species at the polyploid level: *R. arkansana*, *R. carolina*, *R. virginiana*, with evidence of hybridization between them. The diploids that are involved in the origins of the polyploid species in that region were also proposed. For Joly et al. [17], only diploids east of the Rocky Mountains are involved in the origins of polyploids. *Rosa arkansana* is derived from the *blanda-woodsii* group, *R. virginiana* originated from the *foliolosa- nitida-palustris* group, and *R. carolina* is derived from a hybrid between the two diploid groups. Thus, for wild rose species domestication and commercial production purposes in the Canadian Maritimes where both North American native wild species of the *R. carolina* complex grow in sympatry and also along with naturalized species such as *R. rugosa* or other members of dogroses (Figure 1), a careful species determination as well as genotypic identification of collected germplasm for propagation are of critical importance to ensure, genetic purity and traceability.

http://dx.doi.org/10.5772/54688

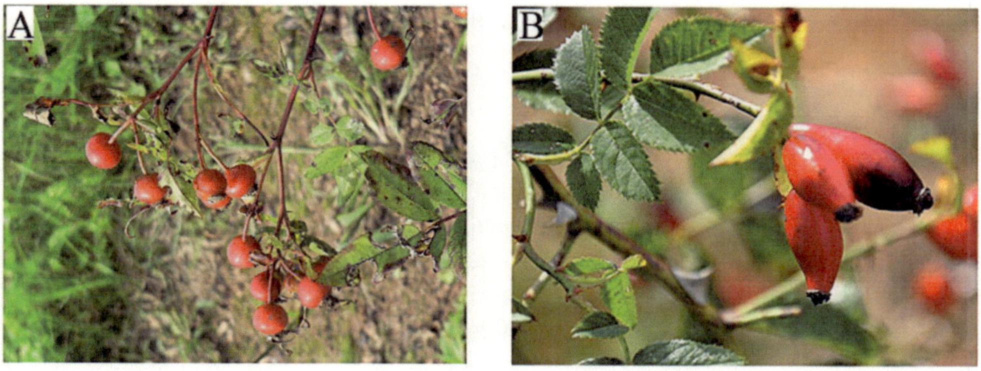

Figure 1. Diversity of rosehip morphology in the Atlantic Canada landscape. A, typical morphology PEI grown rosehip. B, morphological feature of a naturalized rosehip to Atlantic Canada.

3.2.3. Genetic and Metabolite diversity within the Prince Edward Island's field collection

Using SSR markers [20] and single nucleotide polymorphisms analysis, our group has assessed the genetic diversity within 30 ecotypes under cultivation and identified three major clusters, with cluster 2 and 3 showing 2 and 3 sub-clusters, respectively [65, 73]. The metabolite profiles in the flesh, seed, and fuzz for anthocyanins, flavonols, tilirosides which is a potent antidiabetic compound, tannins and fatty acids were also determined from the 30 ecotypes [65, 73]. The level of anthocyanin was very low in all ecotypes, with only one ecotype showing a level that was 30-40 % higher compared to the average. A large diversity was observed for flavonols and tiliroside among ecotypes. Only 4 ecotypes had a high content for both flavonols and tiliroside in the analyzed tissues (Ghose et al, submitted). One ecotype showed 18:3 level as high as 41.2%. The data suggests that it is possible to select and propagate a given ecotype for its unique metabolite profile for commercial and drug production [65, 73].

3.3. Domestication and end uses

Roses have been domesticated by man first for the beauty of their flower and incorporated in many cultural and political practices [74] and are now encountered on all continents, climates, and market places. Nonetheless, the medicinal uses of rose leaves, flowers and fruits were also widespread in human history [13, 54, 75-78].

3.3.1. Flower roses

The best known uses for roses are their flowers as ornamental on tables, in home backyards, public gardens and spaces. Historically, only very few wild rose species (at most 5 to 11 species) have been involved as parents in the today flower roses. One example of using native rose species in North America is related to the Parkland Rose series developed at AAFC in Morden, Manitoba. These flower roses are hardy, winter resistant and some of these rose varieties involve in their pedigree *R. Arkansana* which is encountered east of the Rocky Mountain in Canada. Beside, its ornamental features, rose flowers are valuable for the cosmetic industry [75, 76, 78].

3.3.2. Wild rosehips

The fruits of roses, the hips, have been highly regarded as important food and medicinal sources [13, 54, 79]. Rosehip is appreciated as traditional vitamin C rich soup in Sweden where the demand is particularly high [80]. Its flesh and seeds have been used in concoctions and tonics for various ailments, including the use as laxative and diuretic, against common cold, gastroinstestinal disorders, gastric ulcers [77, 81, 82], and anti-inflammatory diseases such as arthritis [83]. A review on the major chemical components of dogrose hips from was recently made by Werlemark [13]. However, a marked variation in chemical composition is associated with species, genotypes, and environments in which the plants evolve. For example, Melville and Pyke [84] found a weak correlation between latitude and vitamin C content of British rosehip populations from Scotland and England. Similarly, Werlemark [13] hypothesised that rosehips produced in a colder climate, especially with colder summer, may have higher vitamin C content compared to those that have been maturing in a warmer climate and also anticipated that local variations in precipitations and temperatures during summer may affect the chemical content of rosehips. It is reasonable to assume that, with different species and cooler summer and fall (Table 2), the Canadian Maritime wild rose species would show different chemical composition, especially in terms of relative amount when compared to their European and South American counterparts. By comparing some rosehip samples from Prince Edward Island, Denmark, Chile and South Africa, our group observed differences between origins, especially with regards to total oil content and fatty acid profiles (Figure 2). Nonetheless, sample preparation (harvesting time and conditioning) can also be a major source of variation. It will be of interest to compare the chemical composition of rosehips collected in each of these regions during the same summer or fall for obtaining factual and conclusive answers to these assumptions.

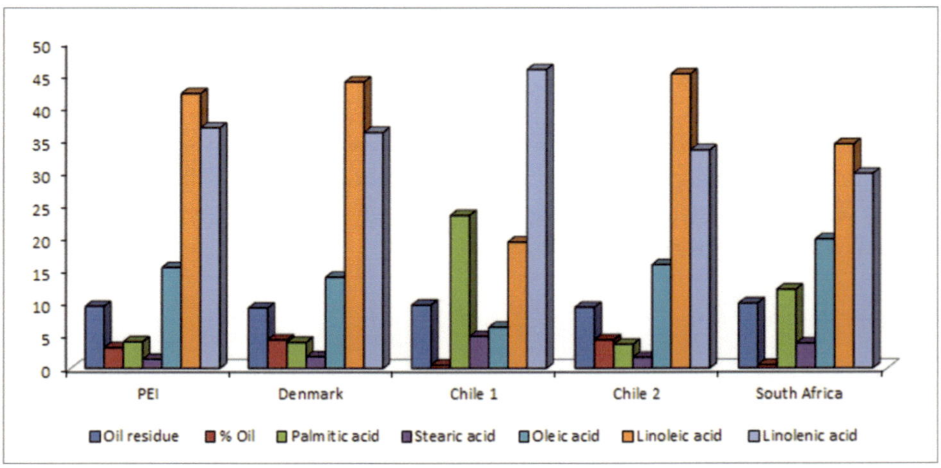

Figure 2. Comparative study of rosehip samples from Prince Edward Island, Denmark, Chile, and South Africa.

Rosehip seed contains pretty well balanced omega-6 (18:2) / omega-3 (18:3) fatty acid ratio and also shows relatively high level of oleic acid as compared to olive and canola oils that are rich in oleic acid but low in both linoleic and linolenic acids (Figure 3). As genetic variability for fatty acid composition has been observed in PEI wild roses (Ghose et al, submitted) and the seed oil content is relatively low, breeding efforts could contribute to increase the oil content.

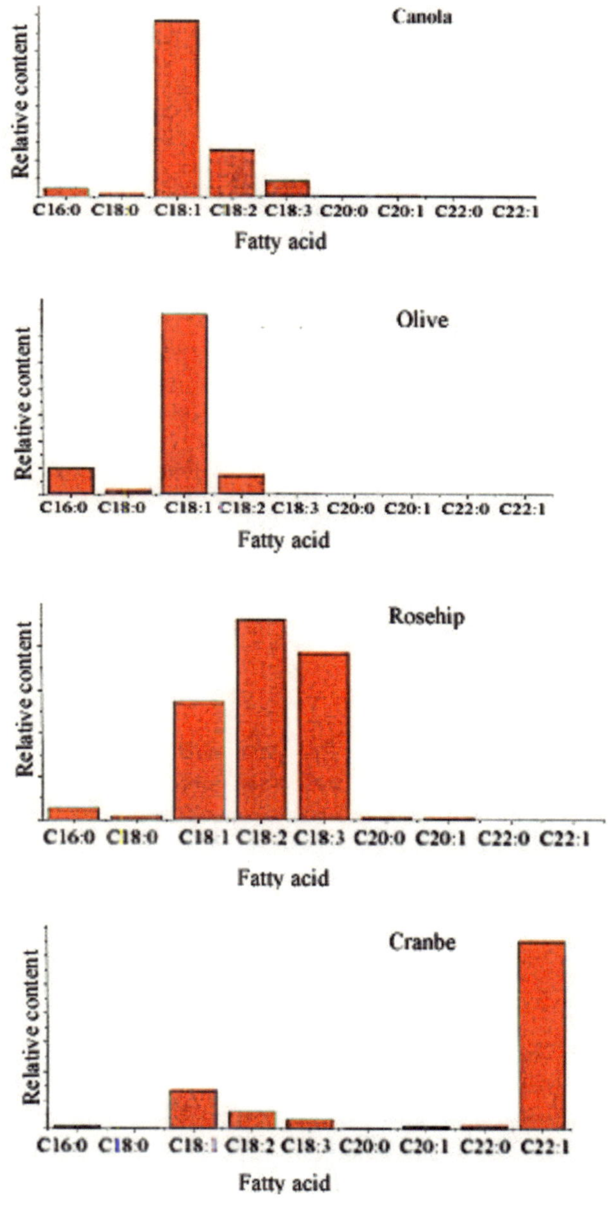

Figure 3. Comparative fatty acid profile of rosehip with three oilseed crops.

3.3.2.1. Agronomy

Although a high value was recognized to rosehip throughout centuries, it is only recently that the wild roses are being domesticated and cultivated for their fruits and to develop agronomic practices that ensure an economic production of the hips [28, 51, 52, 56, 77, 85]. However, due to the diversity of species, genotypes, soils and climates, different agronomic practices are being implemented and tested in different regions, including Denmark, Turkey, Bulgaria, Chile and Canada. Whereas Chilean started their trials by developing a nursery built on the "Tunnel" greenhouse model with a capacity to accommodate 15.000 cuttings, under an irrigation system with nebulizers to reduce temperature and humidification before a developmental stage in the fields, the Danish, Swedish and Canadian choose to established field trials using wild cutting, spacing, density and nutrient management trials [28, 55]. In Sweden, the germplasm used were mostly concentrated on the Scandinavian *Rosa* species of section *Caninae* especially, *R. dumalis, R. rubiginosa* and their interspecific hybrids [86] whereas Danish rosehips are produced mainly from *R. canina* (www.hyben-vital.com) although it may also involve other Scandinavian species. In Chile, the current production is mainly focused on wild hand-harvested hips from uncharacterized and naturalized species introduced to south America by Spanish and is mostly a mixture of *R. rubiginosa, R. canina, R. moschata* and many other species found in western Europe [66]. In Prince Edwards Island, (Canada), current recent genetic study based on 30 wild ecotypes collected from this province suggested that all accessions currently under field trial are from *R. virginiana* and its natural hybrids with *R. Carolina* (Ghose et al, submitted). At present, very few cultivars have been named and released for commercial fruit production. One cultivar, the cultivar "Mechthilde von Neuerburg" derived from *R. rubiginosa* was reported in Germany. Two cultivars (Sylwia and Sylwana) derived from *R. canina* were reported in Poland, whereas cultivar Plovdiv 1 from *R. canina,* and cultivar Karpatia from *R. villosa* were reported in Bulgaria and Slovakia, respectively [13]. For all of these semi-domesticated wild rosehips, it is not known or reported whether the ongoing domestication process has already impacted on some of the phenotypic traits such fruit size, fruit setting or metabolite profile. By comparing the pomology characteristics of 5 wild rosehip ecotypes growing in the wild or in the field settings, we observed that the field setting contributed to increase the fruits size and delayed the maturity when compared with growing in the wild, suggesting an occurrence of a domestication syndrome for these traits (Fofana, personal observation). However, no significant difference was found between the two environments for the number of seed in each of the ecotype.

3.3.2.1.1. Soils and climates

Although originally native to temperate regions of the globe, roses have adapted to warmer regions and grow well now in very diversified habitats and soil types [13, 79]. The soil should be well drained though and not heavy. Species preference for soil type has nonetheless been reported. *R. villosa* was reported to grow better in a dry soil with low calcium content whereas *R. canina* and *R. dumalis* prefer more calcareous soil. *R. rubiginosa* also prefers more calcium and grows well in a relatively heavy soil [13]. *R. palustris* grows in marshes and *R. nitida* in bogs. Similarly, *R. virginiana* likes salt marshes and salty soils (Joly, personal communications).

In Prince Edwards Island province (Canada), wild rosehips are found in a variety of habitats including hedgerows, wet and dry pastures, thickets, swamps and uplands in dry orthic humo-ferric Podzol sandy soils [55]. In hard winter climates such as Canada, plant survival rate in the field setting can vary from genotype to genotype and for the same genotype, plastic coverage has been shown to increase the winter survival rate (Figure 4).

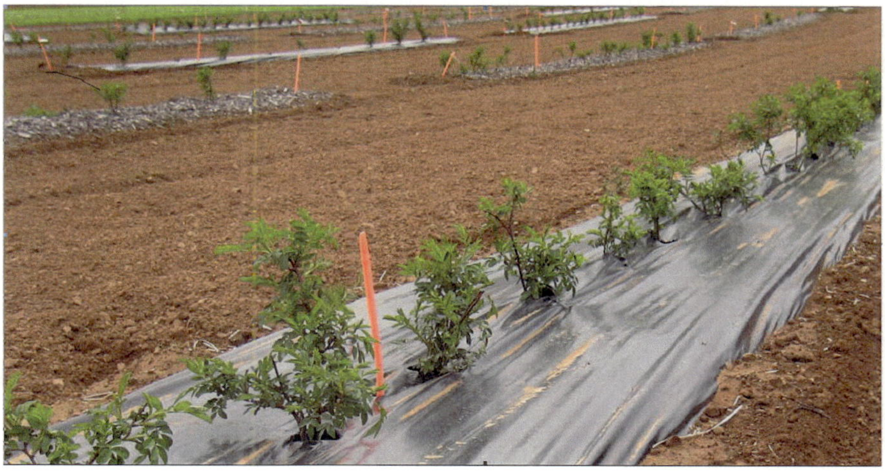

Figure 4. Effect of planting beds coverage with plastic on winter survival.

	Temperature (°C)		Precipitations (mm)		Soil type	Latitude
	Summer	Fall	Summer	Fall		
PEI Canada	16 – 22	7 – 18	270	300	Orthic humo-ferric Podzol with sandy loam	46.04 – 46.57
Denmark	17	9	170	150	Typic Fragiudalf	55 – 57.4
Sweden	13	5	180	120- 140	Aeric Endoaquept	55 – 68 N
Turkey	17 – 29	6 – 7	50	70	Typic Haploxeroll	36 – 42 N
Bulgaria	25	14	180	120	pseudopodzolic- podzolic	41 – 43 N
Chile	17 – 28	8 - 20	350- 500	200 -300	Andisol - Ultisol	18 – 58 S

Table 2. Comparison of average temperature and precipitations during summer and fall in major rosehip production countries.

3.3.2.1.2. Fertilization

Barry et al [55] described the first time the establishment of field trial for North American wild roses belonging to the *R. carolina* complex, with as an objective to investigate the effects of several field management practices on commercial rosehip production in Atlantic Canada. Treatments were applied at planting in a factorial randomized complete block design in June 2004 and included three in-row mulch (none, bark, and straw) treatments, three in-row fertility (none, compost, and fertilizer) treatments, and two interrow management (tilled and sod) treatments. The compost consisted of an initial mix of softwood sawdust, lobster waste, and old hay. Prior to planting, compost was applied at 60 t ha−1 (54 kg plot−1) in a 1-m band over the row and was incorporated by hand raking. The fertilizer used was a commercial grade (5N-20P-20K). This fertilizer formulation was chosen for use during the first year to promote root development and plant establishment. During the second year (2005), compost was reapplied as top-dress on 22 June 2005 and the fertilizer used was a commercial grade (10N-10P-10K), which was applied as top-dress on 25 May 2005. A fertilizer with higher nitrogen content was chosen with the aim of improving overall plant health and yield during the second growing season. Fertilizer was applied at a rate of 800 kg ha−1 (648 g plot−1) in a 1-m band over the planting row. In Dogroses, Werlemark and Nybom [13] reported 50 g NPK for each plant at planting and 300 kg/ha of organic-mineral NKP in the subsequent year, with additional calcium amendment depending on soil types and species. In Prince Edwards Island, mulching increased nutrient uptake of N and P and increased plant growth. Fertilizer increased plant growth and yield of rose hips compared to no fertilizer or compost treatments. Tilled interrow treatment increased in shoot lengths, diameters, and plant spreads compared to interrow sod. The study indicated that during the early establishment years of a rose hip plantation in Atlantic Canada, wild roses grow best with the use of mulch, fertilizer, and tillage between the rows [55].

3.3.2.1.3. Pests and diseases management

Traditionally, fungal diseases such as black spot caused by *Diplocarpon rosae*, powdery mildew (*Podosphaera pannosa*) rusts (*Phargmidium spp*) and leaf spot *(Sphaceloma rosarum)* have been reported to be problematic in ornamental roses [87-90] and field-grown dogroses [13, 48, 91, 92]. These fungal diseases management is carried through fungicide treatment [93] and selection of genetic resistance [94-96]. Genetic resistance sources within wild rose species within *Caninae* section have been investigated for field rosehip production. Fungal disease tolerance characteristics were identified in *R. rubiginosa* and in interspecific hybrids involving species from *Caninae* and *Cinnamomae* sections [48]. Up to date, no such disease resistance screening has been performed within the *R. carolina* complex for a commercial wild rosehips production in North American. However, our observations in the field showed evidence of these diseases on PEI wild roses (Figure 5). Research in this field should be carried to mitigate the disease incidence in their new field environment. As for any crop, introduction of elite genotypes in cropping systems for rosehips production will lead to a decreased genetic diversity of the cultigens. It is thus anticipated that more susceptibility to major diseases could be observed in the field as compared to the wild populations from which they derive. The preservation of natural habitats hosting the wild populations is of great importance to ensure an availability of genetic stocks to be used in the introgression of disease resistance genes from the wild types to the cultigens.

Insects such aphids (*Aphidina*), grasshoppers (*Orthoptera*), mites (*Tetranychidae*), sawflies (*Tenthredinidae*), gall-making cynipids (*Diplolepis*) as well as the rosehip fly (*Rhagoletis alternate*) have also been reported in dogrose orchards and to cause severe damage in some cases

[13]. Nematode (*Pratylenchus penetrans*) is causal pests of severe lesions to roots in a wide range of ornamental hosts, including roses, mainly in temperate regions. Peng [97] reported that *R. virginiana* is a good nematode resistance source. Because Prince Edwards Island is world leading potato producing area with prevalence of nematodes in the agricultural landscape, development of rosehips orchards with *R. virginiana* genetic background could be a mean for reducing nematode populations in highly infested fields.

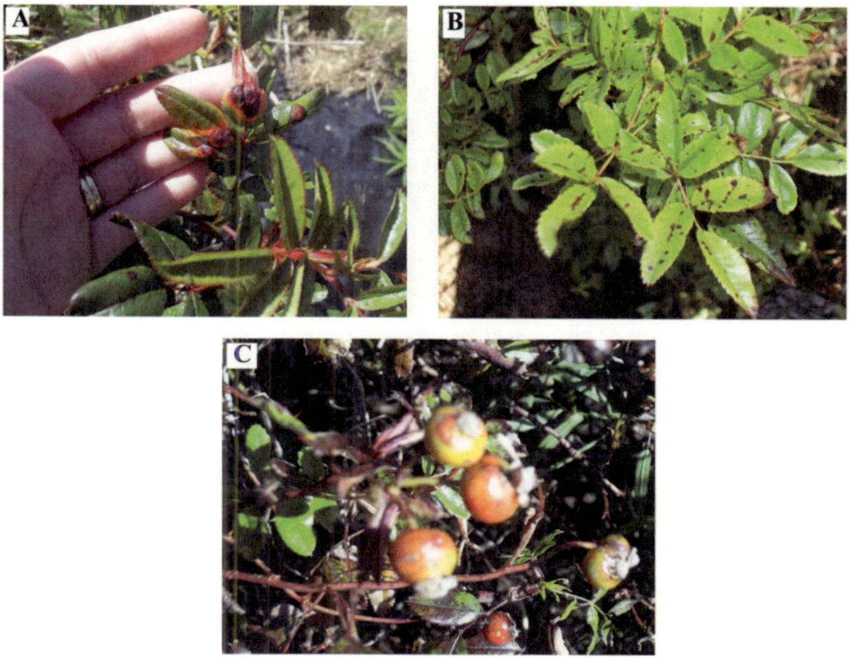

Figure 5. Foliar and fruits diseases in wild roses. A, powdery mildew; B, leaf spot; C, lesions on immature rosehips probably caused by *Phargmidium spp* (Rust) or *Sphaceloma rosarum* (leaf spot).

3.3.2.1.4. Yield and storage

Rosehip yield vary considerably depending on the plant material, cultivation procedures, age of orchard, and harvesting methods. Werlemark and Nybom [13] reported that up to 8 kg of rosehips per bush could be harvested by hand in commercial planting of dogrose hybrid PiRo 3. Similarly up to 3 t/ha could be obtained from *R. dumalis* and *R. rubiginosa* with mechanical harvesting in Sweden. In these cases however, no mention is made about the age of the orchards as yield increases markedly several years after planting. In contrast, Sanderson and Fillmore [56], reported in 14 rosehip ecotypes of the *R. Carolina* complex grown in field condition an average rosehip yield ranging between 411 and 2000 kg/ha, with a fruit mean weight of 1.01 – 1.62 g, over the first four hand harvesting years. The lowest and highest yielding selections showed 910 and 3634 kg/ha in the fourth years, respectively (Table 3).

Compared with reports by Ercisli and Guleryuz [98], Dogan and Kazankaya [99], Güneş and Dölek [100], the fruit weight reported by Sanderson is lower but showed relatively narrow range of variation between ecotypes, reflecting the relatively narrow genetic diversity among these ecotypes. Joly (personal communication) reported that *R. virginiana* and *R. Arkansana* are the two species with the greatest number of fruits per flowering branches. They have more fruits than *R. carolina* and the height of *R. virginiana* makes it one of the most productive North American roses. To preserve the integrity of rosehip bioactives, the postharvest handling and storage conditions are key factors. Both sun-drying and mechanical dryers are being used at commercial scale and the reader can see more details in Werlemark and Nybom [13].

	Biological yield					Mean fruit
Selection	2006	2007	2008	2009	Mean	weight
			(kg ha^{-1})			(g)
s26	877	1413	2368	3634	2000	1.62
s30	347	569	1557	2676	1431	1.31
s28	498	335	1136	1759	946	1.57
s22	416	422	831	1464	783	1.29
s67	270	338	910	1440	740	1.39
s25	355	116	562	1725	719	1.29
s57	195	371	941	1178	675	1.03
s33	395	330	654	1227	657	1.33
s55	313	384	679	1167	638	1.42
s36	181	166	862	1307	622	1.01
s140	300	186	576	1342	610	1.21
s142	406	430	464	956	568	1.17
s68	284	281	430	1092	514	1.21
s122	246	83	416	910	411	1.12
Grand mean	363	387	885	1563	808	1.28

Table 3. Yield progression over four years after plantation and mean fruit weight of 14 rosehip ecotypes grown in field (2006-2009)

3.3.2.2. Biotechnology

One of the shortcoming issues for the establishment of commercial rosehip production orchard is the availability plant materials for large acreages. So far, all established fields are based on cuttings or seedlings obtained from wild selections. Because of the genetic diversity within the genus *Rosa* and morphological similarities between species, hybrids (interspecific and intraspecific) and their parental species at the collection sites, an accurate identification at the collection site and the traceability of the putative cultivars under development is challenging and not guaranteed. This issue will become major issues in a near future as rosehip provenances will increase and the bioactive metabolites that are associated to each species, provenance, and ecotypes are made available for marketing purposes. Thus, the use of combined morphological, cytological, and molecular biology tools for assigning a genetic identity, and the use of regeneration technologies that ensure mass plant production and ensuring the genetic integrity of clones is a research direction that should be undertaken similarly to the ornamental flower industry.

3.3.2.2.1. Regeneration and propagation

3.3.2.2.1.1. Regeneration by seed

The use of plant regeneration from seed for commercial production has been reported [85, 101]. It ensures the production of higher number of plants for field planting in a relatively short period of time. However, the mating system of *Rosa* species is a major source of genetic variability between plant materials obtained using such an approach, especially when the seed is collected from uncontrolled sources like wild plants.

3.3.2.2.1.2. Cutting and explants

Cuttings and explants are currently the materials of choice in commercial wild rose production [64, 86, 101], and most, if not all, of these explants (Figure 6) are derived from wild plants. Wild rose plants grow in the nature as populations that can involve different species, interspecific and intraspecifc hybrids, parental and sibling all growing in a confined area. Collecting cuttings in such an environment, even from the same patch, does not ensure the genetic integrity of the collected material for propagation. Once collected, the material should be well characterized and identified. Now, remains our ability to get enough characterized plant materials for large field planting. We believe that the well characterized plant material should be used as starting point for plant regeneration and mass production in the form of rooted seedling or cuttings. This is the approach we pursue in Canada for commercial wild rose production (Figure 7).

3.3.2.2.1.3. Tissue culture

Tissue protocols have been developed and available for flower roses [102-104] and could be applied to rosehip production. Once elite genotypes such as those reported by Sanderson and Fillmore [56] are identified, tissue culture should be able to ensure a sustainable plant production or field planting by growers (Figure 7).

3.3.2.2.2. Cell culture

Similar to tissue culture, rose plants can be regenerated by cell culture. Contrary to tissue culture however, the new plants are obtained from callus generated from sterile explants. This method leads to pure line but can also create new lines different from the mother plant from which the explant was obtained because of somaclonal variations that may occur during the induction of callus and regeneration processes. Thus, for the production of mass plant production from a selected elite wild ecotype, tissue culture appears more appropriate as it minimizes the risk of somaclonal variations while showing high rate of plant multiplication.

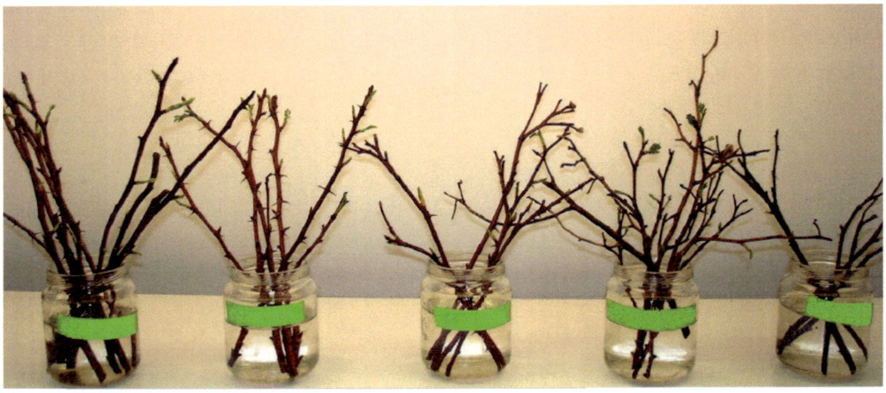

Figure 6. Rose cuttings for multiplication. Sterile rose dormant stems were conditioned to break dormancy. Note the active buds sprouting.

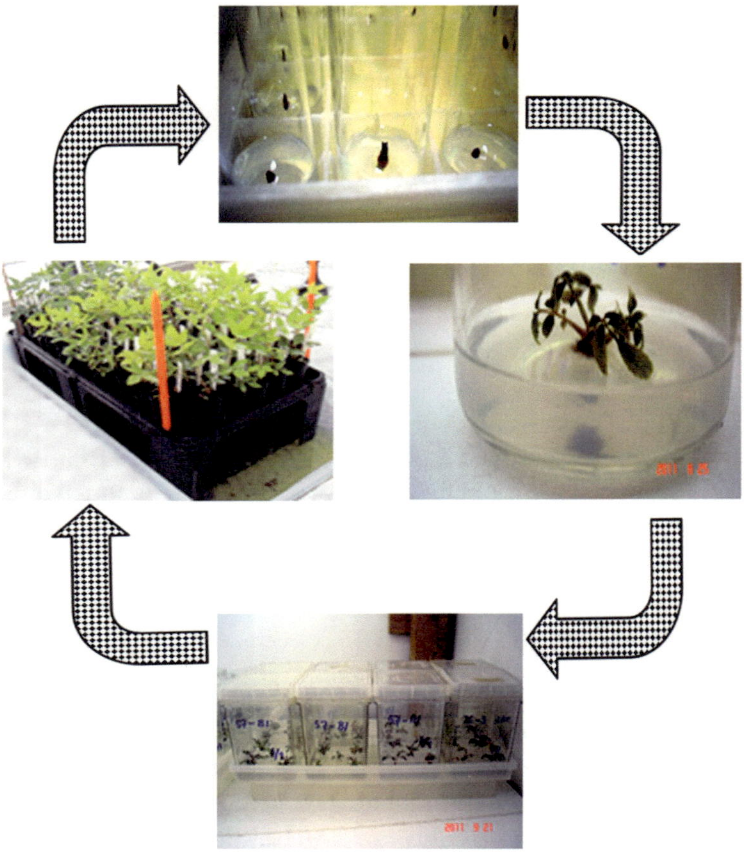

Figure 7. Mass rosehip plant regeneration from active buds of well characterized rosehip genotypes. A, active buds in regeneration media; B, regenerated rose plant; C, plant multiplication in rooting media; and D, acclimation in greenhouse.

4. Conclusions

With the increasing demands for natural heath products, plant biodiversity is being thoroughly revisited. The genus *Rosa* has a complex taxonomy that is still being investigated with scrutiny. East of the Rocky Mountain, *Rosa* species belonging to *R. carolina* complex in the *Cinnamomae* section include five diploid species, three tetraploid species and their natural hybrid. Several of these species as well as their interspecific hybrids are encountered on Prince Edwards Islands, Canada. A commercial rosehip production program using wild selected ecotypes has been developed and elite selections with high yielding potential have been identified and agronomic practices set for field management. The collection has been characterised using a combined morphological, cytological and molecular tools and appears to be made of *R. virginina* and its natural hybrids with *R. carolina*. Genetic and metabolite diversity among these wild ecotypes was observed and could be of high potential for large field production and breeding programs. However, the disease resistance status in this complex is unknown. As for any new crop, increased incidence of exiting diseases and recruitment of new diseases is anticipated in the field setting as compared to the wild populations from which they derive. The preservation of natural habitats hosting the wild populations as source of genetic stocks is critical to ensure gene transfer from the wild types to the cultigens through breeding. Future works should also aim at developing mass plant production to ensure sustainable plant material supply from the elite selections.

Acknowledgements

Rosehip research by BF and KS was partly supported by AAFC start-up fund to BF, A-base to KS, and an AIF fund received by BF and KS from University of Prince Edward Island (UPEI) through the Innovative Canadian bioActives and Nutraceuticals (ICAN) project. The authors warmly thank Dr. Simon Joly (University of Montreal) for his kind willingness to proof read this manuscript; David Main, Sylvia Wyand (Crops and Livestock Research Centre, Charlottetown), Nicholas Kaye, Stephen Locke, and Ningzhang Zhou (NRC, Charlottetown) for their technical assistance.

Author details

Bourlaye Fofana[1*], Kaushik Ghose[1,2], Bob Chapman[1] and Kevin Sanderson[1]

1 Crops and Livestock Research Centre, Agriculture and Agri-Food Canada, Charlottetown, PEI, Canada

2 University of Prince Edwards Island and National Research Council, Charlottetown, PEI, Canada

References

[1] Erickson DL, Smith BD, Clarke AC, Sandweiss DH, Tuross N. An Asian origin for a 10,000-year-old domesticated plant in the Americas. Proc Natl Acad Sci USA 2005;102:18315-18320.

[2] Beja-Pereira A, England PR, Ferrand N, ordan S, Bakhiet AO, Mohammed A. Abdalla MA, Marjan Mashkour M, Jordana J, Taberlet P, LuikartG. African Origins of the Domestic Donkey. Science 2004;304:1781.

[3] Pickersgill B. Domestication of plants in the Americas: insights from Mendelian and molecular genetics. Ann Bot 2007;100:925-940.

[4] Pigershill B. Taxonomy and the origin and evolution of cultivated plants in the New World. Nature 1977;268:591-595.

[5] Vaughan DA, Balazs E, Heslop-Harrison JS. From Crop Domestication to Super-domestication. Ann Bot 2007;100:893-901.

[6] Simmonds NW. Principles of crop improvement. N.Y.: Longman; 1979. p. 408.

[7] Van Raamsdonk LWD. The cytological and genetical mechanisms of plant domestication exemplified by four crop models. Botanical review 1995;61:367-399.

[8] de Wet JMJ. Species concepts and systematics of domesticated cereals. Die Kutturpflanze 1981;29:177-198.

[9] Yamasaki M. Maize domestication and breeding based on genomic variation. Tanpakushitsu Kakusan Koso 2007;52:1942-1946.

[10] Yamasaki M, Wright SI, McMullen MD. Genomic screening for artificial selection during domestication and improvement in maize. Ann Bot 2007;100:967-973.

[11] Casas A, Caballero J, Valiente-Banuet A, Soriano JA, Davila P. Morphological variation and the process of domestication of *Stenocereus stellatus* (*Cactaceae*) in Central Mexico. American Journal of Botany 1999;86:522.

[12] Gepts P. Crop domestication as a long-term selection experiment. Plant Breeding 2004;24:1-44.

[13] Werlemark G, Nybom H. Dogroses: Botany, Horticulture, genetics, and Breeding. Willey Blackwell; 2010. p. 199-255.

[14] Office of the gene technology regulator. The biology and Ecology of *Rosa x hybrida* (Rose). In: D. o. H. a. a. Australlian Government editor; 2005. p. 19.

[15] Linnaeus C. editor. Species plantarum. Laurentus salvius; 1753. p. 1200.

[16] Bruneau A, Starr JR, Joly S. Phylogenetic relationships in the genus *Rosa*: new evidence from chloroplast DNA sequences and an appraisal of current knowledge. Systematic Botany 2007;32.

[17] Joly S, Starr JR, Lewis WH, Bruneau A. Polyploid and hybrid evolution in roses east of the Rocky Mountains. American Journal of Botany 2006;93:412-425.

[18] Khaitova L, Werlemark G, Nybom H, Kovarik A. Frequent silencing of rDNA loci on the univalent-forming genomes contrasts with their stable expression on the bivalent-forming genomes in polyploid dogroses (*Rosa* sect. Caninae). Heredity 2010;104:113-120.

[19] Millan T, Osuna F, Cobos S, Torres AM, Cubero JI. Using RAPDs to study phylogenetic relationships in *Rosa*. Theor Appl Genet 1996;92:273-277.

[20] Esselink GD, Smulders MJM, Vosman B. Identification of cut rose (*Rosa hybrida*) and rootstock varieties using robust sequence tagged microsatellite site markers. Theoretical and Applied Genetics 2003;106:277-286.

[21] Macphail VJ, Kevan PG. Review of the breeding systems of wild roses (*Rosa spp.*). Floriculture and Ornemental Biotechnology 2009;3:1-13.

[22] de Vries DP, Dubois LAM. Rose breeding: Past, present and prospects. Acta Horticulturae 1996;424:241-248.

[23] Ercisli S, Guleryuz M. Rose hip utilization in Turkey. Acta Horticulturae 2005;690:77-81.

[24] Gudin S. Rose breeding technologies. Acta Horticulturae 2001;547:23-33.

[25] Gustafsson A. The constitution of the *Rosa canina* complex. Hereditas 1944;30:405-428.

[26] Leus L, Van Huylenbroeck J, Van Bockstaele E, Höfte M. Bioassays for screening resistance in commercial rose breeding. Acta Horticulturae 2003;612:39-45.

[27] Lundin H. The ascorbic acid content in certain agricultural products. Breeding experiments with wild rose bushes to obtain hips with a high ascorbic acid content suitable for industrial use. Nordisk Jordbrugsforskning 1946;3-4:65-85.

[28] Uggla M, Nybom H. Domestication of a new crop in Sweden - Dogroses (*Rosa* sect. Caninae) for commercial rose hip production. Acta Horticulturae 1998;484:147-152.

[29] Parra F, Casas A, Penaloza-Ramirez JM, Cortes-Palomec AC, Rocha-Ramirez V, Gonzalez-Rodriguez A. Evolution under domestication: ongoing artificial selection and divergence of wild and managed *Stenocereus pruinosus* (*Cactaceae*) populations in the Tehuacan Valley, Mexico. Ann Bot 2010;106:483-496.

[30] Kovacs S, Facsar G, Udvardy L, Toth M. Phenological, morphological and pomological characteristics of some rose species found in Hungary. Acta Horticulturae 2005;690:71-76.

[31] Nybom H, Carlson-Nilsson U, Werlemark G, Uggla M. Different levels of morphometric variation in three heterogamous dogrose species (*Rosa* sect. Caninae, *Rosaceae*). Plant Systematics and Evolution 1997;204:207-224.

[32] Nybom H, Olsson A, Werlemark G. Morphometirc variation in Nordic dogroses (*Rosa* sect. Caninae, *Rosaceae*). Symb Bot Ups 1996;31:59-68.

[33] Raymond O, Fiasson JL, Jay M. Synthetic taxonomy of *Rosa* races using ACT-STATIS. Zeitschrift fur Naturforschung Section C, Biosciences 2000;55:399-409.

[34] Uggla M, Gao X, Werlemark G. Variation among and within dogrose taxa (*Rosa* sect. caninae) in fruit weight, percentages of fruit flesh and dry matter, and vitamin C content. Acta agriculturae Scandinavica Section B, Soil and plant science 2003;53:147-155.

[35] Ma Y, Crane CF, Byrne DH. Karyotypic relationships among some *Rosa* species. Caryologia 1997;50:317-326.

[36] Mullis K, Faloona F, Sharf S, Saiki R, Horn G, Erlich H. Specific enzymatic amplification of DNA in vitro: The polymerase chain reaction. Cold Spring Harb Symp Quant Biol 1986;51:263-273.

[37] Wu S, Ueda Y, He H, Nishihara S, Matsumoto S. Phylogenetic analysis of Japanese *Rosa* species using matK sequences. Breeding Science 2000;50:275-281.

[38] Wu S, Ueda Y, Nishihara S, Matsumoto S. Phylogenetic analysis of Japanese *Rosa* species using DNA sequences of nuclear ribosomal internal transcribed spacers (ITS). Journal of Horticultural Science and Biotechnology 2001;76:127-132.

[39] Joly S, Bruneau A. Incorporating allelic variation for reconstructing the evolutionary history of organisms from multiple genes: An example from *Rosa* in North America. Syst Biol 2006;55:623-636.

[40] Joly S, Bruneau A. Measuring branch support in species trees obtained by gene tree parsimony. Syst Biol 2009;58:100-113.

[41] Kimura T, Nishitani C, Iketani H, Ban Y, Yamamoto T. Development of microsatellite markers in rose. Molecular Ecology Notes 2006;6:810-812.

[42] Nybom H, Esselink GD, Werlemark G, Vosman B. Microsatellite DNA marker inheritance indicates preferential pairing between two highly homologous genomes in polyploid and hemisexual dog-roses, *Rosa* L. sect. Caninae DC. Heredity 2004;92:139-150.

[43] Rusanov K, Kovacheva N, Vosman B, Zhang L, Rajapakse S, Atanassov A, Atanassov I. Microsatellite analysis of *Rosa damascena* Mill. accessions reveals genetic similarity between genotypes used for rose oil production and old Damask rose varieties. Theor Appl Genet 2005;111:804-809.

[44] Joly S, Bruneau A. Delimiting species boundaries in *Rosa* Sect. Cinnamomeae (*Rosaceae*) in Eastern North America. Syst Bot 2007;32:819-836.

[45] Werlemark G, Uggla M, Nybom H. Morphological and RAPD markers show a highly skewed distribution in a pair of reciprocal crosses between hemisexual dog rose species, *Rosa* sect. Caninae. Theoretical and Applied Genetics 1999;98:557-563.

[46] Werlemark G, Nybom H. Skewed distribution of morphological character scores and molecular markers in three interspecific crosses in *Rosa* section Caninae. Hereditas (Lund) 2001;134:1-13.

[47] Mercure M, Bruneau A. Hybridization between the escaped *Rosa rugosa* (*Rosaceae*) and the native *R. Blanda* in Eastern North America. American Journal of Botany 2008;95:597-607.

[48] Carlson-Nilsson BU, Uggla M. Can wild dogroses tame the fungal beast? Acta Horticulturae 2005;690:181-187.

[49] Rehder A. Manual of cultivated trees and shrubs hardy in North America. New York; 1940. p. 996.

[50] Koopman WJ, Wissemann V, De Cock K, Van Huylenbroeck J, De Riek J, Sabatino GJ, Visser D, Vosman B, Ritz CM, Maes B, Werlemark G, Nybom H, Debener T, Linde M, Smulders MJ. AFLP markers as a tool to reconstruct complex relationships: A case study in *Rosa* (*Rosaceae*). American Journal of Botany 2008;95:353-366.

[51] Ercisli s. Rose (*Rosa spp*) germplasm resources of Turkey. Genet Res Crop Evol 2005;52:787-795.

[52] Nybom H, Werlemark G, Carlson-Nilsson U, Olsson, Uggla M. Genetic variation in a new crop - Dogroses Dogroses (*Rosa* sect. Caninae) for commercial rosehip production. Acta Horticulturae 1998;484:139-146.

[53] Bradshaw HDJ, Strauss SH. Breeding strategies for 21st century: domestication of poplar. . In: J. G. I. D.I. Dickmann, J.H. Eckenwalder, J. Richardson editor. Poplar culture in North America. Ottawa: NRC Press; 2001. p. 383-394.

[54] Ocksook YI, Jovel EM, Towers GHN, Wahbe TR, Cho D. Antioxidant and antimicrobial activities of native *Rosa sp.* from British Columbia, Canada. Inter J Food Sci and Nutr 2007;53:178-189.

[55] Barry R, Sanderson K, Fillmore S. Establishment of wild roses for commercial rose hip production in Atlantic Canada. International Journal of Fruit Science 2008;8:266-281.

[56] Sanderson K, Fillmore S. Evaluation of native rose selections for rose hip production in Prince Edward Island. International Journal of Fruit Science 2010;10:379-389.

[57] Bai D, Brandle J, Reeleder R. Genetic diversity in North American ginseng (*Panax quinquefolius* L.) grown in Ontario detected by RAPD analysis. Genome 1997;40:111-115.

[58] Melville R, Pyke M. The effect of specific variability and the environment on the vitamin C content of British rose hips. Proceedings of the Linnean Society of London 1947;159:5-16.

[59] Pyke M, Melville R. Vitamin C in rose hips. Biochemical Journal 1942;36:336.

[60] Salashinskii NA, Bersheda NA. Vitamin C retention in quick frozen rose hips during prolonged storage. Tovarovedenie 1991;24:20-22.

[61] Tuba J, Hunter G, Hutchinson MJ, Kennedy LL. On sources of vitamin C. 1. Rose hips. Canadian Journal of Research, Section Botanical Sciences 1943;2:363-373.

[62] Grossi C, Raymond O, Jay M. Flavonoid and enzyme polymorphisms and taxonomic organisation of *Rosa* sections: *Carolinae, Cinnamomeae, Pimpinellifoliae* and *Synstylae*. Biochemical Systematics and Ecology 1998;26:857-871.

[63] Wissemann V. Evolution by hybridisation. The influence of reticulate evolution on biosymmetrical patterns and processes in plants. Theory in Biosciences 2005;123:223-233.

[64] Ercişli S, Güleryüz M. A study of the propagation of the hardwood cuttings of some rose hips. Turkish Journal of Agriculture & Forestry 1999;23:305-310.

[65] Ghose K, McCallum B, Kirby C, Sanderson K, Fofana B. Genetic and metabolite diversity in Atlantic Canada wild roses and its implications in drug and cultivar development. Plant Biology 2010 Meeting. Montreal Convention Centre, Montreal, July 31-August 4, 2010; 2010.

[66] Joublan JP, Rios D. Rose culture and industry in Chile. Acta Horticulturae 2005;690:65-69.

[67] Nybom H, Werlemark G, Carlson-Nilsson U, Olsson A, Uggla M. Genetic variation in a new crop - dogroses (*Rosa* sect. *Caninae*) for commercial rosehip production. Acta Horticulturae 1999;484:139-145.

[68] Watson S. Contributions to American botany. I. A history and revision of the roses of North America. Proceedings of the American Academy of Arts and Sciences 1885;20:324-352.

[69] Crepin F. Rosae Americanae. I. Observations upon the genus *Rosa* in North America. Botanical Gazette 1896;22:1-34.

[70] Crepin F. Sketch of a new classification of roses. Journal of the Royal Horticultural Society 1889;11:217-228.

[71] Erlanson MacFarlane EW. The old problem of sepcies in *Rosa* with special reference to north America. America Rose Annual 1966;51:150-160.

[72] Erlanson MacFarlane EW. A self-polination mechanism and other Items in Rose species. America Rose Annual 1961;48:188-193.

[73] Ghose K, McCallum J, Kirby C, Sanderson K, Fofana B. Genetic and metabolite diversity in Atlantic Canada wild roses and its implications in drug and cultivar development. 2nd Maritime Natural Products Conference. Charlottetown, Aug.31-Sept 2, 2010 PE, Canada; 2010.

[74] De pronville m. Monographie du genre Rosier. Paris: Audot; 1824.

[75] Bayrak A, Akguel A. Volatile oil composition of Turkish rose (*Rosa damascena*). Journal of the Science of Food and Agriculture 1994;64:441-448.

[76] Hashidoko Y. The phytochemistry of *Rosa rugosa*. Phytochemistry 1996;43:535-549.

[77] Turkben C, Barut E, Copur OU, Durgut E, Himelrick DG. Evaluation of rose hips (*Rosa* spp.) selections. International Journal of Fruit Science 2005;5:113-121.

[78] Velioglu YS, Mazza G. Characterization of flavonoids in petals of *Rosa damascena* by HPLC and spectral analysis Journal of Agricultural and Food Chemistry 1991;39:463-467.

[79] Celik F, Kazankayan A, Ercisli S. Fruit characteristics of some selected promising rose hip (*Rosa* spp.) genotypes from Van region of Turkey. African Journal of Agricultural Research 2009;4:236-240.

[80] Uggla M, Nybom H. Domestication of a new crop in Sweden - dogroses (*Rosa* sect. Caninae) for commercial rose hip production. Acta Horticulturae 1999;484:147-151.

[81] Gurbuz I, Ustun O, Yesilada E, Sezik E, Kutsal O. Anti-ulcerogenic activity of some plants used as folk remedy in Turkey. Journal of Ethnopharmacology 2003;88:93-97.

[82] Yeslada E, Gurbuz I. A compilation of the studies on the anti-ulcerogenic effects of medicinal plants. (Recent Progress in Medicinal Plants. Vol. 2). Phytochemistry and pharmacology 2003.

[83] Winther K, Apel K, Thamsborg G. A powder made from seeds and shells of a rose-hip subspecies (*Rosa canina*) reduces symptoms of knee and hip osteoarthritis: a randomized, double-blind, placebo-controlled clinical trial. Scandinavian journal of rheumatology 2005;34:302-308.

[84] Melville R, Pyke M. the effect of specific variability and the environment on the vitamin C content of British rosehips. Biological Journal of the Linnean Society 1947;1:5-16.

[85] Uggla M. Domestication of wild roses for fruit production.Alnarp, Sweden: Swedish University of Agricultural Sciences; Doctoral thesis; 2004.

[86] Uggla M, Martinsson M. Cultivate the wild roses - experiences from rose hip production in Sweden. Acta Horticulturae 2005;690:83-89.

[87] Gachomo EW, Kotchoni SO. Microscopic and biochemical evidence of differentially virulent field isolates of *Diplocarpon rosae* causing black spot disease of roses. Plant Physiol Biochem 2010;48:167-175.

[88] Gachomo EW, Seufferheld MJ, Kotchoni SO. Melanization of appressoria is critical for the pathogenicity of *Diplocarpon rosae*. Mol Biol Rep 2010;37:3583-3591.

[89] Semina SN, Timoshenko NM. The resistance of species of wild rose to powdery mildew. Mikologiya i Fitopatologiya 1979;13:496-500.

[90] Wojdyla AT. Chitosan (biochikol 020 PC) in the control of some ornamental foliage diseases. Commun Agric Appl Biol Sci 2004;69:705-715.

[91] Uggla M, Carlson-Nilsson BU. Screening of fungal diseases in offspring from crosses between *Rosa* sections Caninae and Cinnamomeae. Scientia Horticulturae 2005;104:493-504.

[92] Uggla M, Carlson-Nilsson BU. Rose hip fly (*Rhagoletis alternata* Fallen) and leaf spot fungus (*Sphaceloma rosarum* (Pass.) Jenkins)-possible threats against rose hip production? Acta Horticulturae 2009;814:857-862.

[93] Margina A, Zheljazkov V. Studies of the influences of some systemic fungicides on the yields and quality of essential oil from Bulgarian oil-bearing rose. Acta Horticulturae 1996;426:355-364.

[94] Hattendorf A, Debener T. NBS-LRR-RGAS in roses: Diversity, genomic organization, expression and chromosomal location. Acta Horticulturae 2007;751:151-162.

[95] Ritz CM, Maier WFA, Oberwinkler F, Wissemann V. Different evolutionary histories of two *Phragmidium* species infecting the same dog rose hosts. Mycological Research 2005;109:603-609.

[96] Uggla M, Gustavsson KE, Olsson ME, Nybom H. Changes in colour and sugar content in rose hips (*Rosa dumalis* L. and *R. rubiginosa* L.) during ripening. Journal of Horticultural Science and Biotechnology 2005;80:204-208.

[97] Peng Y, Chen W, Moens M. Resistance of *Rosa* species and cultivars to *Pratylenchus penetrans*. HortScience 2003;38:560-564.

[98] Ercisli S, Guleryuz M. Fruit properties of promising rose hips (*Rosa spp.*) from the North-eastern Anatolia Region of Turkey. Asian Journal of Chemistry 2006;18:239-242.

[99] Dogan A, Kazankaya A. Fruit properties of rose hip species grown in Lake Van Basin (Eastern Anatolia Region). Asian Journal of Plant Sciences 2006;5:120-122.

[100] Güneş M, Dölek Ü. Fruit characteristics of promising native rose hip genotypes grown in Mid-North Anatolia Region of Turkey. Journal of Food, Agriculture and Environment 2010;8:460-463.

[101] Hosafc H, Arslan N, Sarhan EO. Propagation of dog roses (*Rosa canina* L.) by seed. Acta Horticulturae 2005;690:159-164.

[102] Datta SK, Chakrabarty D, Deepti, Mandal AKA, Misra P, Saxena M. In-vitro petal culture and callus formation in *Rosa* species. Indian Journal of Agricultural Sciences 2002;72:271-276.

[103] Dohm A, Ludwig C, Nehring K, Debener T. Somatic embryogenegis in roses. Acta Horticulturae 2001;547:341-347.

[104] Lauzer D, Laberge C. Establishment of a collection of *Rosa* species through in vitro embryo culture. HortScience 1996;31:458-459.

Chapter 3

Magnetic Resonance Technologies: Molecules to Medicine

Nadine Merkley, Ian Burton, Tobias Karakach and
Raymond T. Syvitski

Additional information is available at the end of the chapter

http://dx.doi.org/10.5772/54231

1. Introduction

Since the discovery of Electron Paramagnetic Resonance (EPR) spectroscopy in 1944 by Zavoisky[1], and the realization of the Nuclear Magnetic Resonance (NMR) spectroscopic signal in the mid 1940's by Bloch and Purcell[2,3], the capabilities and applications of the technology have continued to advance at an enormous rate particularly after the implementation of Fourier transform NMR in the mid 1960's by Ernst[4]. Magnetic Resonance (MR) spectroscopy was initially utilized to characterize the structure of matter.[1,5] Through the early to mid 1970's, the development of multidimensional (nD) methods and more powerful instruments opened the door for the detailed atomistic characterization of small molecules culminating in structural elucidation of proteins by the mid 1980's.[6] At about the same time, it was proposed that a magnetic field gradient could be applied to obtain a 3-dimensional (3D) image leading to the invention of nuclear Magnetic Resonance Imaging (MRI) with, among other capabilities, the potential to monitor the bio-distribution and bio-accumulation of molecules *in vivo*.[7] Beyond the 1980's MR technologies were mixing with other technologies and evolving to play an integral role for advancing pharmaceuticals and becoming indispensable tools for drug discovery, design and diagnostics.

1.1. Capabilities

Early on it was recognized (see Ref. 8 and references therein) that MR techniques can offer a variety of unique advantages over other spectroscopic techniques such as MR is completely non-destructive and non-invasive. Thus, MR technologies can be utilized with inanimate samples or living organisms with no obvious detrimental or destructive effects. In addition, MR techniques can be applied to a variety of states of matter including solution, semi-solids,

solids and mixtures obtaining comprehensive information of the chemical and physical properties. In addition to the typical static structural information, one can also detail dynamic processes. NMR measurements provide information about dynamic processes with rates in the range from 10^{-2} to 10^{-10} sec^{-1}. Furthermore, many nuclei possess magnetic moments, and with the availability of more sensitive spectrometers, chemists are beginning to take greater advantage of the technique for structure/bonding information for organometallic compounds (for example see Ref. 9).

An important application, although commonly overlooked, is the accurate quantitative information that can be obtained without the need for laborious calibrations. Under quantitative conditions and for all practical purposes with semi-solid or solution state samples, NMR spectroscopy has the unique distinction of having a uniform molar response for all nuclei of the same type *i.e.* all ^1H nuclei have the same integrated intensity and thus, a single calibrated (internal or more significantly external) standard can be used for accurate quantitation.[10] For the aforementioned reasons NMR is a valuable tool for providing atomistic structural, dynamic and quantitative information on natural products such as small molecules, metabolites, peptides, proteins, complex mixtures, and molecular assemblies such as lipid bilayers or tissues.

Nuclear MRI, on-the-other-hand, can provide 3D images of macroscopic matter, and monitor the bio-accumulation and bio-distribution of MRI tagged natural products *in vivo*. Ultimately MR technologies can be used at almost every stage along the natural product discovery pipeline – from discovery to implementation, from molecules to medicine.

1.2. Scope and limitations

MR technologies encompass a range of techniques including electron or nuclear MR spectroscopy, MR time domain, and nuclear or electron MRI. Herein, this chapter focuses on the nuclear MR technologies of spectroscopy and imaging for solution and semi-solid states. We provide a general overview of techniques and methodologies applicable throughout the development pipeline for natural products, as well as some potential impacts the information has for product development. It is well beyond the scope of a chapter (or in fact an entire book) to be a comprehensive description of all applicable MR methodologies. Thus within each section, the reader is directed to review articles, books, *etc.*

2. NMR spectroscopy

NMR is a technique that detects electrical currents induced by precessing nuclear magnetic moments within a uniform static magnetic field.[11] Nuclei with non-zero spin moments are MR active and in principle are detectable. Each individual type of spin-active nucleus has a unique precessional frequency dependent upon the strength of the static magnetic field, the magnetic properties of the isotope and the local electronic environment of the nucleus. The general precessional frequency is dependent upon the type of nucleus and thus NMR can readily distinguish among for example ^{13}C, ^1H, ^2H or ^3H. The applications and significance

http://dx.doi.org/10.5772/54231

of NMR has exploded because the exact precessional frequency (*i.e.* the chemical shift) within a group of the same nuclei is influenced by the local electronic environment of the nuclei and thus, NMR can readily distinguish (for example) a ^1H nuclei that is chemically bound to different nuclei (*e.g.* carbon vs. nitrogen, *etc.*), is chemically bound to different oxidation states of the same nuclei (*e.g.* methyl vs. methylene carbon), and/or are in identical bonding environments (*e.g.* methyl ^1H nuclei) but in different electronic environments induced by surrounding functional groups (*e.g.* aromatic vs. carbonyl groups). In addition, if a nucleus is influenced by another spin active nucleus either through a bond connection or in spatial proximity, a correlation exists that may be NMR detectable. In this way atomistic properties (such as the 3D spatial arrangement of nuclei and dynamics) can be determined.[12]

In addition to the distinct nuclear chemical shift, data from MR can be further separated based upon relaxation and/or diffusion properties of a nucleus or molecule.[12,13] Thus, MR technologies can discriminate among large molecules like peptides, proteins and macromolecular assemblies, and small molecules like metabolites or synthetic organic molecules. The relaxation time (influenced by the rotational correlation time and molecular fluctuations) of a molecule plays an important role in distinguishing among small drug molecules and large proteins, or between a single lipid molecule that behaves as a small molecule and an assembly of lipid molecules that, as a collective, behave as large molecules.

One drawback is that under typical conditions MR techniques are sample intensive requiring µM to mM concentrations translating to µg to g quantities of material. For natural product discovery, the sample intensive requirement can be an issue as extracts may only contain nano to micro gram quantities of material.[14] A number of methods have been proposed to overcome the mass demand with the most significant for general applications being the invention of cryogenically helium cooled detection systems that substantially reduce thermal noise ultimately improving the signal-to-noise ratio by up to 10 fold and reducing data acquisition times by up to 100 times.[15,16] A next generation improvement is cryogenically cooled probes that require smaller sample volumes. Currently the combination of the 700 MHz NMR spectrometer and new detection technologies requiring only 35 µl of sample affords the Biomolecular Magnetic Resonance Facility at NRC-Halifax one of the world's most sensitive instruments for mass-limited samples reducing the typical quantities by up to 50 times.[17] The limits of detection for this instrument can be as low as 10 nano-grams for small molecules (IWB, NM, TK and RTS unpublished).

Although to some extent the sample intensive nature of NMR can be addressed, a second drawback for larger proteins and macromolecular assemblies (>40 kDa) is the loss of peak resolution due to spectral overlap, broad line-widths, reduced signal-to-noise ratios and increased spectral complexity[12]. There have been efforts to address this issue however, these efforts are limited in scope and application.[18-20]

2.1. Structure elucidation

After a natural product or extract has been verified to be biologically active, an essential component within the discovery pipeline is to identify compound(s) and determine structure(s). Structural elucidation is essential if chemical modifications are to be made, if the product is for human consumption and/or if a patent application is to be filed as it will distinguish the uniqueness of the compound as well as help identify relationships with pre-existing compounds. Structural characterization is somewhat different between small and large molecules; the distinction between the two regimes is defined by the Nuclear Overhauser Effect (nOe) cross-relaxation rate which is positive or negative depending upon the spectrometer frequency and the overall molecular tumbling time.[12] Generally, "small molecules" are regarded as molecules that do not aggregate and have a molecular mass of <1 000 atomic mass units.

2.1.1. Small molecules

The advent of nD experiments propelled NMR to be a leading tool for natural product characterization. Previously natural products were degraded into fragments, chemically derivatized and/or completely synthesised to confirm the structure. It is still valuable for structure elucidation using NMR to obtain information from the aforementioned techniques as well as other techniques such as mass spectrometry (MS; for exact mass, functional groups and connectivities), infra-red spectroscopy (for functional groups), and separation techniques (for classes of compound *e.g.* phenolic, steroid, protein, *etc.*).

The initial NMR spectroscopic assessment as outlined in Scheme 1, typically begins with 1-dimensional (1D) ^{1}H spectra to determine purity, confirm the compound class, and examine the general appearance of the peaks. A spectrum with sharp well resolved peaks and the anticipated ratio of integrated intensities is indicative of a pure sample dissolved in an appropriate solvent. Broad peaks or peaks that are of fractional ratio could indicate an impure sample, however, they could also be an indication of chemical exchange or limited solubility. The preliminary information gained from other techniques is important when ascertaining if the spectral appearance is appropriate. From 1D data the splitting patterns from J-(*i.e.* scalar)-couplings provide information on the pattern of covalent bonding as well as the torsional angle distributions between spin active nuclei 3-bonds apart.[21]

^{1}H detected 2-dimensional (2D) experiments in which magnetic coherence is propagated through J-couplings or magnetization is transferred through dipole-dipole cross-relaxation interactions, reduce the overlap complexity of 1D spectra and provide correlations to other ^{1}H nuclei or heteronuclei most commonly ^{13}C or ^{15}N. Common homonuclear ^{1}H-^{1}H 2D experiments based on J-couplings are TOtal Correlation SpectroscopY (TOCSY)[22], and COrrelation SpectroscopY (COSY)[23]. Both of these experiments provide information on individual spin systems and chemical bonding. COSY experiments are used to connect ^{1}H nuclei that are within 3-bonds of each other whereas TOCSY experiments can connect all spins belonging to a J-coupled network *e.g.* the entire spin system connected through 3-bond correlations. Analysis of COSY data can provide J-coupling constants which can be related *via* the Karplus curve[24] to torsional angle restraints.[21]

Homonuclear 2D ^{1}H-^{1}H nOe SpectroscopY (NOESY)[25] and Rotating frame Overhauser Effect SpectroscopY (ROESY)[26] experiments are based on dipolar cross-relaxation interactions providing distance information between nuclei that are physically close (up to ≈5 Å) in space. It is noteworthy to mention that for NOESY and ROESY spectra to have correlations, nuclei do not have to be on the same molecule. This aspect of the nOe provides the basis for determining ligand/receptor interaction characteristics (see Section 2.2). The sign and intensity of NOESY cross-peaks are dependent upon the main static magnetic field ($\omega_0 = B_0$) and the rotational correlation time of the molecule (τ_c); for small molecules (<1 kDa) the nOe cross-relaxation rate is positive whereas for larger molecules (>2 kDa) the nOe is negative. ROESY are best suited for medium size molecules of ~1 kDa where for NOESY the nOe becomes zero (*i.e.* $\omega_0\tau_c \approx 1.12$)[26]. Analysis of the NOESY and/or ROESY data is important for determining the configuration/conformation of the compound and for connecting individual spin systems determined from the TOCSY and/or COSY data. Another aspect of nD NMR techniques is the addition of ^{13}C editing to the spectra. These heteronuclear experiments are ^{1}H detected increasing the sensitivity and indirectly providing ^{13}C shifts especially important for mass limited samples. Standard heteronuclear experiments are ^{1}H-^{13}C-HSQC[27-29], ^{1}H-^{13}C-HMBC[30], and ^{1}H-^{13}C-H2BC[31]. Strategies for selecting the proper pulse sequences, acquisition and processing parameters for natural product elucidation has been previously reviewed.[32] Implementing higher-dimensional experiments, for example, HSQC-TOCSY, HSQC-NOESY, provides valuable information for complex natural products on the through bond or space connections by exploiting the heteronuclei chemical shift for further separation.

When assessing the structure of a chemically modified molecule or a molecule for which minor structural changes are suspected, acquiring a complete structural suite of experiments may not be necessary. In such circumstances, a series of edited 1D and 2D experiments have been developed that can isolate the chemical modification of interest and express only correlations to the modification. Isolating a particular peak of interest reduces the time required for data acquisition, simplifies analysis and can help to quickly confirm modifications; valuable tools for isolating information from complex molecules are reviewed in Ref. 33.

A standard approach for small molecule structure elucidation involves identification of the individual fragments or spin systems followed by their assembly.[34] This approach outlined in Scheme 1 uses 1D data to assess purity, classify the compound type and compare with NMR chemical shift databases. Analysis of the 2D homonuclear data (COSY and TOCSY) identifies the individual short spin systems in the compound. Heteronuclear HSQC data provides ^{13}C chemical shift information and direct H-C links. HMBC data links distant H-C spin systems that help link molecular fragments. Data from the NOESY and ROESY spectra also aid in linking spins systems, and determining relative configuration and conformation, for example, relative stereochemistry, ring junctions, and double bond regiochemistry. The final step is confirming that proposed shift assignments and structural characteristics agree with coupling constants and splitting patterns among spectra, along with other data collected. There are numerous books detailing the specifics for analyzing NMR data of small molecules, see for example Refs. 35-38.

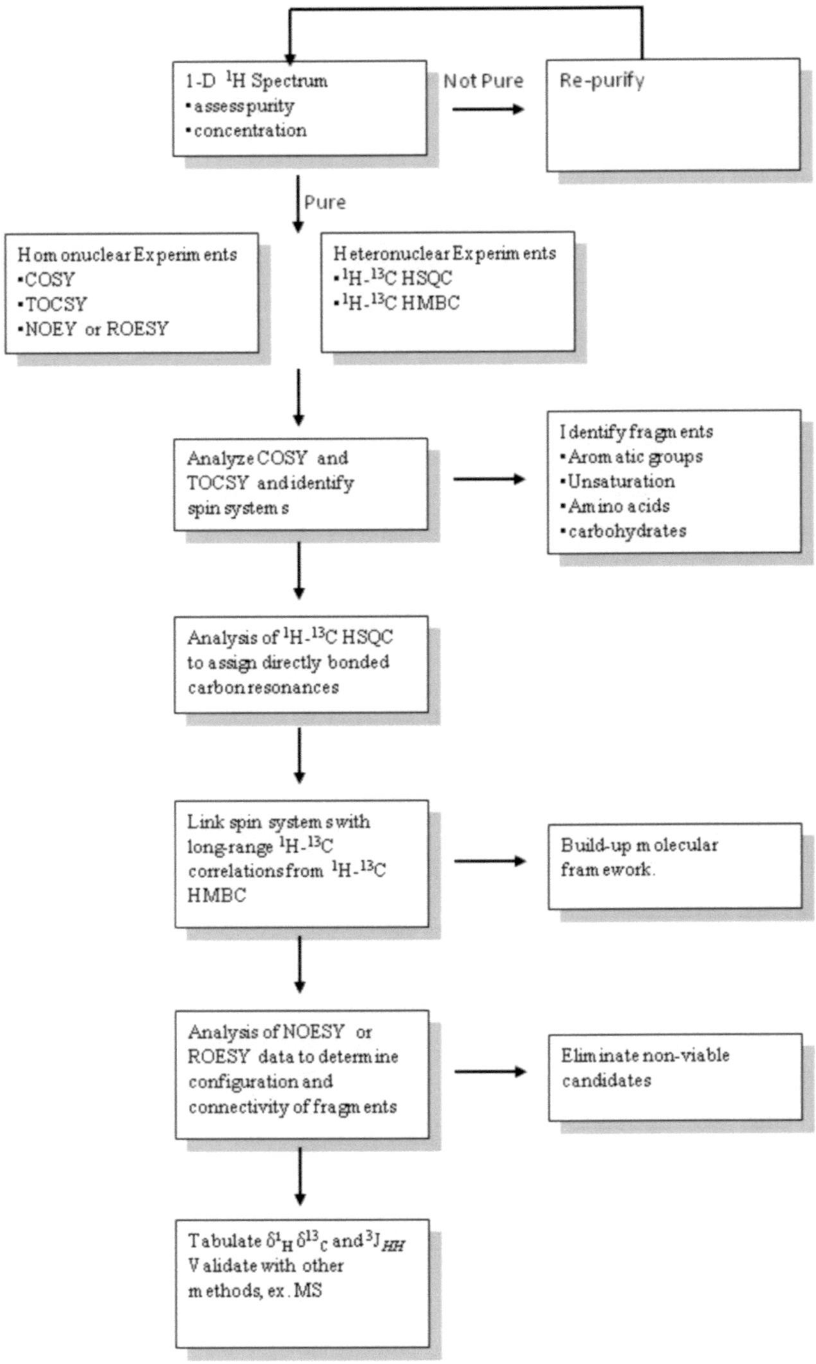

Scheme 1. The flowchart can be utilized as a general scheme for small natural product structural elucidation. Typically, a series of ^{1}H and ^{13}C NMR experiments are required in order to fully confirm the structure.

http://dx.doi.org/10.5772/54231

2.1.2. Proteins & peptides

MR allows for structural characterization of moderately sized proteins or peptides.[12,39] Since the line width of the NMR signal depends upon the rotational correlation time τ_c, the resultant signal intensity reduction and decreased spectral resolution typically precludes detailed analysis of large proteins. To date the largest protein to be structurally characterized by NMR is the 82 kDa or 723 amino acid malate synthase G.[40] In contrast, X-ray techniques in principle have no size limit however, not all proteins are amenable to crystallization esp. membrane-associated proteins and crystallization can alter the protein structure[41] making NMR attractive for elucidating structures in "native" solution environments. "Non-native" conditions can also be applicable for protein folding/unfolding or temperature stability. Initial investigation into biomolecular structure elucidation typically requires information from other techniques such as MS, circular dichroism, micro-array for initial determination of the amino acid sequence. A general scheme for the elucidation of a protein 3D structure (Scheme 2) involves initial production of the protein either by synthesis and refolding, or by recombinant expression, and followed by acquisition and data analysis. From the analysis through bond backbone and side-chain connections, through space nOe connections and additional constraints are utilized as restraints within simulated annealing protocols that calculate superimposable ensembles of lowest-energy structures.[42]

NMR is a sample intensive technique requiring milligrams of the biomolecule. For small peptides, synthesis (mg quantities) is typical and offers the possibility of selective isotopic labelling with the preferred spin active nuclei ^{13}C (over the 98% natural abundant spin-inactive ^{12}C) and/or ^{15}N (over the 99% natural abundance quadrupole and difficult to observe ^{14}N). However for large proteins, synthesis is too onerous and costly. Therefore development of a recombinant expression protocol capable of producing bacterial, mammalian or other proteins with the correct folding and linkages (in the case of lipoproteins or polysaccharide proteins) is required. In addition, expression systems allow for point mutations. For proteins >50 amino acids it is advantageous to label the protein with the isotopes ^{13}C and ^{15}N. Alternatively, structure elucidation of small monomeric peptides of <50 amino acids does not necessarily require labelling and the experiments and strategies outlined in Section 2.1.1 can be utilized. Isotopically labelled proteins can be achieved by growing *E. coli* with the particular expression gene on minimal media supplemented with $^{13}C_6$-glucose and/or ^{15}N ammonium chloride. Although *E. coli* is widely used for its low cost, the high productivity yields depend upon the plasmid, host and tags.[43] In addition with prokaryotic systems, protein re-folding can be a potential bottle neck along with failure to express toxic proteins, degradation and the absence of post-modification. Other non-*E. coli* prokaryotic and eukaryotic cell-lines that have been used for labelling, such as insect cells[44], are reviewed in Ref. 45. Eukaroytic *Pichia pastoris* has been widely and successfully used for labelling using minimal media,[46] and cell-free expression allows for high yields with relatively small reaction volumes[47]. With cell-free, any combination of labelled and unlabelled amino acids can be incorporated into the protein without isotopic scrambling.[47] An advantage of the cell-free system is that reagents, that stabilize expression, can be added. For example, protease inhibitors, detergents or membrane mimetics for insoluble or membrane associated proteins.[48]

However, each amino acid is added to the medium which can become costly for uniform ^{15}N and/or ^{13}C labelling. Overall, the particular expression system used depends upon such factors as post-translational modifications, the labelling scheme, membrane association, total cost and expression efficiency.

Over the past decade specialized isotope labelling strategies have been developed for biomolecular NMR, including full or partial deuteration, specific amino acid labelling and regiospecific labelling.[49] Labelling proteins with deuterium is practical for simplifying complex NMR spectra or for studying protein-substrate complexes. Furthermore, as the molecular weight of the biomolecule increases the spin-spin relaxation time (T_2) decreases considerably, inhibiting coherence transfer along amino acid side-chains. Substitution of ^{2}H for ^{1}H nuclei increases T_2 enhancing the coherence transfer. Perdeuteration of the backbone prevents connection to the side-chain ^{1}H nuclei, whereas a random, uniform deuteration level between 50% and 90% is most desirable. [50,51] Nevertheless, perdeuteration is beneficial for studying protein-substrate or protein-protein complexes, in which one portion of the complex is "invisible" reducing the overlap and spectral complexity allowing information of conformational changes to be more readily identified. In the pursuit of NMR information of larger proteins, labelling strategies have been developed for selective methyl labelling of alanine, leucine, valine and isoleucine ($H_{\gamma}1$) residues with perdeuteration of the backbone. This labelling scheme allowed for the analysis of relaxation dynamics of a 1 MDa protein complex.[52,53] Site specific information on protein conformational changes upon substrate binding can be obtained from selective amino acid labelling of the backbone. Within the protocol, media is supplemented with isotopically labelled amino acids, isotopic scrambling may result in instances where the supplemented amino acids are precursors to other amino acids. Scrambling of the isotope labels can be overcome by using *E. coli* strains with lesions in their biosynthetic pathways,[54] and recently demonstrated with a prototphic strain.[55] Contrary to selective amino acid labelling it has been proposed that unlabelling specific amino acids against a uniformly $^{13}C/^{15}N$ labelled background is beneficial.[56] Selective unlabelling of the protein still allows for sequential assignment of regions of the protein. Segmental labelling of individual domains or portions of large proteins has been established in which labelled segments of the protein are ligated together.[57,58] Segmental labelling of a large protein is useful for studying domain-domain interactions[59], conformational changes and substrate binding studies.

Preparation of protein samples is straightforward for soluble monomeric proteins at concentrations >1 mM. A wide range of deuterated buffers are available for controlling the pH of the sample. Deuterated or an inorganic buffer are desirable to minimize interference within ^{1}H spectra. The pH requires consideration as at pH > 8.0 labile amide ^{1}H nuclei can rapidly exchange with water becoming invisible. This can be utilized to reduce spectral complexity; however, it may also affect residues of interest. Approximately one-third of human genes code for membrane-associated proteins and to utilize NMR for studying the structure/function relationship of these proteins requires the protein to be folded in a membrane environment.[60] A range of membrane mimetics are available for solution and solid state NMR.[61]

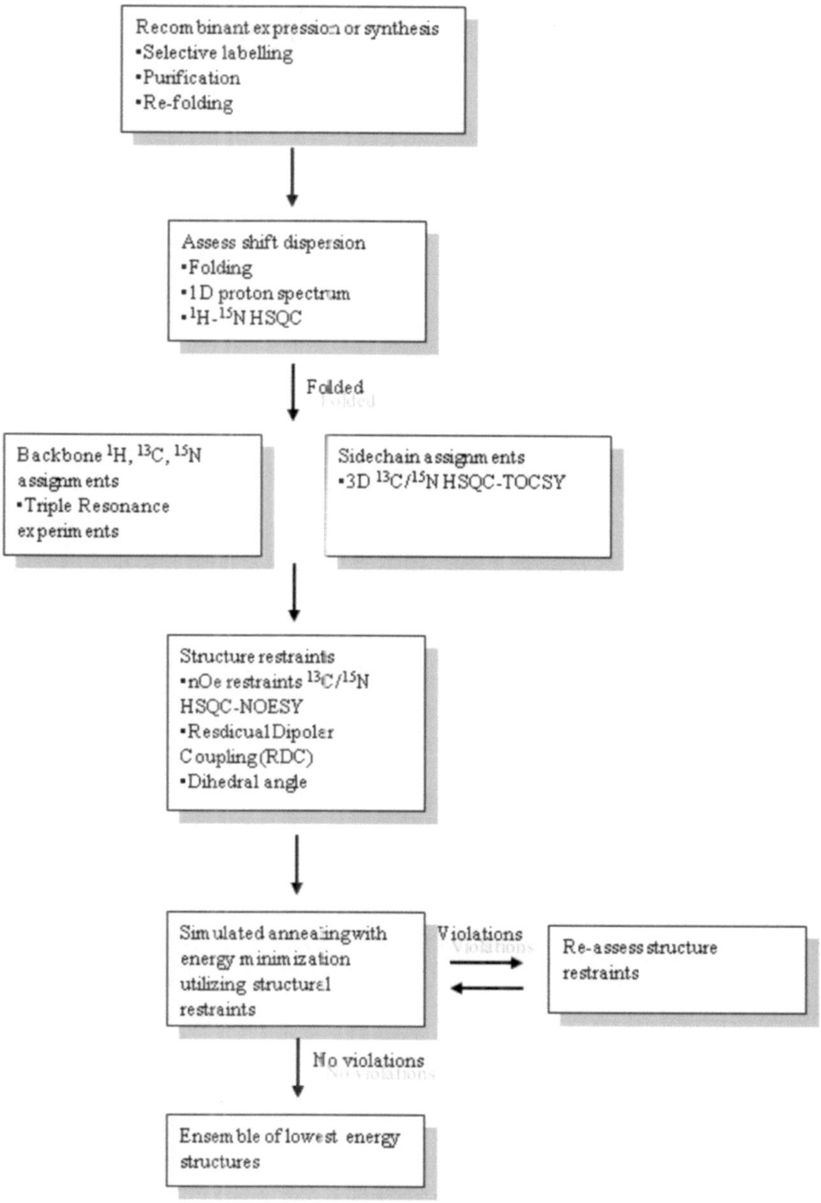

Scheme 2. The flowchart can be utilized as a general scheme for protein structural elucidation. Successful structural elucidation for proteins relies on elaborate but well established ^{1}H, ^{15}N and ^{13}C NMR experiments.

With the advent of 2D NMR experiments a strategy for the 3D structure determination of small proteins utilizing homonuclear NMR spectra was established.[39] Extension of the 2D NMR experiments to nD experiments along with isotopic labelling allowed for the 3D structure determination of much larger proteins including membrane proteins.[12,62] 3D and 4D

NMR techniques allow NMR data to be filtered by the ^{13}C or ^{15}N nuclei thus, reducing spectral overlap especially important for large proteins. In the past decade data on larger proteins has been facilitated with the development of Transverse Relaxation Optimized SpectroscopY (TROSY) experiments.[63,64] NMR structural and dynamic analysis of a supra-molecular systems of 1 MDa has been achieved in combination with selective methyl labelling.[65,66]

Typical NMR structure determination involves manual assignment of the backbone and side-chain chemical shifts. Extensive assignment of the ^1H-^1H nOe from NOESY experiments yields distance restraints as the volumes of the NOESY peaks are proportional to the average of $1/r^6$ distance between the ^1H nuclei. More recently routines for automatic resonance and nOe assignments have been developed.[67,68] However, these methods require labelled proteins and high-quality data to be effective. Regardless, protein structures are calculated using a molecular dynamics computer simulation program with predefined *a priori* bond connectivities, lengths and angles, and NMR derived restraints.

NMR restraints are most commonly from nOe experiments but may also include dihedral angles, hydrogen bonding information and residual dipolar couplings.[69] Dihedral angles can be calculated from measured/fitted[70] J-couplings or predicted from backbone chemical shifts of the $^1H_{\alpha}$, $^{13}C_{\alpha}$, $^{13}C_{\beta}$, ^{13}CO and ^{15}N resonances.[42,71] ^1H nuclei exchange rates are reduced in protein domains which are structured, or can be used to identify binding domains. Residual dipolar couplings are valuable for identifying angular constraints for large domains and structural changes in substrate binding.[72,73]

An ensemble of lowest energy structures that satisfy the NMR derived restraints is calculated. Quality of the calculated structures is based on the consistency of the experimental data compared to the inputted restraints. Agreement of the structures among each other is evaluated with the RMSD to the lowest energy structure. In addition, NMR quality assessment scores, recall, precision and F-measures (RPF scores) have been developed to directly measure the quality of structures compared to the NOESY peak list.[74] Structural calculations are an iterative process as not all restraints will be satisfied during the first simulated annealing calculation. It is typical for misassignments to occur due to spectral overlap or poor volume calculations. In principle the number of correctly assigned and integrated restraints should out-weigh the incorrectly assigned restraints. Thus during the calculations, a set of restraints could be identified as being violated regularly. From the identification, the NMR data is re-examined and the restraints corrected. Calculations are re-run and violations checked iteratively until well defined structures with minimal restraint violations obtained.

Tertiary/quaternary structural aspects can be confirmed with NMR through diffusion experiments. NMR is one of the most accurate and precise methods for determining diffusion constants.[13,75] Diffusion constants are related to the hydrodynamic radius through the Stoke-Einstein equation and thus can be indirectly used to determine the mass of the diffusing species.[13,76] Of particular importance for proteins is determining the aggregation number.[77]

http://dx.doi.org/10.5772/54231

2.2. Pharmacophore identification & binding characterization

Natural products have a diverse range of mechanisms for eliciting a biological response. Some natural products act as free-radical scavengers never directly interacting with the organism, whereas other compounds bind to molecular targets triggering a signaling cascade and altering the physiological state. Determining the mode of action of a small natural product molecule and where necessary the biological target requires extensive micro-biological investigations. NMR can play a role within these investigations in particular by identifying the pharmacophore of the natural product. The pharmacophore is the constituent of the molecule that binds to a biological receptor to modify its biological response.[78] Identifying the pharmacophore is an important aspect for drug discovery and understanding the mechanism of action as it assists with "intelligent" design of drugs through modifications that change binding characteristics (*e.g.* modifying the pharmacophore region) or solubility/permeability properties (*e.g.* modifying sites distant from the pharmacophore).[79,80]

The difference in the NMR nOe response between a small molecule rapidly tumbling in solution and a small molecule that is bound to a slowly tumbling large protein (see Section 2.1.1) is exploited to isolate and identify the pharmacophore (see chapter 14 of Ref. 81 and Refs. 82,83). In order to clearly define the pharmacophore complete structural analysis of the molecule is required (see Section 2.1.1); in order to sequence identify the active site within the receptor, complete structural analysis of the protein (preferably including ^{15}N and ^{13}C chemical shifts and connectivities) is required (see Section 2.1.2). A number of these techniques require mg quantities of purified ligand, receptor or both. Purifying compounds can be a detrimental drawback especially if the receptor is a membrane bound protein that is difficult to express and purify. Nevertheless, if the receptor is highly over-expressed within a cell (*e.g.* cancer cell that over-expresses a particular protein) the possibility exists for the experiment to be performed *in vivo*.[84] Essentially 6 fundamental methods are available for pharmacophore/binding characterization:[81,82] chemical-shift perturbations[85], saturation transfer difference (STD)[86], water-logsy (wLogsy)[87,88], transfer-NOESY (tr-NOESY)[89], selective relaxation[90] and diffusion editing[90]. Selective relaxation, diffusion editing and tr-NOESY experiments in principle can be used for nM to mM binding constants (K_D) whereas chemical shift perturbations, STD and wLogsy are valuable for pM to mM K_D ranges with the concentration of receptor in the nM range. It is well beyond the scope of this chapter to describe these experiments in detail especially since these experiments can be combined to provide further characterization such as combining diffusion editing with STD to simultaneously determine the pharmacophore and binding constant.[91] There are numerous reviews that provided explicit details (see Refs. 82,92-94).

With these tools both the ligand and receptor can be characterized. Typically chemical shift perturbation or mapping methods helps to characterize the active site of the receptor. A series of ^{1}H-^{15}N or ^{1}H-^{13}C HSQC spectra of the labelled receptor are collected as the ligand is titrated. Changes in chemical shifts of the receptor are indicative of ^{1}H nuclei that are perturbed during binding, although care must be taken as to not over-interpret data as this could also be indicative of structural alterations distant from the binding site. In cases where the receptor is large (*i.e.* > 30 kDa) extensive resonance overlap may preclude unambiguous interpretation of the HSQC data. Expression techniques to isolate particular amino acids or regions of the receptor are valuable for these experiments (see Section 2.1.2). One disadvantage of this technique is the necessity of a complete resonance assignment of the target or at least the active site.

Diffusion editing is a technique that can be used to determine the K_D by examining the change in diffusion properties of the ligand (typically < 2 kDa) upon titration to the receptor (typically > 100 kDa). Although limited with pharmacophore and binding pocket identification, it is nevertheless a valuable tool to identify binding events from a mixture of possible small ligands or to combine with other techniques.

The most often utilized techniques are the STD, wLogsy, tr-NOESY and selective relaxation.[95] These techniques are used when the target is too large for chemical shift perturbations, is not available with the desired isotopic labelling scheme or the target aggregates/precipitates at high concentrations. For these techniques, non-specific binding events in the nM-μM range may be difficult to rule out unless compared with a known binder or used with a competitive binder.[96] Regardless, these techniques are invaluable for specifically observing resonances of a low-affinity ligands that bind to a receptor. With selective relaxation experiments, differences in relaxation properties of the ligand between a free and bound state help identify interacting ^{1}H nuclei that are in close proximity to the receptor. The relaxation properties of the free ligand (*i.e.* no receptor) are compared to the relaxation properties for the ligand at various receptor titers and mixing times. Changes within the relaxation values can distinguish ^{1}H nuclei that are in direct contact with the receptor from ^{1}H nuclei that show magnetization relay or ^{1}H nuclei distant from the receptor. For wLogsy experiments, ^{1}H resonances arising from ^{1}H nuclei in close proximity to the receptor (*i.e.* are part of the pharmacophore) are opposite sign to ^{1}H resonances arising from ^{1}H nuclei that are distant from the receptor or are on a ligand that does not bind to the receptor (Fig. 1A). The wLogsy also has the advantage of identifying ^{1}H nuclei that are part of salt bridges between the ligand and receptor. For STD experiments, small molecules that do not bind to the receptor show a zero response (Fig. 1B) whereas the ^{1}H nuclei of the pharmacophore show a response. Because the wLogsy is a direct observation technique whereas the STD is generated from a difference of spectra, the wLogsy tends to have fewer artifacts and can be more sensitive. The tr-NOESY experiments can provide structural information about the ligand in the bound state as well as potentially information on the type of amino acids on the receptor involved in binding; typically no information regarding the sequence specificity of the amino acids is gleaned. The tr-NOESY is advantageous if the ligand changes conformation upon binding as it can be utilized to determine the bound state structure of the ligand which is a valuable asset for understanding the mode of action. The tr-NOESY is a 2D technique and as such requires mg quantities of ligand and substantially more time to acquire the data. For rapid screening of natural products the STD and wLogsy are the experiments of choice.

Beyond the individual experiments, combinations of these various experiments are possible. For example, to investigate the folding/unfolding properties of a peptide the combination of a ^{1}H-^{15}N HSQC and wLogsy can be used to monitor amide ^{1}H nuclei exchange rates valuable for identifying H-bonding and buried residues.[77,97] This experimental combination can also be utilized with/without ligand to identify amide ^1H nuclei that are involved with ligand binding. Using the wLogsy to saturate the water signal avoids the challenges of the typical methods of monitoring exchange by addition of D_2O such as protein precipitation, conformational changes induced by concentrating/diluting or complete loss of signal due to rapid deuterium exchange.[77,98]

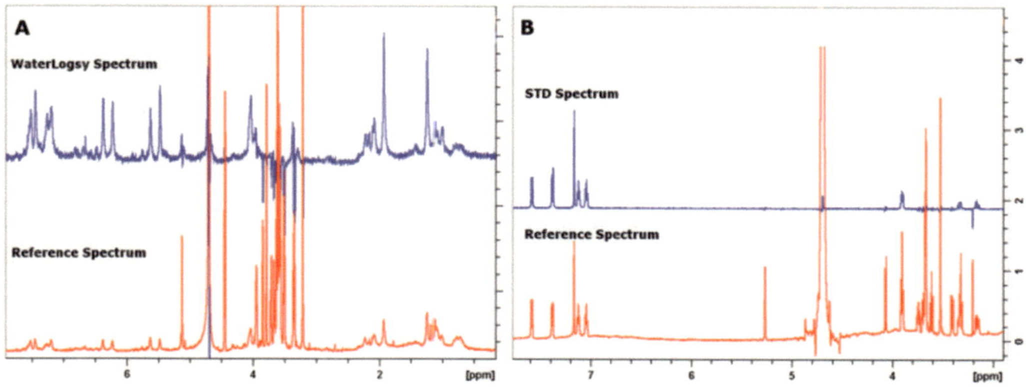

Figure 1. STD and wLogsy experiments can be utilized for identifying the pharmacophore of a small natural product molecule. Panel **A** represents a wLogsy experiment (blue spectrum) of a compound that binds (positive peaks) to an enzyme and a compound that does not bind (negative peaks). The positive peaks are of ^1H nuclei that are adjacent or in proximity to a salt bridge involving water. The negative peaks are from either the binding compound that are not within the binding pocket, or from the control non-binder compound. The red spectrum is the reference spectrum. Panel **B** represents the STD experiment (blue) of human serum albumin, a binder tryptophan and a non-binder sucrose. The positive peaks are from ^1H nuclei on the tryptophan that are within the binding pocket. Peaks that are not observed compared to the reference spectrum (red) represent either the control compound, or ^1H nuclei on the tryptophan that are distant to the binding pocket.

2.3. Quantitative analysis & QA/QC

Nuclear MR technologies have traditionally been associated with molecular characterization. The quantitative nature has been acknowledged from integration of signals to distinguish between for example methyl and methylene ^1H nuclei; however, it has rarely been exploited for absolute quantitative analysis (qNMR) or quality assurance/quality control (QA/QC).[10] MR techniques are capable of accurately and precisely determining the concentration of molecules within a purified sample or complex mixture without the need for elaborate calibrations.[99] In addition samples can be in solution or semi-solid states.[100] Relatively simple protocols have been developed that use a single certified external standard to calibrate the instrument. From the calibrated system, other samples can be rapidly quantitated.[10,99]

MR technologies have the unique distinction of having a uniform molar response for all nuclei of the same type, *i.e.*, the NMR signals are proportional to the molar concentration of the nuclei allowing for a direct comparison of the concentration of all compounds within a mixture. Thus for example, for all organic molecules regardless of the concentration, the intensity of each signal within the NMR spectrum is a direct measure of the number of ^{1}H nuclei that contribute to that signal. Furthermore, spectra can be recorded in such a manner as to allow for accurate comparison between different samples within different sample tubes and different solvents; the implications are far reaching for qNMR and QA/QC. For example, concentrations of natural products or impurities can be determined for samples within sealed tubes reducing the handling requirements of toxic or precious samples, or rapid crude or refined product profiling ensuring purity, integrity and consistency with applications to fractionation or end-product QA/QC.[99] Fully automated protocols have been developed that have been coupled with metabolomics investigations providing absolute scaling for temporal data.

2.4. Metabolomics analysis

Analysis of metabolites and metabolic flux can help ascertain the effects of a particular natural product or extract on an organism. Metabolic analysis can be utilized while identifying biological activity *in vitro*, or during *in vivo* investigations. Perhaps one of the best practical definitions of metabolomics was offered by Oliver describing it as an approach for simultaneously measuring the complete set of metabolites (low molecular weight intermediates) that are context dependent and which vary according to the physiological, developmental or pathological state of an organism.[101] From the perspective of natural products, such a definition fits in the framework of extracts from plants, fungi and secretions from microorganisms such as bacteria. When metabolomics is viewed from context dependence, only those metabolites that vary according to environmental, biochemical, and/or physiological fluctuations are important. In this regard, there are a vast number of metabolites present in botanical extracts and secretions from organisms that are useful for inducing biological responses in organisms including humans. For instance, ginseng has been argued to induce biochemical changes in humans that lead to anti-tumor, antioxidant, anti-fatigue and anti-stress activities while *Streptomyces coelicolor* secrete therapeutic natural products during their quiescent growth phase.[102,103] The discussion within this section follows the aforementioned definition and is restricted to metabolomics applied to botanical natural products since it is one of the fastest growing subsections established as "plant metabolomics."[104-106] NMR is a suitable method for such analyses since it allows simultaneous detection of a diverse group of both primary metabolites (sugars, organic acids, amino acids *etc.*) and secondary ones (flavonoids, alkaloids tri-terpenes *etc.*) Nevertheless, the applications are extensible to the "animal kingdom" metabolomics since the underlying sample composition is similar and characterized by large heterogeneity exhibiting vast dynamic range in concentration.

The numerous advantages of NMR have been a major driver for developing NMR based metabolomics technologies. NMR is ideal for resolving the complexity of metabolomics samples given that methods exist for compounds with nuclei such as ^{1}H, ^{13}C, ^{15}N and ^{31}P to provide spectral fingerprints with compound specificity and quantitative accuracy even within complex matrices. For example, from the un-annotated 1D ^{1}H NMR spectra of seaweed extracts, visible differences in chemical composition are observed (Fig. 2). NMR signals have a uniform molar response (see Section 2.3). This property has particularly been important

http://dx.doi.org/10.5772/54231

with propelling NMR metabolomics as a technology. NMR is a non-destructive technique ideal suited because many of these samples are difficult to obtain and may be precious. The stability of many NMR instrumentation allows for repeated measures (often years apart) of a sample with accurate reproducibly. This advantage also lends the technology to inter-laboratory studies that are important for establishing the robustness of a given measurement and technique.[52] Advances in technology now allow for high throughput analysis with automated, temperature controlled sample changers such as Bruker's SampleJet®.

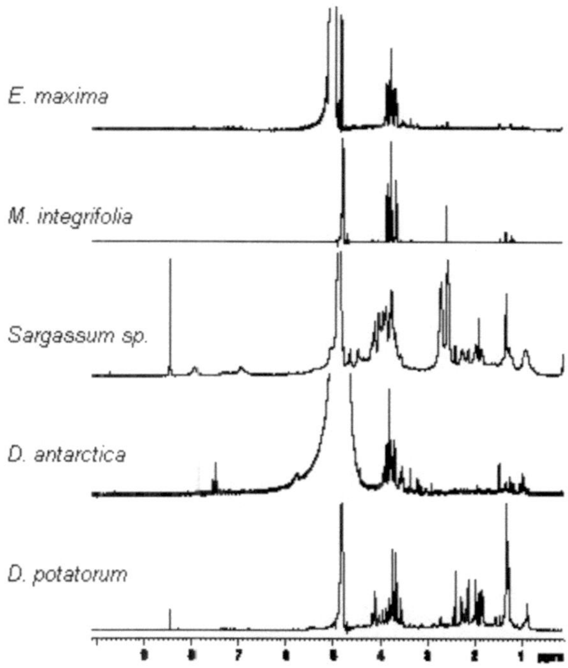

Figure 2. NMR spectra of aqueous extracts from various strains of brown seaweeds showing distinct differences within the spectral features.

The most commonly cited disadvantage of NMR for metabolomics is the lack of sensitivity.[106] This is a major hindrance given that in typical sample matrices, the concentration of constituent metabolites often exhibits a large dynamic range in concentration. Low abundance metabolites will invariantly be overlapped by highly abundant ones. Furthermore, in some applications such low level metabolites maybe of high value. For instance a phytochemical preparation may exhibit activity in a biological readout but such activity is induced by the low level metabolites which are undetectable *via* NMR. Approaches for simplifying sample matrices have been developed in order to separate, for instance, lipophilic from hydrophilic metabolites.[107] In addition, recent advances in NMR hardware have significantly improved sensitivity, especially with the advent of cryogenic probes and microprobes.

NMR-based metabolomics applications have been in the literature for over two decades, [108,109] but the technology only realized widespread acceptance and application in the later part of the last decade.[105,110-112] This shift is attributed to the utility of pattern recognition methods for analysis of multiple spectra, allowing the visualization of patterns corresponding to differences among samples and identification of chemical shifts responsible for eliciting such differences.[113] Specifically, principal component analysis (PCA) has been a significant driver as it allows patterns associated with the variability in the relative concentrations of metabolites to be assessed by the human eye, often in two dimensions. PCA analysis assisted with the classification of different extracts of the sea weed *Ascophyllum nodosum* (Fig. 3).[114] In recent years, many other pattern recognition methods (classified either as supervised or unsupervised) have been developed and applied to data. Unsupervised methods do not include *a priori* knowledge of the class memberships of a given sample. Such methods include PCA, SIMCA, independent component analysis (ICA) and the so called machine learning methods such as neural networks and self organizing maps (SOM). On the other hand, supervised methods use information about the samples in order to build models that can later be used to predict the class to which an unknown sample belongs. Such methods include partial least squares discriminant analysis (PLS-DA).

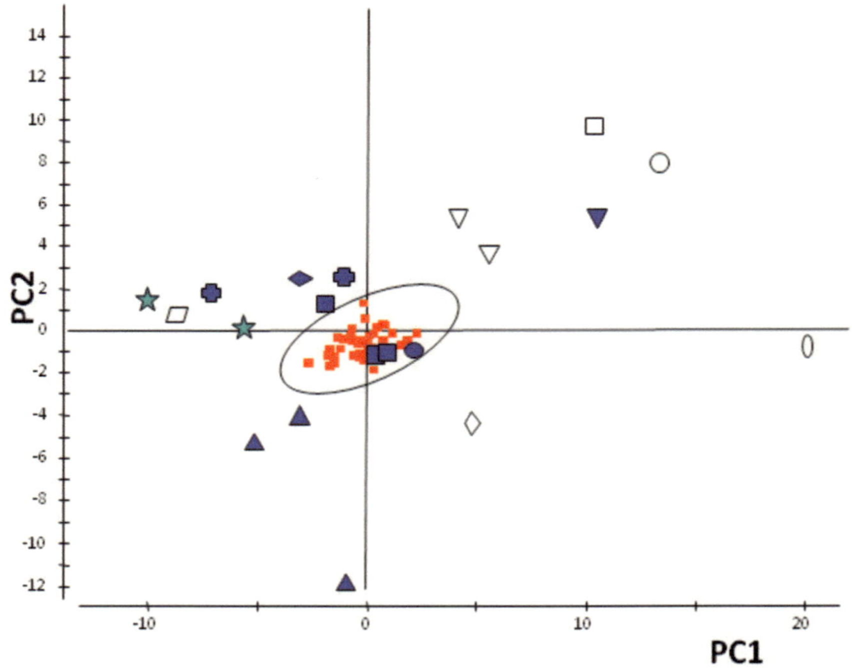

Figure 3. A principal component scores plot of a product characterization study showing similar samples from one manufacturer tightly clustered in the center (solid red squares); the ellipse encloses these samples plus two others that are known to incorporate that manufacturer's samples (solid blue squares and circle). Competitors' samples are distributed throughout the plot with each symbol representing products from a single manufacturer. Unfilled symbols represent samples recorded under acidic conditions.

http://dx.doi.org/10.5772/54231

Ultimately, the impetus for natural product metabolomics analyses is the need for high throughput screening to determine biological activity and the requirements from the nutraceutical industry to purport therapeutic health benefits from unprocessed foods. Traditional approaches with the development of novel drugs are difficult, expensive and time consuming. It is estimated that over $800 million and an average of 14.2 years are spent before a novel drug application is approved. Because natural products are a rich source of lead compounds in the drug discovery pipeline, the metabolomics approach provides an avenue for a systematic characterization of complex mixtures such as phytochemical extracts linking observations made via biological assays without the need for isolation. This promises to complement high throughput screening of compounds in order to shorten the drug discovery process. Indirectly, NMR has been used in metabolomics to measure the fate of consumed natural products and their effects on human physiology. One study has shown that the consumption of dark chocolate, for instance, affects energy homeostasis in humans.[115] In another study, differences in metabolic profiles were observed in human urine following consumption of black compared to green tea specifically increases in urinary hippuric acid and 1,3-dihydroxyphenyl-2-O-sulfate, which are end products of tea flavonoid degradation.[116] Several other studies exist in the literature and have been reviewed for instance within Ref. 117.

Perhaps one of the biggest gaps with metabolomics developments for natural products is the lack of certified reference materials for quantification of analytes. Such reference materials would enhance product characterization and validation of biological observations, especially with studies of bioactivity assessment. Those studies are often inconsistent due to inadequate chemical characterization of complex botanical mixtures, making comparison of results across studies difficult. Fortunately, it is possible to determine the concentration of 'active' compounds using external standards, *via* NMR, as long as both the external standard and the compound of interest are of the same nuclei type (see Section 2.3).[10]

2.5. Semi-solid state & macromolecular assemblies

In addition to studying soluble molecules or extracts dissolved in solution state, it can be advantageous and/or necessary to study semi-solids such as intact tissues, cells, raw materials or product formulations; metabolites or components are in their native environment *i.e.* potentially time consuming and disrupting/degrading extractions, or chemical modifications are not required in order to obtain valuable information. Semi-solid materials require specialized NMR probes to overcome sever spectral line-broadening as result of the restricted molecular mobility. To acquire a high-resolution spectrum of a semi-solid, High Resolution Magic Angle Spinning (HR-MAS) was developed in the late 1990's as a hybrid between solid and solution state NMR.[118] Similar to solid state NMR the spinning of the sample at the "magic angle" (54.7°) to the applied magnetic field reduces line broadening effects. Spinning speeds are typically between 3 to 5 kHz and cells remain intact and viable.[119] HR-MAS requires <100 uL of the semi-solid. HR-MAS does not require the high powered pulses that solid state NMR requires and many of the nD experiments that are utilized for structural biology can be applied, although stable isotope labelling is preferred for the less abundant ^{13}C, and ^{15}N nuclei. HR-MAS can be applied for many natural product studies[118,120] commonly used to study metabolic changes in diseased and treated tissues,[121,122] metabolism,[123] combinatorial chemistry[124] and whole cells[125]. Intensities in the HR-MAS NMR spectra are dependent on the environment of the analyte and as such molecules that are in rigid environments with completely restricted mobility are not detected. Macro molecular assemblies on-the-other-hand can be examined for profiling and quantitation of algae lipid content and polysaccharides or metabolites.[100]

3. MRI

MRI is a nuclear MR technique applicable for natural product development in particular during *in vivo* testing and diagnostic stages. MRI is capable of producing 3D images that can be used to monitor changes in brain activity in response to application of a natural product *via* fMRI techniques[126-128], indirectly monitor the effects of a natural product on tumours[129], or directly monitor the bio-distribution and bio-accumulation of a natural product by tagging the compound with an MRI contrast agent.[130-133].

Direct monitoring of the natural product is one of the most typical methods for drug development. For direct monitoring however, the molecules should be tagged with a MRI contrast agent which contains a paramagnetic centre causing ^{1}H nuclei on water in close proximity to "relax" much faster than ^{1}H nuclei distant from the paramagnetic centre. [134] This rapid relaxation is exploited with MRI and is depicted as "dark spots" within the image whereas unaffected water molecules remain as bright areas. In order to "tag" a natural product with a MRI contrast agent such as super-paramagnetic iron oxide (SPIO), the complete structure and pharmacophore identification is valuable (see Section 2.2) as it allows one to pick a functional group distant from the active site that can be chemically coupled to the contrast agent. Many SPIO contrast agents are commercially available with a variety of functional groups amenable to chemical coupling under aqueous conditions.[134]

Once the natural product is conjugated to the paramagnetic particle, it can be administered to an organism and imaged. The bio-distribution and bio-accumulation of the tagged molecule is monitored and compared against a control particle that does not contain the active natural product.[133,135-137] The difference in clearance time is considered as conformation that the molecule is associated with the tissue being examined. As an example the peptide SOR-C27, a 27 amino acid fragment of the paralytic natural product peptide SOR-54 from the Northern Short Tail shrew (*Blarina brevicauda*) was found to bind the calcium ion channel TRPV6 which is highly over-expressed by breast, prostate and ovarian cancers.[138,139] The SOR-C27 peptide was chemically bonded to a maleimide functionalized SPIO particle through the sulfur centre of the Cys-14 residue. From MRI investigations on an ovarian cancer xenograft mouse model, the SPIO-peptide particle persisted at the tumour site 24 hours post injection whereas the control SPIO particle rapidly cleared. The persistence of the SPIO-peptide particle at the tumour site is conformation that the peptide is associated with the tumour[139].

4. Summary

A comprehensive overview of MR techniques for natural product development is well beyond the scope of a single chapter or book. The fundamental experiments have been briefly outlined and the typical information that is gleaned from the experiments presented. Many other opportunities were not covered such as determining equilibrium dissociating constants, or use of spin labels for lead drug optimization. MRI has tremendous application for later stage *in vivo* applications of the drug development pipeline. Together the MR technologies of NMR and MRI can cover the full range of natural product drug development from discovery through to clinical testing (Fig. 4).

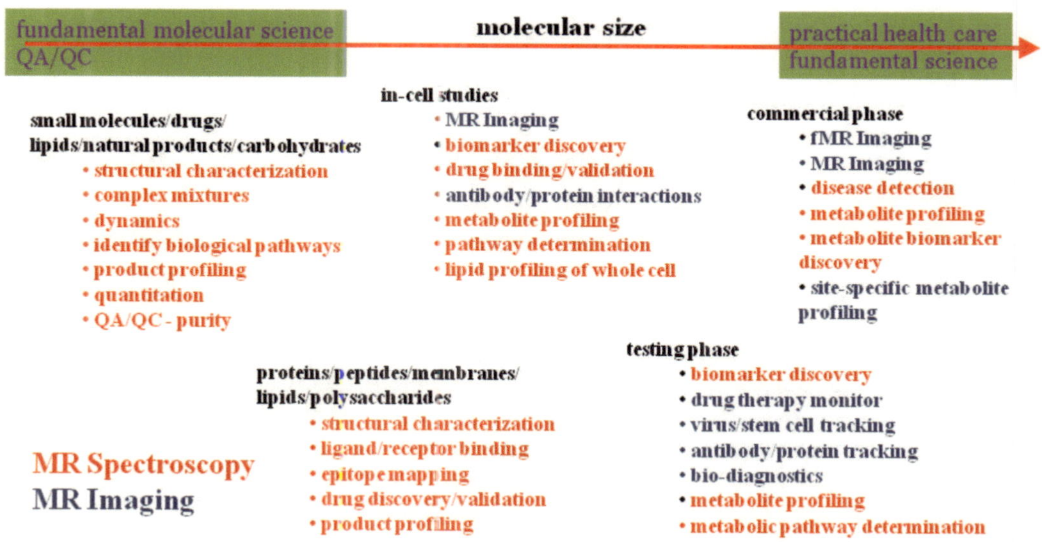

Figure 4. Applications for nuclear MR technologies cover the entire range of natural product development from fundamental molecular sciences through to practical health care. Spectroscopic applications (red) are delineated from imaging applications (blue).

Acknowledgements

Dr. John Walter (retired) has assisted with discussions during the writing of this review and was instrumental with establishing the Biomolecular Magnetic Resonance Facility (BMRF), housed at the National Research Council of Canada's Oxford St. Institute.

Author details

Nadine Merkley, Ian Burton, Tobias Karakach and Raymond T. Syvitski*

*Address all correspondence to: Ray.Syvitski@nrc-cnrc.gc.ca

Biomolecular Magnetic Resonance Facility (BMRF), National Research Council of Canada, Canada

References

[1] Zavoisky YK. Relaxation of liquid solutions for perpendicular fields. J Phys USSR 1945;9:211-216.

[2] Bloch F, Hansen WW, Packard M. Nuclear Induction. Phys Rev 1946;69(3-4):127.

[3] Purcell EM, Torrey HC, Pound RV. Resonance Absorption by Nuclear Magnetic Moments in a Solid. Phys Rev 1946;69(1-2):37-38.

[4] Ernst RR, Anderson WA. Application of fourier transform spectroscopy to magnetic resonance. Rev Sci Instrum 1966;37(1):93-102.

[5] Gutowsky HS. Nuclear Magnetic Resonance. Annu Rev Phys Chem 1954;5(1): 333-356.

[6] Williamson MP, Havel TF, Wuthrich K. Solution conformation of proteinase inhibitor IIA from bull seminal plasma by 1H nuclear magnetic resonance and distance geometry. J Mol Biol 1985;182(2):295-315.

[7] P Mansfield and PKG. NMR 'diffraction' in solids? Journal of Physics C: Solid State Physics 1973;6(22):L422.

[8] Jonas J, Gutowsky HS. NMR in Chemistry--An Evergreen. Annu Rev Phys Chem 1980;31(1):1-28.

[9] Gielen M, Willem R, Wrackmeyer B. Advanced applications of NMR to organometallic chemistry. Chichester ; New York: Wiley; 1996.

[10] Burton IW, Quilliam MA, Walter JA. Quantitative 1H NMR with external standards: use in preparation of calibration solutions for algal toxins and other natural products. Anal Chem 2005;77(10):3123-3131.

[11] Rabi II, Cohen VW. The Nuclear Spin of Sodium. Phys Rev 1933;43(7):582.

[12] Cavanagh J, Fairbrother WJ, Palmer III AG, Skelton NJ. Protein NMR Spectroscopy: Principles and Practice. New York: Academic Press; 1996.

[13] Johnson CS. Diffusion ordered nuclear magnetic resonance spectroscopy: principles and applications. Prog Nucl Mag Res Sp 1999;34(3-4):203-256.

[14] Hu T, Burton IW, Cembella AD, Curtis JM, Quilliam MA, Walter JA, et al. Characterization of Spirolides A, C, and 13-Desmethyl C, New Marine Toxins Isolated from Toxic Plankton and Contaminated Shellfish. J Nat Prod 2001;64(3):308-312.

[15] Kovacs H, Moskau D, Spraul M. Cryogenically cooled probes - a leap in NMR technology. Prog Nucl Magn Reson Spectrosc 2005;46(2-3):131-155.

[16] Molinski TF. NMR of natural products at the 'nanomole-scale'. Nat Prod Rep 2010;27(3):321-329.

[17] Hilton BD, Martin GE. Investigation of the experimental limits of small-sample heteronuclear 2D NMR. J Nat Prod 2010;73(9):1465-1469.

[18] Wand AJ, Ehrhardt MR, Flynn PF. High-resolution NMR of encapsulated proteins dissolved in low-viscosity fluids. Proceedings of the National Academy of Sciences 1998;95(26):15299-15302.

[19] Grzesiek S, Anglister J, Ren H, Bax A. Carbon-13 line narrowing by deuterium decoupling in deuterium/carbon-13/nitrogen-15 enriched proteins. Application to triple resonance 4D J connectivity of sequential amides. J Am Chem Soc 1993;115(10): 4369-4370.

[20] Pervushin K, Riek R, Wider G, Wuthrich K. Attenuated T2 relaxation by mutual cancellation of dipole-dipole coupling and chemical shift anisotropy indicates an avenue to NMR structures of very large biological macromolecules in solution. Proceedings of the National Academy of Sciences 1997;94(23):12366-12371.

[21] Karplus M. Vicinal proton coupling in nuclear magnetic resonance. J Amer Chem Soc 1963;85:2870-2871.

[22] Braunschweiler L, Ernst RR. Coherence transfer by isotropic mixing: Application to proton correlation spectroscopy. Journal of Magnetic Resonance (1969) 1983;53(3): 521-528.

[23] Jeener J. Lecture, Ampere Summer School. 1971.

[24] Karplus M. Contact electron-spin coupling of nuclear magnetic moments. J Chem Phys 1959;30:11-15.

[25] Jeener J, Meier BH, Bachmann P, Ernst RR. Investigation of exchange processes by two-dimensional NMR spectroscopy. J Chem Phys 1979;71:4546-4553.

[26] Bothner-By A, Stephens RL, Lee J, Warren CD, Jeanloz RW. Structure determination of a tetrasaccharide: transient nuclear Overhauser effects in the rotating frame. J Am Chem Soc 1984;106(3):811-813.

[27] Mueller L. Sensitivity enhanced detection of weak nuclei using heteronuclear multiple quantum coherence. J Am Chem Soc 1979;101(16):4481-4484.

[28] Bodenhausen G, Ruben DJ. Natural abundance nitrogen-15 NMR by enhanced heteronuclear spectroscopy. Chemical Physics Letters 1980;69(1):185-189.

[29] Bax A, Ikura M, Kay LE, Torchia DA, Tschudin R. Comparison of different modes of two-dimensional reverse-correlation NMR for the study of proteins. Journal of Magnetic Resonance (1969) 1990;86(2):304-318.

[30] Bax A, Summers MF. Proton and carbon-13 assignments from sensitivity-enhanced detection of heteronuclear multiple-bond connectivity by 2D multiple quantum NMR. J Am Chem Soc 1986;108(8):2093-2094.

[31] Nyberg NT, Duus JÃ, SÃ¸rensen OW. Heteronuclear Two-Bond Correlation: Suppressing Heteronuclear Three-Bond or Higher NMR Correlations while Enhancing Two-Bond Correlations Even for Vanishing 2JCH. J Am Chem Soc 2005;127(17): 6154-6155.

[32] Reynolds WF, Enriquez RG. Choosing the best pulse sequences, acquisition parameters, postacquisition processing strategies, and probes for natural product structure elucidation by NMR spectroscopy. J Nat Prod 2002;65(2):221-244.

[33] Fukushi E. Advanced NMR approaches for a detailed structure analysis of natural products. Biosci Biotechnol Biochem 2006;70(8):1803-1812.

[34] Bross-Walch N, Kuhn T, Moskau D, Zerbe O. Strategies and tools for structure determination of natural products using modern methods of NMR spectroscopy. Chem Biodivers 2005;2(2):147-177.

[35] Claridge TDW, ScienceDirect. High-resolution NMR techniques in organic chemistry. 2009:383.

[36] Jacobsen NE, Ebooks Corporation. NMR Spectroscopy Explained. 2007:686.

[37] Noda I, Ozaki Y, Ebooks Corporation. Two-Dimensional Correlation Spectroscopy. 2005:311.

[38] Richards S, Hollerton J, Ebooks Corporation. Essential Practical NMR for Organic Chemistry. 2010:230.

[39] Wuthrich K. Nuclear Magnetic Resonance (NMR) Spectroscopy of Proteins. eLS: John Wiley & Sons, Ltd; 2001.

[40] Tugarinov V, Muhandiram R, Ayed A, Kay LE. Four-dimensional NMR spectroscopy of a 723-residue protein: chemical shift assignments and secondary structure of malate synthase g. J Am Chem Soc 2002;124(34):10025-10035.

[41] Sikic K, Tomic S, Carugo O. Systematic comparison of crystal and NMR protein structures deposited in the protein data bank. Open Biochem J 2010;4:83-95.

[42] Shin J, Lee W, Lee W. Structural proteomics by NMR spectroscopy. Expert Rev Proteomics 2008;5(4):589-601.

[43] Acton TB, Xiao R, Anderson S, Aramini J, Buchwald WA, Ciccosanti C, et al. Preparation of protein samples for NMR structure, function, and small-molecule screening studies. Methods Enzymol 2011;493:21-60.

[44] Insect cell media - BioExpress 2000: New results from CIL. ; 05//; Providence, RI; 2005.

[45] Saxena K, Dutta A, Klein-Seetharaman J, Schwalbe H. Isotope labeling in insect cells. Methods in Molecular Biology 2012;831:37-54.

[46] Wood MJ, Komives EA. Production of large quantities of isotopically labeled protein in Pichia pastoris by fermentation. J Biomol NMR 1999;13(2):149-159.

[47] Staunton D, Schlinkert R, Zanetti G, Colebrook SA, Campbell ID. Cell-free expression and selective isotope labelling in protein NMR. Magn Reson Chem 2006;44 Spec No:S2-9.

[48] Sobhanifar S, Reckel S, Junge F, Schwarz D, Kai L, Karbyshev M, et al. Cell-free expression and stable isotope labelling strategies for membrane proteins. J Biomol NMR 2010;46(1):33-43.

[49] Ohki S, Kainosho M. Stable isotope labeling methods for protein NMR spectroscopy. Prog Nucl Magn Reson Spectrosc 2008;53(4):208-226.

[50] Fiaux J, Bertelsen EB, Horwich AL, Wuthrich K. Uniform and residue-specific 15N-labeling of proteins on a highly deuterated background. J Biomol NMR 2004;29(3): 289-297.

[51] Murray V, Huang Y, Chen J, Wang J, Li Q. A Novel bacterial expression method with optimized parameters for very high yield production of triple-labeled proteins. Methods in Molecular Biology 2012;831:1-18.

[52] Religa TL, Ruschak AM, Rosenzweig R, Kay LE. Site-directed methyl group labeling as an NMR probe of structure and dynamics in supramolecular protein systems: applications to the proteasome and to the ClpP protease. J Am Chem Soc 2011;133(23): 9063-9068.

[53] Ruschak AM, Kay LE. Methyl groups as probes of supra-molecular structure, dynamics and function. J Biomol NMR 2010;46(1):75-87.

[54] Waugh DS. Genetic tools for selective labeling of proteins with alpha-15N-amino acids. J Biomol NMR 1996;8(2):184-192.

[55] O'Grady C, Rempel BL, Sokaribo A, Nokhrin S, Dmitriev OY. One-step amino acid selective isotope labeling of proteins in prototrophic Escherichia coli strains. Anal Biochem 2012;426(2):126-128.

[56] Krishnarjuna B, Jaipuria G, Thakur A, D'Silva P, Atreya HS. Amino acid selective unlabeling for sequence specific resonance assignments in proteins. J Biomol NMR 2011;49(1):39-51.

[57] Skrisovska L, Schubert M, Allain FH. Recent advances in segmental isotope labeling of proteins: NMR applications to large proteins and glycoproteins. J Biomol NMR 2010;46(1):51-65.

[58] Muona M, Aranko AS, Raulinaitis V, Iwai H. Segmental isotopic labeling of multi-domain and fusion proteins by protein trans-splicing in vivo and in vitro. Nat Protoc 2010;5(3):574-587.

[59] Chen J, Wang J. A segmental labeling strategy for unambiguous determination of domain–domain interactions of large multi-domain proteins. J Biomol NMR 2011;50(4): 403-410.

[60] Fagerberg L, Jonasson K, von Heijne G, Uhlen M, Berglund L. Prediction of the human membrane proteome. Proteomics 2010;10(6):1141-1149.

[61] Warschawski DE, Arnold AA, Beaugrand M, Gravel A, Chartrand E, Marcotte I. Choosing membrane mimetics for NMR structural studies of transmembrane proteins. Biochim Biophys Acta 2011;1808(8):1957-1974.

[62] Qureshi T, Goto NK. Contemporary methods in structure determination of membrane proteins by solution NMR. Top Curr Chem 2012;326:123-186.

[63] Zhu G, Yao X. TROSY-based NMR experiments for NMR studies of large biomolecules. Prog Nucl Magn Reson Spectrosc 2008;52(1):49-68.

[64] Tzeng S-, Pai M-, Kalodimos CG. NMR studies of large protein systems. Methods in Molecular Biology 2012;831:133-140.

[65] Kay LE. Solution NMR spectroscopy of supra-molecular systems, why bother? A methyl-TROSY view. J Magn Reson 2011;210(2):159-170.

[66] Sprangers R, Kay LE. Quantitative dynamics and binding studies of the 20S proteasome by NMR. Nature 2007;445(7128):618-622.

[67] Guntert P. Automated structure determination from NMR spectra. Eur Biophys J 2009;38(2):129-143.

[68] Gronwald W, Kalbitzer HR. Automated structure determination of proteins by NMR spectroscopy. Prog Nucl Magn Reson Spectrosc 2004;44(1-2):33-96.

[69] Banci L, Bertini I, Luchinat C, Mori M. NMR in structural proteomics and beyond. Prog Nucl Magn Reson Spectrosc 2010;56(3):247-266.

[70] Delaglio F, Wu Z, Bax A. Measurement of Homonuclear Proton Couplings from Regular 2D COSY Spectra. Journal of Magnetic Resonance 2001;149(2):276-281.

[71] Shen Y, Delaglio F, Cornilescu G, Bax A. TALOS+: a hybrid method for predicting protein backbone torsion angles from NMR chemical shifts. J Biomol NMR 2009;44(4):213-223.

[72] Jain NU. Use of residual dipolar couplings in structural analysis of protein-ligand complexes by solution NMR spectroscopy. Methods Mol Biol 2009;544:231-252.

[73] Chen K, Tjandra N. The use of residual dipolar coupling in studying proteins by NMR. Top Curr Chem 2012;326:47-67.

[74] Huang YJ, Powers R, Montelione GT. Protein NMR recall, precision, and F-measure scores (RPF scores): structure quality assessment measures based on information retrieval statistics. J Am Chem Soc 2005;127(6):1665-1674.

[75] Wu DH, Chen AD, Johnson CS. An improved diffusion-ordered spectroscopy experiment incorporating bipolar-gradient pulses. J Magn Reson Ser A 1995;115(2):260-264.

[76] Harpaz Y, Gerstein M, Chothia C. Volume changes on protein-folding. Structure 1994;2(7):641-649.

[77] Syvitski RT, Burton I, Mattatall NR, Douglas SE, Jakeman DL. Structural characterization of the antimicrobial Peptide pleurocidin from winter flounder. Biochemistry 2005;44(19):7282-7293.

[78] Kier LB. Molecular Orbital Calculation of Preferred Conformations of Acetylcholine, Muscarine, and Muscarone. Mol Pharmacol 1967;3(5):487-494.

[79] Guener OF, Editor. Pharmacophore: Perception, Development, and Use in Drug Design. [In: IUL Biotechnol. Ser., 2000; 2]. : International University Line; 2000.

[80] Guccione S, Editor. Pharmacophores Elucidation and Their Use in Drug Design. [In: Curr. Pharm. Des., 2001; 7(7)]. : Bentham Sci Publ; 2001.

[81] Marchioro C, Davalli S, Provera S, Heller M, Ross A, Senn H. Experiments in NMR-based screening. Methods Princ Med Chem 2003;16:321-340.

[82] Meyer B, Peters T. NMR spectroscopy techniques for screening and identifying ligand binding to protein receptors. Angew Chem , Int Ed 2003;42(8):864-890.

[83] Meyer B, Weimar T, Peters T. Screening mixtures for biological activity by NMR. Eur J Biochem 1997;246(3):705-709.

[84] Claasen B, Axmann M, Meinecke R, Meyer B. Direct observation of ligand binding to membrane proteins in living cells by a saturation transfer double difference (STDD) NMR spectroscopy method shows a significantly higher affinity of integrin alpha(IIb)beta3 in native platelets than in liposomes. J Am Chem Soc 2005;127(3): 916-919.

[85] Feeney J, Batchelor JG, Albrand JP, Roberts GCK. The effects of intermediate exchange processes on the estimation of equilibrium constants by NMR. Journal of Magnetic Resonance (1969) 1979;33(3):519-529.

[86] Keller RM, WÃ¼thrich K. Assignment of the heme c resonances in the 360 MHz 1H NMR spectra of cytochrome c. Biochimica et Biophysica Acta (BBA) - Protein Structure 1978;533(1):195-208.

[87] Ludwig C, Michiels PJ, Wu X, Kavanagh KL, Pilka E, Jansson A, et al. SALMON: solvent accessibility, ligand binding, and mapping of ligand orientation by NMR spectroscopy. J Med Chem 2008;51(1):1-3.

[88] Dalvit C, Fogliatto G, Stewart A, Veronesi M, Stockman B. WaterLOGSY as a method for primary NMR screening: practical aspects and range of applicability. J Biomol NMR 2001;21(4):349-359.

[89] Balaram P, Bothner-By A, Breslow E. Localization of tyrosine at the binding site of neurophysin II by negative nuclear Overhouser effects. J Am Chem Soc 1972;94(11): 4017-4018.

[90] Hajduk PJ, Olejniczak ET, Fesik SW. One-Dimensional Relaxation- and Diffusion-Edited NMR Methods for Screening Compounds That Bind to Macromolecules. J Am Chem Soc 1997;119(50):12257-12261.

[91] Kramer M, Kleinpeter E. STD-DOSY: A new NMR method to analyze multi-component enzyme/substrate systems. J Magn Reson 2010;202(2):245-249.

[92] Fejzo J, Lepre C, Xie X. Application of NMR screening in drug discovery. Curr Top Med Chem (Hilversum, Neth) 2003;3(1):81-97.

[93] Lepre CA. Strategies for NMR screening and library design. Methods Princ Med Chem 2003;16:391-415.

[94] Carlomagno T. Ligand-target interactions: what can we learn from NMR? Annu Rev Biophys Biomol Struct 2005;34:245-266.

[95] Klages J, Coles M, Kessler H. NMR-based screening: a powerful tool in fragment-based drug discovery. Analyst 2007;132(7):693-705.

[96] Murali N, Jarori GK, Landy SB, Rao BD. Two-dimensional transferred nuclear Overhauser effect spectroscopy (TRNOESY) studies of nucleotide conformations in creatine kinase complexes: effects due to weak nonspecific binding. Biochemistry 1993;32(47):12941-12948.

[97] Koskela H, Heikkinen O, Kilpelainen I, Heikkinen S. Rapid and accurate processing method for amide proton exchange rate measurement in proteins. J Biomol NMR 2007;37(4):313-320.

[98] Howard GC, Brown WE, Editors. Modern Protein Chemistry: Practical Aspects. : CRC; 2002.

[99] Pauli GF, Jaki B, Lankin D, Burton I, Walter J. Quantitative NMR (qNMR) of Bioactive Natural Products. In: Colegate S, Molyneux R, editors. Bioactive Natural Products: Detection, Isolation and Structural Determination. 2nd ed. Boca Raton, Florida: CRC Press; scheduled 2007.

[100] Merkley N, Syvitski RT. Profiling whole microalgal cells by high-resolution magic angle spinning (HR-MAS) magnetic resonance spectroscopy. J Appl Phycol 2012;24(3):535-540.

[101] Oliver SG. Functional genomics: lessons from yeast. Philos Trans R Soc Lond B Biol Sci 2002;357(1417):17-23.

[102] Wang H, Peng D, Xie J. Ginseng leaf-stem: bioactive constituents and pharmacological functions. Chin Med 2009;4:20.

[103] Jayapal KP, Philp RJ, Kok YJ, Yap MG, Sherman DH, Griffin TJ, et al. Uncovering genes with divergent mRNA-protein dynamics in Streptomyces coelicolor. PLoS One 2008;3(5):e2097.

[104] Krishnan P, Kruger NJ, Ratcliffe RG. Metabolite fingerprinting and profiling in plants using NMR. J Exp Bot 2005;56(410):255-265.

[105] Fiehn O. Metabolomics--the link between genotypes and phenotypes. Plant Mol Biol 2002;48(1-2):155-171.

[106] Sumner LW, Mendes P, Dixon RA. Plant metabolomics: large-scale phytochemistry in the functional genomics era. Phytochemistry 2003;62(6):817-836.

[107] Wu H, Southam AD, Hines A, Viant MR. High-throughput tissue extraction protocol for NMR- and MS-based metabolomics. Anal Biochem 2008;372(2):204-212.

[108] Iles RA, Chalmers RA. Nuclear magnetic resonance spectroscopy in the study of inborn errors of metabolism. Clin Sci (Lond) 1988;74(1):1-10.

[109] Schripsema J, Verpoorte R. Investigation of extracts of plant cell cultures by proton nuclear magnetic resonance spectroscopy. Phytochem Anal 1991;2(4):155-162.

[110] Nicholson JK, Lindon JC, Holmes E. 'Metabonomics': understanding the metabolic responses of living systems to pathophysiological stimuli via multivariate statistical analysis of biological NMR spectroscopic data. Xenobiotica 1999;29(11):1181-1189.

[111] Nicholson JK, Connelly J, Lindon JC, Holmes E. Metabonomics: a platform for studying drug toxicity and gene function. Nat Rev Drug Discov 2002;1(2):153-161.

[112] Verpoorte R, Choi Y, Kim H. NMR-based metabolomics at work in phytochemistry. Phytochemistry Reviews 2007;6(1):3-14.

[113] Holmes E, Antti H. Chemometric contributions to the evolution of metabonomics: mathematical solutions to characterising and interpreting complex biological NMR spectra. Analyst 2002;127(12):1549-1557.

[114] Craigie J, MacKinnon S, Walter J. Liquid seaweed extracts identified using ^{1}H NMR profiles. J Appl Phycol 2008;20(5):665-671.

[115] Martin FP, Rezzi S, Pere-Trepat E, Kamlage B, Collino S, Leibold E, et al. Metabolic effects of dark chocolate consumption on energy, gut microbiota, and stress-related metabolism in free-living subjects. J Proteome Res 2009;8(12):5568-5579.

[116] Van Dorsten FA, Daykin CA, Mulder TP, Van Duynhoven JP. Metabonomics approach to determine metabolic differences between green tea and black tea consumption. J Agric Food Chem 2006;54(18):6929-6938.

[117] Manach C, Hubert J, Llorach R, Scalbert A. The complex links between dietary phytochemicals and human health deciphered by metabolomics. Mol Nutr Food Res 2009;53(10):1303-1315.

[118] Power WP. High-resolution magic angle spinning-enabling applications of NMR spectroscopy to semi-solid phases. Annu Rep NMR Spectrosc 2011;72:111-156.

[119] Weybright P, Millis K, Campbell N, Cory DG, Singer S. Gradient, high-resolution, magic angle spinning 1H nuclear magnetic resonance spectroscopy of intact cells. Magn Reson Med 1998;39(3):337-345.

[120] Lindon JC, Beckonert OP, Holmes E, Nicholson JK. High-resolution magic angle spinning NMR spectroscopy: Application to biomedical studies. Prog Nucl Magn Reson Spectrosc 2009;55(2):79-100.

[121] Beckonert O, Coen M, Keun HC, Wang Y, Ebbels TM, Holmes E, et al. High-resolution magic-angle-spinning NMR spectroscopy for metabolic profiling of intact tissues. Nat Protoc 2010;5(6):1019-1032.

[122] Sitter B, Bathen TF, Tessem M, Gribbestad IS. High-resolution magic angle spinning (HR MAS) MR spectroscopy in metabolic characterization of human cancer. Prog Nucl Magn Reson Spectrosc 2009;54(3-4):239-254.

[123] Hanoulle X, Wieruszeski JM, Rousselot-Pailley P, Landrieu I, Baulard AR, Lippens G. Monitoring of the ethionamide pro-drug activation in mycobacteria by (1)H high resolution magic angle spinning NMR. Biochem Biophys Res Commun 2005;331(2): 452-458.

[124] Schroder H. High resolution magic angle spinning NMR for analyzing small molecules attached to solid support. Comb Chem High Throughput Screen 2003;6(7): 741-753.

[125] Li W. Multidimensional HRMAS NMR: a platform for in vivo studies using intact bacterial cells. Analyst 2006;131(7):777-781.

[126] Thongsaard W, Marsden C, Morris P, Prior M, Shah Y. Effect of Thunbergia laurifolia , a Thai natural product used to treat drug addiction, on cerebral activity detected by functional magnetic resonance imaging in the rat. Psychopharmacology (Berl) 2005;180(4):1-9.

[127] Miskowiak KW, Favaron E, Hafizi S, Inkster B, Goodwin GM, Cowen PJ, et al. Erythropoietin modulates neural and cognitive processing of emotional information in biomarker models of antidepressant drug action in depressed patients. Psychopharmacology (Berl) 2010;210(3):419-428.

[128] Miskowiak KW, Favaron E, Hafizi S, Inkster B, Goodwin GM, Cowen PJ, et al. Effects of erythropoietin on emotional processing biases in patients with major depression: an exploratory fMRI study. Psychopharmacology (Berl) 2009;207(1):133-142.

[129] Rudin M, McSheehy PM, Allegrini PR, Rausch M, Baumann D, Becquet M, et al. PTK787/ZK222584, a tyrosine kinase inhibitor of vascular endothelial growth factor

http://dx.doi.org/10.5772/54231

receptor, reduces uptake of the contrast agent GdDOTA by murine orthotopic B16/BL6 melanoma tumours and inhibits their growth in vivo. NMR Biomed 2005;18(5):308-321.

[130] Rudin M, Allegrini P, Beckmann N, Gremlich HU, Kneuer R, Laurent D, et al. Noninvasive imaging in drug discovery and development. Ernst Schering Res Found Workshop 2004;(48)(48):47-75.

[131] Islam T, Josephson L. Current state and future applications of active targeting in malignancies using superparamagnetic iron oxide nanoparticles. Cancer Biomarkers 2009;5(2):99-107.

[132] Kiessling F. Noninvasive cell tracking. Handb Exp Pharmacol 2008;185:305-321.

[133] Bio-Accumulation of a TRPV-6 Binding Peptide SOR-C27 in an Ovarian Cancer Mouse Model by Magnetic Resonance Imaging (MRI). BHCRI 3rd Annual Cancer Conference Halifax, Canada.

[134] Gruettner C, Mueller K, Teller J, Westphal F, Foreman A, Ivkov R. Synthesis and antibody conjugation of magnetic nanoparticles with improved specific power absorption rates for alternating magnetic field cancer therapy. J Magn Magn Mater 2007;311(1):181-186.

[135] Kinoshita M, Yoshioka Y, Okita Y, Hashimoto N, Yoshimine T. MR molecular imaging of HER-2 in a murine tumor xenograft by SPIO labeling of anti-HER-2 affibody. Contrast Media Mol Imaging 2010;5(1):18-22.

[136] Thorek DL, Chen AK, Czupryna J, Tsourkas A. Superparamagnetic iron oxide nanoparticle probes for molecular imaging. Ann Biomed Eng 2006;34(1):23-38.

[137] Hung Y, Sava VM, Juang C, Yeh T, Shen W, Huang GS. Gastrointestinal enhancement of MRI with melanin derived from tea leaves (Thea sinensis Linn.). J Ethnopharmacol 2002;79(1):75-79.

[138] Stewart JM, inventor. AnonymousPeptide composition for cancer treatment by inhibiting trpv6 calcium channel activity. US20110071089A1. 2011 03/24.

[139] Stewart JM, inventor. AnonymousSoricidin derived peptides and methods for the detection of TRPV-6 cancers and drug delivery. WO2010148501A1. 2010 12/29.

Section 2

Bioactive Proteins from Natural Sources

Chapter 4

Marine Natural Products for Protein Misfolding Modulation

James C. Giffin and Kathryn Varya Ewart

Additional information is available at the end of the chapter

http://dx.doi.org/10.5772/54585

1. Introduction

Proteins are linear covalent chains of amino acids. In most proteins, the chain winds in a specific way to adopt a set fold, or "conformation", that is stable and that allows it to function. A number of proteins remain unfolded in their native state and these are referred to as intrinsically disordered proteins. These unfolded proteins remain soluble and functional and some exhibit specific ligand binding capability, which can cause them to adopt an induced fold. In contrast to these two functional situations of natively folded and disordered proteins, proteins that are normally folded or disordered can misfold, that is, to fold incorrectly.

Proteins may misfold as a result of enzymatic cleavage, post-translational modification, mutation, overabundance or structural destabilization due to alteration in the tissue environment. Accumulation of misfolded proteins can occur more readily when proteostasis mechanisms that foster correct folding of proteins, such as the chaperone system, and that clear the cell of misfolded proteins, such as the ubiquitin-proteasome system, are compromised [1]. A subset of human proteins appears to have an unusual tendency to misfold and this is recognized as a central event in a number of human diseases (reviewed by [2]). Improper folding often leads to problems because the misfolded protein cannot perform its normal role (loss of essential function) and because it assembles into oligomeric forms or larger aggregates that are toxic to the cell (gain of harmful function) [3]. The most recognized misfolded conformation is a stacking of β-sheets forming a crossed-β secondary structure that assembles into a linear multimeric fiber called amyloid (reviewed in [2]).

Several neurodegenerative diseases share protein misfolding as an underlying cause [4, 5]. These diseases can be classified based upon the proteins affected [3] while sharing a common mechanism of emergence. Protein misfolding in neurodegenerative diseases has been the focus of many reviews; excellent examples are in [5-9]. Therefore, a comprehensive review will not be undertaken here. The canonical neurodegenerative diseases are Alzheimer's disease (AD), Parkinson's disease (PD), Huntington's disease, amyotrophic lateral sclerosis and the prion diseases. Although each involves distinct proteins, misfolding has a common role. Huntington's disease is caused by an excessive number of sequential glutamines near the N terminus of the protein huntingtin. An expansion of the natural glutamine stretch exceeding approximately 33 residues results in Huntington's symptoms and the age of onset of the disease declines with increasing residue number [10-12]. A likely reason for this is the increased propensity for aggregation with increasing polyglutamine length [13]. Amyotrophic lateral sclerosis is a disease associated with the death of the upper and lower motor neurons in the spinal cord, brain stem and motor cortex. The affected neurons accumulate aggregate protein inclusions that may be causing the cells to die. Mutations in genes encoding superoxide dismutase-1, TAR DNA binding protein 43 and fused in sarcoma/ translation in liposarcoma (FUS/TLS) are implicated in ALS (reviewed in [14]). Prion diseases display several interesting commonalities with these other neurodegenerative diseases. Prion diseases emerge from misfolded prion protein, which serves as a template for subsequent misfolding of native prion protein with ensuing aggregation and neuron loss. The propagation of pathogenic misfolding from one protein molecule to its healthy neighbours by templating was long considered to be unique to prions; however, recent studies have suggested that molecular templating of misfolded proteins occurs with other neurodegenerative diseases as well. Furthermore, templating is inferred by observation of their spatial spread from select foci in the brain [5, 15, 16]. It is notable that prion diseases, which are infectious, may occur in animals or humans of all ages, whereas the apparently non-transmissible protein folding diseases occur mainly with ageing. This implies that a key step in all protein folding disease may be the initial establishment of a misfolded protein in a neuron, whether it is a misfolded protein taken in at any age by infection or misfolding that emerges in a susceptible endogenous protein due to faltering proteostasis with ageing. Therefore, the prevention of misfolding and/or the promotion of disaggregation and refolding of misfolded proteins *in vivo* appear to be the most direct means of dealing with all these diseases.

In this chapter, the focus is on AD and PD, as these are the two most prevalent neurodegenerative diseases, and the proteins that misfold in these diseases are well studied. AD accounts for approximately two thirds of all cases of dementia [17]; it leads to cognitive deficits in reasoning, memory, abstraction and motor skills, with eventual death. It is characterized at the molecular level by extracellular aggregates of a short peptide called amyloid beta (Aβ, and also called beta amyloid), which can form oligomers and larger fibrils with amyloid structure and later emerging intracellular neurofibrillary tangles that are composed of hyperphosphorylated tau protein (reviewed in [18]). In this chapter, Aβ normally refers to $A\beta_{42}$, which is the 42-residue peptide and also appears to be most toxic form. There is increasing evidence that the Aβ oligomers have a key and likely causative role in AD. Most compelling are studies showing mutations in the regulatory region or encoded protein sequence in amyloid precursor gene in families predisposed to AD [19-21]. In contrast to AD, PD has been found to involve the misfolding of α–synuclein (αS) into aggregates found in Lewy bodies and Lewy neurites. PD affects the *substantia nigra*, a region of the brain in-

http://dx.doi.org/10.5772/54585

volved with reward, addiction and movement. Many of the onset symptoms of PD reflect this, and the diagnosis is based on resting tremor, slowness of movement, rigidity and postural instability [22]. These two proteins are unrelated in sequence and they have distinct structures in their native form, with Aβ a short mainly unstructured peptide and αS a larger 140-residue protein that is post-translationally modified and that can exist in alternative conformations including a largely α-helical form and a disordered state [23, 24]. In spite of these differences, both proteins misfold and aggregate, and the aggregates of each can be detected and measured using assays that will be discussed in the section below.

There is growing interest in the development of protein folding modulators that would offer to prevent or alleviate misfolding and to avoid the damage that occurs in neurodegenerative diseases. There has been progress along several avenues, but no magic bullet to date. Nonetheless, there remains substantial untapped diversity among natural products and notably in marine resources. With a focus on Aβ and αS, which are implicated in AD and PD, respectively, this chapter will examine natural agents that may prevent or ameliorate protein misfolding diseases, with particular attention to the potential of marine resources for possible discovery and development.

2. Screening and evaluation for action on protein folding

With the recognition that protein misfolding is a cause of several neurodegenerative diseases and a common mechanism of their progression, promising developments have begun to emerge (reviewed in the next section). These have relied upon the measurement of protein misfolding modulation as an early step in screening and evaluation of new active molecules or as a follow-up step in the evaluation of known and promising candidates because of their suspected effects on the diseases. Identification of a molecule as a folding modulator raises the possibility that it could address the cause of AD or PD, rather than only addressing their symptoms, which makes products identified in this way potentially valuable in prevention as well as in amelioration of existing disease.

2.1. *In vitro* analysis of protein misfolding modulation

For both Aβ and αS, the transition from the native state to an amyloid conformation is not direct, but involves steps or stages. These may include unfolding, oligomerization and further aggregation into amyloid fibrils, with the possibility of off-pathway aggregation or reversal of these processes [25, 26]. This is summarized in Fig. 1. Compounds may prevent misfolding and/or templating by inhibiting the unfolding of a natively folded protein, by promoting the folding of an unfolded form, by preventing amyloid formation or by diverting the protein toward an alternative aggregation pathway leading to a less harmful aggregate. A selection of assay approaches to misfolding evaluation will be compared here in terms of information value, throughput and versatility.

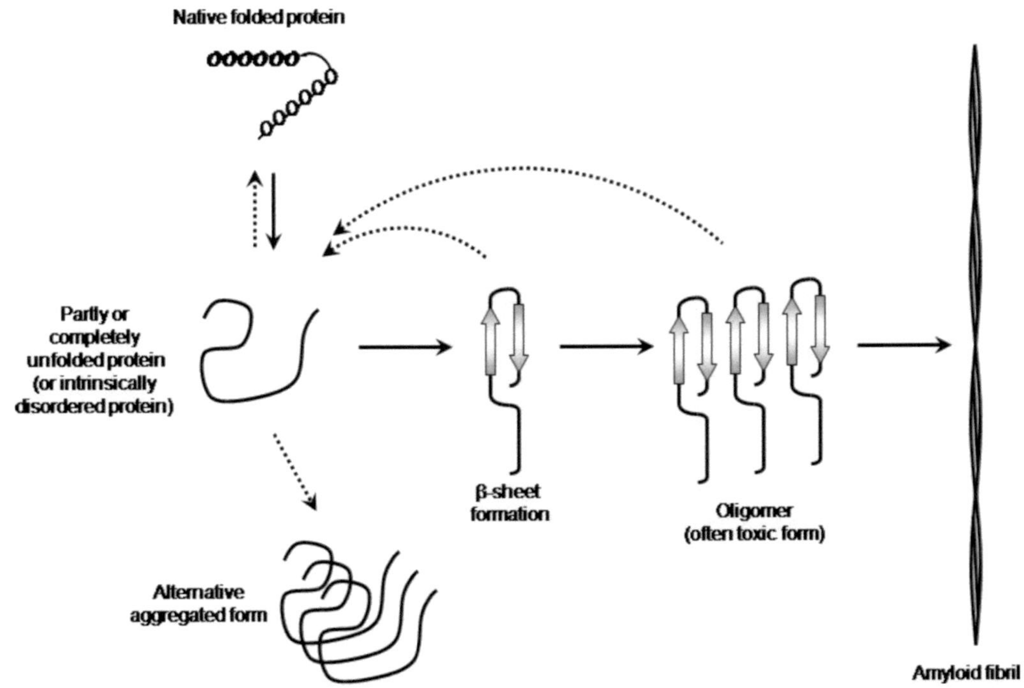

Figure 1. Overview of the general trajectory of protein misfolding with amyloid formation. Solid black arrows show pathway toward amyloid formation and stippled arrows show pathways of prevention or reversal of amyloid and related oligomers. This is an original diagram based upon information in reviews [2, 23].

2.1.1. Protein unfolding

For the discovery and development of novel agents against diseases such as AD and PD, a fuller picture of the action of a compound can be obtained by investigating the distinct steps of unfolding, aggregation, misfolding and amyloid formation. Proteins may remain largely folded and still produce amyloid or similar aggregates, provided that a local aggregation-prone sequence is exposed [27]. Nonetheless, for most proteins that readily form amyloid, it appears that that the loss of native folding is a required step [27]. Both Aβ and αS appear to have some unfolded or disordered character, but with regions that can become helical under appropriate conditions [28-30]. Inducing or preserving this helical conformation is a rational approach to preventing amyloid formation [29, 31, 32].

Folded and unfolded proteins differ in several characteristics that can be easily measured and that would allow folding modulators to be detected and evaluated. Some of the most common methods are summarized here. For example, proteins absorb right and left-circularly polarized light differently; this circular dichroism (CD) can be measured over a series of wavelengths to give informative spectra. The CD spectra of unfolded and folded proteins differ and those of proteins with predominantly α-helix and β-sheet secondary structure can be easily distinguished. In more detailed studies, the proportion of each major secondary structure in a protein can be calculated from the spectrum using software such as DICHRO-WEB [33]. Moreover, diagnostic features such as minima at wavelengths of 208 and 222 nm for α-helical proteins can be monitored in order to quantify changes in fold in response to temperature, solution components or other factors. To date, CD has been used for small-scale studies on protein folding and protein-ligand interaction because throughput is limited to a single sample at a time. The recent development of a high-speed automated CD spectrometer (ACD, Applied Photophysics) may allow this approach to be employed more broadly in sample screening. An advantage of CD measurement is that it is an intrinsic property of a protein; thus, the spectra require no additive and the protein can be measured directly without accessory molecules or modifications. Another intrinsic feature of proteins that can be measured directly is fluorescence. Proteins with aromatic side chains fluoresce when exposed to UV light and this can undergo a shift in intensity or wavelength of intensity maximum with folding. Fluorescence can also be measured using new devices that allow miniaturized measurements in a parallel manner using a similar rapid-throughput approach (e.g. the Optim 1000, Avacta Innovative Analysis). Likewise, differential binding of dyes such as SYPRO Orange allow protein forms with different exposure of hydrophobic residues to solvent to be distinguished. In the case of SYPRO Orange, the dye is quenched when free in an aqueous solution, but it becomes unquenched when it interacts with the hydrophobic regions that are exposed upon protein unfolding and its fluorescence increases as a consequence. This measurement can be performed efficiently on large numbers of samples using devices designed for quantitative PCR [34]. Measurements by these approaches allow protein folding to be assessed and changes in fold and/or fold stability to be examined. An informative and frequently employed measure of fold stability is the melting temperature (Tm), as proteins with more stable folds normally melt at higher temperatures. The Tm can be determined by any of the above techniques. A compound that stabilizes the folded conformation of a protein would raise its Tm and this change can be easily quantified by the above approaches. A caveat with amyloid-forming proteins is that stabilized folding, as exhibited by a higher Tm, may not necessarily represent the native folding that is assumed to preclude amyloid formation. For this reason, CD is particularly valuable, as it also allows the secondary structure to be determined; a spectrum distinct from that of β-sheet would provide a reasonable indication that the stable form is native and unrelated to amyloid.

2.1.2. Amyloid-like structure

It was through dye binding that amyloid plaques were first discovered. Fibrous aggregates in tissues stained blue when treated with acid followed by iodine and the aggregates were termed amyloid because they were believed to be starch based upon the colour development (reviewed in [35]). Although it is a misnomer, the name amyloid has endured and several different dyes have become invaluable in the study of protein misfolding and amyloid formation *in vitro*.

Thioflavin T (ThT), a benzothiazole dye, and Congo red, a diazobenzidine dye, are both commonly used to quantify the amount of amyloid protein present in a solution. ThT was first described to have amyloid-binding ability over 50 years ago [36] and it has since been in widespread use in the study of amyloidosis and the search for possible binding molecules. Congo red has also been in use for amyloid detection and quantification for several decades since its first description in that role [37]. Both of these dyes undergo a red shift in their fluorescence emission when they interact with amyloid fibrils. They cannot be used to distinguish between amyloid fibrils and smaller aggregates; however, they allow quantitative analysis and they continue to find wide use in amyloid analysis. Thioflavin S is a mixture of components derived from ThT and it has no spectral shift in absorbance or emission, which makes it suitable only for imaging and not for quantitation in solution because of high background [35]. Derivatives of N-arylaminonaphtalene including ANS and bis-ANS bind primarily to early stage aggregation in amyloid formation [38, 39]. They have not been as widely used as ThT and Congo Red, but they may find greater use with the increasing focus on aggregation pathways (see section 3 below).

Recently, there has been interest in identifying newer binding fluorophores that allow oligomeric aggregates to be distinguished from fibrils. An example is the indole compound tryptophanol. It allows specific detection and quantitation of prefibrillar oligomeric Aβ because its fluorescence is quenched only in the presence of that form of Aβ with no similar quenching in the presence of Aβ fibrils [40]. Another is the carbocyanine dye JC-1 that distinguishes different aggregation states of αS [41]. JC-1 allows real-time tracking of αS aggregation, as different fluorescent signals are emitted for monomer and fibrillar binding and the ratio of the two signals allows for real-time visualization of αS aggregation [41].

Another recent development is the elaboration of antibodies and related agents that recognize proteins exclusively in their amyloid conformation, allowing the amyloid portion of the protein in question to be detected and quantified. A monoclonal antibody raised against αS was shown to recognize the protein in its amyloid form and, although the anticipated use is mainly *in vivo*, it showed effective recognition in an *in vitro* ELISA format [42]. Novel antibodies, termed gammabodies, were engineered by grafting a series of peptide sequences from Aβ into immunoglobulin variable regions [43]. These have found use in distinguishing oligomeric and amyloid forms of Aβ and this technology would be expected to be applicable to other aggregating proteins [43]. Since an amyloid-like structure is relevant to many diseases, a new capture and detection peptoid that behaves in a manner similar to an antibody offers unusual versatility. This peptoid, based upon a 6-amino acid stretch in the human PrP sequence, binds to the amyloid forms of Aβ, αS, amylin and serpin [44].

Model proteins that undergo transition to an amyloid-like conformation may also offer alternatives for amyloid formation-related studies [45]. For example, the 37-residue natively α-helical winter flounder (*Pseudopleuronectes americanus*) antifreeze protein wflAFP-6 (HPLC-6) adopts an amyloid-like structure during the freeze-thaw process [46, 47]. This may offer an interesting model system for the study of the conversion of a protein from its native form into amyloid fibrils [47, 48]. The ability to generate rapid amyloid formation in wflAFP-6 using the freeze-thaw process would offer low background compared with Aβ assays and the consistent α-helical nature of the native AFP may also allow initial unfolding steps to be more clearly evidenced than in proteins with less defined native structure. Nonetheless, a molecule found to be an amyloid-relevant folding modulator using AFP amyloid-like transition assays may be universal or nearly so, as in the case of the peptoid detection system described above, or it may be specific to the wflAFP-6 and have no effect on other amyloid-forming proteins. Therefore, in spite of its potential advantages, further study of the antifreeze protein model would be required before its adoption in an assay platform.

2.1.3. Protein interaction during amyloid formation

As the interaction between locally or entirely misfolded monomers appears critical to non-native protein association, there is interest in identifying molecules that directly interfere with that process. Therefore, assays for binding competition or impedance have been developed. A convenient new microplate assay employs fluorescently labelled Aβ. Unlabelled Aβ is coated onto the plate surface and then the labelled Aβ is applied in solution and allowed to bind [49]. After unbound material is washed off, the fluorescence remaining can be used to determine the level of interaction of Aβ [49]. Although the aggregation state of the Aβ in solution or on the plate is not indicated, the assay indicates the interaction between in-solution and on-plate Aβ that is inhibitable, which can be taken to represent either oligomer formation or assembly into larger fibrils. Thus, molecules that affect any part of this process can be readily identified. Nonetheless, with the aggregation state of the binding units unclear except where Aβ fragments are used, this assay does not indicate which step(s) in assembly of the monomer-oligomer-fibril are being affected.

Aβ oligomerization and fibril formation can be challenging to study *in vitro* using dyes and other methods because of spurious background oligomer formation and the difficulty in determining how much oligomer may already have formed in a starting sample [50]. For these reasons, assays that avoid these problems have garnered interest. In one example, a procedure was developed involving a semi-denaturing detergent-agarose gel electrophoresis followed by blotting and immunological detection with an appropriate antibody recognizing the protein in all its forms [51]. The method allows amyloid aggregate size distributions to be determined and the user can distinguish among the monomeric, oligomeric and large aggregated (likely fibril) forms. A drawback is that it involves a vacuum transfer of proteins from the gel to a PVDF membrane. A derived method employing capillary blotting to a nitrocellulose membrane, reminiscent of nucleic acid blotting, has made the assay more precise and scaleable for screening purposes [52]. These methods allow the association state of the starting material to be determined and the effect of any product to be evaluated in comparison. Another approach is to eliminate the possibility of aggregates in the starting solution. An example is an assay based upon the expression of the Aβ sequence in tandem with green fluorescent protein (GFP) as a fusion within a bacterial cell [53]. Aggregation of Aβ precludes GFP folding and so there is no fluorescence, whereas addition of a molecule impeding the aggregation of Aβ results in GFP folding to its native structure with consequent fluorescence. A more directly quantifiable *in vitro* form of this assay was developed using the Venus yellow fluorescent protein (vYFP) instead of GFP, which allows denaturation and refolding under precisely controlled conditions to detect molecules that promote or inhibit aggregation [50].

2.2. Cell- and organism-based analyses

Once an active extract is identified by efficient *in vitro* assay and similar assay-guided fractionation has revealed the class of molecules or the molecule that is responsible, determination of effects *in vivo* is of interest. Using culture models such as the PC12 primary neuronal cells or the SH-SY5Y neuroblastoma cell line, effects of active molecules can be determined. In a first approach, cells can be treated by transfection or other means to harbour high levels of the protein of interest and then the effect of active molecules on cell survival can be measured using one of several commercially available assays for dead cells, which measure lactate dehydrogenase leakage or other indicative parameters. However, more precise information can be gleaned by histological analysis using stains such as Congo red or thioflavin S, described above, that reveal the presence of amyloid accumulation. Immunohistochemistry using appropriate antibodies against Aβ or αS can be even more informative, as some allow distinction of oligomeric denatured forms from amyloid fibrils.

Cell-based assays can also provide an indication of the possibility of a molecule crossing the blood-brain barrier. Although Aβ circulates in the serum [54] and αS is expressed in red blood cells [55], it is considered preferable for a compound to have direct access to the brain where the pathology takes place. Therefore, blood-brain barrier models in cell culture, such as the MDR-MCCK monolayer [56], are available to predict the permeability for specific substances. Nonetheless, blood brain barrier physiology is more complex than the models or direct plasma/brain ratio determinations would predict [57]. For that reason, results must be interpreted with care.

Animal models provide critical understanding in terms of the distribution, mode of action and effectiveness of an active molecule. Besides the well-known mouse models for many neurodegenerative diseases, there are valuable invertebrate and fish models. An αS-transgenic *Drosophila* fly model is available for PD [58] and an Aβ-transgenic model for AD [59] The nematode worm, *Caenorhabditis elegans,* can be used to study AD and PD [60, 61]. Zebrafish (*Danio rerio*) have an Aβ protein precursor-encoding gene [62] and synuclein genes have been identified in this species [63]. Zebrafish may also become informative for studies of αS once the encoded proteins in this organism are better understood.

3. Protein folding modulators from common terrestrial natural products

A large number of molecules have been shown to influence the aggregation of Aβ [18] and a growing number have shown effects on αS (discussed below). Although no effective therapy for PD or AD has emerged to date, progress on a number of natural products is encouraging. This situation is not surprising, as synthetic and combinatorial chemistry normally rely on a limited number of structural scaffolds and random permutations of structures and synthesizable units [64]. In contrast, natural molecules are highly diverse and they have been subject to evolutionary pressure under distinct conditions in which valuable activities have been selected. Therefore, they may offer a combination of variety and biological pre-selection that may make a therapeutic activity more likely [64].

3.1. Natural protein folding modulators from terrestrial sources

Several natural molecules have garnered interest because they modulate amyloid formation by Aβ (reviewed in [18, 65, 66]). A number of salient examples involving Aβ and αS are presented here.

3.1.1. Curcumin

Curcumin is a natural polyphenol found in the traditional Indian spice turmeric. This molecule has been extensively investigated, in part because of its role in traditional Ayurvedic medicine [67]. Numerous studies have shown curcumin to have wide ranging biological activities, including Aβ folding modulation. Curcumin shows promising interaction with Aβ. For example, using an oligomer-specific antibody for immunoblotting, cucurmin was found prevent Aβ oligomerization and toxicity *in vitro*. In the same study, curcumin was shown to bind to amyloid plaques in brain sections of mice transgenic for the human amyloid precursor protein [68]. In addition, mature fibrils of the slightly shorter $A\beta_{40}$ peptide were destabilized by curcumin [68]. Curcumin and other polyphenols, including tannic acid, rosmarinic acid, and myricetin, were shown to inhibit fibril formation and destabilized mature fibrils for both Aβ and αS [69]. As a result, curcumin has been a component of interest in clinical trials and, most recently the exclusive molecule in a trial for prevention of early cognitive decline and abnormal Aβ accumulation in the brain [70]. If an effect is observed, it would be interesting to see if it acts directly upon misfolding at the dosage used in subjects.

3.1.2. Epigallocatechin-3-gallate

In terms of bioactive molecules in traditional medicine, perhaps the most recognized is (-)-epigallocatechin 3-gallate (EGCG) that is found in unfermented (green) tea (*Camellia sinensis*). EGCG is a pleiotropic polyphenolic molecule with interesting protein folding modulation activity. In *C. elegans* expressing human Aβ in muscle cells, western blotting analysis using an anti-Aβ antibody showed EGCG to inhibit Aβ oligomerization [71]. Studies of Aβ and αS using ThT fluorescence, electron microscopy and other biophysical methods showed interaction with EGCG and ensuing "off-pathway" aggregation into spherical oligomers, which thereby prevented the formation of typical aggregation intermediates and amyloid fibrils by both proteins [25]. Further investigation revealed EGCG to bind directly to the β-sheet structure in the amyloid fibrils formed by Aβ and by αS and to direct their rearrangement into smaller non-toxic protein aggregates [26]. A clinical trial is planned to examine the effect of EGCG on early stage AD [72] and this may have effects based upon the protein folding modulation described here, other properties of the molecule, or a combination thereof if adequate levels are attained in the brain. Other tea compounds may offer similar protection. Theaflavins are formed by oxidation of EGCG during the fermentation process to produce black tea. These derivatives were shown to have similar activity to EGCG in modulating the polymerization of Aβ and αS [73].

3.1.3. Carotenoids and related molecules

Carotenoids (pro-vitamin A) and vitamin A are present in many commonly consumed foods. The *in vitro* examination of vitamin A and β-carotene activity on AB fibril formation, as measured using dye binding and electron microscopy suggest protective effects that appear to result from binding to a region in the C-terminal half of the peptide [74, 75]. This is consistent with reports that vitamin A and related molecules inhibit the progression of AD symptoms [76]. Also using dye binding and electron microscopy, vitamin A and β-carotene were shown to inhibit the formation of αS amyloid fibrils and to destabilize existing fibrils [77].

3.1.4. Scyllo-inositol

Another natural molecule that has garnered interest is scyllo-inositol, which is abundant in the coconut palm (*Cocos nucifera*) [78]. Scyllo-inositol is a stereoisomer of myo-inositol that stabilizes a non-toxic oligomeric aggregate of Aβ [78-80]. This is in contrast to phosphatidylinositol, which was found to promote fibrillogenesis and membrane insertion of Aβ [78]. Scyllo-inositol also protected against Aβ oligomer-induced inhibition of long-term potentiation [80]. A clinical trial of scyllo-inositol was inconclusive after the highest doses were discontinued [81]. Nonetheless, it remains a compound of interest provided that drawbacks can be addressed.

3.1.5. Emerging sources

In addition to the well-studied molecules above, there are growing possibilities for other sources of folding modulators. For example, another source of interesting polyphenols is the wolf berry, *Lycium barbarum,* which is used in traditional Chinese medicine and was shown to protect against Aβ-related cell death [82]. Extracts obtained from other species used in traditional Chinese medicine, including cat's claw (*Uncaria rhynchophylla*) and tree peony (*Paeonia suffruticosa*) have shown relevant activity [83-85]. The tree peony contains 1,2,3,4,6-penta-O-galloyl-beta-D-glucopyranose, which prevented Aβ fiber formation and reversed the process in existing fibers [84]. In addition, other polyphenols procyanidins from apple (*Malus domestica*), silymarin from thistle (*Carduus marianus*) and reservatrol from red grapes (*Vitis sp.*) show interesting activities that may warrant further study [86-88].

3.2. Challenges with natural folding modulators

Although much attention has been brought to the natural folding modulators present in various terrestrial species, none have yet translated into meaningful therapies. The best prospect currently appears to be EGCG [89], which nonetheless presents challenges.

3.2.1. Challenges in delivery of natural products

EGCG is susceptible to decomposition during storage prior to being consumed, much of it may be destroyed by normal stomach acid during digestion, it is not highly bioavailable and it carries the possibility of hepatotoxicity (reviewed in [90]). Therefore, ideal handling, delivery and dosage would need to be determined before this molecule could be employed successfully to manage disease-related misfolding in animals or humans. Nonetheless, studies have suggested that the use of green tea is negatively correlated to the prevalence of cognitive impairment [91] and that tea shows a dose-dependent effect in protection from PD [92]. Therefore, even with regular storage, preparation and consumption of tea as part of a normal diet, it appears that tea components, and likely EGCG or its derived theaflavins, have a measure of benefit. It is not yet clear whether the reported benefits involve the modulation of protein misfolding, and this would be an area for future study. Curcumin presents challenges similar to those of EGCG and derivatives. Dietary ingestion of curcumin appears sufficient to offer some measure of protection from neurodegenerative diseases in populations that consume it (reviewed in [93]), suggesting its bioavailability. Yet, bioavailability was found to be limiting and work has been undertaken toward improving delivery of curcumin by combining it with phosphatidyl choline, olive oil and stearic acid [94]. Similarly, plasma levels of EGCG following oral consumption were higher when the product was encapsulated in chitosan nanoparticles [95]. The promising suggestion is that formulation and delivery may be optimized to enhance availability of these protein folding modulators *in vivo*. Other compounds such as carotenoids are bioavailable and cross the blood-brain barrier as well, possibly making them convenient for the establishment of protein folding modulators [96].

3.2.2. *Requirement for crossing the blood-brain barrier*

It is widely accepted that molecules must cross the blood-brain barrier in order to have relevant biological effects on neurodegenerative diseases; however, interesting new findings are suggesting that this may not always be the case. In a study using radiolabeled $A\beta_{40}$ administered to the brains of rats, elevated peripheral $A\beta_{40}$ levels reduced protein clearance from the brain [97]. Conversely, a decline of Aβ levels in blood plasma can lead to cognitive improvement, presumably by reducing Aβ levels in the brain [98, 99]. Furthermore, genetic study of the presenilin gene encoding a secretase with a role in Aβ synthesis revealed a heritable expression level in the liver, suggesting a role of liver-expressed protein in brain Aβ levels [100]. Follow-up investigation using ST571, a drug that lowers peripheral Aβ levels but that does not cross the blood-brain barrier, showed reduction in brain Aβ [100]. Although these were studies of complete Aβ levels rather than the different conformations and aggregates, together they do imply that modulation of peripheral oligomerized and fibrillar forms of Aβ, which would facilitate clearance, could affect the brain ratios of differently associated Aβ forms. Therefore, protein folding modulators that do not cross the blood-brain barrier may still be worth considering in the prevention and treatment of disease. These studies have the drawback of assuming a stable and functional blood-brain barrier over the course of these diseases; however, other findings suggest that functioning of the blood-brain barrier may become compromised over the course of AD and other neurodegenerative diseases (reviewed in [101]), which may result in inappropriate dosages of molecules from plasma. Therefore, the prevention phase may be critical to the benefit of any molecule that acts peripherally to modulate Aβ, as that is the point at which normal transfer of molecules such as Aβ across the barrier can occur. Alternatively, the compromised blood-brain-barrier during the disease phase may allow therapeutic molecules to reach the brain more efficiently. These possibilities require further study.

4. Marine possibilities for natural protein folding modulators

Natural products from the land include promising as sources of novel protein folding modulators for the reasons outlined earlier. By extension, marine sources may hold proportionally greater opportunity for discovery than their terrestrial counterparts because, until this decade, much of the ocean biota was unexplored. The Census of Marine Life uncovered remarkable and previously unknown plant and animal biodiversity in the oceans (reviewed in [102]). In the Gulf of Maine alone, the current species count identifies at least 652 fish species, 184 species of birds, 733 different species of microscopic plants and algae and 32 mammalian species [103]. Microbial diversity is also extensive worldwide, as inferred from the large number of new protein families uncovered from marine microbes [104].

Marine resources offer largely untapped diversity that may offer new options for natural product development [105]. Only six marine natural products and 14 synthetic compounds based upon the structures of natural marine products are FDA-approved agents or in clinical trial (reviewed in [106]). However, this list is likely to grow. In 2010, 895 new citations were reported on marine-derived compounds [107]. Marine species are already being examined for molecules that inhibit β-secretase 1, an enzyme that processes the amyloid precursor protein to give Aβ and other fragments [108]. Nonetheless, the development of inhibitors has been very difficult elsewhere [108] and there may be other biological consequences to the modulation of this enzyme. Therefore, it is ideal to focus more specifically on protein misfolding, which appears to be the linchpin in most of the neurodegenerative diseases. There is a wide variety of challenging and variable marine environments that would naturally select for traits that include protein folding modulation due to temperature or pressure, chemical defense molecules and other products that may be undersampled or undiscovered because of accessibility. Marine plants and sessile marine animals may produce chemical defenses that are remarkable in comparison to those of species that can move away from danger. In addition, species that inhabit highly variable or extreme environments, such as freezing waters, have adaptations to maintain proteostasis during exposure to extreme temperatures and solution properties [109-111]. For these reasons, they may represent ideal sources of natural molecules to prevent or ameliorate protein misfolding.

The discovery, characterization and production of marine-derived molecules appears promising, but with complexity and risk, nonetheless. A general overview of the process is shown in Fig. 2.

4.1. Natural protein folding modulators from marine sources

4.1.1. Marine polyphenols

Polyphenols are abundant and varied in marine algal species (reviewed in [112]). Like their terrestrial counterparts, algal polyphenols have shown folding modulation of Aβ. The brown seaweed (macroalgae) *Ecklonia cava* is found in the waters around Japan and Korea, where it is used as a herbal remedy. A butanol extract from *E. cava* has been shown to prevent production and aggregation of Aβ and to reduce amyloid plaques [113]. Electron microscopy showed the Aβ oligomers to be reduced and dye binding as well, indicating an inhibition of fibril formation. The polyphenolic phlorotannins are considered to be the active compounds responsible for the biological activities of *E. cava* [114, 115]. Nonetheless, other molecules cannot be strictly ruled out [113].

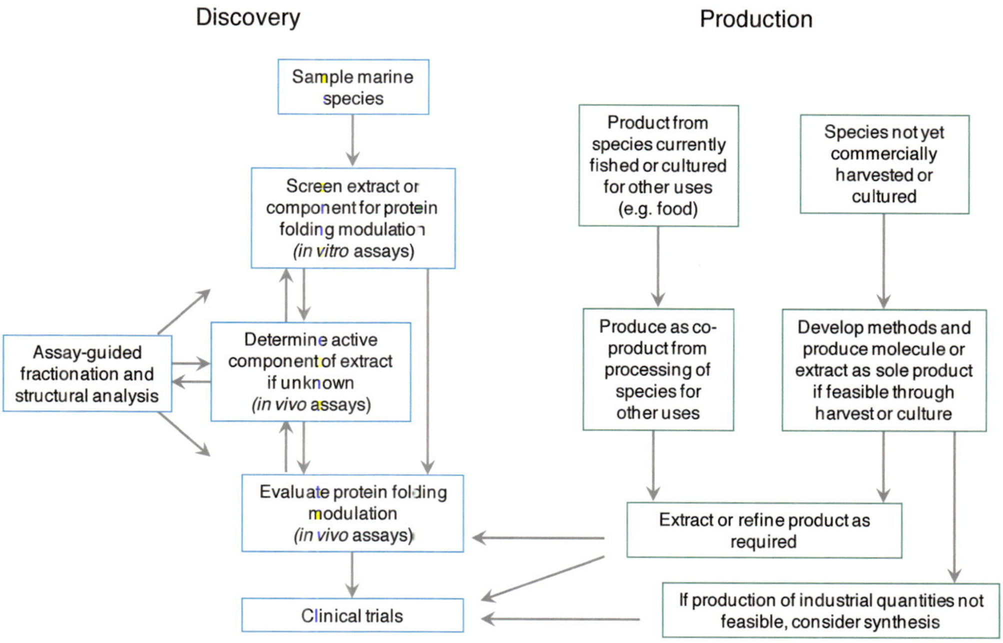

Figure 2. Schematic summary of key steps in the identification and development of marine-sourced protein folding modulators. Blue boxes are steps involved in discovery and characterization of protein folding modulation and the molecule responsible. Green boxes are steps involved in production of the molecule (or of an extract containing it). For more detail, see chapter text. Structural elucidation is not included here as it is not covered in this chapter; it is covered in another chapter of this book.

4.1.2. Marine carotenoids

Marine algae and invertebrates harbour large quantities of carotenoids. This is of interest because, as noted above, carotenoids are among the molecules showing promise in modulation of protein misfolding. Algal carotenoids are widely varied (reviewed in [112]). These appear to be particularly accessible through enzyme-assisted extraction (reviewed in [116]) and they may have interesting activities. Shrimp and crab processing wastes are also excellent sources of carotenoids. Crustacean shells left over during processing contain the carotenoid astaxanthin (reviewed in [112]), which gives them their striking colour. This is in addition to the chitin in the shells, and its component glucosamine, which is well known in other contexts. There are no reports of evaluation of marine-derived carotenoids in protein folding modulation, as there are for terrestrial counterparts. With the numerous and varied sources of marine carotenoids, these could be compared with terrestrial versions previously reported to modulate protein folding.

4.1.3. Marine toxins

There is a plethora of marine toxins with distinctive neurological effects. These toxins are mainly known for the poisoning risk they carry. Nonetheless, a few of them have valuable biological activities as research chemicals and one has intriguing effects relative to AD. Using cell-based assays, the toxin 13-desmethyl spirolide C from the dinoflagellate *Alexandrium ostenfeldii* was shown to reduce Aβ accumulation in cells by just over 40% [117]. The antibody used (6E10, Covance) detects Aβ without distinguishing between monomeric or oligomeric or fibril forms. It would therefore be valuable to repeat these analyses using fold-specific anti-Aβ antibodies or another fold-sensitive method to see if any effect there could be detected. Otherwise, it may act on Aβ in other beneficial ways that would also be of interest.

4.1.4. Marine-sourced chemical chaperones and conflicting results

A variety of chemical chaperones, which are loosely defined as small molecules that promote folding of many proteins, have gained interest in terms of wide-spectrum protection of proteins from misfolding (reviewed in [118]). In marine species faced with protein misfolding risk, the accumulation of one or more chemical chaperones is a common adaptation because these small chaperoning molecules promote general proteostasis [111, 119]. Therefore, at first glance, these molecules would appear to be ideal in terms of proteins such as Aβ and αS. They could be produced naturally or synthetically, depending upon their molecular features, and they may stabilize many different proteins. However, some chemical chaperones may have problematic effects with respect to amyloidotic protein misfolding. Glycerol at supraphysiological concentrations (molar range) and trimethylamine oxide (TMAO) at moderate concentrations were both shown to favour the transition of Aβ from its unfolded conformation to the β-sheet form requisite for fiber formation [120]. Protofibril to fibril conversion was also enhanced [120]. The situation appears more complex for αS, with elevated concentrations (molar range) of TMAO favouring a partially folded form with high propensity for fibril formation and even higher concentrations of TMAO favouring an oligomeric α-helical conformation [121], which may be consistent with a native α-helical form of the protein that resists misfolding [29]. Although these chaperone concentrations used were far in excess of those that would be reached *in vivo*, the effects suggest a possibility to be aware of if a novel folding modulator appears to be non-specific. Stabilization by chemical chaperones may bring an increased risk of aggregation for some proteins [119]. Furthermore, stabilization of a wider range of cell proteins or protein complexes may cause unanticipated problems. Therefore, examination of unusual and off-target effects would be prudent in the evaluation of chemical chaperones.

4.2. Sources for marine products

A challenge presented by many rare or remote marine species that may produce pharmaceutical or nutraceutical molecules is the difficulty in obtaining sufficient product in a sustainable manner, from both the environmental and economic standpoints [122]. Options for these products include the development of culture methods for the species or synthesis of the molecule, although in many cases the molecules are too complex to be efficiently synthesized [122, 123]. In contrast, an advantage for nutraceutical or drug development from many

http://dx.doi.org/10.5772/54585

accessible marine species, both plant and animal, is that they are already supplied as human food sources. Additionally, a large number of marine species are currently farmed, and availability of a standard supply for natural product development would be more straightforward and predictable than it would be for their wild counterparts. Sustainable production or harvesting of species for natural marine products would be a key consideration in production of folding modulators, just as it is for the production of foods.

In the case of some seaweeds, marine harvesting can be carried out. However, on-land cultivation offers the additional benefits of ideal traceability and process control, albeit with substantial costs [124]. For microalgae, this would be the only option. Algal processing wastes are significant and they are of interest for the development of by-products [125].

For commercially fished animal species, processing for food production is a frequent practice. These wild finfish and shellfish species, as well as those grown in aquaculture, can generate substantial waste during processing for food production and this waste often go to landfills or composting. The identification of valuable properties or activities in waste materials allows them to be used to produce co-products and, with green chemistry initiatives, these could be produced in a sustainable fashion from a healthy wild harvesting or aquaculture operation. There is growing interest in co-product development, as highlighted by two contrasting examples. Snow crab (*Chionoecetes opilio*) are fished across the Maritime provinces of Canada. Crab processing waste currently contributes to landfills, but the potential for additional product development with the identification of sufficiently valuable uses is being considered [126] as is the case elsewhere, likely based upon chitin but possibly upon other products as well. Innovative solutions to waste challenges are also being pursued in salmon aquaculture. Integrated multi-trophic aquaculture of Atlantic salmon (*Salmo salar*) with macroalgal species and mussels (*Mytilus edulis*) in the Bay of Fundy, Canada, minimizes waste accumulation by allowing nutrient and resource recovery with diminished impact on the local environment and this process is advancing toward commercial production [127]. The economic viability of this integration initiative will rely upon the development of foods along with other high-value products from the cultured species [128]. A neuroprotective protein folding modulator from such a resource could enhance markets for the food, while offering the possibility of producing sustainable nutraceuticals and eventual pharmaceuticals as co-products if appropriate.

5. Conclusions

With protein misfolding identified as a causative event in multiple neurodegenerative diseases and with no definitive means of prevention or cure in place, the progress being made in the discovery and development of natural protein misfolding modulators is of great interest. Although several promising leads from terrestrial sources have been identified, none have been shown to provide a clear result in disease outcome to date. Therefore, while current products are being developed and refined, it would be logical to investigate a wider range of sources for protein folding modulators. In this context, marine species deserve a second (or, in some cases, a first) look.

There has already been extensive work on marine molecules from some sources, but crucial to the proposed endeavour is screening for the most relevant activities. For example, testing marine molecules or extracts for effects in model Aβ or αS cell survival assays may not indicate protein folding modulation. However, the reverse is likely to be true in most cases. In other words, appropriate protein folding modulation activity should lead to enhanced cell survival. It is also important to be mindful of assay subtleties. Testing for anti-fibrillization activity may uncover molecules that cause toxic oligomers to accumulate instead of amyloid fibrils, leading to increased pathology instead of amelioration. Similarly, searching for molecules that bring about a reduction in total Aβ (or αS) may not be prudent, as we have little understanding of the normal roles of these proteins in the brain and therefore drastic reduction in levels may have undesirable consequences [18]. For these reasons, an assay suite that allows determination of toxic oligomers as well as other (non-toxic) oligmers, monomers, amyloid fibrils and other aggregates would be ideal. In order to identify a marine extract or molecule that provides protective protein folding modulation, the spectrum of its effects on protein misfolding and association protein would need to be investigated. Furthermore, because a number of natural molecules appear to affect the misfolding trajectories of both Aβ and αS, these would be of particular interest because of the potential for wider-ranging protection from toxic misfolding.

In closing, examination of marine biota for protein folding modulators using a suitable suite of assays may offer a promising opportunity to identify a safe, effective and sustainable protein folding modulator that addresses the cause of a neurodegenerative disease. The untapped diversity of marine species combined with a rational selection of assays for folding modulator identification based upon examples used in terrestrial investigations and coupled with appropriate downstream *in vivo* analysis would be ideal. For proteins such as Aβ and αS, which form similar amyloids and can even cross-seed in spite of their structural differences [129], a further tantalizing prospect would be the identification of a molecule that would be effective for both AD and PD. Given the paucity of treatments currently available, discovery of an active molecule from a marine resource could bring hope at this time.

Acknowledgements

We thank Dr. Stephen Ewart (Novaceutics Consulting) for his helpful review of the manuscript. Research on protein misfolding in the laboratory of K.V. Ewart is supported by the National Research Council of Canada and by an NSERC Discovery grant.

Author details

James C. Giffin[1] and Kathryn Vanya Ewart[2]

1 Department of Biology, Dalhousie University, Halifax, Canada

2 National Research Council Aquatic and Crop Resource Development, Halifax, Canada

http://dx.doi.org/10.5772/54585

References

[1] Chen B, Retzlaff M, Roos T, Frydman J. Cellular strategies of protein quality control. Cold Spring Harb Perspect Biol 2011; 3 a004374.

[2] Herczenik E, Gebbink MF. Molecular and cellular aspects of protein misfolding and disease. Faseb J 2008; 22 2115-2133.

[3] Uversky VN. Intrinsic disorder in proteins associated with neurodegenerative diseases. Front Biosci 2009; 14 5188-5238.

[4] Rakhit R, Cunningham P, Furtos-Matei A, Dahan S, Qi XF, Crow JP, Cashman NR, Kondejewski LH, Chakrabartty A. Oxidation-induced misfolding and aggregation of superoxide dismutase and its implications for amyotrophic lateral sclerosis. J Biol Chem 2002; 277 47551-47556.

[5] Guest WC, Silverman JM, Pokrishevsky E, O'Neill MA, Grad LI, Cashman NR. Generalization of the prion hypothesis to other neurodegenerative diseases: an imperfect fit. J Toxicol Environ Health A 2011; 74 1433-1459.

[6] Harrison RS, Sharpe PC, Singh Y, Fairlie DP. Amyloid peptides and proteins in review. Rev Physiol Biochem Pharmacol 2007; 159 1-77.

[7] Morales R, Green KM, Soto C. Cross currents in protein misfolding disorders: interactions and therapy. CNS Neurol Disord Drug Targets 2009; 8 363-371.

[8] Aguzzi A, O'Connor T. Protein aggregation diseases: pathogenicity and therapeutic perspectives. Nat Rev Drug Discov 2010; 9 237-248.

[9] Lee SJ, Lim HS, Masliah E, Lee HJ. Protein aggregate spreading in neurodegenerative diseases: problems and perspectives. Neurosci Res 2011; 70 339-348.

[10] Andrew SE, Goldberg YP, Kremer B, Telenius H, Theilmann J, Adam S, Starr E, Squitieri F, Lin B, Kalchman MA, et al. The relationship between trinucleotide (CAG) repeat length and clinical features of Huntington's disease. Nat Genet 1993; 4 398-403.

[11] Duyao M, Ambrose C, Myers R, Novelletto A, Persichetti F, Frontali M, Folstein S, Ross C, Franz M, Abbott M, et al. Trinucleotide repeat length instability and age of onset in Huntington's disease. Nat Genet 1993; 4 387-392.

[12] Snell RG, MacMillan JC, Cheadle JP, Fenton I, Lazarou LP, Davies P, MacDonald ME, Gusella JF, Harper PS, Shaw DJ. Relationship between trinucleotide repeat expansion and phenotypic variation in Huntington's disease. Nat Genet 1993; 4 393-397.

[13] Walters RH, Murphy RM. Examining polyglutamine peptide length: a connection between collapsed conformations and increased aggregation. J Mol Biol 2009; 393 978-992.

[14] Liscic RM, Breljak D. Molecular basis of amyotrophic lateral sclerosis. Prog Neuropsychopharmacol Biol Psychiatry 2011; 35 370-372.

[15] Brundin P, Melki R, Kopito R. Prion-like transmission of protein aggregates in neurodegenerative diseases. Nat Rev Mol Cell Biol 2010; 11 301-307.

[16] Jucker M, Walker LC. Pathogenic protein seeding in Alzheimer disease and other neurodegenerative disorders. Ann Neurol 2011; 70 532-540.

[17] Nussbaum RL, Ellis CE. Alzheimer's disease and Parkinson's disease. N Engl J Med 2003; 348 1356-1364.

[18] Carter MD, Simms GA, Weaver DF. The development of new therapeutics for Alzheimer's disease. Clin Pharmacol Ther 2010; 88 475-486.

[19] Goate A, Chartier-Harlin MC, Mullan M, Brown J, Crawford F, Fidani L, Giuffra L, Haynes A, Irving N, James L, et al. Segregation of a missense mutation in the amyloid precursor protein gene with familial Alzheimer's disease. Nature 1991; 349 704-706.

[20] Sherrington R, Rogaev EI, Liang Y, Rogaeva EA, Levesque G, Ikeda M, Chi H, Lin C, Li G, Holman K, Tsuda T, Mar L, Foncin JF, Bruni AC, Montesi MP, Sorbi S, Rainero I, Pinessi L, Nee L, Chumakov I, Pollen D, Brookes A, Sanseau P, Polinsky RJ, Wasco W, Da Silva HA, Haines JL, Perkicak-Vance MA, Tanzi RE, Roses AD, Fraser PE, Rommens JM, St George-Hyslop PH. Cloning of a gene bearing missense mutations in early-onset familial Alzheimer's disease. Nature 1995; 375 754-760.

[21] Hutton M, Perez-Tur J, Hardy J. Genetics of Alzheimer's disease. Essays Biochem 1998; 33 117-131.

[22] Hoehn MM, Yahr MD. Parkinsonism: onset, progression and mortality. Neurology 1967; 17 427-442.

[23] Breydo L, Wu JW, Uversky VN. α-synuclein misfolding and Parkinson's disease. Biochim Biophys Acta 2012; 1822 261-285.

[24] Stefanis L. α-Synuclein in Parkinson's disease. Cold Spring Harb Perspect Med 2012; 2 a009399.

[25] Ehrnhoefer DE, Bieschke J, Boeddrich A, Herbst M, Masino L, Lurz R, Engemann S, Pastore A, Wanker EE. EGCG redirects amyloidogenic polypeptides into unstructured, off-pathway oligomers. Nat Struct Mol Biol 2008; 15 558-566.

[26] Bieschke J, Russ J, Friedrich RP, Ehrnhoefer DE, Wobst H, Neugebauer K, Wanker EE. EGCG remodels mature α-synuclein and amyloid-β fibrils and reduces cellular toxicity. Proc Natl Acad Sci U S A 2010; 107 7710-7715.

[27] Nelson R, Eisenberg D. Structural models of amyloid-like fibrils. Adv Protein Chem 2006; 73 235-282.

[28] Jarvet J, Danielsson J, Damberg P, Oleszczuk M, Graslund A. Positioning of the Alzheimer Aβ(1-40) peptide in SDS micelles using NMR and paramagnetic probes. J Biomol NMR 2007; 39 63-72.

[29] Bartels T, Choi JG, Selkoe DJ. alpha-Synuclein occurs physiologically as a helically folded tetramer that resists aggregation. Nature 2011; 477 107-110.

[30] Wang W, Perovic I, Chittuluru J, Kaganovich A, Nguyen LT, Liao J, Auclair JR, Johnson D, Landeru A, Simorellis AK, Ju S, Cookson MR, Asturias FJ, Agar JN, Webb BN, Kang C, Ringe D, Petsko GA, Pochapsky TC, Hoang QQ. A soluble α-synuclein construct forms a dynamic tetramer. Proc Natl Acad Sci U S A 2011; 108 17797-17802.

[31] Nerelius C, Sandegren A, Sargsyan H, Raunak R, Leijonmarck H, Chatterjee U, Fisahn A, Imarisio S, Lomas DA, Crowther DC, Stromberg R, Johansson J. Alpha-helix targeting reduces amyloid-β peptide toxicity. Proc Natl Acad Sci U S A 2009; 106 9191-9196.

[32] Ito M, Johansson J, Stromberg R, Nilsson L. Unfolding of the amyloid β-peptide central helix: mechanistic insights from molecular dynamics simulations. PLoS One 2011; 6 e17587.

[33] Whitmore L, Wallace BA. DICHROWEB, an online server for protein secondary structure analyses from circular dichroism spectroscopic data. Nucleic Acids Res 2004; 32 W668-673.

[34] Nettleship JE, Brown J, Groves MR, Geerlof A. Methods for protein characterization by mass spectrometry, thermal shift (ThermoFluor) assay, and multiangle or static light scattering. Methods Mol Biol 2008; 426 299-318.

[35] LeVine H, 3rd. Quantification of β-sheet amyloid fibril structures with thioflavin T. Methods Enzymol 1999; 309 274-284.

[36] Vassar PS, Culling CF. Fluorescent stains, with special reference to amyloid and connective tissues. Arch Pathol 1959; 68 487-498.

[37] Puchtler H, Sweat F, Levine M. On the binding of Congo red by amyloid. J Histochem Cytochem 1962; 10 355-364.

[38] Hawe A, Sutter M, Jiskoot W. Extrinsic fluorescent dyes as tools for protein characterization. Pharm Res 2008; 25 1487-1499.

[39] Bertoncini CW, Celej MS. Small molecule fluorescent probes for the detection of amyloid self-assembly *in vitro* and *in vivo*. Curr Protein Pept Sci 2011; 12 205-220.

[40] Reinke AA, Abulwerdi GA, Gestwicki JE. Quantifying prefibrillar amyloids *in vitro* by using a "thioflavin-like" spectroscopic method. Chembiochem 2010; 11 1889-1895.

[41] Lee JH, Lee IH, Choe YJ, Kang S, Kim HY, Gai WP, Hahn JS, Paik SR. Real-time analysis of amyloid fibril formation of α-synuclein using a fibrillation-state-specific fluorescent probe of JC-1. Biochem J 2009; 418 311-323.

[42] Kovacs GG, Wagner U, Dumont B, Pikkarainen M, Osman AA, Streichenberger N, Leisser I, Verchere J, Baron T, Alafuzoff I, Budka H, Perret-Liaudet A, Lachmann I. An antibody with high reactivity for disease-associated α-synuclein reveals extensive brain pathology. Acta Neuropathol 2012; 124 37-50.

[43] Perchiacca JM, Ladiwala AR, Bhattacharya M, Tessier PM. Structure-based design of conformation- and sequence-specific antibodies against amyloid β. Proc Natl Acad Sci U S A 2012; 109 84-89.

[44] Yam AY, Wang X, Gao CM, Connolly MD, Zuckermann RN, Bleu T, Hall J, Fedynyshyn JP, Allauzen S, Peretz D, Salisbury CM. A universal method for detection of amyloidogenic misfolded proteins. Biochemistry 2011; 50 4322-4329.

[45] Zurdo J. Polypeptide models to understand misfolding and amyloidogenesis and their relevance in protein design and therapeutics. Protein Pept Lett 2005; 12 171-187.

[46] Graether SP, Slupsky CM, Sykes BD. Freezing of a fish antifreeze protein results in amyloid fibril formation. Biophys J 2003; 84 552-557.

[47] Graether SP, Sykes BD. Structural characterization of amyloidotic antifreeze protein fibrils and intermediates. J Toxicol Environ Health A 2009; 72 1030-1033.

[48] Dube A, Investigation of antifreeze protein activity in blue mussels and amyloid-like transition in a predominant winter flounder serum antifreeze protein, Graduate thesis, Dalhousie University, Halifax, Canada, 2012; 224 p.

[49] Guo JP, Yu S, McGeer PL. Simple *in vitro* assays to identify amyloid-β aggregation blockers for Alzheimer's disease therapy. J Alzheimers Dis 2010; 19 1359-1370.

[50] Arslan PE, Chakrabartty A. Probing Alzheimer amyloid peptide aggregation using a cell-free fluorescent protein refolding method. Biochem Cell Biol 2009; 87 631-639.

[51] Kryndushkin DS, Alexandrov IM, Ter-Avanesyan MD, Kushnirov VV. Yeast [PSI+] prion aggregates are formed by small Sup35 polymers fragmented by Hsp104. J Biol Chem 2003; 278 49636-49643.

[52] Halfmann R, Lindquist S. Screening for amyloid aggregation by semi-denaturing detergent-agarose gel electrophoresis. J Vis Exp 2008; 16 838.

[53] Kim W, Kim Y, Min J, Kim DJ, Chang YT, Hecht MH. A high-throughput screen for compounds that inhibit aggregation of the Alzheimer's peptide. ACS Chem Biol 2006; 1 461-469.

[54] Seeman P, Seeman N. Alzheimer's disease: β-amyloid plaque formation in human brain. Synapse 2011; 65 1289-1297.

[55] Barbour R, Kling K, Anderson JP, Banducci K, Cole T, Diep L, Fox M, Goldstein JM, Soriano F, Seubert P, Chilcote TJ. Red blood cells are the major source of alpha-synuclein in blood. Neurodegener Dis 2008; 5 55-59.

[56] Wang Q, Rager JD, Weinstein K, Kardos PS, Dobson GL, Li J, Hidalgo IJ. Evaluation of the MDR-MDCK cell line as a permeability screen for the blood-brain barrier. Int J Pharm 2005; 288 349-359.

[57] Jeffrey P, Summerfield SG. Challenges for blood-brain barrier (BBB) screening. Xenobiotica 2007; 37 1135-1151.

[58] Mizuno H, Fujikake N, Wada K, Nagai Y. α-Synuclein Transgenic *Drosophila* As a Model of Parkinson's Disease and Related Synucleinopathies. Parkinsons Dis 2010; 2011 212706.

[59] Iijima-Ando K, Iijima K. Transgenic *Drosophila* models of Alzheimer's disease and tauopathies. Brain Struct Funct 2010; 214 245-262.

[60] Kuwahara T, Koyama A, Gengyo-Ando K, Masuda M, Kowa H, Tsunoda M, Mitani S, Iwatsubo T. Familial Parkinson mutant alpha-synuclein causes dopamine neuron dysfunction in transgenic *Caenorhabditis elegans*. J Biol Chem 2006; 281 334-340.

[61] Link CD. C. elegans models of age-associated neurodegenerative diseases: lessons from transgenic worm models of Alzheimer's disease. Exp Gerontol 2006; 41 1007-1013.

[62] Xia W. Exploring Alzheimer's disease in zebrafish. J Alzheimers Dis 2010; 20 981-990.

[63] Sun Z, Gitler AD. Discovery and characterization of three novel synuclein genes in zebrafish. Dev Dyn 2008; 237 2490-2495.

[64] Hunter P. Harnessing nature's wisdom. turning to nature for inspiration and avoiding her follies. EMBO Rep 2008; 9 838-840.

[65] Kim J, Lee HJ, Lee KW. Naturally occurring phytochemicals for the prevention of Alzheimer's disease. J Neurochem 2010; 112 1415-1430.

[66] Park SY. Potential therapeutic agents against Alzheimer's disease from natural sources. Arch Pharm Res 2010; 33 1589-1609.

[67] Aggarwal BB, Sundaram C, Malani N, Ichikawa H. Curcumin: the Indian solid gold. Adv Exp Med Biol 2007; 595 1-75.

[68] Yang F, Lim GP, Begum AN, Ubeda OJ, Simmons MR, Ambegaokar SS, Chen PP, Kayed R, Glabe CG, Frautschy SA, Cole GM. Curcumin inhibits formation of amyloid β oligomers and fibrils, binds plaques, and reduces amyloid *in vivo*. J Biol Chem 2005; 280 5892-5901.

[69] Ono K, Yamada M. Antioxidant compounds have potent anti-fibrillogenic and fibril-destabilizing effects for α-synuclein fibrils *in vitro*. J Neurochem 2006; 97 105-115.

[70] Small G. Clinical Trial: 18-months study of curcumin. (http://clinicaltrials.gov/ct2/show/study/NCT01383161?term=curcumin+alzheimer%27s&rank=5).

[71] Abbas S, Wink M. Epigallocatechin gallate inhibits beta amyloid oligomerization in *Caenorhabditis elegans* and affects the daf-2/insulin-like signaling pathway. Phytomedicine 2010; 17 902-909.

[72] Friedemann P. Clinical trial: Sunphenon EGCG (epigallocatechin-gallate) in the early stage of Alzheimer´s disease (SUN-AK). (http://clinicaltrials.gov/ct2/show/NCT00951834).

[73] Grelle G, Otto A, Lorenz M, Frank RF, Wanker EE, Bieschke J. Black tea theaflavins inhibit formation of toxic amyloid-β and α-synuclein fibrils. Biochemistry 2011; 50 10624-10636.

[74] Ono K, Yoshiike Y, Takashima A, Hasegawa K, Naiki H, Yamada M. Vitamin A exhibits potent antiamyloidogenic and fibril-destabilizing effects *in vitro*. Exp Neurol 2004; 189 380-392.

[75] Takasaki J, Ono K, Yoshiike Y, Hirohata M, Ikeda T, Morinaga A, Takashima A, Yamada M. Vitamin A has anti-oligomerization effects on amyloid-β *in vitro*. J Alzheimers Dis 2011; 27 271-280.

[76] Ono K, Yamada M. Vitamin A and Alzheimer's disease. Geriatr Gerontol Int 2012; 12 180-188.

[77] Ono K, Yamada M. Vitamin A potently destabilizes preformed alpha-synuclein fibrils *in vitro*: implications for Lewy body diseases. Neurobiol Dis 2007; 25 446-454.

[78] Dasilva KA, Shaw JE, McLaurin J. Amyloid-β fibrillogenesis: structural insight and therapeutic intervention. Exp Neurol 2010; 223 311-321.

[79] McLaurin J, Golomb R, Jurewicz A, Antel JP, Fraser PE. Inositol stereoisomers stabilize an oligomeric aggregate of Alzheimer amyloid β peptide and inhibit Aβ -induced toxicity. J Biol Chem 2000; 275 18495-18502.

[80] Townsend M, Shankar GM, Mehta T, Walsh DM, Selkoe DJ. Effects of secreted oligomers of amyloid β-protein on hippocampal synaptic plasticity: a potent role for trimers. J Physiol 2006; 572 477-492.

[81] Salloway S, Sperling R, Keren R, Porsteinsson AP, van Dyck CH, Tariot PN, Gilman S, Arnold D, Abushakra S, Hernandez C, Crans G, Liang E, Quinn G, Bairu M, Pastrak A, Cedarbaum JM. A phase 2 randomized trial of ELND005, scyllo-inositol, in mild to moderate Alzheimer disease. Neurology 2011; 77 1253-1262.

[82] Chang RC, So KF. Use of anti-aging herbal medicine, *Lycium barbarum*, against aging-associated diseases. What do we know so far? Cell Mol Neurobiol 2008; 28 643-652.

[83] Fujiwara H, Iwasaki K, Furukawa K, Seki T, He M, Maruyama M, Tomita N, Kudo Y, Higuchi M, Saido TC, Maeda S, Takashima A, Hara M, Ohizumi Y, Arai H. *Uncaria rhynchophylla*, a Chinese medicinal herb, has potent antiaggregation effects on Alzheimer's β-amyloid proteins. J Neurosci Res 2006; 84 427-433.

[84] Fujiwara H, Tabuchi M, Yamaguchi T, Iwasaki K, Furukawa K, Sekiguchi K, Ikarashi Y, Kudo Y, Higuchi M, Saido TC, Maeda S, Takashima A, Hara M, Yaegashi N, Kase Y, Arai H. A traditional medicinal herb Paeonia suffruticosa and its active constituent 1,2,3,4,6-penta-O-galloyl-beta-D-glucopyranose have potent anti-aggregation effects on Alzheimer's amyloid beta proteins in vitro and in vivo. J Neurochem 2009; 109 1648-1657.

[85] Xian YF, Lin ZX, Mao QQ, Hu Z, Zhao M, Che CT, Ip SP. Bioassay-Guided Isolation of Neuroprotective Compounds from *Uncaria rhynchophylla* against Beta-Amyloid-Induced Neurotoxicity. Evid Based Complement Alternat Med 2012; 2012 802625.

[86] Feng Y, Wang XP, Yang SG, Wang YJ, Zhang X, Du XT, Sun XX, Zhao M, Huang L, Liu RT. Resveratrol inhibits beta-amyloid oligomeric cytotoxicity but does not prevent oligomer formation. Neurotoxicology 2009; 30 986-995.

[87] Murata N, Murakami K, Ozawa Y, Kinoshita N, Irie K, Shirasawa T, Shimizu T. Silymarin attenuated the amyloid β plaque burden and improved behavioral abnormalities in an Alzheimer's disease mouse model. Biosci Biotechnol Biochem 2010; 74 2299-2306.

[88] Toda T, Sunagawa T, Kanda T, Tagashira M, Shirasawa T, Shimizu T. Apple Procyanidins Suppress Amyloid β-protein aggregation. Biochem Res Int 2011; 2011 784698.

[89] Roberts BE, Shorter J. Escaping amyloid fate. Nat Struct Mol Biol 2008; 15 544-546.

[90] Mereles D, Hunstein W. Epigallocatechin-3-gallate (EGCG) for clinical trials: more pitfalls than promises? Int J Mol Sci 12 5592-5603.

[91] Kuriyama S, Hozawa A, Ohmori K, Shimazu T, Matsui T, Ebihara S, Awata S, Nagatomi R, Arai H, Tsuji I. Green tea consumption and cognitive function: a cross-sectional study from the Tsurugaya Project 1. Am J Clin Nutr 2006; 83 355-361.

[92] Tan EK, Tan C, Fook-Chong SM, Lum SY, Chai A, Chung H, Shen H, Zhao Y, Teoh ML, Yih Y, Pavanni R, Chandran VR, Wong MC. Dose-dependent protective effect of coffee, tea, and smoking in Parkinson's disease: a study in ethnic Chinese. J Neurol Sci 2003; 216 163-167.

[93] Scapagnini G, Caruso C, Calabrese V. Therapeutic potential of dietary polyphenols against brain ageing and neurodegenerative disorders. Adv Exp Med Biol 2010; 698 27-35.

[94] Begum AN, Jones MR, Lim GP, Morihara T, Kim P, Heath DD, Rock CL, Pruitt MA, Yang F, Hudspeth B, Hu S, Faull KF, Teter B, Cole GM, Frautschy SA. Curcumin structure-function, bioavailability, and efficacy in models of neuroinflammation and Alzheimer's disease. J Pharmacol Exp Ther 2008; 326 196-208.

[95] Dube A, Nicolazzo JA, Larson I. Chitosan nanoparticles enhance the plasma exposure of (-)-epigallocatechin gallate in mice through an enhancement in intestinal stability. Eur J Pharm Sci 2011; 44 422-426.

[96] Werner EA, Deluca HF. Retinoic acid is detected at relatively high levels in the CNS of adult rats. Am J Physiol Endocrinol Metab 2002; 282 E672-678.

[97] Marques MA, Kulstad JJ, Savard CE, Green PS, Lee SP, Craft S, Watson GS, Cook DG. Peripheral amyloid-β levels regulate amyloid-β clearance from the central nervous system. J Alzheimers Dis 2009; 16 325-329.

[98] Boada M, Ortiz P, Anaya F, Hernandez I, Munoz J, Nunez L, Olazaran J, Roca I, Cuberas G, Tarraga L, Buendia M, Pla RP, Ferrer I, Paez A. Amyloid-targeted therapeutics in Alzheimer's disease: use of human albumin in plasma exchange as a novel approach for Aβ mobilization. Drug News Perspect 2009; 22 325-339.

[99] Kato M, Kawaguchi K, Nakai S, Murakami K, Hori H, Ohashi A, Hiki Y, Ito S, Shimano Y, Suzuki N, Sugiyama S, Ogawa H, Kusimoto H, Mutoh T, Yuzawa Y, Kitaguchi N. Potential therapeutic system for Alzheimer's disease: removal of blood Aβs by hemodialzyers and its effect on the cognitive functions of renal-failure patients. J Neural Transm 2012; .

[100] Sutcliffe JG, Hedlund PB, Thomas EA, Bloom FE, Hilbush BS. Peripheral reduction of β-amyloid is sufficient to reduce brain β-amyloid: implications for Alzheimer's disease. J Neurosci Res 2011; 89 808-814.

[101] Bell RD, Zlokovic BV. Neurovascular mechanisms and blood-brain barrier disorder in Alzheimer's disease. Acta Neuropathol 2009; 118 103-113.

[102] O'Dor R, Miloslavich P, Yarincik K. Marine biodiversity and biogeography--regional comparisons of global issues, an introduction. PLoS One 2010; 5 e11871.

[103] Gulf of Maine Biodiversity (http://www.coml.org/discoveries/ecology/gulf_of_maine_biodiversity).

[104] Yooseph S, Sutton G, Rusch DB, Halpern AL, Williamson SJ, Remington K, Eisen JA, Heidelberg KB, Manning G, Li W, Jaroszewski L, Cieplak P, Miller CS, Li H, Mashiyama ST, Joachimiak MP, van Belle C, Chandonia JM, Soergel DA, Zhai Y, Natarajan K, Lee S, Raphael BJ, Bafna V, Friedman R, Brenner SE, Godzik A, Eisenberg D, Dixon JE, Taylor SS, Strausberg RL, Frazier M, Venter JC. The Sorcerer II Global Ocean Sampling expedition: expanding the universe of protein families. PLoS Biol 2007; 5 e16.

[105] Montaser R, Luesch H. Marine natural products: a new wave of drugs? Future Med Chem 2011; 3 1475-1489.

[106] Gerwick WH, Moore BS. Lessons from the past and charting the future of marine natural products drug discovery and chemical biology. Chem Biol 2012; 19 85-98.

[107] Blunt JW, Copp BR, Keyzers RA, Munro MH, Prinsep MR. Marine natural products. Nat Prod Rep 2012; 29 144-222.

[108] Williams P, Sorribas A, Liang Z. New methods to explore marine resources for Alzheimer's therapeutics. Curr Alzheimer Res 2010; 7 210-213.

[109] Todgham AE, Hoaglund EA, Hofmann GE. Is cold the new hot? Elevated ubiquitin-conjugated protein levels in tissues of Antarctic fish as evidence for cold-denaturation of proteins *in vivo*. J Comp Physiol B 2007; 177 857-866.

[110] Chen Z, Cheng CH, Zhang J, Cao L, Chen L, Zhou L, Jin Y, Ye H, Deng C, Dai Z, Xu Q, Hu P, Sun S, Shen Y, Chen L. Transcriptomic and genomic evolution under constant cold in Antarctic notothenioid fish. Proc Natl Acad Sci U S A 2008; 105 12944-12949.

[111] Gong Z, Croft K, Driedzic WR, Ewart KV. Chemical chaperoning action of glycerol on the antifreeze protein of rainbow smelt. J Therm Biol 2010; 36 78-83.

[112] Lordan S, Ross RP, Stanton C. Marine bioactives as functional food ingredients: potential to reduce the incidence of chronic diseases. Mar Drugs 2011; 9 1056-1100.

[113] Kang IJ, Jeon YE, Yin XF, Nam JS, You SG, Hong MS, Jang BG, Kim MJ. Butanol extract of *Ecklonia cava* prevents production and aggregation of beta-amyloid, and reduces beta-amyloid mediated neuronal death. Food Chem Toxicol 2011; 49 2252-2259.

[114] Jung WK, Ahn YW, Lee SH, Choi YH, Kim SK, Yea SS, Choi I, Park SG, Seo SK, Lee SW, Choi IW. *Ecklonia cava* ethanolic extracts inhibit lipopolysaccharide-induced cyclooxygenase-2 and inducible nitric oxide synthase expression in BV2 microglia via the MAP kinase and NF-kappaB pathways. Food Chem Toxicol 2009; 47 410-417.

[115] Wijesekara I, Yoon NY, Kim SK. Phlorotannins from *Ecklonia cava* (Phaeophyceae): biological activities and potential health benefits. Biofactors 2010; 36 408-414.

[116] Wijesinghe WA, Jeon YJ. Enzyme-assistant extraction (EAE) of bioactive components: a useful approach for recovery of industrially important metabolites from seaweeds: a review. Fitoterapia 2012; 83 6-12.

[117] Alonso E, Vale C, Vieytes MR, Laferla FM, Gimenez-Llort L, Botana LM. 13-Desmethyl spirolide-C is neuroprotective and reduces intracellular Aβ and hyperphosphorylated tau *in vitro*. Neurochem Int 2011; 59 1056-1065.

[118] Papp E, Csermely P. Chemical chaperones: mechanisms of action and potential use. Handb Exp Pharmacol 2006; 405-416.

[119] Yancey PH. Organic osmolytes as compatible, metabolic and counteracting cytoprotectants in high osmolarity and other stresses. J Exp Biol 2005; 208 2819-2830.

[120] Yang DS, Yip CM, Huang TH, Chakrabartty A, Fraser PE. Manipulating the amyloid-β aggregation pathway with chemical chaperones. J Biol Chem 1999; 274 32970-32974.

[121] Uversky VN, Li J, Fink AL. Trimethylamine-N-oxide-induced folding of α-synuclein. FEBS Lett 2001; 509 31-35.

[122] Benkendorff K. Aquaculture and the production of pharmaceuticals and nutraceuticals. In: Burnell G, G. A (Eds.), New technologies in aquaculture: improving production efficiency, quality and environmental management, Woodhead Publishing, Cambridge, U.K., 2009, pp. 866-892.

[123] Faulkner DJ. Marine pharmacology. Antonie Van Leeuwenhoek 2000; 77 135-145.

[124] Hafting JT, Critchley AT, Cornish ML, Hubley SA, Archibald AF. On-land cultivation of functional seaweed products for human usage. J Appl Phycol 2012; 24 385-392.

[125] Subhadra B. Algal biorefinery-based industry: an approach to address fuel and food insecurity for a carbon-smart world. J Sci Food Agric 2010; 91 2-13.

[126] Stewart G, Noyes-Hull G, Feasibility of producing value added products from snow crab processing waste in Cape Breton, Nova Scotia, Gulf Aquarium and Marine Station Cooperative, Cheticamp, Canada, 2010; 44 p.

[127] Reid GK, Robinson SMC, Chopin T, Mullen J, Lander T, Sawhney M, MacDonald B, Haya K, Burridge L, Page F, Ridler N, Boyne-Travis S, Sewuster J, Marvin R, Szemerda M, Powell F. Recent developments and challenges for open-water, integrated multi-trophic aquaculture (IMTA) in the Bay of Fundy, Canada. AAC Special Publication 2011; 13 43-47.

[128] Chopin T, Neori A, Buschmann A, Pang S, Sawhney M. Diversification of the aquaculture sector: seaweed cultivation, integrated multi-trophic aquaculture,integrated sequential biorefineries. Global Aquaculture Advocate 2011; 14 58-60.

[129] Ono K, Takahashi R, Ikeda T, Yamada M. Cross-seeding effects of amyloid β-protein and α-synuclein. J Neurochem 2012; e-publication in press (doi: 10.1111/j. 1471-4159.2012.07847.x)

Chapter 5

Marine Flatfish-Derived Bioactive Peptides: From the Ocean to the Bedside

Susan Douglas

Additional information is available at the end of the chapter

http://dx.doi.org/10.5772/51124

1. Introduction and Relevance

Infectious diseases and cancer are leading causes of mortality and our ability to combat them is compromised due to the emergence of antibiotic-resistant strains of bacteria and chemotherapy-resistant cancer cells. Combined with the scarcity of new classes of antibiotics due to the abandonment of antibacterial research by pharmaceutical companies (Williams and Bax, 2009) and the lengthy development time lines to market (Projan and Bradford, 2007), there is an urgent need for alternative therapeutics. Cationic antimicrobial peptides (CAPs) have emerged as a promising source of novel therapeutics. Not only do they rapidly kill microbes and cancer cells, they also can modulate host innate immunity to augment clearance of microbes and promote tissue healing resulting from inflammation. Furthermore, they are less prone to resistance than traditional antibiotics (McPhee and Hancock, 2005). Synthetic variants of naturally occurring CAPs, have been designed that exhibit greater selectivity and stability. Here I summarize some of the key features of CAPs, directing the reader to recent pertinent reviews, and focus on characteristics of pleurocidin CAPs that make them attractive for clinical applications.

2. Physical properties of cationic antimicrobial peptides

2.1. Classes

CAPs are small peptides (10-50 amino acids) with a high content of positively charged (net charge +2 to +9) and hydrophobic (up to 50%) amino acids. Currently over 1800 naturally occurring CAPs from almost all forms of life are annotated in the Antimicrobial Peptide Database (http://aps.unmc.edu/AP/main.php). They can be classified into four structural groups: linear α-helical, β-sheet, loop, and extended structures enriched in certain amino acids such as Arg, Phe, Pro, Gly, Trp and His (Zasloff, 2002). Linear α-helical CAPs such as magainin, LL-37 and pleurocidin are usually unstructured in aqueous solution but adopt an α-helical conformation upon interaction with lipids, thereby acquiring antimicrobial activity. They often contain a hinge in the middle, due to Gly or Pro residues, which enhances the ability of the peptide to enter the cell (Park et al., 2000). CAPs that form stable β-sheet structures contain cysteine residues that are able to form disulphide bonds (usually 1-4 depending on the type of CAP). These include the protegrins, defensins and drosomycins. Looped CAPs, thanatin and brevinin, contain a C-terminal loop carrying a strong positive charge (Fehlbaum et al., 1996). CAPs such as bactenecin, prophenin and indolicidin are enriched in specific amino acids, usually lack cysteines, and form linear or extended coils. CAPs are usually produced as inactive pre-pro-peptides and proteolytically cleaved to release the mature biologically active peptide.

2.2. Pleurocidin

Pleurocidins comprise a family of linear α-helical CAPs consisting of a highly conserved amino-terminal signal sequence and a carboxy-terminal anionic segment flanking the more variable mature peptide of approximately 25 amino acids (Douglas et al., 2001; Patrzykat et al., 2003). This anionic portion may counteract the positively charged mature peptide, thereby keeping it inactive until cleaved. They show some sequence similarity to other fish CAPs, including piscidin, moronecidin and the recently discovered gaduscidin (Browne et al., 2011; Sun et al., 2007). Pleurocidins are encoded as clusters of genes comprised of four exons, and binding sites for transcription factors involved in host defense are located upstream of the promoters (Douglas et al., 2003).

Pleurocidin variant NRC-04 is the best-studied of this family of peptides. Early studies showed that in 25% dodecylphosphatidylcholine (DOPC)/ dodecylphosphatidyl-ethanolamine (DOPE) vesicles, it forms a structure containing between 12% and 24% α-helical content (Yoshida et al., 2001). Supporting this, it was only weakly incorporated into neutral bilayers composed of a 7:3 mixture of DOPC and DOPE; however, it strongly associated with a slightly anionic bilayer of 7:3:1 DOPC, DOPE, and dodecylphosphatidylserine (DOPS), forming well-defined single ion channels (Saint et al., 2002). NMR studies have shown that in 0% DPC, pleurocidin has no identifiable well-defined secondary structure but in 30% TFE and in 10 mM DOPC micelles, it was 25% α-helical and this increased to 95% in 140 mM DOPC (Syvitski et al., 2005). The hydrophobic amino acids residues clustered on approximately 2/3 of the helix and hydrophilic residues on the remaining 1/3 of the helix.

3. Distribution and expression of cationic antimicrobial peptides

3.1. Organismal distribution

CAPs are ubiquitous in nature and play a crucial role in first-line host defense against pathogens. Fish and marine invertebrates, because of their diversity and reliance on nonspecific innate immune defenses, have proved to be a particularly good source of novel CAPs with therapeutic potential (Otero-González, 2010; Smith and Fernandes, 2009).

3.2. Expression

3.2.1. Tissue specificity

In mammals, CAPs are expressed in cells of the skin and mucosal surfaces, as well as blood cells such as platelets, monocytes/macropages, neutrophils, and mast cells (Guaní-Guerra et al., 2010). Tissues often express a cocktail of different CAPs with varying activities and the expression of a given CAP variant may be restricted to a specific cell type (see Wiesner and Vilcinskas, 2010). For example, of the six different α-defensins, four are produced predominantly in neutrophils whereas two are secreted from Paneth cells of the small intestine.

Fish CAPs such as pleurocidin are expressed in a broad range of tissues and cell types including epithelial, immune and blood cells (Browne et al., 2011). Pleurocidin is produced by epithelial cells of the skin and gut (Cole et al., 1997; Douglas et al., 2001) as well as circulating immune cells (Murray et al., 2007). Interestingly, different pleurocidin variants are produced by different cell types (Douglas et al., 2003), underscoring the importance of screening multiple tissues to uncover the true diversity of CAPs.

3.2.2. Developmental stage

The presence of CAPs in neonates, who have yet to develop adaptive immunity, provides enteric protection and impacts the composition of the commensal microflora. Milk lactoferrin, from which the CAP lactoferricin is produced by pepsin cleavage in the stomach, plays a major role in maternal and innate immunity (Jenssen and Hancock, 2009). Dermicidin YP-30 is important for maternal and early post-natal protection (Wiesner and Vilcinskas, 2010). Mouse cathelin-related antimicrobial peptide undergoes a developmental switch from constitutive intestinal epithelial expression in neonates to Paneth cell expression in adult intestinal crypts (Menard et al., 2008).

Pleurocidin transcripts were detected early in development of winter flounder, when larvae are most susceptible to pathogen-induced mortality, and showed a progressive increase as development proceeded to adulthood (Douglas et al., 2001). Furthermore, different pleurocidin variants were present at different stages of development, indicating that screening of CAP production from various developmental stages of an organism is an excellent means of discovering novel peptide variants.

3.2.3. Constitutive or inducible

CAPs may be expressed constitutively or inducibly in response to stress, poor nutrition, inflammation (Wehkamp et al., 2003), injury or microbial infection (Redfern et al., 2011; Zasloff, 2006), and exposure to environmental factors such as zinc (Talukder et al., 2011) or vitamin D (White, 2010). For example, hCAP-18/LL-37 protein and mRNA expression was up-regulated in neutrophils that had migrated to the inflamed gingival tissues of patients with chronic periodontitis (Turkoglu et al., 2011) and mycoplasma infection induces cathelicidin expression in neutrophils of infected mice (Tani et al., 2011). Interestingly, increased endogenous glucocorticoid levels induced by psychological stress reduce CAP expression in mice, leading to increased susceptibility to infection (Aberg et al., 2007).

Expression of fish CAPs is also regulated in response to stress and disease (Douglas et al., 2003a; Sun et al., 2007), and novel variants are often induced by such stressors. Monitoring levels of CAPs in aquaculture settings provides early warning of immunosuppression due to chronic stress, and conversely induction of CAPs provides protection against anticipated stressful situations such as handling (Noga et al., 2011).

4. Mode of action of cationic antimicrobial peptides

4.1. Membrane effects

CAPs can cause lysis of biological membranes or cross membranes by spontaneous lipid-assisted translocation. The initial interaction is electrostatic between the cationic residues of the peptide and the negatively charged constituents of the target cell, whether they are in an outer bacterial envelope, a viral envelope or a eukaryotic cell membrane. Because of the high proportion of uncharged zwitterionic lipids and sterols in normal eukaryotic membranes, however, these membranes are not as susceptible as negatively charged bacterial membranes or cancer cell membranes, which contain elevated levels of negatively charged sialylated glycoproteins (van Beek et al., 1973), *O*-glycosylated mucins (Yoon et al., 1996) and phosphatidylserine (Riedl et al., 2011).

Upon binding, the peptide assumes an amphipathic secondary structure that facilitates membrane disruption. A number of mechanisms have been proposed including micelle formation by the carpet model (Shai, 2002) and pore formation by the barrel-stave and toroidal pore models (Brogden, 2005; Hadley and Hancock, 2010). Additional variations on these initial models for bacterial membrane interactions have been proposed including localized membrane disorganization by the aggregate model (Hancock and Rozek, 2002), the formation of disordered toroidal pores, charged lipid clustering, membrane thinning, electroporation, non-lytic membrane depolarization, anion carriers and oxidized lipid targeting (Nguyen et al., 2011).

Pleurocidin has been proposed to act via the toroidal pore model, based on its interactions with model membranes (Saint et al., 2002). This finding is supported by NMR studies that show that in DOPC pleurocidin exists as a very large species, probably composed of 20-25 aggregating molecules (Syvitski et al., 2005), indicating that at high concentrations pleurocidin forms pores within the membrane environment or disrupts the membrane by aggregation. A more recent study proposed that CAPS similar to pleurocidin such as magainin 2 adopt a surface alignment in mixed zwitterionic/anionic membranes and forms disordered toroidal pores (Leontiadou et al., 2006). The interaction of pleurocidin with the anionic lipid phosphatidylglycerol (PG) rather than the zwitterionic lipid phosphatidylethanolamine (PE) in mixed membranes, resulting in disruption of membrane integrity, was confirmed using NMR (Mason et al., 2006). Interestingly, the three His residues, which become protonated at acidic pH, play no role in membrane disruption, most likely due to their position along the spine of the helix where they would be unlikely to interact with lipid head groups.

The Gly13 residue in the middle of pleurocidin confers flexibility between a longer α-helix at the amino terminus and a shorter α-helix at the carboxy terminus allowing it to interact with the negatively charged phospholipid membranes (Yang et al., 2006). Replacing Gly13 with Ala removes this hinge region, resulting in a much higher α-helical content and loss of cell selectivity. This analog is hemolytic and interacts with both negatively charged (mimicking bacterial and cancer cell membranes) and zwitterionic (mimicking erythrocyte and normal mammalian cell membranes) phospholipids. Similarly, substitution of both Gly13 and Gly17 by Ala results in a large increase in α-helicity and a correspondingly dramatic increase in hemolytic activity, indicating that the hinge region facilitates flexibility and confers bacterial cell selectivity (Lim et al., 2004a). It is interesting that Gly13 is conserved in 15 of the 26 identified pleurocidin variants whereas Gly17 is conserved in only 6, indicating that Gly13 plays the more important role in peptide function.

Sterols are commonly found in eukaryotic but not bacterial cell membranes, and their presence in anionic mixed membranes reduces the ability of pleurocidin to insert even though the peptide maintains its α-helical configuration (Mason et al., 2007). Cholesterol, found in membranes of higher eukaryotes, was shown to be more effective than ergosterol, commonly found in those of fungi and certain protozoa, in reducing insertion of CAPs. These differences in membrane sterol content explain the differential sensitivity of bacteria, lower eukaryotes and higher eukaryotes to CAPs such as pleurocidin. Using a fluorescent membrane probe, pleurocidin has been shown to structurally perturb the plasma membrane of the fungal pathogen *Candida albicans* (Jung et al., 2007), confirming earlier killing assay results (Patrzykat et al., 2003).

Structural modelling predicted that only 12 of the 26 described pleurocidin variants formed amphipathic α-helices and killing assays showed that these were cytotoxic to HL-60 human leukemia cells, resulting in rapid and complete killing (Morash et al., 2011). Cell death was non-apoptotic and probably occurred by the formation of ion channels that dissipated the membrane potential and led to cell lysis. The active pleurocidin variants were the more highly charged (>+6.5) members of the family; interestingly only one of them was also hemolytic. The anti-cancer activities of two pleurocidin variants (NRC-03 and NRC-07) against breast cancer cells involve binding to negatively charged cell-surface molecules (Hilchie et al., 2011).

4.2. Intracellular effects

A number of CAPs, when administered at low doses, are able to penetrate the bacterial membrane and disrupt metabolic processes (see Marcos and Gandia, 2009; Nicolas, 2009). CAPs can assume different structures whilst exerting their inhibitory effects. For example, when bound to DNA, buforin II assumes an extended form whereas magainin and pleurocidin assume an α-helical form and bind DNA less effectively (Lan et al., 2010). Combinations of CAPs that exert their effects on different targets may exhibit synergy, and provide more potent killing activity.

Pleurocidin usually causes membrane disruption at high concentrations whereas at low concentrations, it can translocate into the cytoplasm without causing cell lysis and exert its effects intracellularly, inhibiting DNA, RNA and protein synthesis (Patrzykat et al., 2002). The intracellular effect of pleurocidin NRC-03 has since been probed using zebrafish embryos, and shown to target the mitochondria and generate superoxide (Morash et al., 2011). TUNEL staining indicates that the DNA of some cells becomes degraded, whereas other cells undergo rapid lysis and cell death without DNA fragmentation. Pleurocidin variants NRC-03 and NRC-07 cause mitochondrial membrane damage and production of reactive oxygen species (ROS) in MDA-MB-231 breast cancer cells (Hilchie et al., 2011).

4.3. Receptors and binding proteins

In most cases, killing is by nonreceptor-mediated mechanisms since all D-amino acid enantiomers are generally as active as the natural L-amino acid peptides. However, stereospecific receptor-mediated translocation has been described (Nicolas, 2009) and some CAPs transduce their effects via signaling networks upon interaction with receptors. Quite a diversity of receptors have been described, possibly reflecting the diversity in peptide structures. Uptake of apidaecin into Gram negative bacteria is proposed to by an energy-dependent mechanism involving a permease or transporter (Castle et al., 1999). The detection of peptide:receptor complexes is technically very difficult but some receptors have been identified. For example, the outer membrane protein OprI from *P. aeruginosa* (Lin et al., 2010) and the outer membrane lipoprotein Lpp in Enterobacteriaceae (Chang et al., 2012) have been shown to serve as receptors for α-helical CAPs. Histatin 5 and some defensins bind Ssa1/2 proteins on the cell surface of *C. albicans* in order to exert their activity, and the potassium transporter TRK1 is also required for histatin5 fungicidal activity (Vylkova et al., 2007). In eukaryotic cells, formyl peptide receptor-like 1 (FPRL1) is used as a receptor for LL-37 to act as a chemoattractant (Yang et al., 2000) and induce angiogenesis (Koczulla et al., 2003). LL-37 has also been shown to mediate keratinocyte migration and cytokine release by transactivation of the epidermal growth factor receptor (Tokumaru et al., 2005) and P2X7 receptor (Elssner et al., 2004), respectively. However, activation of receptors could be via CAP-induced changes in membrane fluidity, ion transport and/or receptor aggregation (Braff et al., 2005) rather than direct binding.

Activation of mast cells by pleurocidin is G protein-dependent and proposed to involve FPRL1 and G protein coupled receptor signaling pathway (Kulka, unpub). The observation that pleurocidin can bind and activate FPRL1 has some important implications for human disease. The FPRL1 receptor subtype is also a receptor for the bacterially-derived peptide fMLP (N-formyl-L-methionyl-L-leucyl-L-phenylalanine) making it an important innate immune receptor (Selvatici et al., 2006). FPRL1 activates key components of the innate immune system and is responsible for chemotactic responses, superoxide anion production and degranulation by neutrophils, macrophages and mast cells. FPRL function has been shown to be important in chronic obstructive pulmonary disease (COPD) due to cigarette smoking (Cardini et al., 2012). FPRL1 can also transactivate epidermal growth factor receptors (EGFR) making them a potentially important target in lung cancer (Cattaneo et al., 2011).

5. Biological activities and therapeutic applications of cationic antimicrobial peptides

5.1. Antibacterial

Because of their rapid, broad spectrum bactericidal action, potency, and low host cytotoxicity, CAPs have elicited much excitement as alternatives to current antibiotics, particularly in the fight against antibiotic-resistant pathogens (Nijnik and Hancock, 2009). CAPs can cause bacterial cell death by disrupting the bacterial membrane, by entering the cell and inhibiting intracellular targets, or by stimulating the immune system to eliminate an infection. They can be used alone or together with other antibacterial agents, with which they frequently synergize.

Pleurocidins show broad-spectrum antimicrobial activity at micromolar concentrations and also show synergistic activity with several antibiotics (Cole et al., 2000; Douglas et al., 2003; Patrzykat et al., 2003). In contrast to many CAPs, pleurocidin is insensitive to NaCl concentrations up to 150 mM, and may therefore have application in relatively high-salt bodily fluids and in treatment of lung infections in patients with cystic fibrosis, who have even higher NaCl content (Goldman et al., 1997).

Recent studies have shown that pleurocidin possesses considerable activity against oral microorganisms growing both planktonically and as a biofilm, even in the presence of saliva (Tao et al., 2011). Incorporation of a targeting moiety to pleurocidin NRC-04 has significantly increased its specificity towards *S. mutans*, the main cause of dental caries, relative to other oral bacteria (Mai et al., 2011). Addition of 5 mM EDTA or 10 ppm sodium fluoride, two compounds commonly used in oral treatments, resulted in increased killing of *S. mutans*. Replacement of Ser14 by His improved the activity of the targeted peptide at low pH similar to that found in the oral cavity, showing that this targeted pleurocidin has good potential as an anticaries agent.

Foodborne infections, especially those of seafood are a major health problem, yet only one CAP, nisin, has been approved by the FDA for use as a food preservative and it has only limited activity against Gram-negative bacteria or fungi (Burrowes et al., 2004).

Pleurocidin was tested against Gram-positive and Gram-negative bacteria of interest in food safety and shown to be highly effective against 17 of 18 strains, particularly the fish spoilage bacterium *Vibrio alginolyticus* (Burrowes et al., 2004). In addition, it was active against the yeasts *S. cerevisiae* and *P. pastoris*, and the mold *P. expansum*, but was not detrimental to human red blood cells or intestinal epithelial cells, indicating that it would be safe to use as a food preservative. Furthermore, since pleurocidin is produced naturally by an edible fish, there are fewer concerns over its use in food preservation.

5.2. Antifungal

The antifungal properties of CAPs have been recognized for some time (De Lucca and Walsh, 1999); however, it is only recently that the mechanism of action has been elucidated. While some CAPs such as LL-37 kill fungal cells by lysing the cell membrane, others such as histatin and defensins 2 and 3 kill in an energy-dependent and salt-sensitive fashion without cell lysis (den Hertog et al., 2005; Vylkova et al., 2007). Magainin 2 and dermaseptin S3(1-16) also cross the cell membrane and interfere with DNA integrity (Morton et al., 2007a; Morton et al., 2007b). Histatin 5, lactoferrin, arenicin-1 and several other CAPs inhibit mitochondrial respiration and induce the formation of ROS and subsequent apoptosis in *C. albicans* (Andres et al., 2008; Cho and Lee, 2011b; Helmerhorst et al., 2001; Hwang et al., 2011a; Hwang et al., 2011b).

Attempts to improve antifungal activity of CAPs have resulted in structural analogs with increased selectivity towards fungi and less host cytotoxicity. Hydrophobicity was shown to be a crucial factor in the antifungal activity of a series of CAP analogs against zygomycetes vs ascomycetes (Jiang et al., 2008). Synthetic, non-peptidic analogs of naturally-occurring CAPs have shown potent activity as anti-*Candida* agents against biofilms in the oral cavity, and reduced mammalian cytotoxicity (Hua et al., 2010).

Pleurocidin also possesses activity against *C. albicans* (Cole et al., 2000; Douglas et al., 2003; Patrzykat et al., 2003) and various derivatives truncated at the amino or carboxy-termini show reduced hemolytic activity although they are generally less potent (Lee and Lee, 2010). Modification of pleurocidin to decrease hydrophobicity and α-helicity also resulted in active peptides with reduced hemolytic activity (Sung and Lee, 2008). A synthetic all-D amino acid entantiomer of pleurocidin has also been designed that showed resistance to trypsin, plasmin and carboxypeptidase B proteases *in vitro* with no loss in antifungal activity (Jung et al., 2007). Pleurocidin induces ROS, oxidative stress, mitochondrial depolarization, caspase activation, and apoptosis in *C. albicans* with concomitant membrane phosphatidylserine externalization, cell shrinkage, DNA fragmentation and nuclear condensation (Cho and Lee, 2011a).

5.3. Antiviral

Enveloped viruses are often susceptible to attack by CAPs. Four different linear CAPs were shown to inactivate vaccinia virus by removal of the outer membrane, thereby rendering the inner membrane susceptible to neutralizing antibody against the exposed antigens (Dean et al., 2010). Novel HIV-1-inhibitory peptides have recently been identified by screening the APD Antimicrobial Peptide Database for CAPs with promising antiviral properties. This uncovered 30 candidate CAPs which, when synthesized and tested, resulted in 11 peptides with EC_{50}<10 μM against HIV-1 (Wang et al., 2010). Some CAPs are able to exert antiviral effects by blocking cell surface receptors used for viral entry. For example, the polyphemusin analog T22 binds CXCR4 on T cells and prevents T cell line-tropic HIV-1 entry (Murakami et al., 1997).

The antiviral activity of pleurocidin variants has been tested against vaccinia virus grown in HeLa cells and four lead candidates were identified based on viral inhibition without HeLa cytotoxicity at both high and low multiplicity of infection (MOI) (Johnston, pers. comm.). At the more biologically relevant low MOI, two peptides were inhibitory with an IC_{50}< 1 μg/ml. Further studies are required to determine the mechanism by which pleurocidin exerts its antiviral effect.

5.4. Anti-parasitic

The anti-parasitic properties of magainins and cecropins have been known for over twenty years and have subsequently been reported for many other CAPs (Harrington, 2011; Mor, 2009). CAPs are able to traverse the membranes of parasite-infected erythrocytes and are proposed to change the properties of the parasite cell membrane, cause membrane lysis, or become internalized and interfere with biological processes. BMAP-28, BMAP-27 and the less cytotoxic truncated derivative BMAP-18 have recently been shown to possess excellent *in vitro* activity against *Leishmania* and African trypanosomes growing both in mammalian cells and in cells of the insect vector (Haines et al., 2009; Lynn et al., 2011). Importantly, BMAP-18 was also able to inhibit release of leukocyte LPS-induced TNF-α associated with inflammation and cachexia in patients with sleeping sickness. Further *in vivo* studies of naturally-occurring and engineered CAPs are needed to demonstrate their potential in the treatment of serious parasite diseases of humans.

Pleurocidin inhibited the bloodstream form of *Trypanosoma brucei* at low concentration but was not effective against the procyclic culture form or the tsetse symbiont (Haines et al., 2003).

5.5. Anticancer

In contrast to conventional chemotherapy drugs that target all actively proliferating cells, CAPs can show selective cytotoxicity towards cancer cells including dormant, slow-growing, and multidrug resistant cells (see Hoskin and Ramamoorthy, 2008)). Both apoptotic (Jin et al., 2010) and non-apoptotic (Ceron et al., 2010; Hilchie et al., 2011; Morash et al., 2011) mechanisms have been proposed. The α-helical CAP, temporin-1CEa, exhibits cytotoxicity towards all of 12 tested human carcinoma cell lines in a concentration-dependent manner, yet no significant cytotoxicity to normal human umbilical vein smooth muscle cells at concentrations that showed potent antitumor activity (Wang et al., 2011). The basis for selectivity is thought to be the presence of phosphatidylserine, which is exposed on non-apoptotic tumor cells including malignant metastatic cells and primary cell cultures. Susceptibility of metastatic cells suggests that CAPs may be useful in treating metastatic as well as primary cancers (Riedl et al., 2011).

In addition to direct killing of cancer cells, CAPs can affect T-cell dependent tumor regulation. Recently, intratumoral administration of a lactoferricin derivative into lymphomas established in mice resulted in tumor necrosis, infiltration of inflammatory cells, and regression of tumors. Transfer of spleen cells from treated mice provided long-term, specific T cell-dependent immunity against the lymphoma, suggesting therapeutic vaccination against cancer using CAPs may be possible (Berge et al., 2010). In contrast, LL-37 was able to induce apoptosis of T regulatory cells, thus inhibiting their immune suppressor activity and thereby enhancing the anti-tumor response (Mader et al., 2011).

Pleurocidins selectively killed human leukemia cells at low concentrations (<32 μg/mL) (Morash et al., 2011) as well as multiple breast cancer cell lines (Hilchie et al., 2011) by a predominantly membranolytic mechanism. Disruption of the cell membrane also augmented the activity of the chemotherapeutic cisplatin, presumably by enhancing access to the nucleus. Furthermore, when administered intratumorally into breast cancer xenografts in mice, pleurocidin inhibited tumor growth and induced tumor necrosis, while not causing observable adverse effects on the mice (Hilchie et al., 2011). These advantageous properties indicate that pleurocidins should be pursued as novel anticancer agents.

5.6. Immunomodulatory

CAPs show multiple activities associated with modulation of the immune system (Jenssen and Hancock, 2010; Yeung et al., 2011) and have been postulated to represent an evolutionary link bridging innate and adaptive immune responses (Selsted and Ouellette, 2005). CAPs are directly chemotactic for immune cells and also stimulate chemokine and cytokine secretion (Lai and Gallo, 2009). Some CAPs are able to boost protein antigens and vaccines that have low immunogenicity by inducing proinflammatory cytokines such as TNF, IFN and IL-1β (Kindrachuk et al., 2009; Mutwiri et al., 2007; Tavano et al., 2011), suggesting that they would be good adjuvants (Huang et al., 2011; Li et al., 2008). CAPs play a critical role in wound healing (Steinstraesser et al., 2008), promoting keratinocyte migration (Aung et al., 2011a), re-epithelialization (Hirsch et al., 2009), deposition of extracellular matrix (Oono et al., 2002), and angiogenesis (Koczulla et al., 2003). Human β-defensins and LL-37 are able to stimulate mast cells, and recently the neuroendocrine CAP catestatin has been reported to induce migration and degranulation of mast cells, release of lipid mediators and production of cytokines and chemokines (Aung et al., 2011b). CAPs also show promise in counteracting sepsis, a major cause of morbidity and mortality in hospitalized patients. For example, intraperitoneal injection of LPS-sensitized mice with S-thanatin reduced serum endotoxin and TNF-α levels, resulting in 100% survival (Wu et al., 2011).

Pleurocidin has a proinflammatory effect in fish cells *in vitro*, inducing expression of IL-1β and COX-2 (Chiou et al., 2006). In addition, pleurocidin variant NRC-08, which has no antibacterial activity, induced the expression of the co-stimulatory marker CD40 as well as IL-12p40, TNF, and TGF from mouse bone marrow-derived immature dendritic cells (Phillips, Lee & Douglas, pers. comm.). The potential immunomodulating effects of this particular pleurocidin variant, which promotes the maturation of DCs, suggest that it could be further explored as a candidate adjuvant for a Th1 response to vaccine antigens.

Pleurocidins activate human mast cells to release granule contents such as histamine and proteases (Kulka, per. comm.) both of which are important in allergic inflammation and tissue hometostasis. Mast cells are critical regulators of the tissue microenvironment capable of responding to many different stimuli including allergens and releasing a huge variety of pro-inflammatory and immunomodulatory mediators. Interestingly, pleurocidin activation of mast cells is unique from that of allergens. Allergens bind to and crosslink surface high affinity immunoglobulin E receptors (FcεRI), which activates increases in intracellular calcium and initiates several signaling pathways. Whereas FcεRI activation results in degranulation, arachidonic acid metabolite release and pro-inflammatory mediator production, pleurocidin activation of FPRL1 initiates degranulation and production of relatively small amounts of chemokines. Furthermore, whereas FcεRI engagement does not activate mast cell chemotaxis, pleurocidins modify adhesion via the fibronectin receptor (CD29) and promote mast cell migration. This suggests that pleurocidins activate selective signaling pathways in mast cells and may be useful tools in targeted mast cell-dependent therapy.

5.7. Cytotoxic

5.7.1. Hemolysis and host cell lysis

Although most CAPs are not hemolytic or cytolytic at the concentrations used for killing microbes or cancer cells, some do exhibit that characteristic, melittin being the most notorious (Tosteson et al., 1985). Magainin also forms pores in human cell membranes and enters the cell within minutes, accumulating in the nucleus and mitochondrion (Imura et al., 2008). Bovine myeloid antimicrobial peptides BMAP-27 and BMAP-28 at 10 times minimal inhibitory concentration (MIC) are toxic towards human erythrocytes and polymorphonuclear cells and induce apoptosis in transformed cell lines and *in vitro*-activated lymphocytes at concentrations near MIC (Risso et al., 1998). A recent high-throughput method to assess cytotoxicity of melittin and structural variants differing in hydrophobicity, amphipathicity and helicity, showed it to be more sensitive than standard tests such as erythrocyte lysis and MTT assay and holds promise for identifying CAP variants with non-hemolytic properties (Walsh et al., 2011).

Hemolysis assays of 26 variants of pleurocidin showed that only one, a histidine-rich variant NRC-19, showed any ability to lyse red blood cells up to a concentration of 128 μg/mL, well above the concentrations required to kill bacterial and cancer cells (Morash et al., 2011). The selectivity of these peptides indicates that they would be excellent candidates as antibacterial and anti-cancer agents.

5.7.2. Sepsis

While many CAPs can reduce sepsis, some actually exacerbate the problem. This is because they are so effective at killing bacterial cells that they cause the release of endotoxin from lysed cells, eliciting an excessive inflammatory response (Risso et al., 1998; Steinstraesser et al., 2003).

Preliminary studies using a mouse cytokine array showed that pleurocidin variants NRC-03 and NRC-08 are able to repress LPS-induced TNF-α and IL-10 secretion from mouse RAW264.7 macrophages, indicating that they may be considered for the control of sepsis (Carroll, Patrzykat & Douglas, pers. comm.).

6. Isolation and discovery of cationic antimicrobial peptides

6.1. Traditional biochemical purification

Standard biochemical techniques for isolation of small peptides have been used to isolate CAPs from tissues, skin secretions and other biological fluids. Briefly, tissue lysates or fluids are diluted in 0.1% trifluoroacetic acid (TFA) and extracted under ice-cold acid conditions. After centrifugation, the acidic supernatant is loaded on a C18 column and the peptide eluted with increasing acetonitrile (5-80%) in 0.05% TFA. Those fractions with antimicrobial activity are pooled and further purified by reverse-phase HPLC with increasing acetonitrile (5-55%) in 0.05% TFA. The material in absorbance peaks is then pooled, dried under vacuum and reconstituted in MilliQ water for mass and sequence analysis using mass spectrometry and automated Edman degradation.

Pleurocidin was originally isolated from homogenates of the skin and mucus secretions of winter flounder using C18 chromatography followed by size fractionation on Sephadex G-50 (Cole et al., 1997). Biologically active fractions were pooled and subjected to strong cation exchange HPLC and then reversed phase HPLC.

6.2.Genomics approaches to antimicrobial peptide discovery

Once even a partial amino acid sequence of a CAP is known, genomic strategies can be employed to identify and isolate DNA sequences encoding CAPs. This can involve screening of cDNA and genomic libraries using oligonucleotide probes or amplification of CAP-encoding sequences from genomic or cDNA by PCR (Iwamuro and Kobayashi, 2010). CAP-encoding sequences can also be identified in genomic and EST sequencing databases by similarity searching using bioinformatics search engines such as BLAST (Browne et al., 2011; Fernandes et al., 2010). Full-length cDNA sequences can then be obtained by 5′- and 3′-RACE. The identification of 28 new human and 43 new mouse β-defensin genes was achieved using a computational search tool to find conserved motifs in draft genome sequences (Schutte et al., 2002).

Pleurocidin was originally cloned from cDNA and genomic libraries using degenerate oligonucleotide probes (Cole et al., 2000; Douglas et al., 2001) or PCR amplicons encoding individual pleurocidin variants (Douglas et al., 2003). Additional pleurocidin variants were amplified by PCR from cDNA of different flatfish species using primers corresponding to the conserved amino-terminal signal peptide and carboxy-terminal anionic propiece (Patrzykat et al., 2003). At least 30 variants have now been cloned (Figure 3).

6.3. *In silico* discovery and rational peptide design

Various *in silico* methods have been used to rationally design CAPs and predict their biological activity (Hadley and Hancock, 2010). These include the use of artificial neural networks, support vector machines and quantitative structure activity relationship (QSAR) modeling (Fjell et al., 2011; Torrent et al., 2011). Combinatorial synthesis and high throughput peptide synthesis using SPOT technology (Hilpert et al., 2007) together with a QSAR-based artificial neural network system (Fjell et al., 2009) have also been used to design active synthetic CAPs. This approach, coupled with high-throughput screening assays using peptide arrays, is invaluable for inexpensively generating large numbers of potential candidates for clinical assessment (Cherkasov et al., 2009).

7. Production of cationic antimicrobial peptides

7.1. Peptide synthesis

Isolation of CAPs from the native producer is not feasible on the scale necessary for investigating therapeutic value and pharmaceutical potential. Therefore, CAPs are usually synthesized by standard solid-phase methods using 9-fluorenyl-methoxycarbonyl (F-moc) protecting groups, cleaved from the resin with 95% trifluoroacetic acid, purified by reverse-phase high performance liquid chromatography using an acetonitrile gradient, and the mass is verified by mass spectrometry. Although synthesis of linear α-helical peptides is fairly routine, good yields of CAPs that require cysteine oxidation to form the correct disulphide bonding pattern are rarely obtained (Tay et al., 2011). Modifications such as carboxy-terminal amidation, biotinylation, fluorescent labeling, incorporation of D-amino acids, acylation, etc. are available for synthetic peptides.

7.2. Fermentation

7.2.1. Bacteria

Production of CAPs in bacteria using recombinant technology, by definition, is a challenge as they inhibit or kill the host bacteria and bacterial proteases can degrade them. Recombinant technology, particularly of tagged fusion peptides, has been used successfully to produce high yields of pure CAP at relatively low cost (Ingham and Moore, 2007). Factors to be considered include optimization of promoter sequence and codon usage from the source organism to bacterial host, signal peptide, tag, fusion partner, ease and cost of cleavage, and cost of subsequent purification steps. A recent approach involving secretion of the tagged SUMO-CAP hybrid into the medium followed by removal of the mature CAP by sumoase protease has been particularly successful in large-scale production of several CAPs (Bommarius et al., 2010; Li et al., 2009). In general, production of α-helical CAPs without disulfide bonds and easily cleavable from their fusion partner has proved to be the most straightforward and cost-effective. A recent report of expression of human β-defensin 28 in *E. coli* is encouraging, however (Tay et al., 2011). By using a construct with both a His-tag and maltose binding protein and including the site for cleavage by TeV, an inexpensive and efficient protease for releasing the mature CAP, large-scale production of correctly folded defensin was achieved.

Pleurocidin has been successfully expressed as a PurF fusion peptide in inclusion bodies, generating milligram quantities of pure peptide (Bryksa et al., 2006). By incorporating

$(^{15}NH_4)_2$-SO_4 as the sole nitrogen source in the growth medium, structural elucidation of the uniformly ^{15}N-labelled peptide by NMR was greatly facilitated (Syvitski et al., 2005).

7.2.2. Fungi

Fungi such as *Saccharomyces cerevisiae* and *Pichia pastoris* represent alternative systems for recombinant expression of CAPs. *P. pastoris* is a methylotrophic yeast that is capable of producing 10-100 times more recombinant protein than *S. cerevisiae.* However, successful production of small proteins less than 10 kDa in *P. pastoris* can be problematic due to low expression, RNA instability or translational blocks. Low amounts (~1 mg/100 mL) of recombinant cecropin were produced in *P. pastoris* (Jin et al., 2006), and recently, high-level production (>200 mg/L) of active recombinant hPAB-β (Chen et al., 2011) and plectasin (Zhang et al., 2011) was achieved in this system.

Production of pleurocidin was attempted using this system; however, no recombinant peptide was recovered, despite correct integration of the pleurocidin sequence into the yeast genome and normal transcription (Burrowes et al., 2005).

7.2.3. Animal cells

Production of CAPs in animal cells has the advantage of accurate processing of the recombinant peptide and addition of post-translational modifications. However, there are few reports of CAP production using this approach. The insect cell/baculovirus system has been used to produce recombinant human β-defensins (Feng et al., 2005) and biologically active hepcidin was successfully expressed, processed and secreted in human embryonic kidney cells (Wallace et al., 2006). The complete pleurocidin pre-pro-peptide gene was cloned into a carp cell line under the control of the carp β-actin promoter. The precursor peptide was expressed continuously for over two years and the mature peptide was secreted into the medium (Brocal et al., 2006).

7.3. Transgenic organisms

Early attempts were made to express CAPs in the milk of transgenic mice (Yarus et al., 1996), tissues of catfish (Dunham et al., 2002), and leaves of tobacco (Yevtushenko et al., 2005) and rice (Imamura et al., 2010); however, while the recombinant CAPs were able to confer pathogen resistance to the host organism, these systems are not designed for large-scale production of CAPs for human applications.

8. Modifications to enhance biological activity and stability

8.1. Amino acid substitutions, additions and deletions

Modification of the amino acid sequence of CAPs to change the charge, hydrophobicity and bulkiness can have dramatic effects on their ability to interact with membranes and exert their biological activity. Amidation of the carboxy terminus usually results in enhanced activity by increasing the net positive charge but has a negligible effect on protease susceptibility. On the other hand, N-terminal acetylation significantly increases resistance to aminopeptidases but decreases antimicrobial activity (Nguyen et al., 2010). In general, high hydrophobicity confers hemolytic and cytotoxic properties on CAPs (McPhee and Hancock, 2005). The effect of amino acid substitutions on antimicrobial vs hemolytic activity has been comprehensively evaluated using a series of rationally designed CAPs of 20 amino acids that differ in charge, polar angle, hydrophobicity and hydrophobic moment (Chou et al., 2008). Increasing the His content of clavanin resulted in an acid-activated CAP that showed enhanced activity against the caries-producing pathogen, *S. mutans*, at low pH (Li et al., 2010). Substitution of Lys by His in a 15-mer CAP resulted in a peptide that was cationic only in the acidic microenvironment found in tumors, and exhibited enhanced anti-tumor activity and reduced systemic toxicity (Makovitzki et al., 2009). Addition of hydrophobic amino acids to the termini of CAPs can also increase potency, although reduced solubility and increased production cost present important drawbacks (Hadley and Hancock, 2010). Recent reports of a truncated frog gaegurin (Won et al., 2011b) and the naturally short bee anoplin (Won et al., 2011a) CAPs emphasize the enhanced antimicrobial effects of such modifications on bacteria and model membranes.

Naturally occurring pleurocidins have variable amino acid sequences that confer different activities against microbes and cancer cells (Morash et al., 2011; Patrzykat et al., 2003). Alignment of the amino acid sequences of the mature peptides revealed conserved positions that could be of importance in bioactivity. For example, the highly conserved Gly13 residue in the middle hinge region is important for α-helicity (Lim et al., 2004b) and the hydrophobic amino acids in the N-terminal region are more crucial for antifungal activity than those in the C-terminal region (Lee and Lee, 2010). Replacement of Ser14 by His improved the activity of a targeted pleurocidin towards *S. mutans* at low pH, which is often found in the oral cavity (Mai et al., 2011).

8.2. Non-natural amino acids and enantiomers

Replacement of L-amino acids by their D counterparts generally does not diminish biological activity but does confer protease resistance on the peptide (Lee and Lee, 2008; Park et al., 2010). Retro-inversion, in which amino acid stereochemistry is changed as well as peptide bond direction yielding isomers with similar side chain topology to the native peptide, has generally met with limited success although partially modified retro-inverso peptides show more promise (Fischer, 2003). Incorporation of non-natural amino acid analogs (Knappe et al., 2010; Marsh et al., 2009) is also effective. Recently, a series of CAPs containing Tic-Oic dipeptide analogues was developed to combat 11 potential bio-terrorism and drug-resistant strains of bacteria (Venugopal, 2010). These CAPs were metabolically stable, potent, and showed selectivity for bacterial relative to host cell membranes.

Replacement of L-Lys and L-Arg residues with D-Lys and D-Arg in pleurocidin conferred resistance to digestion by trypsin but also abolished activity, presumably because the α-helical structure was disrupted by the inclusion of just a subset of amino acids (Douglas, unpub.). In support of this, an all D-amino acid analog of pleurocidin showed proteolytic resistance and double the antifungal (Jung et al., 2007) and antibacterial (Lee and Lee, 2008) potency. Similarly, an all D-amino acid analog of pleurocidin NRC-03, showed improved activity against breast cancer cells compared to the natural L-form peptide (Hilchie, Hoskin, unpub).

8.3. Peptidomimetics

Peptidomimetics such as β-peptides and peptoids have been designed that maintain the amphiphilic structure and antimicrobial activity and are resistant to protease degradation; these abiotic structures exhibit *in vivo* stability and enhanced bioavailability (Rotem and Mor, 2009; Scott et al., 2008). Synthetic mimics of antimicrobial peptides (SMAMPs) that adopt amphiphilic secondary structures and possess potent and selective antimicrobial activity have been inexpensively synthesized from small synthetic oligomers (Lienkamp et al., 2008; Scott et al., 2008). Another novel technique is hydrocarbon stapling (Sa'adedin and Bradshaw, 2010) in which an α-helical peptide is chemically modified to generate a relatively protease resistant, cell-permeable peptide that binds its target with increased binding affinity.

8.4. Acylation

Addition of fatty acid chains to the termini of CAPs can increase their antibacterial activity or endow them with antifungal activity. Linear oligomers consisting of alternating uncharged and cationic Lys residues displayed varying degrees of antibacterial, antifungal and hemolytic activity when they were N-acylated, depending on the length of the acyl group and the different degrees of oligomerization that were induced (Shai et al., 2006). Addition of fatty acids of increasing lengths to magainin increased the extent of oligomerization of the resulting lipopeptide, and concurrently the antifungal activity.

8.5. Cyclisation

Cyclisation by, for example, disulfide bridge formation or head-to-tail backbone cyclization, results in a more constrained peptide structure that is less susceptible to protease degradation (Nguyen et al., 2010). Cyclisation of two cationic hexapeptides, including the active portion of lactoferricin, was found to be highly effective for both serum stability and antimicrobial activity. Interestingly, disulfide cyclization resulted in more active peptides while backbone cyclization resulted in more proteolytically stable peptides. The modifications did not result in hemolytic activity, thereby making them attractive therapeutic candidates. Dendrimers of CAPs have enhanced ability to permeabilize membranes and are stabler than monomeric forms (Pieters et al., 2009).

8.6. Targeted and hybrid peptides

One of the drawbacks of antibiotic use is the deleterious effect broad spectrum antibiotics have on the normal microflora, which often allows opportunistic pathogens such as *C. albicans* and *S. aureus* to overgrow after treatment. Selectively targeted antimicrobial peptides (STAMPs) can overcome this problem and can selectively kill the target species while leaving the benign commensals largely unaffected. This effect was first demonstrated using a STAMP consisting of a competence stimulating peptide (CSP) moiety targeting the caries-causing pathogen *Streptococcus mutans* attached to a killing moiety derived from novispirin G10 (Eckert et al., 2006). Incorporation of such a STAMP into an oral rinse resulted in reduction in salivary *S. mutans*, plaque, lactic acid and enamel demineralization, suggesting further clinical evaluation is warranted (Sullivan et al., 2011). Targeting of tumor cells has also been achieved and addition of the tumor-homing peptide bombesin to the amino terminus of magainin 2 resulted in tenfold enhanced killing *in vitro* and decrease in the size of tumor xenografts in mice (Liu et al., 2011).

We have used this approach to combine the minimal targeting portion of CSP with the killing domain of pleurocidin variant NRC-04 to treat *S. mutans* in both planktonic and biofilm conditions. The hybrid peptide was selectively active against *S. mutans* in the presence of saliva and physiological or higher salt concentration and was non-hemolytic (Mai et al., 2011). Furthermore, activity was augmented by a preventative dose of 1 mM NaF, a compound commonly used in oral care. The development of such targeted peptides paves the way for their use as a probiotic treatment to prevent dental caries.

9. Advantages and limitations of cationic antimicrobial peptides

9.1. Bioactivity

CAPs exert rapid, broad spectrum, bactericidal activity at micromolar concentrations and are valuable weapons in the fight against antibiotic-resistant microbes e.g. MRSA. In addition, targeted CAPs may be used as probiotics to eradicate pathogenic bacteria while leaving normal flora unaffected. Their ability to kill fungi, viruses and parasites is also beneficial clinically. Many CAPs neutralize endotoxin and can be used to counteract sepsis or to enhance host defenses through immunomodulatory effects. Increased innate clearance of microbes results in less bacterial debris (van der Does et al., 2010) and ensuing inflammation (Andra et al., 2006). Their application both in killing tumor cells and in enhancing host antitumor responses is gaining momentum (Yeung et al., 2011).

9.2. Resistance

CAPs have a low propensity to induce microbial resistance, mainly due to their multiple targets and mechanisms of action. CAPs are usually expressed in high concentrations only at sites of infection; continuous exposure of microbes, which often leads to resistance, is therefore minimized. In addition, cocktails of several different CAPs are often produced simultaneously, leading to increased microbial killing.

Despite this, some reports on the emergence of resistance have appeared. These include reduction in bacterial cell surface negative charge, secretion of exoproteases and induction of transporters (see Nizet, 2006; Peschel and Sahl, 2006), all of which require significant expenditure of metabolic energy by the microbe. In most cases, the resistance that arises is very low compared to conventional antibiotics.

In Gram negative organisms such as *Salmonella* and *Pseudomonas*, the PhoP-PhoQ two component sensor system has been shown to control resistance to aminoglycosides, polymyxin B, and cationic antimicrobial peptides (Macfarlane et al., 1999; Macfarlane et al., 2000; Groisman, 2001). In *Pseudomonas*, CAPs and the polymyxins are capable of inducing the pmrA-pmr genes and the putative LPS modification operon, thus increasing resistance to these agents (McPhee et al., 2003). The homologous basR-basS system of *E. coli* is also induced by exposure to sublethal concentrations of the proline-rich CAP, Bac7(1-35), suggesting that it may also mediate resistance (Tomasinsig et al., 2004). Resistance to Gram positive organisms such as *Staphylococcus* is mediated by the Aps three component sensor system, and interestingly, some CAPs are inducers of this system (Li et al., 2007). Recently, additional resistance genes in other bacteria such as *Clostridium difficile* (McBride and Sonenshein, 2011) and *Vibrio* (Shen et al., 2010) have been discovered, emphasizing the importance of this phenomenon.

9.3. Cost

Solid phase peptide synthesis is expensive and companies seeking regulatory approval for peptides in their pipelines require suppliers that adhere to good manufacturing practice (GMP) regulations, which also adds to the cost. However, there have been many advances in synthetic chemistry that have significantly reduced the cost of not only peptides but also non-peptide mimics and peptoids, and the lower operating costs of suppliers in Asia has resulted in more affordable peptides (Eckert, 2011).

9.4. Stability

Although CAPs represent a promising class of therapeutics, they have several *in vivo* drawbacks such as salt inactivation, protease degradation, and poor bioavailability. As described above, a number of approaches can be used to mitigate these limitations. Serum stability can be overcome by cyclisation or incorporation of amino acid analogs and some CAPs, particularly those such as pleurocidin that originated from marine sources, are active at physiological salt concentrations (Mai et al., 2011; Patrzykat et al., 2003).

9.5. Side effects

Some CAPs exhibit *in vivo* toxicity and for others there are unknown toxicity profiles (see section 5.7). Nephrotoxicity has been associated with polymixin cyclic peptides (Mogi and Kita, 2009). Since some CAPs can stimulate growth factor receptors, induction of tumorigenesis must be considered. Similarly, excessive release of histamine from mast cells must be avoided to minimize adverse reactions.

10.Clinical use and commercialization

10.1. Companies

A number of CAPs and synthetic CAP analogs such as pexiganan™ (magainin derivative), omiganan™ (indolicidin derivative), novispirin™ (cathelicidin derivative) and iseganan™ (protegrin-1 derivative) are now in commercial development. Several recent reviews describe the companies, their products and their progression through clinical trials (Eckert, 2011; Kindrachuk and Napper, 2010; Yeung et al., 2011; Zhang and Falla, 2010). Some candidates show great promise in the treatment of such disorders as HIV-associated oral candidiasis, acne, wound infections, diabetic foot ulcers, and oral biofilms. However, the inability to demonstrate advantage over existing therapeutics has resulted in failure of a number of CAPs at Phase III clinical trials. As appropriate formulations, bioassays and endpoints are established, the probability that these promising products will receive regulatory approval will improve.

10.2. Formulations

Because of systemic toxicity and bioavailability issues as well as the diverse and complex mechanisms of action, the majority of CAPs have been developed as topical formulations e.g. for diabetic foot ulcers (Lipsky et al., 2008) and skin infections (Falla and Zhang, 2010). Depending on the application, a number of different ways of formulating CAPs can be envisioned (Eckert, 2011). CAPs have been incorporated into lens preservation and artificial tear solutions (Huang et al., 2005) and aerosols (Lange et al., 2001). Inclusion of CAPs in coatings (Kazemzadeh-Narbat et al., 2010), polymers (Gao et al., 2011), hydrogels (Roy and Das, 2008), liposomes (Lange et al., 2001), micro- and nanoparticles (Bi et al., 2011; Garlapati et al., 2011) and even chewing gum (Faraj et al., 2007) also represent promising formulations. Long-term activity has been achieved by covalent immobilization of gramicidin A on functionalized gold surfaces and resulted in inhibition of Gram-positive and Gram-negative bacteria and the yeast *Candida albicans* for up to 6 months as well as delayed development of bacterial biofilm for 24 hours (Yala et al., 2011). Surface modifications by CAPs will be important in preventing colonization of medical devices such as catheters and bioimplants.

CAPs can also be used in combination therapies with each other or with approved antibiotics. For example, cecropin B enhanced the activities of beta lactams in rat septic shock models (Ghiselli et al., 2004). Cecropin A and magainin 2 administered together showed *in vitro* synergy against *S. aureus* in a mouse sepsis model (Cirioni et al., 2006). Magainin 2 administered with vancomycin showed the highest efficacy in this model.

Pleurocidin showed synergistic activity with inducible histone peptides and lysozyme in a salmonid *in vivo* infection model (Patrzykat et al., 2001). Studies with *S. mutans* showed that the efficacy of a targeted pleurocidin was increased in the presence of EDTA and sodium fluoride, two commonly used components of oral rinses (Mai et al., 2011).

10.3. Targeted delivery

CAPs with cell-penetrating properties are under development as vectors for translocation of bioactive cargos with inherently poor membrane-crossing abilities into eukaryotic cells (Splith and Neundorf, 2011). Delivery of CAP-modified liposomes containing therapeutics to bacteria has also been reported, e. g. bacteria-targeted delivery of photodynamic antimicrobial chemotherapy to improve efficiency against MRSA and *P. aeruguinosa* in local infections (Yang et al., 2011).

11.Conclusions

CAPs show exciting promise as novel therapeutic agents, particularly in the fight against antibiotic-resistant bacteria and cancer and as immunostimulants. However, translation to clinical use has been hampered by concerns over stability, cost, systemic administration, known toxicity, and unknown long-term toxicity. The applications that show the most promise are those involving topical applications, particularly in combination with established antibiotics. Deeper understanding of the varied mechanisms of action of these diverse peptides and the production of cost-effective, stable, and highly selective CAPs will aid in bringing these molecules closer to the clinic.

Author details

Susan Douglas*

Address all correspondence to: susan.douglas@nrc.ca

Institute for Marine Biosciences, Canada

References

[1] Aberg, K. M., Radek, K. A., Choi, E. H., Kim, D. K., Demerjian, M., Hupe, M., Kerbleski, J., Gallo, R. L., Ganz, T., Mauro, T., et al. (2007). Psychological stress downregulates epidermal antimicrobial peptide expression and increases severity of cutaneous infections in mice. *J Clin Invest*, 117, 3339-3349.

[2] Andra, J., Gutsmann, T., Garidel, P., & Brandenburg, K. (2006). Mechanisms of endotoxin neutralization by synthetic cationic compounds. *J Endotoxin Res*, 12, 261-277.

[3] Andres, M. T., Viejo-Diaz, M., & Fierro, J. F. (2008). Human lactoferrin induces apoptosis-like cell death in Candida albicans: critical role of K+-channel-mediated K+ efflux. *Antimicrob Ag Chemother*, 52, 4081-4088.

[4] Aung, G., Niyonsaba, F., Ushio, H., Hoq, M. I., Ikeda, S., Ogawa, H., & Okumura, K. (2011a). A neuroendocrine antimicrobial peptide, catestatin, stimulates interleukin-8 production from human keratinocytes via activation of mitogen-activated protein kinases. *J Dermatol Sci*, 61, 142-144.

[5] Aung, G., Niyonsaba, F., Ushio, H., Kajiwara, N., Saito, H., Ikeda, S., Ogawa, H., & Okumura, K. (2011b). Catestatin, a neuroendocrine antimicrobial peptide, induces human mast cell migration, degranulation and production of cytokines and chemokines. *Immunology*, 132, 527-539.

[6] Berge, G., Eliassen, L. T., Camilio, K. A., Bartnes, K., Sveinbjornsson, B., & Rekdal, O. (2010). Therapeutic vaccination against a murine lymphoma by intratumoral injection of a cationic anticancer peptide. *Cancer Immunol Immunother*, 59, 1285-1294.

[7] Bi, L., Yang, L., Narsimhan, G., Bhunia, A. K., & Yao, Y. (2011). Designing carbohydrate nanoparticles for prolonged efficacy of antimicrobial peptide. *J Control Release*, 150, 150-156.

[8] Bommarius, B., Jenssen, H., Elliott, M., Kindrachuk, J., Pasupuleti, M., Gieren, H., Jaeger, K. E., Hancock, R. E., & Kalman, D. (2010). Cost-effective expression and purification of antimicrobial and host defense peptides in Escherichia coli. *Peptides*, 31, 1957-1965.

[9] Braff, M. H., Hawkins, M. A., Di Nardo, A., Lopez-Garcia, B., Howell, M. D., Wong, C., Lin, K., Streib, J. E., Dorschner, R., Leung, D. Y., et al. (2005). Structure-function relationships among human cathelicidin peptides: dissociation of antimicrobial properties from host immunostimulatory activities. *J Immunol*, 174, 4271-4278.

[10] Brocal, I., Falco, A., Mas, V., Rocha, A., Perez, L., Coll, J. M., & Estepa, A. (2006). Stable expression of bioactive recombinant pleurocidin in a fish cell line. *Appl Microbiol Biotechnol*, 72, 1217-1228.

[11] Brogden, K. A. (2005). Antimicrobial peptides: pore formers or metabolic inhibitors in bacteria? *Nat Rev Microbiol*, 3, 238-250.

[12] Browne, M. J., Feng, C. Y., Booth, V., & Rise, M. L. (2011). Characterization and expression studies of Gaduscidin-1 and Gaduscidin-2; paralogous antimicrobial peptide-like transcripts from Atlantic cod (Gadus morhua). *Dev Comp Immunol*, 35, 399-408.

[13] Bryksa, B. C., Mac, Donald. L. D., Patrzykat, A., Douglas, S. E., & Mattatall, N. R. (2006). A C-terminal glycine suppresses production of pleurocidin as a fusion peptide in Escherichia coli. *Prot Expr Purif*, 45, 88-98.

[14] Burrowes, O. J., Diamond, G., & Lee, T. C. (2005). Recombinant expression of pleurocidin cDNA using the Pichia pastoris expression system. *J Biomed Biotechnol*, 3, 74-384.

[15] Burrowes, O. J., Hadjicharalambous, C., Diamond, G., & Lee, T. C. (2004). Evaluation of antimicrobial spectrum and cytotoxic activity of pleurocidin for food applications. *J Food Sci*, 63, 66-71.

[16] Cardini, S., Dalli, J., Fineschi, S., Perretti, M., Lungarella, G., & Lucattelli, M. (2012). Genetic ablation of the Fpr1 gene confers protection from smoking-induced lung emphysema in mice. *Am J Respir Cell Mol Biol*, PMID 22461430.

[17] Castle, M., Nazarian, A., Yi, S. S., & Tempst, P. (1999). Lethal effects of apidaecin on Escherichia coli involve sequential molecular interactions with diverse targets. *J Biol Chem*, 274, 32555-32564.

[18] Cattaneo, F., Iaccio, A., Guerra, G., Montagnani, S., & Ammendola, R. (2011). NADPH-oxidase-dependent reactive oxygen species mediate EGFR transactivation by FPRL1 in WKYMVm-stimulated human lung cancer cells. *Free Radic Biol Med*, 51, 1126-1136.

[19] Ceron, J. M., Contreras-Moreno, J., Puertollano, E., de Cienfuegos, G. A., Puertollano, M. A., & de Pablo, M. A. (2010). The antimicrobial peptide cecropin A induces caspase-independent cell death in human promyelocytic leukemia cells. *Peptides*, 31, 1494-1503.

[20] Chang, T. W., Lin, Y. M., Wang, C. F., & Liao, Y. D. (2012). Outer membrane lipoprotein Lpp is Gram-negative bacterial cell surface receptor for cationic antimicrobial peptides. *J Biol Chem*, 287, 418-428.

[21] Chen, Z., Wang, D., Cong, Y., Wang, J., Zhu, J., Yang, J., Hu, Z., Hu, X., Tan, Y., Hu, F., et al. (2011). Recombinant antimicrobial peptide hPAB-beta expressed in Pichia pastoris, a potential agent active against methicillin-resistant Staphylococcus aureus. *Appl Microbiol Biotechnol*, 89, 281-291.

[22] Cherkasov, A., Hilpert, K., Jenssen, H., Fjell, C. D., Waldbrook, M., Mullaly, S. C., Volkmer, R., & Hancock, R. E. (2009). Use of artificial intelligence in the design of small peptide antibiotics effective against a broad spectrum of highly antibiotic-resistant superbugs. *ACS Chem Biol*, 4, 65-74.

[23] Chiou, P., Khoo, J., Bols, N. C., Douglas, S., & Chen, T. T. (2006). Effects of linear cationic alpha-helical antimicrobial peptides on immune-relevant genes in trout macrophages. *Dev Comp Immunol*, 30, 797-806.

[24] Cho, J., & Lee, D. G. (2011a). Oxidative stress by antimicrobial peptide pleurocidin triggers apoptosis in Candida albicans. *Biochimie*, 93, 1873-1879.

[25] Cho, J., & Lee, D. G. (2011b). The antimicrobial peptide arenicin-1 promotes generation of reactive oxygen species and induction of apoptosis. *Biochim Biophys Acta.*

[26] Chou, H. T., Kuo, T. Y., Chiang, J. C., Pei, M. J., Yang, W. T., Yu, H. C., Lin, S. B., & Chen, W. J. (2008). Design and synthesis of cationic antimicrobial peptides with improved activity and selectivity against Vibrio spp. *Int J Antimicrob Agents*, 32, 130-138.

[27] Cirioni, O., Silvestri, C., Ghiselli, R., Giacometti, A., Orlando, F., Mocchegiani, F., Chiodi, L., Vittoria, A. D., Saba, V., & Scalise, G. (2006). Experimental study on the efficacy of combination of alpha-helical antimicrobial peptides and vancomycin against Staphylococcus aureus with intermediate resistance to glycopeptides. *Peptides* , 27, 2600-2606.

[28] Cole, A. M., Darouiche, R. O., Legarda, D., Connell, N., & Diamond, G. (2000). Characterization of a fish antimicrobial peptide: gene expression, subcellular localization, and spectrum of activity. *Antimicrob Ag Chemother*, 44, 2039-2045.

[29] Cole, A. M., Weis, P., & Diamond, G. (1997). Isolation and characterization of pleurocidin, an antimicrobial peptide in the skin secretions of winter flounder. *J Biol Chem*, 272, 12008-12013.

[30] De Lucca, A. J., & Walsh, T. J. (1999). Antifungal peptides: Novel therapeutic compounds against emerging pathogens. *Antimicrob Ag Chemother*, 43, 1-11.

[31] Dean, R. E., O'Brien, L. M., Thwaite, J. E., Fox, M. A., Atkins, H., & Ulaeto, D. O. (2010). A carpet-based mechanism for direct antimicrobial peptide activity against vaccinia virus membranes. *Peptides*, 31, 1966-1972.

[32] den, Hertog. A. L., van Marle, J., van Veen, H. A., Van't, Hof. W., Bolscher, J. G., Veerman, E. C., & Nieuw, Amerongen. A. V. (2005). Candidacidal effects of two antimicrobial peptides: histatin 5 causes small membrane defects, but LL-37 causes massive disruption of the cell membrane. *Biochem J*, 388, 689-695.

[33] Douglas, S. E., Gallant, J. W., Gong, Z., & Hew, C. (2001). Cloning and developmental expression of a family of pleurocidin-like antimicrobial peptides from winter flounder, Pleuronectes americanus (Walbaum). *Dev Comp Immunol*, 25, 137-147.

[34] Douglas, S. E., Patrzykat, A., Pytyck, J., & Gallant, J. W. (2003). Identification, structure and differential expression of novel pleurocidins clustered on the genome of the winter flounder, Pseudopleuronectes americanus (Walbaum). *Eur J Biochem*, 270, 3720-3730.

[35] Dunham, R. A., Warr, G. W., Nichols, A., Duncan, P. L., Argue, B., Middleton, D., & Kucuktas, H. (2002). Enhanced bacterial disease resistance of transgenic channel catfish Ictalurus punctatus possessing cecropin genes. *Mar Biotechnol*, 4, 338-344.

[36] Eckert, R. (2011). Road to clinical efficacy: challenges and novel strategies for antimicrobial peptide development. *Future Microbiol*, 6, 635-651.

[37] Eckert, R., He, J., Yarbrough, D. K., Qi, F., Anderson, M. H., & Shi, W. (2006). Targeted killing of Streptococcus mutans by a pheromone-guided "smart" antimicrobial peptide. *Antimicrob Ag Chemother*, 50, 3651-3657.

[38] Falla, T. J., & Zhang, L. (2010). Efficacy of hexapeptide-7 on menopausal skin. *J Drugs Dermatol*, 9, 49-54.

[39] Faraj, J. A., Dorati, R., Schoubben, A., Worthen, D., Selmin, F., Capan, Y., Leung, K., & De Luca, P. P. (2007). Development of a peptide-containing chewing gum as a sustained release antiplaque antimicrobial delivery system. *AAPS PharmSciTech*, 26.

[40] Fehlbaum, P., Bulet, P., Chernysh, S., Briand, J. P., Roussel, J. P., Letellier, L., Hetru, C., & Hoffmann, J. A. (1996). Structure-activity analysis of thanatin, a 21-residue inducible insect defense peptide with sequence homology to frog skin antimicrobial peptides. *Proc Natl Acad Sci U S A*, 93, 1221-1225.

[41] Feng, Z., Jiang, B., Chandra, J., Ghannoum, M., Nelson, S., & Weinberg, A. (2005). Human beta-defensins: differential activity against candidal species and regulation by Candida albicans. *J Dent Res*, 84, 445-450.

[42] Fernandes, J. M., Ruangsri, J., & Kiron, V. (2010). Atlantic cod piscidin and its diversification through positive selection. PLoS One , e9501., 5

[43] Fischer, P. M. (2003). The design, synthesis and application of stereochemical and directional peptide isomers: a critical review. *Curr Protein Pept Sci*, 4, 339-356.

[44] Fjell, C. D., Jenssen, H., Cheung, W. A., Hancock, R. E., & Cherkasov, A. (2011). Optimization of antibacterial peptides by genetic algorithms and cheminformatics. *Chem Biol Drug Des*, 77, 48-56.

[45] Fjell, C. D., Jenssen, H., Hilpert, K., Cheung, W. A., Pante, N., Hancock, R. E., & Cherkasov, A. (2009). Identification of novel antibacterial peptides by chemoinformatics and machine learning. *J Med Chem*, 52, 2006-2015.

[46] Gao, G., Lange, D., Hilpert, K., Kindrachuk, J., Zou, Y., Cheng, J. T., Kazemzadeh-Narbat, M., Yu, K., Wang, R., Straus, S. K., et al. (2011). The biocompatibility and biofilm resistance of implant coatings based on hydrophilic polymer brushes conjugated with antimicrobial peptides. *Biomaterials*, 32, 3899-3909.

[47] Garlapati, S., Eng, N. F., Kiros, T. G., Kindrachuk, J., Mutwiri, G. K., Hancock, R. E., Halperin, S. A., Potter, A. A., Babiuk, L. A., & Gerdts, V. (2011). Immunization with PCEP microparticles containing pertussis toxoid, CpG ODN and a synthetic innate defense regulator peptide induces protective immunity against pertussis. *Vaccine*, 29, 6540-6548.

[48] Ghiselli, R., Giacometti, A., Cirioni, O., Mocchegiani, F., Orlando, F., D'Amato, G., Sisti, V., Scalise, G., & Saba, V. (2004). Cecropin B enhances betalactams activities in experimental rat models of gram-negative septic shock. *Ann Surg*, 239, 251-256.

[49] Goldman, M. J., Anderson, G. M., Stolzenberg, E. D., Kari, U. P., Zasloff, M., & Wilson, J. M. (1997). Human beta-defensin-1 is a salt-sensitive antibiotic in lung that is inactivated in cystic fibrosis. *Cell*, 88, 553-560.

[50] Guaní-Guerra, E., Santos-Mendoza, T., Lugo-Reyes, S. O., & Terán, L. M. (2010). Antimicrobial peptides: general overview and clinical implications in human health and disease. *Clin Immunol*, 135, 1-11.

[51] Hadley, E. B., & Hancock, R. E. (2010). Strategies for the discovery and advancement of novel cationic antimicrobial peptides. *Curr Top Med Chem*, 10, 1872-1881.

[52] Haines, L. R., Hancock, R. E. W., & Pearson, T. W. (2003). Cationic antimicrobial peptide killing of African trypanosomes and Sodalis glossinidius, a bacterial symbiont of the insect vector of sleeping sickness. *Vector-borne Zoonotic Dis*, 3, 175-186.

[53] Haines, L. R., Thomas, J. M., Jackson, A. M., Eyford, B. A., Razavi, M., Watson, C. N., Gowen, B., Hancock, R. E., & Pearson, T. W. (2009). Killing of trypanosomatid parasites by a modified bovine host defense peptide, BMAP-18. *PLoS Negl Trop Dis*, 3, e373.

[54] Hancock, R. E., & Rozek, A. (2002). Role of membranes in the activities of antimicrobial cationic peptides. *FEMS Microbiol Lett*, 206, 143-149.

[55] Harrington, J. M. (2011). Antimicrobial peptide killing of African trypanosomes. *Parasite Immunol*, 33, 461-469.

[56] Helmerhorst, E. J., Troxler, R. F., & Oppenheim, F. G. (2001). The human salivary peptide histatin 5 exerts its antifungal activity through the formation of reactive oxygen species. *Proc Natl Acad Sci U S A*, 98, 14637-14642.

[57] Hilchie, A. L., Doucette, C. D., Pinto, D. M., Patrzykat, A., Douglas, S., & Hoskin, D. W. (2011). Pleurocidin-family cationic antimicrobial peptides are cytolytic for breast carcinoma cells and prevent growth of tumor xenografts. *Breast Cancer Res*, 13, R102 .

[58] Hilpert, K., Winkler, D. F., & Hancock, R. E. (2007). Peptide arrays on cellulose support: SPOT synthesis, a time and cost efficient method for synthesis of large numbers of peptides in a parallel and addressable fashion. *Nat Protoc*, 2, 1333-1349.

[59] Hirsch, T., Spielmann, M., Zuhaili, B., Fossum, M., Metzig, M., Koehler, T., Steinau, H. U., Yao, F., Onderdonk, A. B., Steinstraesser, L., et al. (2009). Human beta-defensin-3 promotes wound healing in infected diabetic wounds. *J Gene Med*, 11, 220-228.

[60] Hoskin, D. W., & Ramamoorthy, A. (2008). Studies on anticancer activities of antimicrobial peptides. *Biochim Biophys Acta*, 1778, 357-375.

[61] Hua, J., Yamarthy, R., Felsenstein, S., Scott, R. W., Markowitz, K., & Diamond, G. (2010). Activity of antimicrobial peptide mimetics in the oral cavity: I. Activity against biofilms of Candida albicans. *Mol Oral Microbiol*, 25, 418-425.

[62] Huang, H. N., Pan, C. Y., Rajanbabu, V., Chan, Y. L., Wu, C. J., & Chen, J. Y. (2011). Modulation of immune responses by the antimicrobial peptide, epinecidin (Epi)-1, and establishment of an Epi-1-based inactivated vaccine. *Biomaterials*, 32, 3627-3636.

[63] Huang, L. C., Jean, D., & Mc Dermott, A. M. (2005). Effect of preservative-free artificial tears on the antimicrobial activity of human beta-defensin-2 and cathelicidin LL-37 in vitro. *Eye Contact Lens*, 31, 34-38.

[64] Hwang, B., Hwang, J. S., Lee, J., Kim, J. K., Kim, S. R., Kim, Y., & Lee, D. G. (2011a). Induction of yeast apoptosis by an antimicrobial peptide, Papiliocin. *Biochem Biophys Res Commun*, 408, 89-93.

[65] Hwang, B., Hwang, J. S., Lee, J., & Lee, D. G. (2011b). The antimicrobial peptide, psacotheasin induces reactive oxygen species and triggers apoptosis in Candida albicans. *Biochem Biophys Res Commun*, 405, 267-271.

[66] Imamura, T., Yasuda, M., Kusano, H., Nakashita, H., Ohno, Y., Kamakura, T., Taguchi, S., & Shimada, H. (2010). Acquired resistance to the rice blast in transgenic rice accumulating the antimicrobial peptide thanatin. *Transgenic Res*, 19, 415-424.

[67] Imura, Y., Choda, N., & Matsuzaki, K. (2008). Magainin 2 in action: distinct modes of membrane permeabilization in living bacterial and mammalian cells. *Biophys J*, 95, 5757-5765.

[68] Ingham, A. B., & Moore, R. J. (2007). Recombinant production of antimicrobial peptides in heterologous microbial systems. *Biotechnol Appl Biochem*, 47, 1-9.

[69] Iwamuro, S., & Kobayashi, T. (2010). An efficient protocol for DNA amplification of multiple amphibian skin antimicrobial peptide cDNAs. *Methods Mol Biol*, 615, 159-176.

[70] Jenssen, H., & Hancock, R. E. (2009). Antimicrobial properties of lactoferrin. *Biochimie*, 91, 19-29.

[71] Jenssen, H., & Hancock, R. E. (2010). Therapeutic potential of HDPs as immunomodulatory agents. *Methods Mol Biol*, 618, 329-347.

[72] Jiang, Z., Kullberg, B. J., van der Lee, H., Vasil, A. I., Hale, J. D., Mant, C. T., Hancock, R. E., Vasil, M. L., Netea, M. G., & Hodges, R. S. (2008). Effects of hydrophobicity on the antifungal activity of alpha-helical antimicrobial peptides. *Chem Biol Drug Des*, 72, 483-495.

[73] Jin, F., Xu, X., Zhang, W., & Gu, D. (2006). Expression and characterization of a housefly cecropin gene in the methylotrophic yeast, Pichia pastoris. *Protein Expr Purif*, 49, 39-46.

[74] Jin, X., Mei, H., Li, X., , Y., Zeng, A. H., Wang, Y., Lu, X., Chu, F., Wu, Q., & Zhu, J. (2010). Apoptosis-inducing activity of the antimicrobial peptide cecropin of Musca domestica in human hepatocellular carcinoma cell line BEL-7402 and the possible mechanism. *Acta Biochim Biophys Sin (Shanghai)*, 42, 259-265.

[75] Jung, H. J., Park, Y., Sung, W. S., Suh, B. K., Lee, J., Hahm, K. S., & Lee, D. G. (2007). Fungicidal effect of pleurocidin by membrane-active mechanism and design of enantiomeric analogue for proteolytic resistance. *Biochim Biophys Acta- Biomembranes*, 1768, 1400-1405.

[76] Kazemzadeh-Narbat, M., Kindrachuk, J., Duan, K., Jenssen, H., Hancock, R. E., & Wang, R. (2010). Antimicrobial peptides on calcium phosphate-coated titanium for the prevention of implant-associated infections. *Biomaterials*, 31, 9519-9526.

[77] Kindrachuk, J., Jenssen, H., Elliott, M., Townsend, R., Nijnik, A., Lee, S. F., Gerdts, V., Babiuk, L. A., Halperin, S. A., & Hancock, R. E. (2009). A novel vaccine adjuvant comprised of a synthetic innate defence regulator peptide and CpG oligonucleotide links innate and adaptive immunity. *Vaccine*, 27, 4662-4671.

[78] Kindrachuk, J., & Napper, S. (2010). Structure-activity relationships of multifunctional host defence peptides. *Mini Rev Med Chem*, 10, 596-614.

[79] Knappe, D., Henklein, P., Hoffmann, R., & Hilpert, K. (2010). Easy strategy to protect antimicrobial peptides from fast degradation in serum. *Antimicrob Ag Chemother*, 54, 4003-4005.

[80] Koczulla, R., von, Degenfeld. G., Kupatt, C., Krotz, F., Zahler, S., Gloe, T., Issbrucker, K., Unterberger, P., Zaiou, M., Lebherz, C., et al. (2003). An angiogenic role for the human peptide antibiotic LL-37/hCAP-18. *J Clin Invest*, 111, 1665-1672.

[81] Lai, Y., & Gallo, R. L. (2009). AMPed up immunity: how antimicrobial peptides have multiple roles in immune defense. *Trends Immunol*, 30, 131-141.

[82] Lan, Y., Ye, Y., Kozlowska, J., Lam, J. K., Drake, A. F., & Mason, A. J. (2010). Structural contributions to the intracellular targeting strategies of antimicrobial peptides. *Biochim Biophys Acta*, 1798, 1934-1943.

[83] Lange, C. F., Hancock, R. E., Samuel, J., & Finlay, W. H. (2001). In vitro aerosol delivery and regional airway surface liquid concentration of a liposomal cationic peptide. *J Pharm Sci*, 90, 1647-1657.

[84] Lee, J., & Lee, D. G. (2008). Structure-antimicrobial activity relationship between pleurocidin and its enantiomer. *Exp Mol Med*, 40, 370-376.

[85] Lee, J., & Lee, D. G. (2010). Influence of the hydrophobic amino acids in the N- and C-terminal regions of pleurocidin on antifungal activity. *J Microbiol Biotechnol*, 20, 1192-1195.

[86] Leontiadou, H., Mark, A. E., & Marrink, S. J. (2006). Antimicrobial peptides in action. *J Am Chem Soc*, 128, 12156-12161.

[87] Li, J. F., Zhang, J., Song, R., Zhang, J. X., Shen, Y., & Zhang, S. Q. (2009). Production of a cytotoxic cationic antibacterial peptide in Escherichia coli using SUMO fusion partner. *Appl Microbiol Biotechnol*, 84, 383-388.

[88] Li, L., He, J., Eckert, R., Yarbrough, D., Lux, R., Anderson, M., & Shi, W. (2010). Design and characterization of an acid-activated antimicrobial peptide. *Chem Biol Drug Des*, 75, 127-132.

[89] Li, M., Lai, Y., Villaruz, A. E., Cha, D. J., Sturdevant, D. E., & Otto, M. (2007). Gram-positive three-component antimicrobial peptide-sensing system. *Proc Natl Acad Sci U S A*, 104, 9469-9474.

[90] Li, M., Yu, D. H., & Cai, H. (2008). The synthetic antimicrobial peptide KLKL5KLK enhances the protection and efficacy of the combined DNA vaccine against Mycobacterium tuberculosis. *DNA Cell Biol*, 27, 405-413.

[91] Lienkamp, K., Madkour, A. E., Musante, A., Nelson, C. F., Nusslein, K., & Tew, G. N. (2008). Antimicrobial polymers prepared by ROMP with unprecedented selectivity: a molecular construction kit approach. *J Am Chem Soc*, 130, 9836-9843.

[92] Lim, S. S., Song, Y. M., Jang, M. H., Kim, Y., Hahm, K. S., & Shin, S. Y. (2004a). Effects of two glycine residues in positions 13 and 17 of pleurocidin on structure and bacterial cell selectivity. *Protein Pept Lett*, 11, 35-40.

[93] Lipsky, B. A., Holroyd, K. J., & Zasloff, M. (2008). Topical versus systemic antimicrobial therapy for treating mildly infected diabetic foot ulcers: a randomized, controlled, double-blinded, multicenter trial of pexiganan cream. *Clin Infect Dis*, 47, 1537-1545.

[94] Liu, S., Yang, H., Wan, L., Cai, H. W., Li, S. F., Li, Y. P., Cheng, J. Q., & Lu, X. F. (2011). Enhancement of cytotoxicity of antimicrobial peptide magainin II in tumor cells by bombesin-targeted delivery. *Acta Pharmacol Sin*, 32, 79-88.

[95] Lynn, M. A., Kindrachuk, J., Marr, A. K., Jenssen, H., Pante, N., Elliott, M. R., Napper, S., Hancock, R. E., & Mc Master, W. R. (2011). Effect of BMAP-28 antimicrobial peptides on Leishmania major promastigote and amastigote growth: role of leishmanolysin in parasite survival. *PLoS Negl Trop Dis*, 5, e1141.

[96] Mader, J. S., Ewen, C., Hancock, R. E., & Bleackley, R. C. (2011). The human cathelicidin, LL-37, induces granzyme-mediated apoptosis in regulatory T cells. *J Immunother*, 34, 229-235.

[97] Mai, J., Tian, X. L., Gallant, J. W., Merkley, N., Biswas, Z., Syvitski, R., Douglas, S. E., Ling, J., & Li, Y. H. (2011). A novel target-specific, salt-resistant antimicrobial peptide against the cariogenic pathogen Streptococcus mutans. *Antimicrob Ag Chemother.*

[98] Makovitzki, A., Fink, A., & Shai, Y. (2009). Suppression of human solid tumor growth in mice by intratumor and systemic inoculation of histidine-rich and pH-dependent host defense-like lytic peptides. *Cancer Res*, 69, 3458-3463.

[99] Marcos, J. F., & Gandia, M. (2009). Antimicrobial peptides: to membranes and beyond. *Expert Opin Drug Discov*, 4, 659-671.

[100] Marsh, E. N., Buer, B. C., & Ramamoorthy, A. (2009). Fluorine--a new element in the design of membrane-active peptides. *Mol Biosyst*, 5, 1143-1147.

[101] Mason, A. J., Chotimah, I. N., Bertani, P., & Bechinger, B. (2006). A spectroscopic study of the membrane interaction of the antimicrobial peptide pleurocidin. *Mol Membr Biol*, 23, 185-194.

[102] Mason, A. J., Marquette, A., & Bechinger, B. (2007). Zwitterionic phospholipids and sterols modulate antimicrobial peptide-induced membrane destabilization. *Biophys J*, 93, 4289-4299.

[103] Mc Bride, S. M., & Sonenshein, A. L. (2011). Identification of a genetic locus responsible for antimicrobial peptide resistance in Clostridium difficile. *Infect Immun*, 79, 167-176.

[104] Mc Phee, J. B., & Hancock, R. E. (2005). Function and therapeutic potential of host defence peptides. *J Pept Sci*, 11, 677-687.

[105] Mc Phee, J. B., Lewenza, S., & Hancock, R. E. (2003). Cationic antimicrobial peptides activate a two-component regulatory system, PmrA-PmrB, that regulates resistance to polymyxin B and cationic antimicrobial peptides in Pseudomonas aeruginosa. *Mol Microbiol*, 50, 205-217.

[106] Menard, S., Forster, V., Lotz, M., Gutle, D., Duerr, C. U., Gallo, R. L., Henriques-Normark, B., Putsep, K., Andersson, M., Glocker, E. O., et al. (2008). Developmental switch of intestinal antimicrobial peptide expression. *J Exp Med*, 205, 183-193.

[107] Mogi, T., & Kita, K. (2009). Gramicidin S and polymyxins: the revival of cationic cyclic peptide antibiotics. *Cell Mol Life Sci*, 66, 3821-3826.

[108] Mor, A. (2009). Multifunctional host defense peptides: antiparasitic activities. *FEBS J*, 276, 6474-6482.

[109] Morash, M. G., Douglas, S. E., Robotham, A., Ridley, C. M., Gallant, J. W., & Soanes, K. H. (2011). The zebrafish embryo as a tool for screening and characterizing pleurocidin host-defense peptides as anti-cancer agents. *Dis Model Mech*, 4, 622-633.

[110] Morton, C. O., Dos, Santos. S. C., & Coote, P. (2007a). An amphibian-derived, cationic, alpha-helical antimicrobial peptide kills yeast by caspase-independent but AIF-dependent programmed cell death. *Mol Microbiol*, 65, 494-507.

[111] Morton, C. O., Hayes, A., Wilson, M., Rash, B. M., Oliver, S. G., & Coote, P. (2007b). Global phenotype screening and transcript analysis outlines the inhibitory mode(s) of action of two amphibian-derived, alpha-helical, cationic peptides on Saccharomyces cerevisiae. *Antimicrob Ag Chemother*, 51, 3948-3959.

[112] Murakami, T., Nakajima, T., Koyanagi, Y., Tachibana, K., Fujii, N., Tamamura, H., Yoshida, N., Waki, M., Matsumoto, A., Yoshie, O., et al. (1997). A small molecule CXCR4 inhibitor that blocks T cell line-tropic HIV-1 infection. *J Exp Med*, 186, 1389-1393.

[113] Murray, H. M., Leggiadro, C. T., & Douglas, S. E. (2007). Immunocytochemical localization of pleurocidin to the cytoplasmic granules of eosinophilic granular cells from the winter flounder gill. *J Fish Biol*, 70, 336-345.

[114] Mutwiri, G., Gerdts, V., Lopez, M., & Babiuk, L. A. (2007). Innate immunity and new adjuvants. *Rev Sci Tech*, 26, 147-156.

[115] Nguyen, L. T., Chau, J. K., Perry, N. A., de Boer, L., Zaat, S. A., & Vogel, H. J. (2010). Serum stabilities of short tryptophan- and arginine-rich antimicrobial peptide analogs. *PLoS One*, 5, e12684.

[116] Nguyen, L. T., Haney, E. F., & Vogel, H. J. (2011). The expanding scope of antimicrobial peptide structures and their modes of action. Trends Biotechnol , 29, 464-472.

[117] Nicolas, P. (2009). Multifunctional host defense peptides: intracellular-targeting antimicrobial peptides. *FEBS J*, 276, 6483-6496.

[118] Nijnik, A., & Hancock, R. E. (2009). Host defence peptides: antimicrobial and immunomodulatory activity and potential applications for tackling antibiotic-resistant infections. *Emerg Health Threats J*, 2, e1-7.

[119] Nizet, V. (2006). Antimicrobial peptide resistance mechanisms of human bacterial pathogens. *Curr Issues Mol Biol*, 8, 11-26.

[120] Noga, E. J., Ullal, A. J., Corrales, J., & Fernandes, J. M. (2011). Application of antimicrobial polypeptide host defenses to aquaculture: Exploitation of downregulation and upregulation responses. *Comp Biochem Physiol Part D Genomics Proteomics*, 6, 44-54.

[121] Oono, T., Shirafuji, Y., Huh, W. K., Akiyama, H., & Iwatsuki, K. (2002). Effects of human neutrophil peptide-1 on the expression of interstitial collagenase and type I collagen in human dermal fibroblasts. *Arch Dermatol Res*, 294, 185-189.

[122] Park, C. B., Yi, K. S., Matsuzaki, K., Kim, M. S., & Kim, S. C. (2000). Structure-activity analysis of buforin II, a histone H2A-derived antimicrobial peptide: the proline hinge is responsible for the cell-penetrating ability of buforin II. *Proc Natl Acad Sci U S A*, 97, 8245-8250.

[123] Park, Y., Park, S. C., Kim, J. Y., Park, J. O., Seo, C. H., Nah, J. W., & Hahm, K. S. (2010). In vitro efficacy of a synthetic all-d antimicrobial peptide against clinically isolated drug-resistant strains. *Int J Antimicrob Agents*, 35, 208-209.

[124] Patrzykat, A., Friedrich, C. L., Zhang, L., Mendoza, V., & Hancock, R. E. (2002). Sublethal concentrations of pleurocidin-derived antimicrobial peptides inhibit macromolecular synthesis in Escherichia coli. *Antimicrob Ag Chemother*, 46, 605-614.

[125] Patrzykat, A., Gallant, J. W., Seo, J. K., Pytyck, J., & Douglas, S. E. (2003). Novel antimicrobial peptides derived from flatfish genes. *Antimicrob Ag Chemother*, 47, 2464-2470.

[126] Patrzykat, A., Zhang, L., Mendoza, V., Iwama, G. K., & Hancock, R. E. (2001). Synergy of histone-derived peptides of coho salmon with lysozyme and flounder pleurocidin. *Antimicrob Agents Chemother*, 45, 1337-1342.

[127] Peschel, A., & Sahl, H. G. (2006). The co-evolution of host cationic antimicrobial peptides and microbial resistance. *Nat Rev Microbiol*, 4, 529-536.

[128] Pieters, R. J., Arnusch, C. J., & Breukink, E. (2009). Membrane permeabilization by multivalent anti-microbial peptides. *Protein Pept Lett*, 16, 736-742.

[129] Projan, S. J., & Bradford, P. A. (2007). Late stage antibacterial drugs in the clinical pipeline. *Curr Opin Microbiol*, 10, 441-446.

[130] Redfern, R. L., Reins, R. Y., & Mc Dermott, A. M. (2011). Toll-like receptor activation modulates antimicrobial peptide expression by ocular surface cells. *Exp Eye Res*, 92, 209-220.

[131] Riedl, S., Rinner, B., Asslaber, M., Schaider, H., Walzer, S., Novak, A., Lohner, K., & Zweytick, D. (2011). In search of a novel target- phosphatidylserine exposed by non-apoptotic tumor cells and metastases of malignancies with poor treatment efficacy. *Biochim Biophys Acta*, 1808, 2638-2645.

[132] Risso, A., Zanetti, M., & Gennaro, R. (1998). Cytotoxicity and apoptosis mediated by two peptides of innate immunity. *Cell Immunol*, 189, 107-115.

[133] Rotem, S., & Mor, A. (2009). Antimicrobial peptide mimics for improved therapeutic properties. *Biochim Biophys Acta*, 1788, 1582-1592.

[134] Roy, S., & Das, P. K. (2008). Antibacterial hydrogels of amino acid-based cationic amphiphiles. Biotechnol Bioeng , 100, 756-764.

[135] Sa'adedin, F., & Bradshaw, J. P. (2010). A differential scanning calorimetry study of the effects and interactions of antimicrobial peptide LS3 on phosphatidylethanolamine bilayers. *Protein Pept Lett*. 17, 1345-1350.

[136] Saint, N., Cadiou, H., Bessin, Y., & Molle, G. (2002). Antibacterial peptide pleurocidin forms ion channels in planar lipid bilayers. *Biochim Biophys Acta*, 1564, 359-364.

[137] Schutte, B. C., Mitros, J. P., Bartlett, J. A., Walters, J. D., Jia, H. P., Welsh, M. J., Casavant, T. L., & Mc Cray, P. B., Jr. (2002). Discovery of five conserved beta-defensin gene clusters using a computational search strategy. *Proc Natl Acad Sci U S A*, 99, 2129-2133.

[138] Scott, R. W., De Grado, W. F., & Tew, G. N. (2008). De novo designed synthetic mimics of antimicrobial peptides. *Curr Opin Biotechnol*, 19, 620-627.

[139] Selsted, M. E., & Ouellette, A. J. (2005). Mammalian defensins in the antimicrobial immune response. *Nat Immunol*, 6, 551-557.

[140] Selvatici, R., Falzarano, S., Mollica, A., & Spisani, S. (2006). Signal transduction pathways triggered by selective formylpeptide analogues in human neutrophils. *Eur J Pharmacol*, 534, 1-11.

[141] Shai, Y. (2002). Mode of action of membrane active antimicrobial peptides. *Biopolymers*, 66, 236-248.

[142] Shai, Y., Makovitzky, A., & Avrahami, D. (2006). Host defense peptides and lipopeptides: modes of action and potential candidates for the treatment of bacterial and fungal infections. *Curr Protein Pept Sci*, 7, 479-486.

[143] Shen, C. J., Kuo, T. Y., Lin, C. C., Chow, L. P., & Chen, W. J. (2010). Proteomic identification of membrane proteins regulating antimicrobial peptide resistance in Vibrio parahaemolyticus. *J Appl Microbiol*, 108, 1398-1407.

[144] Splith, K., & Neundorf, I. (2011). Antimicrobial peptides with cell-penetrating peptide properties and vice versa. *Eur Biophys J*, 40, 387-397.

[145] Steinstraesser, L., Burghard, O., Nemzek, J., Fan, M. H., Merry, A., Remick, D. I., Su, G. L., Steinau, H. U., & Wang, S. C. (2003). Protegrin-1 increases bacterial clearance in sepsis but decreases survival. *Crit Care Med*, 31, 221-226.

[146] Steinstraesser, L., Koehler, T., Jacobsen, F., Daigeler, A., Goertz, O., Langer, S., Kesting, M., Steinau, H., Eriksson, E., & Hirsch, T. (2008). Host defense peptides in wound healing. *Mol Med*, 14, 528-537.

[147] Sullivan, R., Santarpia, P., Lavender, S., Gittins, E., Liu, Z., Anderson, M. H., He, J., Shi, W., & Eckert, R. (2011). Clinical efficacy of a specifically targeted antimicrobial peptide mouth rinse: Targeted elimination of Streptococcus mutans and prevention of demineralization. *Caries Res*, 45, 415-428.

[148] Sun, B. J., Xie, H. X., Song, Y., & Nie, P. (2007). Gene structure of an antimicrobial peptide from mandarin fish, Siniperca chuatsi (Basilewsky), suggests that moronecidins and pleurocidins belong in one family: the piscidins. *J Fish Dis*, 30, 335-343.

[149] Sung, W. S., & Lee, D. G. (2008). Pleurocidin-derived antifungal peptides with selective membrane-disruption effect. *Biochem Biophys Res Commun*, 369, 858-861.

[150] Syvitski, R. T., Burton, I., Mattatall, N. R., Douglas, S. E., & Jakeman, D. L. (2005). Structural characterization of the antimicrobial peptide pleurocidin from winter flounder. *Biochemistry*, 44, 7282-7293.

[151] Talukder, P., Satho, T., Irie, K., Sharmin, T., Hamady, D., Nakashima, Y., Kashige, N., & Miake, F. (2011). Trace metal zinc stimulates secretion of antimicrobial peptide LL-37 from Caco-2 cells through ERK and 38MAP kinase. *Int Immunopharmacol 11*, 141-144.

[152] Tani, K., Shimizu, T., Kida, Y., & Kuwano, K. (2011). Mycoplasma pneumoniae infection induces a neutrophil-derived antimicrobial peptide, cathelin-related antimicrobial peptide. *Microbiol Immunol*, 55, 582-588.

[153] Tao, R., Tong, Z., Lin, Y., Xue, Y., Wang, W., Kuang, R., Wang, P., Tian, Y., & Ni, L. (2011). Antimicrobial and antibiofilm activity of pleurocidin against cariogenic microorganisms. *Peptides*, 32, 1748-1754.

[154] Tavano, R., Segat, D., Gobbo, M., & Papini, E. (2011). The honeybee antimicrobial peptide apidaecin differentially immunomodulates human macrophages, monocytes and dendritic cells. *J Innate Immun*.

[155] Tay, D. K., Rajagopalan, G., Li, X., Chen, Y., Lua, L. H., & Leong, S. S. (2011). A new bioproduction route for a novel antimicrobial peptide. *Biotechnol Bioeng*, 108, 572-581.

[156] Tokumaru, S., Sayama, K., Shirakata, Y., Komatsuzawa, H., Ouhara, K., Hanakawa, Y., Yahata, Y., Dai, X., Tohyama, M., Nagai, H., et al. (2005). Induction of keratinocyte migration via transactivation of the epidermal growth factor receptor by the antimicrobial peptide LL-37. *J Immunol*, 175, 4662-4668.

[157] Tomasinsig, L., Scocchi, M., Mettulio, R., & Zanetti, M. (2004). Genome-wide transcriptional profiling of the Escherichia coli response to a proline-rich antimicrobial peptide. *Antimicrob Agents Chemother*, 48, 3260-3267.

[158] Torrent, M., Andreu, D., Nogues, V. M., & Boix, E. (2011). Connecting peptide physicochemical and antimicrobial properties by a rational prediction model. *PLoS One* , 6, e16968.

[159] Tosteson, M. T., Holmes, S. J., Razin, M., & Tosteson, D. C. (1985). Melittin lysis of red cells. *J Membr Biol*, 87, 35-44.

[160] Turkoglu, O., Kandiloglu, G., Berdeli, A., Emingil, G., & Atilla, G. (2011). Antimicrobial peptide hCAP-18/LL-37 protein and mRNA expressions in different periodontal diseases. *Oral Dis*, 17, 60-67.

[161] van Beek, W. P., Smets, L. A., & Emmelot, P. (1973). Increased sialic acid density in surface glycoprotein of transformed and malignant cells--a general phenomenon? *Cancer Res*, 33, 2913-2922.

[162] van der Does, A. M., Bogaards, S. J., Ravensbergen, B., Beekhuizen, H., van Dissel, J. T., & Nibbering, P. H. (2010). Antimicrobial peptide hLF1-11 directs granulocyte-macrophage colony-stimulating factor-driven monocyte differentiation toward macrophages with enhanced recognition and clearance of pathogens. *Antimicrob Ag Chemother*, 54, 811-816.

[163] Venugopal, D. (2010). Novel antimicrobial peptides that exhibit activity against select agents and other drug resistant bacteria. *Bioorg Med Chem*, 18, 5137-5147.

[164] Vylkova, S., Nayyar, N., Li, W., & Edgerton, M. (2007). Human beta-defensins kill Candida albicans in an energy-dependent and salt-sensitive manner without causing membrane disruption. *Antimicrob Agents Chemother*, 51, 154-161.

[165] Wallace, D. F., Jones, M. D., Pedersen, P., Rivas, L., Sly, L. I., & Subramaniam, V. N. (2006). Purification and partial characterisation of recombinant human hepcidin. *Biochimie*, 88, 31-37.

[166] Walsh, E. G., Maher, S., Devocelle, M., O'Brien, P. J., Baird, A. W., & Brayden, D. J. (2011). High content analysis to determine cytotoxicity of the antimicrobial peptide, melittin and selected structural analogs. *Peptides*, 32, 1764-1773.

[167] Wang, C., Li, H. B., Li, S., Tian, L. L., & Shang, D. J. (2011). Antitumor effects and cell selectivity of temporin-1CEa, an antimicrobial peptide from the skin secretions of the Chinese brown frog (Rana chensinensis). *Biochimie*.

[168] Wang, G., Watson, K. M., Peterkofsky, A., & Buckheit, R. W., Jr. (2010). Identification of novel human immunodeficiency virus type 1-inhibitory peptides based on the antimicrobial peptide database. *Antimicrob Ag Chemother*, 54, 1343-1346.

[169] Wehkamp, J., Harder, J., Weichenthal, M., Mueller, O., Herrlinger, K. R., Fellermann, K., Schroeder, J. M., & Stange, E. F. (2003). Inducible and constitutive beta-defensins are differentially expressed in Crohn's disease and ulcerative colitis. *Inflamm Bowel Dis*, 9, 215-223.

[170] White, J. H. (2010). Vitamin D as an inducer of cathelicidin antimicrobial peptide expression: past, present and future. *J Steroid Biochem Mol Biol*, 121, 234-238.

[171] Wiesner, J., & Vilcinskas, A. (2010). Antimicrobial peptides: the ancient arm of the human immune system. *Virulence*, 1, 440-464.

[172] Williams, K. J., & Bax, R. P. (2009). Challenges in developing new antibacterial drugs. *Curr Opin Investig Drugs*, 10, 157-163.

[173] Won, A., Khan, M., Gustin, S., Akpawu, A., Seebun, D., Avis, T. J., Leung, B. O., Hitchcock, A. P., & Ianoul, A. (2011a). Investigating the effects of L- to D-amino acid substitution and deamidation on the activity and membrane interactions of antimicrobial peptide anoplin. *Biochim Biophys Acta*, 1808, 1592-1600.

[174] Won, H. S., Kang, S. J., Choi, W. S., & Lee, B. J. (2011b). Activity optimization of an undecapeptide analogue derived from a frog-skin antimicrobial peptide. *Mol Cells*, 31, 49-54.

[175] Wu, G., Li, X., Deng, X., Fan, X., Wang, S., Shen, Z., & Xi, T. (2011). Protective effects of antimicrobial peptide S-thanatin against endotoxic shock in mice introduced by LPS. *Peptides*, 32, 353-357.

[176] Yala, J. F., Thebault, P., Hequet, A., Humblot, V., Pradier, C. M., & Berjeaud, J. M. (2011). Elaboration of antibiofilm materials by chemical grafting of an antimicrobial peptide. *Appl Microbiol Biotechnol*, 89, 623-634.

[177] Yang, D., Chen, Q., Schmidt, A. P., Anderson, G. M., Wang, J. M., Wooters, J., Oppenheim, J. J., & Chertov, O. (2000). LL-37, the neutrophil granule- and epithelial cell-derived cathelicidin, utilizes formyl peptide receptor-like 1 (FPRL1) as a receptor to

chemoattract human peripheral blood neutrophils, monocytes, and T cells. *J Exp Med,* 192, 1069-1074.

[178] Yang, J. Y., Shin, S. Y., Lim, S. S., Hahm, K. S., & Kim, Y. (2006). Structure and bacterial cell selectivity of a fish-derived antimicrobial peptide, pleurocidin. *J Microbiol Biotechnol,* 16, 880-888.

[179] Yang, K., Gitter, B., Ruger, R., Wieland, G. D., Chen, M., Liu, X., Albrecht, V., & Fahr, A. (2011). Antimicrobial peptide-modified liposomes for bacteria targeted delivery of temoporfin in photodynamic antimicrobial chemotherapy. *Photochem Photobiol Sci,* 10, 1593-1560.

[180] Yarus, S., Rosen, J. M., Cole, A. M., & Diamond, G. (1996). Production of active bovine tracheal antimicrobial peptide in milk of transgenic mice. *Proc Natl Acad Sci U S A,* 93, 14118-14121.

[181] Yeung, A. T., Gellatly, S. L., & Hancock, R. E. (2011). Multifunctional cationic host defence peptides and their clinical applications. *Cell Mol Life Sci,* 68, 2161-2176.

[182] Yevtushenko, D. P., Romero, R., Forward, B. S., Hancock, R. E., Kay, W. W., & Misra, S. (2005). Pathogen-induced expression of a cecropin A-melittin antimicrobial peptide gene confers antifungal resistance in transgenic tobacco. *J Exp Bot,* 56, 1685-1695.

[183] Yoon, W. H., Park, H. D., Lim, K., & Hwang, B. D. (1996). Effect of O-glycosylated mucin on invasion and metastasis of HM7 human colon cancer cells. *Biochem Biophys Res Commun,* 222, 694-699.

[184] Yoshida, K., Mukai, Y., Niidome, T., Takashi, C., Tokunaga, Y., Hatakeyama, Y., & Aoyagi, H. (2001). Interaction of pleurocidin and its analogs with phospholipid membrane and their antibacterial activity. *J Pept Res,* 57, 119-126.

[185] Zasloff, M. (2002). Antimicrobial peptides of multicellular organisms. *Nature,* 415, 389-395.

[186] Zasloff, M. (2006). Inducing endogenous antimicrobial peptides to battle infections. *Proc Natl Acad Sci U S A,* 103, 8913-8914.

[187] Zhang, J., Yang, Y., Teng, D., Tian, Z., Wang, S., & Wang, J. (2011). Expression of plectasin in Pichia pastoris and its characterization as a new antimicrobial peptide against Staphyloccocus and Streptococcus. *Protein Expr Purif,* 78, 189-196.

[188] Zhang, L., & Falla, T. J. (2010). Potential therapeutic application of host defense peptides. *Methods Mol Biol,* 618, 303-327.

Section 3

Bioactive Ingredients in Nutrition

Chapter 6

Anticancer Properties of Phytochemicals Present in Medicinal Plants of North America

Wasundara Fernando and
H. P. Vasantha Rupasinghe

Additional information is available at the end of the chapter

http://dx.doi.org/10.5772/55859

1. Introduction

Cancer is one of the most severe health problems in both developing and developed countries, worldwide. Among the most common (lung, stomach, colorectal, liver, breast) types of cancers, lung cancer has continued to be the most common cancer diagnosed in men and breast cancer is the most common cancer diagnosed in women. An estimated 12.7 million people were diagnosed with cancer across the world in 2008, and 7.6 million people died from the cancer during the same year [1]. Lung cancer, breast cancer, colorectal cancer and stomach cancer accounted for two-fifths of the total cases of cancers diagnosed worldwide [1]. More than 70% of all cancer deaths occurred in low- and middle-income countries. Deaths due to cancer are projected to continuously increase and it has been estimated that there will be 11.5 million deaths in the year 2030 [1] and 27 million new cancer cases and 17.5 million cancer deaths are projected to occur in the world by 2050 [2]. According to Canadian cancer statistics, issued by the Canadian Cancer Society, it is estimated that 186,400 new cases of cancer (excluding 81,300 non-melanoma skin cancers) and 75,700 deaths from cancer will occur in Canada in 2012 [1]. The lowest number of incidences and mortality rate is recorded in British Columbia. Both incidence and mortality rates are higher in Atlantic Canada and Quebec [3].

More than 30% of cancers are caused by modifiable behavioral and environmental risk factors, including tobacco and alcohol use, dietary factors, insufficient regular consumption of fruit and vegetable, overweight and obesity, physical inactivity, chronic infections from *Helicobacter pylori*, hepatitis B virus (HBV), hepatitis C virus (HCV) and some types of human papilloma virus (HPV), environmental and occupational risks including exposure to ionizing and non-ionizing radiation [4].

Conventional treatment of cancer includes interventions such as psychosocial support, surgery, radiotherapy and chemotherapy [4]. Currently, the most commonly use cancer chemotherapy includes mainly alkylating agents, antimetabolites, antitumor antibiotics, platinum analogs and natural anticancer agents. However, due to the increasing rate of mortality associated with cancer and adverse or toxic side effects of cancer chemotherapy and radiation therapy, discovery of new anticancer agents derived from nature, especially plants, is currently under investigation. Screening of medicinal plants as a source of anticancer agents was started in the 1950s, with the discovery and development of vinca alkaloids, vinblastine and vincristine and the isolation of the cytotoxic podophyllotoxins [5] (Figure 01). The cool temperate climate of North America supports the growth of an enormous number of plant species which are important sources of unique phytochemicals having anticancer properties (Table 01). In this chapter, selected medicinal plants grown in the cool climate of North America (mainly Canada and USA) are discussed. The major bioactive phytochemicals and their mechanisms of action are also reviewed.

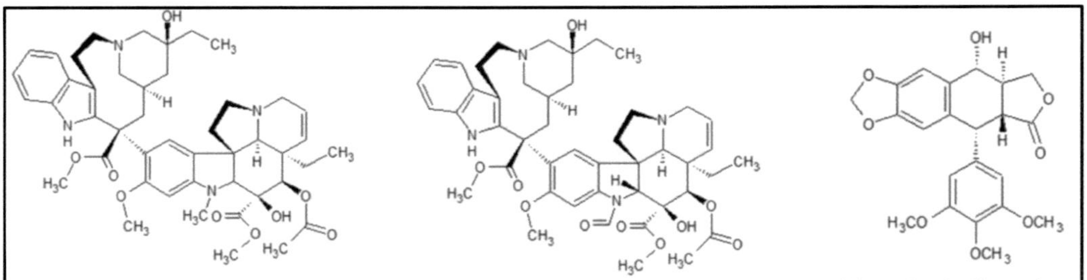

(a) Vinblastine **(b) Vincristine** **(c) Podophyllotoxins**

Metabolite	*Natural source*		*Mode of action*	*Ref*
	Botanical name	*Family*		
Vinblastine	*Catharanthus roseus* (Madagascar periwinkle)	Apocenacea	Inhibition of microtubule assembly	6, 7
Vincristine	*Catharanthus roseus* (Madagascar periwinkle)	Apocenacea	Inhibition of microtubule assembly	6, 7
Podophyllotoxins	*Podophyllum hexandrum* (Himalayan mayapple)	Berberidaceae	Inhibition of microtubule assembly	8, 9

(a) Vinblastine – [dimethyl (2β,3β,4β,5α,12β,19α)- 15-[(5S,9S)- 5-ethyl- 5-hydroxy- 9-(methoxycarbonyl)-1,4,5,6,7,8,9,10-octahydro- 2H- 3,7-methanoazacycloundecino[5,4-b]indol- 9-yl] - 3-hydroxy- 16-methoxy- 1-methyl-6,7-didehydroaspidospermidine- 3,4-dicarboxylate] (b) Vincristin – [(3aR,3a1R,4R,5S,5aR,10bR)-methyl 4-acetoxy-3a-ethyl-9-((5S,7S,9S)-5-ethyl-5-hydroxy-9-(methoxycarbonyl)-2,4,5,6,7,8,9,10-octahydro-1H-3,7-methano[1]azacycloundecino[5,4-b]indol-9-yl)-6-formyl-5-hydroxy-8-methoxy-3a,3a1,4,5,5a,6,11,12-octahydro-1H-indolizino[8,1-cd]carbazole-5-carboxylate] (c) Podophyllotoxin – [(10*R*,11*R*,15*R*,16*R*)-16-hydroxy-10-(3,4,5-trimethoxyphenyl)-4,6,13-trioxatetracyclohexadeca-1,3(7),8-trien-12-one]

Figure 1. Some selected currently used phytochemical-based anticancer agents

Plant	Family	Parts used	Major bioactive compounds	Growing regions	Ref
Achyranthes aspera (Devil's Horsewhip)	Amaranthaceae	Leaf	Triterpenoid saponins	USA	14
Annona glabra (Pond apple)	Annonaceae	Leaf and fruit	Acetogenins	USA	15
Aralia nudicaulis (Wild sarsaparilla)	Araliacea	Whole plant	Steroids, sarsasapogenin, smilagenin, sitosterol, stigmasterol, pollinastrenol, glycosides, saponins, sarsasaponin parillin, smilasaponin, smilacin, sarsaparilloside, and sitosterol glucoside	Mainly Canada	16
Aster brachyactis (Rayless aster)	Asteraceae	Aerial parts	Not known	North America	17
Carduus nutans (Nodding plumeless thistle)	Asteraceae	Aerial parts	Linalool derivatives, aliphatic acids, diacids, aromatic acids, and phenols	North America	18, 19
Erythronium americanum (Adder's tongue)	Liliaceae	Whole plant	Alpha-methylenebutyrolactone	North America	20, 21
Eupatorium cannabinum (Bonesets)	Asteraceae	Whole plant	Sesquiterpene lactone, pyrrolizidine alkaloid, and flavonoid	North America	20, 21,19, 22
Foeniculum vulgare (Wild pepper fennel)	Apiaceae	Seed	α-pinene, anisic aldehyde, cineole, fecchone, limonene, and myrcene	North America	23
Hydrastis canadensis (Orange root)	Ranunculaceae	Whole plant	Isoquinoline alkaloids (hydrastine, berberine, berberastine, candaline), resin and lactone	Canada, USA	20, 21
Hypericum perforatum (St. John's wort)	Clusiaceae	Flower	Hypericin and hyperforin	USA, Canada (British Columbia)	24
Lactuca sativa (Garden lettuce)	Asteraceae	Leaf	Sesquiterpene lactone	USA, Canada	25
Lantana camara (Wild sage)	Verbenaceae	Whole plant	Alkaloids (camerine, isocamerine, micranine, lantanine, lantadene), phenols, flavonoids, tannins, saponins, and phytosterols	USA	26, 27, 28
Larrea tridentate (Creosote bush)	Zygophyllaceae	Whole plant	Resins and lignans	Southwestern USA	18, 29, 30
Linum usitatissimum (Common Flax)	Linaceae	Seed	Enterodiol, enterolactone, lignans, and omega-3 fatty acids	Canada, USA	31, 32

Plant	Family	Parts used	Major bioactive compounds	Growing regions	Ref
Olea europrae (Olive)	Oleaceae	Leaf and oil	Oleuropein, hydroxytyrosol, hydroxytyrosol acetate, luteolin-7-O-glucoside, luteolin-4'-O-glucoside and luteolin, oleic acid and polyphenol	USA	33, 34, 35, 36, 37
Panax quinquefolius (North American Ginseng)	Araliaceae	Root, Leaf	Ginsenosides and saponins	Eastern North America	20, 21
Plantago lanceolata (Ribwort plantain)	Plantaginaceae	Aerial parts	Phenolics and flavonoids	Canada, USA	38
Podophyllum peltatum (Mayapple)	Berberidaceae	Rhizome	Podophyllotoxins	Eastern North America	39
Polygonatum multiflorum (Tuber fleece flower)	Polygonaceae	Whole plant	Saponin and flavonoid and vitamin A	USA	20, 21, 40
Pyrus malus (Apple)	Rosaceae	Bark and fruit	Quercetin, catechin, flavonoid, coumaric and gallic acids, phloridzin and procyanidin	North America	21
Rhodiola rosea (Golden root)	Crassulaceae	Rhizome	Monoterpene alcohols and their glycosides, cyanogenic glycosides, aryl glycosides, phenylethanoids, phenylpropanoids and their glycosides, flavonoids, flavonlignans, proanthocyanidins and gallic acid derivatives	Eastern Canada	41, 42
Saponaria vaccaria (Cowherb)	Caryophyllaceae	Seed	Flavonoids, cyclopeptides, and bisdesmosidic saponins	Western Canada	43
Silybum marianum (Milk thistle)	Asteraceae	Dried fruit, seed	Silymarin-polyphenoic flavolignans (silybin, isosilybin, silychristin, silydianin and taxifoline)	Canada, USA	44, 45
Sonchus arvensis (Perennial sow-thistle)	Asteraceae	Whole plant	Alkanes, n-alkenes, n-aldehydes and n-alcohols, shikimate metabolites, carotenoid-derived compounds, terpenoids, steroids, and phenols	Canada	46, 47
Tanacetum vulgare (Tansy)	Asteraceae	Aerial parts	Monoterpenes, sesqueterpenes, and oxygenated sesqueterpenes	Canada, USA	48
Taraxacum officinale (Dandelions)	Asteraceae	Root and leaf	Sesquiterpene lactones, triterpenoids, sterols, tannins, alkaloids, inulin, caffeic acid, and flavonoids	North America	49

Plant	Family	Parts used	Major bioactive compounds	Growing regions	Ref
Taxus brevifolia (Pacific yew tree)	Taxaceae	Bark	Taxol (diterpene)	Pacific Northwest	50
Thuja occidentalis (White cedar)	Cupressaceae	Whole plant	Flavonoid, tannin, and volatile oil	Northeastern USA, Eastern Canada	13, 51
Xanthium strumarium (Cocklebur)	Asteraceae	Fruit	Sesquiterpene lactones (Xanthatin and Xanthinosin)	Canada	17

Table 1. Medicinal plants with potential anticancer properties grown in North America

2. Pathophysiology of cancer

Cancer is a population of abnormal cells which divide without control, with the ability to invade other tissues. Cancer and some of the other chronic diseases share common pathogenesis mechanisms, such as DNA damage, oxidative stress, and chronic inflammation [10]. It is understood that both environmental factors and chemical carcinogens play a key role in the initiation and progression of cancer. Among the major environmental factors are asbestos, polluted air near industrial emission sources, exposure to secondary tobacco smoke, indoor air pollution such as radon, drinking water containing arsenic, chlorination by-products, and other pollutants [11]. Chemicals with carcinogenic activity can be classified as DNA reactive (e.g.: nitrogen mustards, chlorambucil, epoxides, aliphatic halides, aromatic amines), epigenetic (e.g.: chlordane, pentachlorophenol, hormones, cyclosporin, purine analogs), dichlorodiphenyltrichloroethane, phenobarbital, minerals (e.g.: asbestos), metals (e.g.: arsenic, beryllium, cadmium) and unclassified carcinogens (e.g.: acrylamide, acrylonitrile, dioxane) [12]. DNA-reactive carcinogens act in the target cells of tissue(s) of their carcinogenicity to form DNA adducts that are the basis for neoplastic transformation [12]. Epigenetic carcinogens lack chemical reactivity and hence, do not form DNA adducts. These carcinogens are produced in the target cells of tissue(s) of their carcinogenicity. Effects of epigenetic carcinogens indirectly lead to neoplastic transformation or enhance the development of tumors from cryptogenically transformed cells [12].

Carcinogenesis is a multi-step process consisting of tumor initiation, promotion and progression [13]. Cancer initiation can be blocked by activating protective mechanisms, either in the extracellular environment or intracellular environment by modifying trans-membrane transport, modulating metabolism, blocking reactive oxygen and nitrogen species, maintaining DNA structure, modulating DNA metabolism and repair, and controlling gene expression [10]. Tumor promotion is the second stage of carcinogenesis and is followed by tumor progression. Both stages can be suppressed by inhibiting genotoxic effects, favoring antioxidant and anti-inflammatory activity, inhibiting proteases and cell proliferation, inducing cell differentiation, modulating apoptosis and signal transduction pathways and protecting intercellular communications [10]. In addition, tumor progression can also be inhibited by affecting the hormonal status and the immune system in various ways and by inhibiting tumor angiogenesis [10].

3. In vitro anticancer activity of phytochemicals and extracts of medicinal plants

Cultured cancer-derived cell lines with comparison to normal healthy cell lines are commonly used to assess the anticancer properties of isolated phytochemicals and extracts of medicinal plants (Table 2). The anticancer properties of ethanolic extract of leaves, pulp and seeds of, *Annona glabra* (L.), commonly known as pond apple, were shown, using human drug-sensitive leukemia (CEM) and its multidrug-resistant-derived (CEM/VLB) cell lines [52]. The most potent anticancer activity was shown in the seed extract of *A. glabra* [52]. Both dried rhizome hexane extract and dried fruit hexane extract, partitioned from total methanol extract, of *Aralia nudicaulis* (L.) caused death of cancer cell lines such as human colon cancer cell (WiDr), human leukemia cell (Molt) and human cervix cancer cell (HeLa) at a lower concentration, than that of required for the death of normal cells [53]. Eupatoriopicrin, a sesquiterpene lactone isolated from *Eupatorium cannabinum* (L.) (Bonesets), indicated anticancer properties on FIO 26 (fibrosarcoma) cells with an IC_{50}=1.5 μg/ml [22]. Methanolic extracts of *Hypericum perforatum* (L.) (St. Johns wort) possessed strong antiproliferative activity in the human prostate cell line (PC-3) and the major constituents, hyperforin and hypericin, synergistically contributed to the reduction of the PC-3 cells proliferation [24]. Maslinic acid, (Figure 2(a)) a triterpene from *Olea europaea* (L.) (Olive), has shown to be significantly inhibitory in cell proliferation of the human colorectal adenocarcinoma cell line (HT29) in a dose dependent manner [33]. The major components in the extract were identified to be oleuropein, hydroxytyrosol, hydroxytyrosol acetate, luteolin-7-*O*-glucoside, luteolin-4'-*O*-glucoside and luteolin [34] (Figure 2). All these phytochemicals inhibited the proliferation of cancer and endothelial cells with IC_{50}, at the low micromolar range [37]. Methanolic leaf extract of *Plantago lanceolata* (L.) (Ribwort plantain) inhibited the growth of three different cell lines; human renal adenocarcinoma (TK-10), the human breast adenocarcinoma (MCF-7) and the human melanoma (UACC-62) cell lines and the MCF-7 was totally inhibited [54]. Further, the ethanolic extract of *P. lanceolata* (L.), produced by maceration with ethanol : water, showed significant antiproliferative activity on cervix epithelioid carcinoma (HeLa), breast adenocarcinoma (MCF-7), colon adenocarcinoma (HT-29) and human fetal lung carcinoma (MRC-5) [38]. Several chemical constituents (Figure 3) from *Silybum marianum* (Milkthistle) have been isolated and their cytotoxic and anticancer potential has been investigated, *in vitro*, using both cancer and normal healthy cell lines. Silymarin, isolated from seeds of *S. marianum*, is a mixture of series of flavolignans, major constituents being: silybin A and B, (also known as silibinin), isosilybin A and B, silychristin, and silydianin [55, 56].

http://dx.doi.org/10.5772/55859

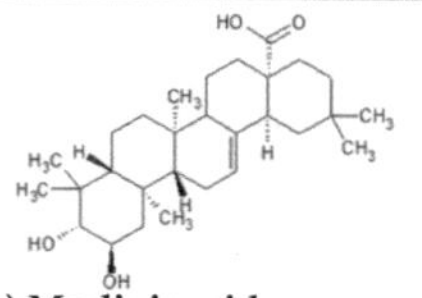

(a) Maslinic acid

IC_{50} (μg/ml)	MOA	Ref
28.8	Bcl-2 inhibition Bax activation	33

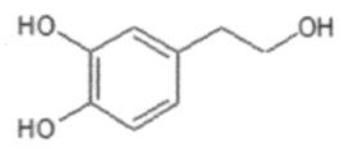

(b) Hydroxytyrosol

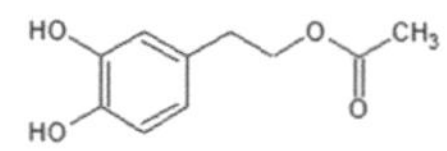

(c) Hydroxytyrosol acetate

Metabolite	IC_{50} (μg/ml)					MOA	Ref
	BBCE	T24	MCF-7	HL60	HT29		
Hydroxytyrosol	2.4	12.4	24.9	50.0	750.0	Cell cycle arrest at G_0/ G_1	34,35,53
Hydroxytyrosol acetate	9.3	23.3	28.7	-	-		34

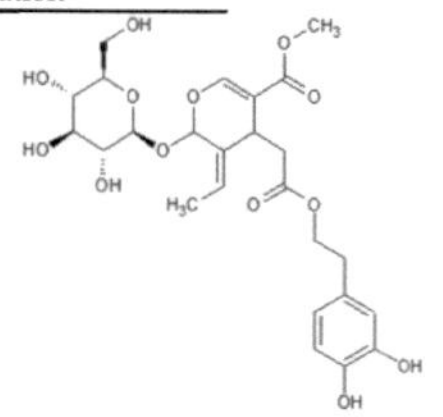

(d) Oleuropein

IC_{50}(μg/ml)			MOA	Ref
BBCE	T24	MCF-7		
2.6	7.6	12.0	Induce G_1 cell cycle arrest	35 37

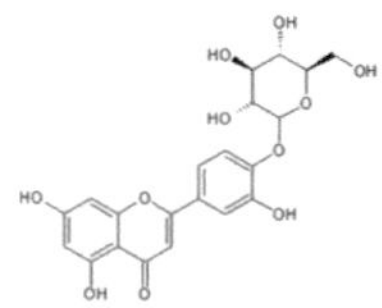

(e) Luteolin-4′-*O*-glucoside

IC_{50} (μg/ml)			MOA	Ref
BBCE	T24	MCF-7		
30.9	31.7	10.8	-	37

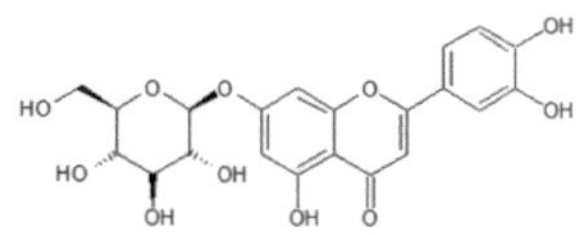

(f) Luteolin-7-*O*-glucoside

IC_{50} (μg/ml)			MOA	Ref
BBCE	T24	MCF-7		
3.9	11.4	40.9	Inhibition of Topoisomerase - 1	37, 55

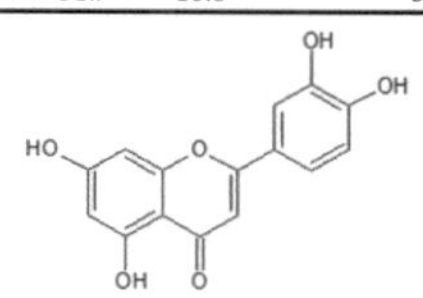

(g) Luteolin

IC_{50} (μg/ml)			MOA	Ref
BBCE	T24	MCF-7		
9.7	28.2	9.1	Inhibition of Topoisomerase - 1	37, 55

IC_{50}: Concentration which inhibited 50% of cell proliferation; **MOA:** Mode of Action; **BBCE:** Bovine Brain Capillary Endothelial cells; **T24:** Human Urinary Bladder Carcinoma cells; **MCF-7:** Human Breast Adenocarcinoma cells; **HL60:** Human Promyelocytic Leukaemia cells; **HT29:** Colon Adenocarcinoma cells

(a) Maslinic acid - [(2a, 3b)-2,3-dihydroxyolean-12-en-28-oic acid]: (b) Oleuropein – [(4S,5E,6S)-4-[2-[2-(3,4-dihydroxyphenyl)ethoxy]-2-oxoethyl]- 5-ethylidene-6-[[(2S,3R,4S,5S,6R)-3,4,5-trihydroxy-6-(hydroxymethyl)- 2-tetrahydropyranyl]oxy]-4H-pyran-3-carboxylic acid, methyl ester] : (c) Hydroxytyrosol – [4-(2-Hydroxyethyl)-1,2-benzenediol]: (d) Hydroxytyrosol acetate – [2-(3,4-dihydroxy)Phenyl ethyl acetate;4-[2-(Acetyloxy)ethyl]-1,2-benzenediol]: (e) Luteolin-7-O-glucoside - [2-(3,4-dihydroxyphenyl)-5-hydroxy-4-oxo-4H-chromen-7-yl beta-D-glucopyranoside; 4H-1-benzopyran-4-one, 2-(3,4-dihydroxyphenyl)-7-(beta-D-glucopyranosyloxy)-5-hydroxy-; 2-(3,4-Dihydroxy-phenyl)-5-hydroxy-7-((2S,3R,4S,5S,6R)-3,4,5-trihydroxy-6-hydroxymethyl-tetrahydro-pyran-2-yloxy)-chromen-4-one] (f) Luteolin-4′-O-glucoside – [3′,5,7-Trihydroxy-4′-(β-D-glucopyranosyloxy)flavone;2-(4-β-D-Glucopyranosyloxy-3-hydroxyphenyl)-5,7-dihydroxy-4H-1-benzopyran-4-one;2-[3-Hydroxy-4-(β-D-glucopyranosyloxy)phenyl]-5,7-dihydroxy-4H-1-benzopyran-4-one] (g) Luteolin - [2-(3,4-Dihydroxyphenyl)- 5,7-dihydroxy-4-chromenone]

Figure 2. Major bio-active compounds present in *Olea europaea* (a,b,c,d,e,f and g) and *Plantago lanceolata* (f and g)

Silybin possessed a dose-dependent growth inhibitory effect on parental ovarian cancer cells (OVCA 433), drug-resistant ovarian cancer cells (A2780 WT) and doxorubicin (DOX)-resistant breast cancer cells (MCF-7) [55]. Both L and D diastereoisomers of silybin inhibited A2780 WT cell growth at low IC_{50} reported with L-diastereoisomer [55]. Furthermore, silybin potentiated the effect of Cisplatin (CDDP, a platinum analog; cis-diamminedichloroplatinum [II]) in inhibiting A2780 WT and CDDP-resistant cell growth. Cisplatin is an inorganic metal complex which acts as an alkylating agent [57]. Similar results recorded with doxorubicin (DOX) on MCF-7 DOX-resistant cells when silybin associated with doxorubicin. Doxorubicin ((7S,9S)-7-[(2R,4S,5S,6S)-4-amino-5-hydroxy-6-methyloxan-2-yl]oxy-6,9,11-trihydroxy-9-(2-hydroxyace tyl)-4-methoxy-8,10-dihydro-7H-tetracene-5,12-dione) is an anthracycline antibiotic isolated from *Streptomyces peucetius* var *caesius* [57]. The effect of silybin-CDDP and silybin-DOX combinations resulted in a synergistic action, as assessed by the Berembaum isobole method [55]. Silymarin demonstrated to have marked inhibition of cell proliferation with almost 50% inhibition in a time dependent manner on the human breast cancer cell line (MDA-MB 468), at 25 μg/ml concentration, after five days of treatment. Its potential anticancer activity was dose dependent and showed a complete inhibition of cancer cells at 50 and 75 μg/ml concentrations at the beginning of Day 2 of exposure [56]. Induction of apoptotic cell death of human prostate cancer (DU145) treated with silibinin is shown to be due to activation of caspase 9 and caspase 3 enzymes [58].

4. Evidence from animal studies for anticancer activity of North American medicinal plants

Anticancer and antiproliferative potential of some North American medicinal plants has also been studied in animal studies (Table 3). *In vivo* antitumor activities of *Achyranthes aspera* (L.) (Devil's Horsewhip) on athymic mice, with are subcutaneous xenograft, harboring human pancreatic tumor were demonstrated, using the leaf extract. The leaf extract significantly reduced both tumor weight and volume in mice treated with leaf extract intraperitonealy [14]. Intravenous administration of 40 mg/kg body weight eupatoriopicrin, a sesquiterpene lactone present in *E. cannabinum,* significantly delayed the growth of tumor in Lewis lung tumour-bearing syngeneic C57B1 female mice [22]. A 70% inhibition of tumor growth in PC-3 cells, orthopedically implanted into the dorsal prostatic lobe in athymic nude mice, was observed, upon their receiving 15 mg/kg intraperitoneal *H. perforatum* methanolic extract [24]. Lantadene A is a pentacyclic triterpenoid, isolated from the weed, *Lantana camara* (L) [59]. Feeding of female Swiss albino mice (LACCA) with a dose of 50 mg/kg body weight of Lantadene A twice a week for 20 weeks, showed potential chemopreventive activity. This chemopreventive activity could be linked to the expression of transcriptional factors and a significant decrease in the mRNA expression of AP-1 and c-fos), NF-kB (p-65) and p53 was observed in Lantadene A treated mice skin tumors [59]. Silibinin decreased tumor multiplicity by 71% ($P < 0.01$) in wild type mice, but did not show any such considerable effect in $iNOS^{-/-}$ mice upon oral feeding of 742 mg/kg body weight silibinin for 5 days per week for 18 weeks [60]. Lesser effects of silibinin in $iNOS^{-/-}$ mice suggested that most of its chemopreventive and angiopreventive effects were through its inhibition of iNOS expression in lung tumors [60]. Treatment of a purified diet, containing 0.5% to 1.0% silibinin on a transgenic adenocarcinoma of are mouse prostate (TRAMP) model, decreased the weight of the tumor in both the prostate and seminal vesicle, when compared with control mice [61].

Treatment of silibinin significantly decreased tumor angiogenesis and proliferation and also there was increased apoptosis in prostate tumor tissue samples in the TRAMP model [61]. The protective effect of silibinin was also demonstrated in mouse skin with tumors caused by acute and chronic UVB-exposure-caused mitogenic and survival signaling and associated biological responses [62]. Mice were treated with silibinin, either topically (9 mg in 200 ml acetone/mouse) or orally (1% of diet), and both administrations strongly inhibited UVB-induced skin tumorigenesis in a long-term study [62]. Thymine dimers are formed in DNA, immediately after UVB irradiation, and are considered as an early and important biomarker for UVB induced DNA damage [62]. A noticeable, 71% reduction ($P < 0.001$) of thymine positive cells was obtained in the mice treated with 1% (w/w) silibinin before the UVB exposure, compared with the UVB alone group [62]. Oral feeding of 200 mg/kg of silibinin for 5 days per week, for 33 days, significantly inhibited human non–small-cell lung cancer cells (NSCLC A549) tumor xenograft growth in nude mice, in a time-dependent manner [63]. This accounted for 58% ($P = 0.003$) reduction in tumor weight per mouse and intraperitoneal administration of 4 mg/kg doxorubicin, once a week for four weeks, showed 61% ($P = 0.005$) reduction in tumor weight. However, interestingly, in silibinin-doxorubicin combination, 76% ($P = 0.002$, versus control) decrease in tumor weight per mouse was observed, that which was significantly different from either treatment alone, showing enhanced efficacy [63].

5. Mode of action of selected phytochemicals of North American medicinal plants

Apoptosis (programmed cell death) is the principal mechanism through which unwanted or damaged cells are safely eliminated from the body. This programmed cell death is mediated via either an extrinsic apoptotic pathway or an intrinsic apoptotic pathway [65]. These two apoptosis signaling pathways differ in the origin of their apoptosis signal, but converge upon a common pathway [66].

The extrinsic pathway is initiated by the stimulation of the cell surface 'death receptor' due to the binding of death ligand and the intrinsic pathway is also known as the mitochondrial pathway in which an intracellular apoptotic signal initiates the process [68]. Various natural extracts, obtained from medicinal plants grown in North America, have been found to induce apoptosis pathways at different levels (Figure 4 and Table 04). Leaf extract of *Achyranthes aspera* activated caspase-3 and induced caspase-3 mRNA in tumor cells. It also decreased Akt-1 transcription, as well its phosphorylation. Suppression of pAkt-1 and a corresponding activation of caspase 3 by the leaf extract, induced apoptosis of tumor cells [14]. It was also found that maslinic acid, isolated from *O. europaea,* inhibited considerably the expression of Bcl-2 (B-cell lymphoma 2), whilst increasing that of Bax. Maslinic acid stimulated the release of mitochondrial cytochrome-c and activated caspase-9 and caspase-3 [33]. These results showed the activation of the mitochondrial apoptotic pathway, in response to the treatment

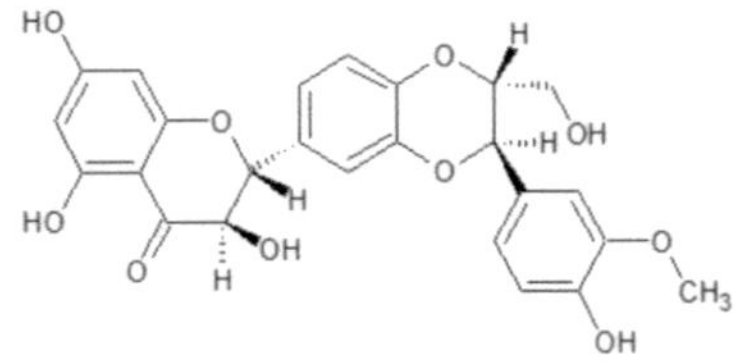

(a) Silybin A

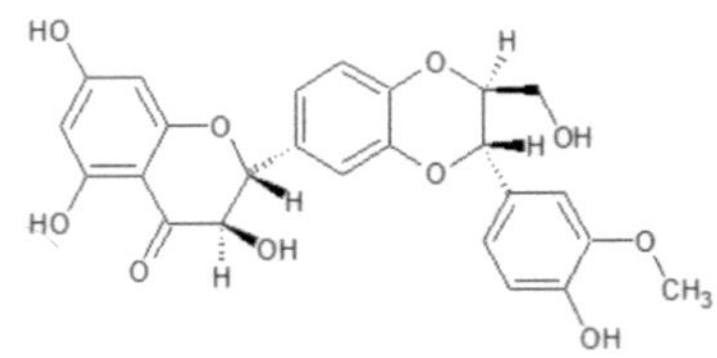

(b) Silybin B

Metabolite	IC_{50}(μg/ml)			MOA	Ref
	MCF7	OVCA 433	A2780		
Silybin	4.8-24	14(L) 20(D)	25	Induce G1 arrest Inhibits STAT3 activation Up-regulates DNA-Protein Kinase-dependent p53 Activation	56 58 67

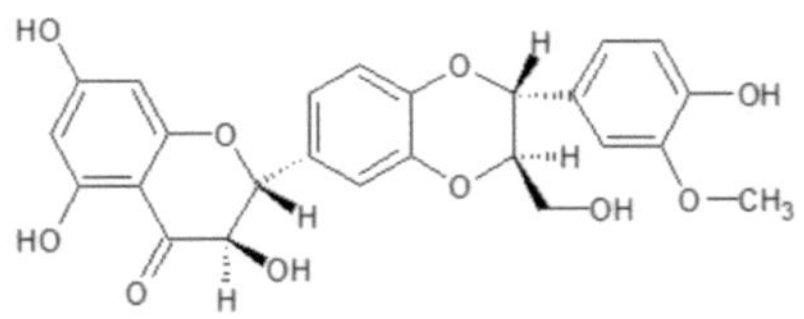

(c) Isosilybin A

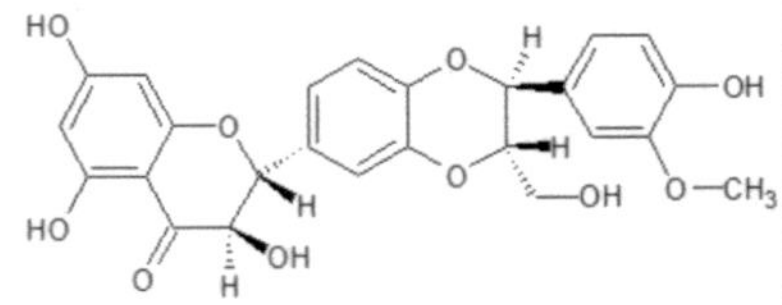

(d) Isosilybin B

Metabolite	IC_{50}(μg/ml)[a] / Apoptosis induction[b]				MOA	Ref
	22Rv1	LAPC4	LNCaP	DU 145		
Isosilybin A	90-180[b]	90-180[b]	90-180[b]	32[a]	Activates Akt–NF-kB–AR axis and increases p53 level	68, 69
Isosilybin B	-	-	-	20.5[a]	Increases p53 level	69

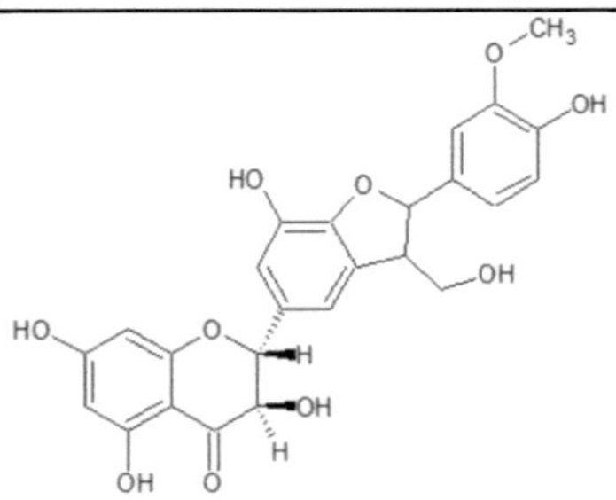

(e) Silychristin

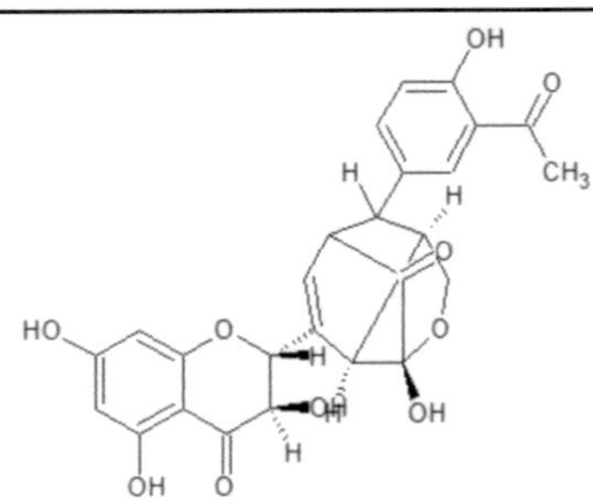

(f) Silydianin

IC_{50}: Concentration which inhibited 50% of cell proliferation; **MOA:** Mode of Action; **MCF-7:** Doxorubicin-resistant breast cancer cells; **OVCA 433:** Parental ovarian cancer cells; **A2780:** Drug-resistant ovarian cancer cells; **22Rv1, LAPC4, LNCaP, DU 145:** Human prostate cancer cells

(a) Silybin A – [(2*R*,3*R*)-3,5,7-trihydroxy-2-[(2*R*,3*R*)-3-(4-hydroxy-3-methoxyphenyl)-2-(hydroxymethyl)-2,3-dihydrobenzo[*b*] [1,4]dioxin-6-yl]chroman-4-one]: (b) Silybin B – [(2*R*,3*R*)-3,5,7-trihydroxy-2-[(2*S*,3*S*)-3-(4-hydroxy-3-methoxyphenyl)-2-(hydroxymethyl)-2,3-dihydrobenzo[*b*] [1,4]dioxin-6-yl]chroman-4-one]: (c) Isosilybin A –[(2*R*,3*R*)-3,5,7-Trihydroxy-2-[(2*R*,3*R*)-2-(4-hydroxy-3-methoxyphenyl)-3-(hydroxymethyl)-2,3-dihydrobenzo[1,4]dioxin-6-yl]-4-chromanone]: (d) (c) Isosilybin B –[(2*R*,3*R*)-3,5,7-Trihydroxy-2-[(2*R*,3*R*)-2-(4-hydroxy-3-methoxyphenyl)-3-(hydroxymethyl)-2,3-dihydrobenzo[1,4]dioxin-6-yl]-4-chromanone]: (e) Silychristin – [(2R,3R)-3,5,7-trihydroxy-2-[(2R, 3S)-7-hydroxy-2-(4-hydroxy-3-methoxyphenyl)-3-(hydroxymethyl)-2,3-dihydro-1-benzofuran-5-yl]-2,3-dihydrochromen-4-one]:

Figure 3. Major bio-active flavonolignans present in *Silybum marianum*

of HT29 colon-cancer cells with maslinic acid. The major flavonoid present in *P. lanceolata,* luteolin-7-*O*-β-glucoside, as well as aglycon luteolin, acted as potent poisons for DNA topoisomerase I on cancer cell lines [54]. Silibinin (major bioactive component from *S. marianum*) markedly activated the DNA-PK-p53 pathway for apoptosis, in response to UVB-induced DNA damage [69]. DNA-PK pull-down assay showed that silibinin pre-treatment strongly increased binding of DNA protein kinase with p53 [69].

Plant	Extraction solvent and concentration	Type of cancer cell line	IC_{50} or growth reduction	Key findings	Ref.
Annona glabra (Pond apple)	Ethanolic extract of lyophilized plant material in powder form	Human drug-sensitive leukemia (CEM) and its multidrug-resistant-derived (CEM/VLB) cell lines	Leaf-1.00 (CEM/ VLB) Pulp-0.65 (CEM/VLB), Seed-0.10 (CEM/VLB) and Leaf-0.30 (CEM), Pulp-0.35 (CEM), Seed-0.07 (CEM) µg/ml	IC_{50} values were significantly lower than Adriamycin (Doxorubicin) (CEM=0.13 µg/ml and CEM/VLB=13.4 µg/ml) indicates its potential for cancer drug discovery programs	52
Aralia nudicaulis (Wild sarsaparilla)	Methanol extracts of rhizome, stem, leaf and fruit were further partitioned with hexane, ethyl acetate, butanol and water	WiDr (colon), Molt (leukemia), HeLa (cervix)	Hexane rhizome extract 30.1 (WiDr), 7.0 (Molt), 33.33 (HeLa) µg/ml	The concentrations of Rhizome hexane and Fruit hexane required for normal cell death was significantly higher than those required for the cancer cells	53
Eupatorium cannabinum (Bonesets)	Eupatoriopicrin concentrations of 0.1 - 50 µg/ml in 96% ethanol	FIO 26 (Fibrosarcoma)	1.5 µg/ml	Possess significant anticancer activity	22
Foeniculum vulgare (Wild pepper fennel)	Not specified	Breast (MCF-7), liver (HepG2)	-	Remarkable anticancer potential	23
Hypericum perforatum (St. John's wort)	Methanolic extract	Prostate (PC-3)	0.42 mg/ml	Extract components synergistically contribute to the	24

Plant	Extraction solvent and concentration	Type of cancer cell line	IC_{50} or growth reduction	Key findings	Ref.
				reduction of the PC-3 cells proliferation	
Linum Usitatissimum (Common flax)	Ethanol extract	Breast (MCF-7, MDA-MB-231)	Growth reduction of 15.8% in MCF-7 and 11.4% in MDA-MB-231	Significantly reduced cell growth and induced apoptotic cell death	31
Olea europrae (Olive)	maslinic acid 0–100 µg/mL	Colon (HT29)	28.8 µg/ml	Cell proliferation inhibition in a dose-dependent manner and causes apoptotic death	33
	Aqueous extract and methanol artificial mixture	Breast (MCF-7), Human urinary bladder (T-24), Bovine brain (BBCE)	72 (MCF-7), 100 (T-24), and 62 (BBCE) for aq. 565 (MCF-7), 135 (T-24), and 42 (BBCE) for methanol µg/ml	Antiproliferative activity of the extracts should mainly be attributed to its identified phytochemicals	34
Plantago lanceolata (Ribwort plantain)	Methanolic extract	Renal (TK-10), breast (MCF-7), melanoma (UACC-62)	"/>250 (TK-10), 47.2 (MCF-7), 50.6 (UACC-62) µg/ml	Growth of MCF-7 was totally inhibited	54
	Extracted by maceration with ethanol/water during 72 hr at room temperature	cervix epitheloid (HeLa),breast (MCF-7), colon (HT-29), fetal lung (MRC-5)	172.3 (HeLa), 142.8 (MCF-7), 405.5 (HT-29), 551.7 (MRC-5) µg/ml	Showed significant antiproliferative activity	38
Rhodiola rosea (Golden root)	Not specified	Urinary bladder (RT4, UMUC-3, T24, 5637, J82)	264 (RT4),100 (UMUC-3), 71 (T24), 151 (5637), 165 (J82) µg/ml	Selectively inhibit the growth of cancer cell lines with minimal effect on nonmalignant cells	41
Saponaria vaccaria (Cowherb)	70% Methanol extract	colon (WiDr), breast (MDA-MB-231), lung (NCI-417), prostate (PC-3),	3.8-9.4 (WiDr), 11.4-19.6 (MDA-MB-231), 12.6-18.4	Dose-dependent growth inhibitory and selective apoptosis-inducing activity. Strong in a breast and a prostate cancer cell lines	43

http://dx.doi.org/10.5772/55859

Plant	Extraction solvent and concentration	Type of cancer cell line	IC_{50} or growth reduction	Key findings	Ref.
		nontumorigenic fibroblast EJ (CRL-2522)	(NCI-417) mg/ml		
Silybum marianum (Milkthistle)	silybin, a flavonoid	Doxorubucin resistant breast (MCF-7), Parental ovarian (OVCA 433), Drug-resistant ovarian (A2780)	4.8-24 µM (MCF-7), 14 & 20 µM - L & D diastereoisomers respectively (A2780) 25 µg/ml	Dose-dependent growth inhibitory effect on all three cell lines	55
	Silymarin at a dosages of 10-75 µg/ml in ethanol	Breast (MDA-MB 468)	- -	Inhibits the cell proliferation in a dose- and time dependent manner	56
	Silibinin in DMSO	Prostate (DU145)	-	Strongly inhibited activation of Stat3 and causes caspase activation and apoptotic death	58
	Isosilybin A and B	Prostate (LNCaP, 22Rv1) Prostate (DU 145)	Iso A:32 µM (DU 145) Iso B:20 µM (DU 145)	Anti-prostate cancer activity mediated via cell cycle arrest and apoptosis induction	69
Taraxacum officinale (Dandelions)	Water (lyophilized or reconstituted)	Acute T-cell leukemia (Jurkat clone E6-1), dominant-negative FADD Jurkat cells (clone I 2.1)	-	Effectively and selectively induced apoptosis in human leukemia cell lines in a dose and time dependent manner	49

Table 2. Anti-cancer properties of phytochemicals and extracts of medicinal plants revealed from *in vitro* studies using cancer cell lines

Plant	Preparation	Animal model used	Dosage	Key findings	Ref.
Achyranthes aspera (Devil's Horsewhip)	5% suspension in hexane followed by extraction in acetone overnight	Athymic nude mice	50, 100 and 200 mg/kg extract in 1 ml PBS administered IP	The tumor weight and volume was significantly reduced in the mice treated for 36 days with 50 mg/kg.	14

Plant	Preparation	Animal model used	Dosage	Key findings	Ref.
	and residue was dissolved in methanol			In one treated mouse tumor completely disappeared	
Eupatorium cannabinum (Bonesets)	Eupatoriopicrin, a sesquiterpene lactone	Syngeneic C57B1 female mice	i.v. injection of 20 or 40 mg/kg	Significantly stronger growth delay of both lung tumours and fibrosarcoma	22
Hypericum perforatum (Orange root)	Methanolic extract	Human prostatic carcinoma cell line orthotopically implanted athymic male nude mice	ip with a dose of 15 mg/kg dissolved in 1% DMSO	Inhibited tumor growth by 70% with no observed side effects	24
Lantana camara (Wild sage)	Lantadene A, pentacyclic triterpenoid	Female Swiss albino mice (LACCA)	50 mg/kg body weight twice a week for 20 weeks	Activity could be linked to the expression of transcriptional factors	59
Silybum marianum (Milkthistle)	Silibinin	Lung - Male B6/129-Nos2tm1Lau ($iNOS^{-/-}$) and B6/129PF2 WT mice	742 mg/kg body weight for 5 d/wk for 18 weeks	Significantly decreases urethane-induced tumor number and size in WT mice. Decreased tumor multiplicity in WT mice, but not in $iNOS^{-/-}$ mice	60
	Silibinin	Prostate - A transgenic adenocarcinoma of mouse prostate (TRAMP) model	Purified diet containing 0% and 1% (w/w) silibinin until	Decreased the weight of tumor + prostate + seminal vesicle. Significantly decreased tumor angiogenesis and proliferation and increased apoptosis also.	61
	Topically applied silibinin in acetone or oral feeding of silibinin	Skin – mouse	9 mg in 200 ml acetone/mouse or 1% in diet	silibinin (both topical and oral) strongly inhibited UVB-induced skin tumorigenesis in long-term study	62
	Silibinin	Skin - SKH-1 hairless mouse	1% (w/w) silibinin in diet for 2 weeks	Strong suppression of UVB-induced damage by dietary feeding of silibinin	63
	Silibinin	Athymic (BALB/c,nu/nu) male nude mice	200 mg/kg body weight, 5 d/wk for 33 days	Significantly inhibits human NSCLC A549 tumor xenograft growth in a time dependent manner	64

Table 3. Anti-cancer properties of medicinal plants revealed from *in vivo* studies using experimental animals

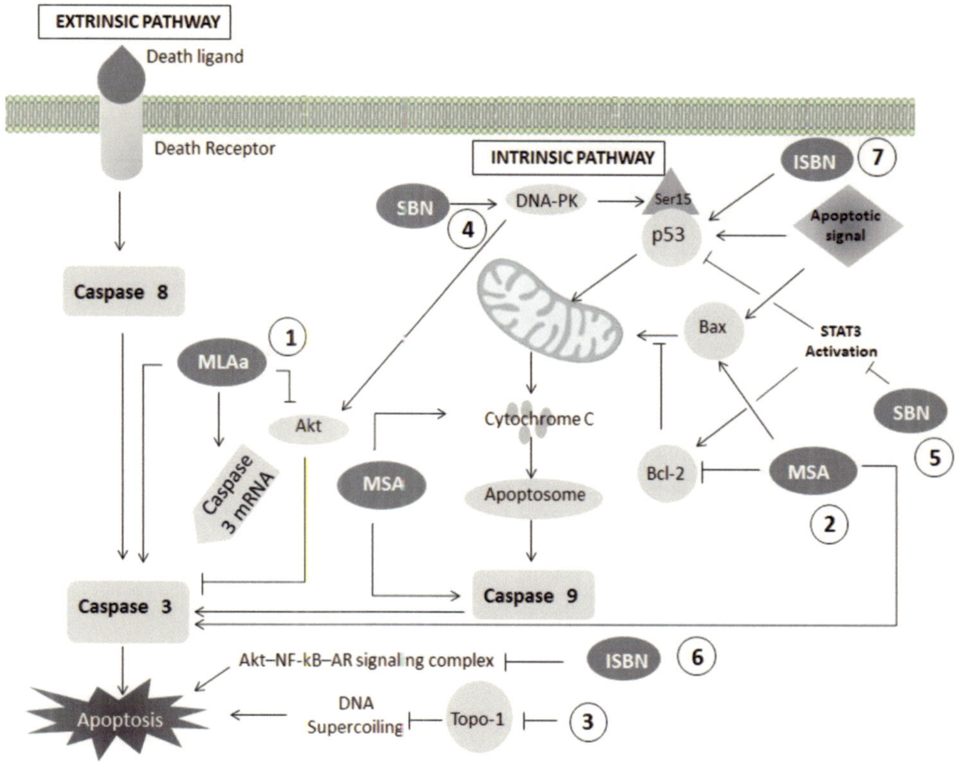

Figure 4. Schematic representation of current knowledge of mode of action of some selected anticancer phytochemicals in North America (in a hypothetical cancer cell).

Akt (Protein kinase B); Bcl-2 (Protein kinase B); Bax (Bcl-2–associated X protein); Topo-1 (Topoisomerase 1); p53 (tumor protein 53); Ser15 (Serine 15); NF-kB (nuclear factor kappa-light-chain-enhancer of activated B cells); AR (Androgen Receptor)

1. Methanolic leaf extract of *Achyranthes aspera* (MLAa) induces caspase -3 mRNA and suppress expression of the kinase Akt-1. Apoptosis is induced by activation of caspase-3 and inhibiting Akt-phosphorylation.

2. The mechanism of Maslinic acid (MSA) (isolated from *Olea europaea*) is regulated via Bcl-2 inhibition and Bax induction, producing mitochondrial disruption, cytochrome-c release, leading finally to the activation of caspases 9 and caspase 3.

3. Luteolin-7-*O*-β-glucoside and its aglycon, luteolin (major bio-active constituents of *Plantago lanceolata*) showed DNA topoisomerase I poison activities and Topoisomerase mediated DNA damage might be the possible mechanism which induce apoptosis.

4. Silibinin (SBN) (extracted from *Silybum marianum*) pretreatment enhance DNA-PK (DNA Protein kinase) associated kinase activity as well as the physical interaction of p53 with DNA-PK and it preferentially activates the DNA-PK-p53 pathway for apoptosis.

5. SBN inhibits active Stat3 phosphorylation, and causes caspase activation and apoptosis.

6. Isosilybin A (ISBN) (extracted from *Silybum marianum*) activates apoptotic machinery in human prostate cancer cells via targeting Akt–NF-kB–AR axis.

7. ISBN increases p53 protein levels.

Plant	Mode of action	References
Achyranthes aspera (Devil's Horsewhip)	Significantly induced caspase-3 mRNA and suppressed expression of the pro survival kinase Akt-1. Apoptosis was induced by activation of caspase-3 and inhibiting Akt phosphorylation.	14
Olea europaea (Olive)	Activation of the mitochondrial apoptotic pathway	33
	Significant block of G_1 to S phase transition manifested by the increase of cell number in G_0/G_1 phase	37
Plantago lanceolata (Ribwort plantain)	The topoisomerase-mediated DNA damage seems to be a candidate mechanism, by which some flavonoids may exert their cytotoxic potential	54
Silybum marianum (Milkthistle)	Induces G_1 arrest in cell cycle progression	56
	Up-regulates DNA-protein kinase-dependent p53 activation to enhance UVB-induced apoptosis	67
	Activates apoptotic machinery in human prostate cancer cells via targeting Akt–NF-kB–AR axis	68
	Inhibits active Stat3 phosphorylation, and causes caspase activation	58
	Increases total p53 levels	69
Podophyllum peltatum (Mayapple)	Inhibition of microtubule assembly	70

Table 4. Mode of action of anticancer activity of phytochemicals present in selected North American medicinal plants

6. Conclusion

Currently, natural products, especially plant secondary metabolites such as isoprenoids, phenolics and alkaloids, have been demonstrated to be the leading providers of novel anticancer agents. Thiese important groups of phytochemicals represent a vast majority of chemical groups, including alkaloids, flavonoids, flavonols, flavanols, terpenes and terpenoids, phenols, flavonolignans and steroids. Potential anticancer properties of these phytochemicals have been shown by both cell culture (*in vitro* methods) and animal (*in vivo* methods) studies. However, *in vitro* and *in vivo* findings should be strengthened by valid human clinical trial data before introducing to the medicine cabinet as natural therapeutics or drugs.

Abbreviations

CEM, Human drug-sensitive leukemia cells; **CEM/VLB**, Human multidrug-resistant-derived leukemia cells; **Jurkat clone E6-1**, Acute T-cell leukemia cells; **WiDr** and **HT29**, Human colon cancer cells; **Molt**, Human leukemia cancer cell; **FIO 26**, Human fibrosarcoma cells; **MCF-7** and **MDA-MB-231**, Human breast cancer cells; **HepG2**, Human hepatocarcinoma cells; **LNCaP**, **22Rv1**, **PC-3** and **DU145**, Human prostate cancer cells; **RT4**, **UMUC-3**, **T24**, **5637** and **J82**, Human urinary bladder cancer cells; **BBCE**, Bovine brain capillary endothelial cells, **TK-10**, Human renal cancer cells; **UACC-62**, Human melanoma cells; **HeLa**, Human cervical epithelioid cells; **MRC-5**, Fetal lung cancer cells; **NCI-417**, Human lung cancer cells; **CRL-2522**, Human nontumorigenic fibroblast cells; **OVCA 433**, Parental ovarian cancer cells; **A2780**, Drug-resistant ovarian cancer cells.

Author details

Wasundara Fernando and H. P. Vasantha Rupasinghe*

*Address all correspondence to: vrupasinghe@dal.ca

Faculty of Agriculture, Dalhousie University, Truro, Nova Scotia, Canada

References

[1] Cancer Research UK and International Agency for Research on Cancer, Cancerstats Cancer Worldwide; 2011.

[2] American cancer society. Global Cancer Facts and Figures 2007. American Cancer Society, Atlanta; 2007.

[3] Canadian Cancer Society's Steering Committee on Cancer Statistics. Canadian Cancer Statistics 2012. Toronto, ON: Canadian Cancer Society; 2012.

[4] Cancers, NMH Facts sheet. World Health Organization; 2010.

[5] Cragg, G. M. and Newman, D. J., Plants as a source of anti-cancer agents, Journal of Ethnopharmacology, 2005; 100: 72-79.

[6] Nobler, L., The discovery of the vinca alkaloids-chemotherapeutic agents against cancer. Biochem. Cell Biol. 1990; 68: 1344-1351.

[7] Jordan, M. A., Thrower, D. and Wilson L., Mechanism of Inhibition of Cell Proliferation by Vinca Alkaloids, Cancer Recearch, 1991; 51: 2212-2222.

[8] Krishan, A., Paika, K. and Frei E., Cytofluorometric Studies on the action of Podophyllotoxin and Epipodophyllotoxins (Vm-26, Vp-16-213) on the Cell Cycle Traverse of Human Lymphoblasts, Journal of Cell Biology, 1975; 66: 521-530.

[9] Nerendra Nagar1*, Rakesh K. Jat1, Rajkumar Saharan1, Sanjay Verma1, Daljeet Sharma1, Kuldeep bansal, Podophyllotoxin and their Glycosidic Derivatives, Pharmacophore, 2011; 2(2): 124-134.

[10] De Flora, S. and Ferguson, L. R., Overview of mechanisms of cancer chemopreventive agents, Mutation Research, 2005; 591: 8–15.

[11] Boffetta, P. and Nyberg, F., Contribution of environmental factors to cancer risk, British Medical Bulletin, 2003; 68: 71–94.

[12] Williams, G. M., Mechanisms of chemical carcinogenesis and application to human cancer risk assessment, Toxicology, 2001; 166: 3–10.

[13] Sebastian, M., Ninan, N., and Elias, E., Nanomedicine and Cancer therapies, Volume 2, Apple Academic Press., 2013.

[14] Subbarayan, P. R., Sarkar, M., Rao, S. N., Philip, S., Kumar, P., Altman, N., Reis, I., Ahmed, M., Ardalan, B. and Lokeshwar. B. L., Achyranthes aspera (Apamarg) leaf extract inhibits human pancreatic tumor growth in athymic mice by apoptosis, Journal of Ethnopharmacology, 2012; 142: 523–530.

[15] Cochrane, C. B., Nair, P. K. R., Melnick, S. J., Resek, A. P. and Ramachandran, C., Anticancer Effects of Annona glabra Plant Extracts in Human Leukemia Cell Lines, Anticancer Research, 2008; 28: 965-972.

[16] Wang, J., Li, Q., Ivanochko, G. and Huang. Y., Anticancer Effect of Extracts from a North American Medicinal Plant – Wild Sarsaparilla, Anticancer Research, 2006; 26: 2157-2164.

[17] Ramirez-Erosa, I., Huang, Y., Hickie, R. A., Sutherland, R. G. and Barl, B., Xanthatin and xanthinosin from the burs of Xanthium strumarium L. as potential anticancer agents, Can. J. Physiol. Pharmacol. 2007; 85: 1160-1172.

[18] Wilkins, A. L., Lu, Y. and Tan, S., Extractives from New Zealand Honeys. 4. Linalool Derivatives and Other Components from Nodding Thistle (Carduus nutans) Honey. J. A. Food Chem. 1993; 41: 873-878.

[19] Woerdenbag, H.J., Lemstra, W., Malingre, T.M. and Konings, A.W.T., Enhanced cytostatic activity of the sesquiterpene lactone eupatoriopicrin by glutathione depletion. Br. J. Cancer. 1989; 59: 68-75.

[20] Jitendra Jena, Rakesh Ranjan, Poonam Ranjan and Manoj Kumar Sarangi. A Study on Natural Anticancer Plants. International Journal of Pharmaceutical and Chemical Sciences 2012; 1 (1): 365 – 368.

[21] S. Madhuri and Govind Pandey. Some anticancer medicinal plants of foreign origin. Current Science 2009; 96(6): 779-78.

[22] Woerdenbag, H.J., Eupatorium cannabinum L. A review emphasizing the sesquiterpene lactones and their biological activity. Pharm Weekbland [Sci], I986; 8: 245-51.

[23] Timsina, B., Shukla, M. and Nadumane, V. K., A review of few essential oils and their anticancer property. Journal of Natural Pharmaceuticals, 2012; 3(1): 1-8.

[24] Martarelli, D., Martarelli, B., Pediconi, D., Nabissi, M. I., Perfumi, M. and Pompei. P., Hypericum perforatum methanolic extract inhibits growth of human prostatic carcinoma cell line orthotopicall yimplanted in nude mice. Cancer Letters, 2004; 210: 27–33.

[25] Han, Y. F., Cao, G. X., Gao X. J., and Xia. M., Isolation and characterisation of the sesquiterpene lactones from Lactuca sativa L var. anagustata. Food Chemistry, 2010; 120: 1083–1088.

[26] Kalita, S., Kumar, G., Karthik, L., Venkata, K. and Rao, B., Phytochemical Composition and In Vitro Hemolytic Activity of Lantana Camara L. (Verbenaceae) Leaves, Pharmacologyonline, 2011; 1: 59-67.

[27] Ghangale, G. D., Tambe, R.Y., Gaykar, A.J. and Dama G.Y., Antimitotic activity of Lantana Camara Flowers, International Journal of Institutional Pharmacy and Life Sciences, 2011; 1(1): 1-6.

[28] Patel, S., A weed with multiple utility: Lantana camara, Rev Environ Sci Biotechnol, 2011; 10: 341–351.

[29] Lambert, J. D., Sang, S., Dougherty, A., Caldwell, C. G., Meyers, R. O., Dorr, R. T. and Timmermann, B. N., Cytotoxic lignans from Larrea tridentate. Phytochemistry, 2005; 66: 811–815.

[30] Arteaga, S., Andrade-Cetto, A. and C′ardenas, R., Larrea tridentata (Creosote bush), an abundant plant of Mexican and US-American deserts and its metabolite nordihydroguaiaretic acid. Journal of Ethnopharmacology, 2005; 98: 231–239.

[31] Lee, J. and Cho, K., Flaxseed sprouts induce apoptosis and inhibit growth in MCF-7 and MDA-MB-231 human breast cancer cells. In Vitro Cell. Dev. Biol.—Animal, 2012; 48: 244–250.

[32] Reuben, S. C., Gopalan, A., Petit, D. M. and Bishayee, A., Modulation of angiogenesis by dietary phytoconstituents in the prevention and intervention of breast cancer. Mol. Nutr. Food Res. 2012; 56: 14–29.

[33] J., Fernando, Eva, R. Z., Rufino-Palomares, E., Lupiáñez, J. A. and Cascante, M., Maslinic acid, a natural triterpene from Olea europaea L., induces apoptosis in HT29 human colon-cancer cells via the mitochondrial apoptotic pathway. Cancer Letters, 2009; 273: 44–54.

[34] Goulas, V., Exarchou, V., Troganis, A. N., Psomiadou, E., Fotsis, T., Briasoulis E. and Gerothanassis. I. P., Phytochemicals in olive-leaf extracts and their antiproliferative activity against cancer and endothelial cells, Mol. Nutr. Food Res. 2009; 53: 600 – 608.

[35] Han, J., Talorete, T. P. N., Yamada P. and Isoda H., Anti-proliferative and apoptotic effects of oleuropein and hydroxytyrosol on human breast cancer MCF-7 cells. Cytotechnology, 2009; 59: 45–53.

[36] Çinar, A., Cansev A. and Şahan. Y., Phenolic Compounds of Olive by-products and Their Function in the Development of Cancer Cells. Biologi Bilimleri Araştırma Dergisi. 2011; 4(2): 55-58.

[37] Goulas, V., Exarchou, V., Troganis, A. N., Psomiadou, E., Fotsis, T., Briasoulis, E. and Gerothanassis, I. P., Phytochemicals in olive-leaf extracts and their antiproliferative activity against cancer and endothelial cells. Mol. Nutr. Food Res. 2009; 53: 600 – 608.

[38] Beara, I. N., Lesjak, M. M., Orcic, D. Z., Simin, N. Đ., Cetojevic-Simin, D. D., Bozin, B. N. and Mimica-Duki, N. M., Comparative analysis of phenolic profile, antioxidant, anti-inflammatory and cytotoxic activity of two closely-related Plantain species: Plantago altissima L. and Plantago lanceolata L. LWT - Food Science and Technology, 2012; 47: 64-70.

[39] Giri A. and Narasu M. L., Production of podophyllotoxin from Podophyllum hexandrum: a potential natural product for clinically useful anticancer drugs. Cytotechnology, 2000; 34: 17–26.

[40] Khan, H., Saeed, M. and Muhammad N., Pharmacological and phytochemical updates of genus Polygonatum. Phytopharmacology. 2012; 3(2): 286-308.

[41] Liu, Z., Li, X., Simoneau, A. R., Jafari, M. and Zi. X., Rhodiola rosea Extracts and Salidroside Decrease the Growth of Bladder Cancer Cell Lines via Inhibition of the mTOR Pathway and Induction of Autophagy. Molecular Carcinogenesis. 2012; 51: 257–267.

[42] Panossian, A., Wikman G. and Sarris. J., Rosenroot (Rhodiola rosea): Traditional use, chemical composition, pharmacology and clinical efficacy. Phytomedicine, 2010; 17: 481–493.

[43] Balsevich, J. J., Ramirez-Erosa, I., Hickie, R. A., Dunlop, D. M., Bishop, G. G. and Deibert, L. K., Antiproliferative activity of Saponaria vaccaria constituents and related compounds. Fitoterapia 2012; 83: 170–181.

[44] Agarwal, R., Agarwal, C., Ichikawa, H., Singh, R. P., and B. B., Aggarwal, Anticancer Potential of Silymarin: From Bench to Bed Side. Anticancer Research, 2006; 26: 4457-4498.

[45] Rnonel, A., Erlini, U. and Narot, A., Constituents of Silybum marianum. Structure of Isosilybin and Stereochemistry of Silybin. J.C.S. Chem. Comm., 1979; 696-697.

[46] Zheng-Xiang, X. and Jing-Yu, L., Steroids and Phenols from Sonchus arvensis. Chin J Nat Med. 2010; 8(4): 267-269.

[47] Radulović, N., Blagojević, P. and Palić, R., Fatty acid derived compounds--the dominant volatile class of the essential oil poor Sonchus arvensis subsp. uliginosus (Bieb.) Nyman. Nat Prod Commun. 2009; 4(3): 405-410.

[48] Mockute, D. and Judzentiene, A., Composition of the Essential Oils of Tanacetum vulgare L. Growing Wild in Vilnius District (Lithuania). Journal of Essential Oil Research, 2004; 16: 550-553.

[49] Ovadje, P., Chatterjee, S., Griffin, C., Tran, C., Hamm C. and Pandey, S., Selective induction of apoptosis through activation of caspase-8 in human leukemia cells (Jurkat) by dandelion root extract. Journal of Ethnopharmacology. 2011; 133: 86–91.

[50] Altmann, K. H. and Gertsch, J., Anticancer drugs from nature—natural products as a unique source of new microtubule-stabilizing agents. Nat. Prod. Rep., 2007; 24: 327–357.

[51] Biswas, R., Mandal, S. K., Dutta, S., Bhattacharyya, S. S., Boujedaini, N. and Khuda-Bukhsh, A. R., Thujone-Rich Fraction of Thuja occidentalis Demonstrates Major Anti-Cancer Potentials: Evidences from In Vitro Studies on A375 Cells. Evidence-Based Complementary and Alternative Medicine, 2011; 1-16.

[52] Wang, J., Li, Q., Ivanochko, G. and Huang, Y., Anticancer Effect of Extracts from a North American Medicinal Plant – Wild Sarsaparilla. Anticancer Research. 2006; 26: 2157-2164.

[53] Babich, H. and Visioli, F., In vitro cytotoxicity to human cells in culture of some phenolics from olive oil, Farmaco, 2003; 58: 403-407.

[54] Gálvez, M., Mart´ın-Cordero, C., López-Lázaro, M., Cortés, F. and Ayuso. M. J., Cytotoxic effect of Plantago spp. on cancer cell lines. Journal of Ethnopharmacology, 2003; 88: 125–130.

[55] Scambia, G., De Vincenzo, R., Ranelletti, F. O., Panici, P.B., Ferrandina, G., D'Agostino, G., Fattorossi, A., Bombardelli, E. and Mancuso, S., Antiproliferative effect of silybin on gynaecological malignancies: synergism with cisplatin and doxorubicin. Eur J Cancer. 1996; 32(5): 877-882.

[56] Zi, X., Feyes, D. K. and R., Agarwal, Human breast cancer cells MDA-MB 468: induction of G1 arrest through an increase in Cip1/p21 concomitant with a decrease in kinase activity of cyclin-dependent kinases and associated cyclins. Clin Cancer Res, 1998; 4: 1055-1064.

[57] Katzung, B.G., Basic and Clinical Pharmacology, 10th Edition, McGraw Hill, 2006.

[58] Agarwal, C., Tyagi, A., Kaur, M. and Agarwal, R., Silibinin inhibits constitutive activation of Stat3, and causes caspase activation and apoptotic death of human prostate carcinoma DU145 cells. Carcinogenesis, 2007; 28(7) 1463–1470.

[59] Kaur, J., Sharma, M., Sharma, P. D. and Bansal, M. P., Antitumor Activity of Lantadenes in DMBA/TPA Induced Skin Tumors in Mice: Expression of Transcription Factors. Am. J. Biomed. Sci. 2010; 2(1): 79-90.

[60] Ramasamy, K., Dwyer-Nield, L. D., Serkova, N. J., Hasebroock, K. M., Tyagi, A., Raina, K., Singh, R. P., Malkinson, A. M. and Agarwal, R., Silibinin Prevents Lung Tumorigenesis in Wild-Type but not in iNOS$^{-/-}$ Mice: Potential of Real-Time Micro-CT in Lung Cancer Chemoprevention Studies. Clin Cancer Res, 2011; 17: 753-761.

[61] Deep, G. and Agarwal, R., Chemopreventive Efficacy of Silymarin in Skin and Prostate Cancer. Integrative Cancer Therapies, 2007; 6(2): 130-145.

[62] Gu, M., Dhanalakshmi, S., Mohan, S., Singh, R. P. and Agarwal, R., Silibinin inhibits ultraviolet B radiation-induced mitogenic and survival signaling, and associated biological responses in SKH-1 mouse skin. Carcinogenesis, 2005; 26(8): 1404—1413.

[63] Gu, M., Dhanalakshmi, S., Singh, R. P. and Agarwal, R., Dietary Feeding of Silibinin Prevents Early Biomarkers of UVB Radiation–Induced Carcinogenesis in SKH-1 Hairless Mouse Epidermis. Cancer Epidemiol Biomarkers Prev, 2005; 14: 1344-1349.

[64] Singh, R. P., Mallikarjuna G. U., and Sharma, G., Oral Silibinin Inhibits Lung Tumor Growth in Athymic Nude Mice and Forms a Novel Chemocombination with Doxorubicin Targeting Nuclear Factor kB- Mediated Inducible Chemoresistance. Clin Cancer Res, 2004; 10: 8641-8647.

[65] Elmore, S., Apoptosis: A Review of Programmed Cell Death. Toxicologic Pathology, 2007; 35:495–516.

[66] Elmorea, S. W., Oostb T. K. and Park, C. M., Inhibitors of Anti-apoptotic Proteins for Cancer Therapy. Annual Reports In Medicinal Chemistry, 2005; 40: 255-270.

[67] Dhanalakshmi, S., Agarwal, C., Singh, R. P. and Agarwal, R., Silibinin Up-regulates DNA-Protein Kinase-dependent p53 Activation to Enhance UVB-induced Apoptosis in Mouse Epithelial JB6 Cells. The Journal of Biological Chemistry, 2005; 280(21) 20375–20383.

[68] Deep, G., Gangar, S. C., Oberlies, N. H., Kroll, D. J. and Agarwal, R., Isosilybin A Induces Apoptosis in Human Prostate Cancer Cells via Targeting Akt, NF-kB, and Androgen Receptor Signaling. Molecular Carcinogenesis, 2010; 49: 902–912.

[69] Deep, G., Oberlies, N. H., Kroll D. J. and Agarwal, R., Isosilybin B and isosilybin A inhibit growth, induce G1 arrest and cause apoptosis in human prostate cancer LNCaP and 22Rv1 cells, Carcinogenesis, 2007; 28: 1533–1542.

[70] Giri, A. and Narasu, M. L., Production of podophyllotoxin from Podophyllum hexandrum: a potential natural product for clinically useful anticancer drugs. Cytotechnology, 2000 34: 17–26.

Chapter 7

A New Perspective on the Development of Cholesterol-Lowering Products

Sandhya V.G. Nair and Yanwen Wang

Additional information is available at the end of the chapter

http://dx.doi.org/10.5772/54729

1. Introduction

1.1. Health impact of cardiovascular disease (CVD)

Cardiovascular disease (CVD) is the principal cause of death worldwide, representing nearly 30% of the annual global mortality and 10% of global health burden [1]. The current status of CVD is now on international scale; which can be considered as the commonest chronic illness in both developed and developing countries, causing the most deaths and the greatest impact on morbidity [2]. In 2006, CVD was the leading cause of death for Canadians, representing 30% of all deaths [3]. A total number of 1.3 million Canadians are diagnosed having heart disease accounting for 5% among those above 12 years and 23% at 75 years and older. The increased rate of obesity and diabetes combined with further aging of the population will likely lead to an increase in the number of people with CVD in the future. This will compromise the health of Canadians, put a strain on the health care system, and have a significant economic impact on Canada [4]. Similarly, over the past five decades the prevalence of CVD has steadily increased in economically developing countries [5]. These countries will account for 76% of an estimated 25 million death due to CVD in 2020 [6]. On an international basis, by 2020 CVD will reach nearly epidemic proportions and become the cause of more deaths, disability and economic loss than any others group of diseases. The number of fatalities by CVD projected to increase to over 20 million a year by 2020 and over 24 million a year by 2030 [7]. Apparently, understanding the aetiology of CVD and accordingly develop preventive and therapeutic approaches to address this health threat continues to be critically important in the next decades although significant achievements have been made in the past decades.

2. Risk factors of CVD

The aetiology of CVD is multifactorial, complex and still not completely understood. However, there is now a general agreement that elevated total cholesterol, LDL-cholesterol and triacylglycerol levels, low HDL-cholesterol concentrations, smoking, high blood pressure, hyperglycemia and diabetes are all risk factors of CVD. Physical inactivity, obesity, diet and low socio-economic status are thought to be predisposing risk factors which work, at least in part, as promoter on other risk factors. These factors predispose to develop syndrome X or metabolic syndrome, which is characterised by obesity, hypertension, dyslipoproteinaemia, and disturbed glucose tolerance [8]. Some other factors such as elevated prothrombotic factors, markers of inflammation, elevated homocysteine, elevated lipoprotein (a) and some psychological factors show associations with CVD [6]. Nevertheless, the aetiology of CVD is far from clear [9], and most factors are unmodifiable while others can be modified through the change of diet habits and lifestyles.

2.1. Unmodifiable risk factors

2.1.1. Ageing

Cardiovascular diseases, such as atherosclerosis, coronary heart disease and resultant heart failure reach epidemic proportions among older persons. Aging leads to arterial stiffening that results in aortic dilation and wall thickening along with increased collagen level. Potential age-associated changes in the tissue levels or responses to growth factors, catecholamines, angiotensin II, endothelin tumor growth factors β (TGF β) or fibroblast growth factors influences myocardial or vascular cells. Deficit in myocardial beta adregenic receptor signalling, decline in omega-3 polyunsaturated fatty acids and increased reactive oxygen species generation occur with aging, which enhances Ca^{2+} influx [10]. The clinical manifestations and prognosis of CVD and resultant heart failure worsen with ageing. Over 83 percent of people who die of coronary heart disease are 65 or older. Thus, age, per se, is the major risk factor for CVD [10].

2.1.2. Gender

There is a marked difference in CVD risk between sexes [11]. Incidence of CVD was approximately 3-fold and mortality about 5-fold greater in men thanin women [12]. Among middle-aged people,incidence of coronary heart disease is 2 to 5 times more in men than in women, and this sexratio varies between populations. The role of major risk factors such as lipid abnormalities, high blood pressure, smoking, obesity and diabetes in the development of CVD is well established amongmen (Jousilahti, Vartiainen et al. 1999). In women, significnat shift in their physiological function and heath profiles occurs during and the postmenopausal. When entering into middle ages, women tend to have lower LDL cholesterol and higher HDL cholesterol values than men of similar age. Following menopause, total cholesterol, LDL cholesterol and triglycerides levels increases while HDL levels remain unchanged or decrease slightly. These alterations in lipid values are thought to be related in part to loss of protective effects of estrogen [13].

2.1.3. Heredity (including race)

The prevalence of CVD considerably varies by race/ ethnicity. Genetic predispositions are a result of gene mutations, which alter the biological function expressed by the original genes (polymorphisms) and increases an individual risk for the disease. Several polymorphism and linkage markers have been identified as being correlated to the onset of CVD. For example, M235T polymorphism of the angiotensinogen gene is linked to hypertension and later to the development of CVD [14]. In many developed countries, racial and ethnic minorities bear disproportionate burden of heart disease. Significant differences in socioeconomic status and conventional heart disease risk factors exist among racial/ethnic groups in the United States, Canada and United Kingdom (Ludwig, Ebbeling et al. 2002). The rate of heart disease among the racial and ethnic group in the United States vary widely, with African Americans having rates a half to three fold greater than Asians, depending on the gender [15]. It is also well documented that the prevalence of CVD is higher in several minority populations (Hispanics and African Americans) in comparison to whites. [16]. However, these differences do not fully account for the observed disparities in disease prevalence, suggesting the presence of other biological factors [17].

2.2. Modifiable risk factors

2.2.1. Obesity

Obesity is an independent risk factor for CVD. It is a chronic metabolic disorder associated with increased morbidity and mortality. Obesity may affect atherosclerosis through many risk factors such as dyslipidemia, hypertension, glucose intolerance, and increased chronic inflammatory and prothrombotic state. Obesity causes a variety of adaptations/ alterations in cardiac structure and function due to excessive adipose tissue accumulation, even in the absence of comorbidities [18]. Thus, it increases cardiac workload that leads to heart failure, coronary heart disease, sudden cardiac death, and arterial fibrillation [19]. In many cases, these events result in mortality and morbidity. By favourably modifying blood lipids, in particular LDL cholesterol, lowering blood pressure, controlling blood sugar, decreasing proinflammatory cytokines and adhesion molecules, weight loss may prevent the progression of atherosclerosis or the occurrence of acute coronary heart events in the obese high-risk populations [18].

2.2.2. High blood cholesterol

A high concentration of serum cholesterol is a major risk factor for coronary heart disease [20]. The relationship between abnormal plasma cholesterol fractions and increased CVD risk was described 60 years ago [21]. The excessive cholesterol, especially cholesterol transported/ carried by low density lipoproteins that contain protein apolipoprotein (apo) B100 contributes to the formation of atherosclerotic plaques in arteries. Accordingly, cholesterol that is carried by LDL particles is called "bad cholesterol". by contrast, HDL cholesterol which transports esterified cholesterol from the periphery to the liver is considered more cardioprotective and sometimes referred to as "good cholesterol" [22]. The ratio of LDL to HDL cholesterol is more important than LDL or HDL cholesterol concentration and has been widely used to evaluate susceptibility to the development of heart disease. For a healthy person, it is recommended to maintain the LDL/HDL ratio below 3.5.

2.2.3. High blood pressure

Hypertension is a highly prevalent major contributor to atherosclerotic cardiovascular disease. It accelerates atherogenesis, imparting a 2- to 3-fold coronary heart disease (CHD) and lethal sequel [23]. In most cases, hypertension results from excessive vasoconstriction of the small arterioles throughout the body, raising the diastolic pressure. Because of high peripheral resistance, the heart needs to generate more force to overcome the resistance created by the constricted arterioles and supply adequate blood to the tissues, which leads to a compensatory rise in systolic blood pressure. This excess of systolic and diastolic blood pressures causes excessive vasoconstriction. Thus, increased levels of systolic and diastolic blood pressure are associated with an increased risk of CVD events [24]. When high blood pressures co-exist with obesity, smoking, hypercholesterolemia, and/or diabetes, the risk of heart attack and stroke increases several times.

2.2.4. Physical inactivity

Sedentary lifestyle is associated with almost twice the risk of developing coronary heart disease compared with their active counterparts. Regular physical activity plays a crucial role in the prevention of CVD. High levels of physical activity are associatedwith substantial reductions in CVD risk, and total mortalitydecreases by 20% to 30% for the increase of every 1000 kcal/wk of energy expenditure resulting from physical activity [25]. Regular exercise has a favourable effect on many of the establishedrisk factors of CVD. Exercisepromotes weight reduction, reduce blood pressure, "bad" cholesterol (LDL level), and total cholesterol,and can raise the "good" cholesterol (HDL) [26].

2.2.5. Diabetes mellitus

Diabetes has long been recognized to be an independent riskfactor for CVD. Type-1 diabetes ortype-2 diabetes is at high risk for several cardiovasculardisorders: coronary heart disease, stroke, peripheral arterialdisease, cardiomyopathy, and congestive heart failure. Closely linked to type-2 diabetes are several metabolic risk factors such as hypertension, atherogenic dyslipidemia which is associated with insulin resistance that relatedto coronary heart disease. Cardiovascularcomplications are now the leading causes of illness and death in the diabetic patient. The incidence of diabetes rises with advancing age, obese and overweight persons and in the populations (race/ethnicity) who areparticularly susceptible to diabetes [27].

http://dx.doi.org/10.5772/54729

2.2.6. Tobacco smoke

Smokingnearly doubles the risk of heart disease. Smoking acts synergisticallywith other risk factors, substantially increasing the risk ofCVD [28]. The exact toxic componentsof cigarette smoke and the mechanisms involved in smoking-relatedcardiovascular dysfunction are notclearly elucidated, but smoking increasesinflammation, thrombosis, and oxidation of LDLcholesterol. Smokers have significantly higherserum total cholesterol, LDL cholesterol and triacylglycerol levels, while having lower blood concentration of HDL cholesterol than non-smokers [29]. Cigarette smoke exposure increases oxidativestress as a potential mechanism for initiating cardiovasculardysfunction. Cigarette smoke exposure decreases the plasma activity of paraoxonase, an enzymethat protects against LDL oxidation. Smoking is also found to be an independent predictor of newcoronary lesion formation and thrombosis [30].

In spite of identification of many unmodifiable and modifiable risk factors, there are still several paradoxes in the pathogenesis of CVD that cannot be sufficiently explained; mortality from CVD is relatively low despite a high intake of saturated fatty acids [31] or a high incidence of CVD without having the expected risk indicators [32]. CVD mortality rate in urban populations is higher compared with rural populations despite a very low fat intake [33]. All these paradoxes support the assumption that some important factors in the aetiology of CVD are currently unknown. However, it has been well established that elevated blood total cholesterol, especially LDL cholesterol levels is one of the primary risk factors that contribute to the development of atherosclerosis and ultimately CVD. Therefore, in the following sections, we focus mainly on the atherosclerosis, cholesterol metabolism and homeostasis, benefits versus side effects of current cholesterol-lowering products, and our perspectives on the development of future cholesterol-lowering products.

3. Atherosclerosis and CVD

Atherosclerosis is a disease of the arterial wall that is characterized by cholesterol accumulation and culminates in potentially life-threatening conditions such as heart attack, stroke and angina. The build-up of cholesterol in the walls of arteries is a hallmark of atherosclerosis. However, the process starts is poorly understood. The atherogenic process starts at an early age with the deposition in blood vessel walls of lipids such as cholesterol, derived from lipoproteins circulating in the bloodstream, which leads to the formation of the characteristic 'fatty streaks'. Inflammatory white blood cells congregate at these damaged areas through their interaction with adhesion molecules expressed by cells in the endothelial layer, which lines the inside of blood vessels. This event then sets off a cascade of inflammatory process and further lipid deposition, leading eventually to full blown atherosclerosis with plaque formation in the artery wall. Atherosclerosis is thus viewed as a chronic inflammatory disease of the blood vessel wall [34], [35]. Oxidized LDL contributes to atherogenesis and is an early event of atherosclerosis. WhenLDL particles become trapped in an artery, they can undergoprogressive oxidation and be internalized by macrophages bymeans of the scavenger receptors on the surfaces of these cells. The internalization leads to the formation of lipid peroxidesand facilitates the accumulation of cholesterol esters, resultingin the formation of foam cells. As the fatty streak progresses, smooth muscle cells (not normally present in the subendothelial space) migrate from the media to the subendothelial space where they proliferate and produce connective tissue to form a fibrous cap, which represents the second phase of atherosclerosis. Finally, complicated lesions occur, which can manifest calcification, hemorrhage, ulceration and thrombosis [35, 36]. All these changes and events lead to the hardening and thickening of artery wall, reducing or blocking blood flow. Atherosclerosis is a silent and asymptomatic disease until complications arise with thrombosis and occurrence of clinical symptoms [37]. The clinical manifestation of atherosclerotic plaque formation is acute vascular occlusion due to the formation of a thrombus or clot which can lead to ischemia of vital organs, such as heart causing myocardial infarction, brain resulting in strokes and lower extremites causing peripheral artery disease. Oxidized LDL contributes to atherothrombosis by inducing endothelial cell apoptosis, and thus plaque erosion, by impairing the anticoagulant balance in endothelium, stimulating tissue factor production by smooth muscle cells, and inducing apoptosis in macrophages [38]. It is reasonably thinking that maintaining a healthy cholesterol or lipid profile is critically important to the health cardiovascular system.

4. Cholesterol homeostasis

Cholesterol, the characteristic steroid alcohol of animal tissues, performs a number of essential functions in the body. For example, cholesterol is a structural component of cell membranes and modulates cell membrane fluidity; cholesterol is a precursor of bile acids, steroid hormones and vitamin D. It is therefore of critical importance that the cells of the body be assured a continuous supply of cholesterol. To meet this need, a complex series of transport, biosynthetic and regulatory mechanism has evolved. The liver plays a central role in the regulation of the body's cholesterol homeostasis. For example, cholesterol enters the liver's cholesterol pool from a number of sources including dietary cholesterol, as well as cholesterol synthesized de novo by extra hepatic tissues as well as by the liver itself. Cholesterol is eliminated from the liver as unmodified cholesterol in the bile or it can be converted to bile acids that are secreted in bile into the intestinal lumen.

Cholesterol, similar with other lipids (triacylglycerols and phospholipids) do not circulate as independent molecules but are carried by specific apolipoproteins to form macromolecular complexes, called lipoproteins. Plasma lipoproteins keep their component lipids soluble during circulation and provide an efficient mechanism for transporting their lipid contents to (and from) the tissues. Four major groups of lipoproteins have been identified and they are important physiologically and in clinical diagnosis. They are chylomicrons, very low density lipoproteins (VLDL or pre β lipoprotein), LDL (β lipoprotein) and HDL (α lipoprotein). They differ in their relative composition of cholesterol, triacylglyceroles, phospholipids and apoproteins.

Chylomicrons, the largest and least dense lipoproteins, predominately transport triacylglycerols to adipose tissue and muscle, but also deliver the absorbed dietary and billiary

http://dx.doi.org/10.5772/54729

cholesterol to the liver. Once most of the triacylglycerols have been delivered to the adipose tissue and muscle, the remnants of the lipoprotein, including cholesterol, apo-E, and apo-B48 are then delivered to and taken up by the liver through interaction with the chylomicron remnant receptor.

VLDL is smaller and more dense than chylomicrons. VLDL contains triacylglycerols, some cholesterol and cholesteryl esters and the apoproteins; apo-B100, apo-CI, apo-CII, apo-CIII, and apoE. VLDL delivers triacylglycerols and cholesteryl esters from the liver and distribute them throughout the body. When VLDL moves into the circulating blood, it is converted first to intermediate density lipoproteins (IDL) and then into low density lipoproteins (LDL). Lipoprotein lipase serves to remove the majority of fatty acids from both the VLDL and IDL, thus increasing the density of the lipoproteins while maintaining cholesterol and cholesteryl ester concentrations. The removal of fatty acids and the loss of all apolipoproteins except apoB-100 and apo(a) results in the formation of LDL.

LDL is the primary blood carrier of cholesterol and delivers cholesterol to all tissues. LDL can be absorbed by the liver and other tissues via receptor mediated endocytosis. The LDL receptor recognizes the main apolipoprotein of LDL, apo-B100, resulting in the intake of LDL and subsequently enzymatic hydrolysis of cholesteryl ester. A positive correlation exists between the incidence of coronary atherosclerosis and the plasma concentration of LDL cholesterol.

High density lipoprotein is the smallest but most dense lipoproteins in the body. Nascent HDL or HDL contains several types of apolipoproteins including apo-AI, II & IV, apo-CI, II & III, apoD and apoE. HDL contains protein, phospholipids, cholesteryl esters, and cholesterol. HDL is produced as a protein-rich particle in the liver and intestine, and serves as a circulating source of Apo-CI & II and ApoE proteins. The HDL protein particle accumulates cholesteryl esters through the esterification of cholesterol by lecithin:cholesterol acyl-transferase (LCAT). LCAT is activated by apo-AI on HDL. HDL returns the liver where cholesterol is removed by reverse cholesterol transport, thus, serving as a scavenger of free cholesterol. Cholesteryl ester transfer protein (CETP) facilitates the transfer of cholesteryl esters from HDL to VLDL, IDL, and LDL in exchange of triacylglycerol, relieving the inhibition of LCAT activity in HDL.

5. Hyperlipidemia and causes

Hyperlipidemia, most common form of dyslipidemia, refers to elevation of lipoproteins and/ or lipids. HDL, LDL, and VLDL vary in their atherogenicities. High levels of cholesterol particularly LDL cholesterol together with low levels ofHDL cholesterol increase the risks for developing atherosclerosis [39]. Hyperlipidemia itself usually causes no symptoms but can lead to the development of symptomatic vascular disease, including coronary artery disease and peripheral arterial disease. There are two different types of hyperlipidemia, primary and secondary hyperlipidemia:

1. Primary hyperlipidemia is generally due to genetic causes, such as a mutation in a receptor or binding protein. This type of hyperlipidemia is often linked to family history. For

instance, defects in the essential components of lipid transportation and metabolism inherited from family. Examples include familial defect in LDL receptor or apo B-100 (diminished LDL clearance and hypercholesterolemia), familial lipoprotein lipase deficiency (hypertriglyceridemia), and combination of multiple unknown defect and known familial defects (combined hyperlipidemia).

2. Secondary hyperlipidemia arises due to other underlying causes, such as sedentary lifestyle coupled with the excessive dietary intakes of saturated fat, cholesterol and trans-fats, in addition to many other disease conditions and drug uses. These factors include obesity, diabetes mellitus, hyperhomocystinemia, smoking, alcohol intake, chronic kidney disease, hypothyroidism, primary biliary cirrhosis and other cholestatic liver diseases, and drugs, such as thiazides, β-blockers, retinoids, estrogen and progesterons, and glucocorticoids.

6. Metabolic pathways involved in cholesterol homeostasis

6.1. Biosynthesis

Cholesterol levels in the body derived from *de novo* biosynthesis and diet. The majority of cholesterol utilized by healthy adults is synthesized in the liver, which accounts for about 70% of the daily cholesterol. Virtually all cells containing nucleus are capable of cholesterol synthesis, which occurs in endoplasmic reticulum and the cytosol. Biosynthesis of cholesterol generally takes place in the endoplasmic reticulum of hepatic cells and begins with acetyl-CoA, which is mainly derived from fatty acid oxidation reaction in the mitochondria. The conversion of 3-hydroxy-3-methylglutaryl-CoA (HMG-CoA) to mevalonate by HMG-CoA reductase is the rate-limiting step of cholesterol biosynthesis and is under strict regulatory control. Thus, HMG-CoA reductase is one of important targets of cholesterol lowering drugs. The development of statin drugs is a very successful story of discovering and applying HMG-CoA reductase inhibitor to lower hypercholesterolemia.

6.2. Absorption

Dietary cholesterol is absorbed within the lumen of the small intestine. Bile salts produced from cholesterol in the liver interact with phospholipids to produce a biliary micelle that is transported via bile into the lumen. Dietary cholesterol in the lumen is easily incorporated into the micelles and together with the biliary cholesterol can be absorbed into the enterocytes. In the enterocytes, absorbed cholesterol is esterified by acyl-coenzyme A:cholesterol acyltransferase 2 (ACAT2), which is found in both the intestine and liver. Reducing the absorption of cholesterol of dietary ad billiary sources has become another key area in cholesterol research and product development. A typical example is plant sterols/stanols that have long found as effective inhibitors of cholesterol absorption. These molecules inhibit cholesterol absorption by competitively inhibiting with cholesterol for incorporation into micelles. Recently, inhibitors, such as ezetimibe, that block the absorption of cholesterol into the enterocytes through suppressing the activity of cholesterol transporters have also been used to reduce absorption of dietary cholesterol.

6.3. Transport

Chylomicrons deliver absorbed dietary and biliary cholesterol from the enterocytes to the liver. During the process, triacylglycerols are released with assistance of lipoprotein lipase and taken up by adipose tissues and muscle, the remnants of the lipoprotein then delivered to, and taken up by, the liver through interaction with the chylomicron remnant receptor. In the liver, absorbed cholesterol, together with synthesized cholesterol and cholesterol transported back from peripheral tissues and LDL receptor-mediated uptake go through several metabolic pathways and secreted out from different outputs. One of them is the secretion in VLDL back into the bloodstream. VLDL removes triacylglycerols and cholesteryl esters from the liver and distributes them throughout the body. Endothelial Lipoprotein lipase remove the majority of fatty acids from both the VLDL and IDL, thus increasing the cholesterol and cholesteryl ester concentrationsand apoB-100 results in LDL. LDL is the primary plasma carrier of cholesterol, which can be taken up by the liver and other tissues via receptor-mediated endocytosis. The cytoplasmic domain of LDL receptor facilitates the formation of coated pits which is the receptor-rich regions of the membrane. The ligand binding domain of the receptor recognizes apo-B100 on LDL, resulting in the formation of a clathrin-coated vesicle that buds from the inner surface of the cell membrane. ATP-dependent proton pumps lower the pH inside the vesicle resulting in dissociation of LDL from its receptor. After loss of the clathrin coat, the vesicles fuse with lysozomes, resulting in peptide and cholesteryl ester enzymatic hydrolysis. On the other hand, HDL is the small and rich in lipoproteins. The HDL protein particle accumulates cholesteryl esters by the esterification of cholesterol with lecithin:cholesterol acyl-transferase (LCAT). In the plasma, these particles undergo aseries of remodeling steps involving two HDL-associated proteins:phospholipid transfer protein (PLTP) and CETP. The primary role of PLTP is in thetransfer of surface remnants, which contain apolipoproteinsand phospholipids originating from triglyceride-rich lipoproteins,to pre-ß–HDL. PLTP has also been implicatedin mediating fusion of HDL particles to generate pre-ß–HDLand CE-rich HDL. CETP promotesboth transfer and exchange of hydrophobic lipids, CE, and triacylglycerols between lipoproteins. HDL can acquire cholesterol from cell membranes and transfer cholesteryl esters to VLDL and LDL via the transferase activity of apoD. More importantly, HDL can return to the liver where cholesterol is removed by reverse cholesterol transport, thus serving as a scavenger of free cholesterol. Scavenging activity of HDL initiates by accepting cholesterol from tissues in smaller HDL_3 via the ATP-binding Cassette transporter -1 (ABC-1). The cholesterol in HDL_3 is then esterified by LCAT, increasing the size of the particles to form the less dense HDL_2. The cycle is completed by the reformation of HDL_3 either after selective delivery of cholesteryl esters to the liver via the scavenger receptor-B1 or by the hydrolysis of HDL_2 phospholipid and triacylglycerol by hepatic lipase. HDL_2 concentration is inversely related to the incidence of coronary atherosclerosis. The enzyme cholesterol esterase controls the hydrolysis of these stored cholesterol esters, yielding bioavailable cholesterol and fatty acids.

6.4. Excretion of cholesterol

About 1 g of cholesterol is eliminated from the body per day, approximately equivalent to the amount that absorbed cholesterol and synthesize cholesterol. Approximately, half is excreted in the feces after conversion to bile acids in liver, and the remainder is excreted as cholesterol. Bile acids serve to remove unwanted cholesterol from the body and to aid in lipid digestion in the intestine. 7α-hydroxylase, the rate limiting enzyme of bile acid biosynthesis converts cholesterol into 7-hydroxycholesterol. 7-hydroxycholesterol is converted to one of the two primary bile acids, cholic acid and chenodeoxycholic acid. Bile acids are then delivered to the intestines where they aid in the absorption of lipids. Some of bile acids are modified to form secondary bile acids (lithocholic acid and deoxycholic acid) in the intestine by intestinal bacteria. However, the majority of bile acids delivered to intestine are recycled by re-absorption in the ileum and returned to the liver by enterohepatic circulation. In liver, glyco- and tauroconjugate bile acids are formed and stored in gall bladder, from where they are released into the intestinal lumen for aid fat/lipids digestion and absorption.

7. Regulation of specific pathways and its influence on cholesterol homeostasis

Blood cholesterol concentration is a result of balance between cholesterol input and cholesterol output. When the input is surpass the output, blood cholesterol increases and by contrast, when cholesterol input is less than the output blood cholesterol levels decrease. Cholesterol input is attributed from the intestinal absorption of dietary and biliary cholesterol and cholesterol biosynthesis. On the other hand, the cholesterol output is mainly from LDL-receptor mediated LDL-cholesterol clearance, reverse transport by HDL, cholesterol catabolism by converting into bile acids, cholesterol and bile acids secretion in bile into the intestine lumen, and fecal excretion.

Metabolic nuclear receptors serve a central role in maintainingcellular and whole-body cholesterol homeostasis [40]. Two important transcriptional mechanisms to regulate cholesterol metabolism are the pathways mediated by sterol responsive element– binding protein (SREBP) and liver X receptor (LXR), which tightly regulate intracellular sterol concentrations. The SREBP pathway ensures that there is sufficientcholesterol to meet cellular requirements by directly activating expression of genesinvolved in the synthesis and uptake of cholesterol, and lipogenesis [41]. In the setting ofexcess free or unesterified cholesterol, SREBP-dependentgene expression is suppressed. LXR and farnesoid X receptor (FXR),together with other members of the nuclear receptor superfamilypromote sterol storage, transport, and catabolism to prevent cholesterol accumulation [42]. LXRs respond to elevated cholesterol levels via transactivationof genes involved in sterol transport (ABCA1, ABCG1, ABCG5,and ABCG8), cholesterol efflux and high-density lipoprotein(HDL) metabolism (ABCA1, APOE, CETP, and

PLTP), and sterol catabolism(CYP7A1) [42]. Other members of metabolicnuclear receptor family include receptors for bile acids (CAR and PXR), and fatty acids (peroxisome prolifer-aotr-activated receptors). Throughthe coordinated regulation of gene transcription, these nuclearreceptors regulate the key aspects of cellular and whole-body sterolhomeostasis, including cholesterol absorption and synthesis, lipoprotein synthesisand remodeling, lipoprotein uptake by peripheral tissues, reversecholesterol transport, and bile acid synthesis and absorption.

The amount of cholesterol that is synthesized in the liver is tightly regulated by dietary cholesterol levels. When dietary intake of cholesterol is high, synthesis is decreased and when dietary intake is low, synthesis is increased. However, cholesterol produced in other tissues is under no such feedback control. Cholesterol and similar oxysterols (the oxygenated derivatives of cholesterol, such as 22(R)-hydroxycholesterol, 2 4(S)-hydroxycholesterol, 27-hydroxycholesterol, and cholestenoic acid) act as regulatory molecules to maintain healthy levels of cholesterol. In tissues, many factor influence cholesterol balance through every cholesterol metabolic pathways.

7.1. LDL receptor-mediated cholesterol clearance

Cellular cholesterol increase is due to the uptake of cholesterol containing lipoproteins by receptors. LDL receptor regulates the cellular transport of LDL particles. One mechanism for regulating LDL receptor expression and controlling the expression of all the enzymes in the cholesterol biosynthetic pathway involves sterol-sensitive response elements (SREs). SREs are found in the promoters of the genes coding for the enzymes of cholesterol biosynthesis pathway and LDL receptors. Transcription factors of SRE activation are SREBPs. Three major SREBP isoforms, SREBP-1a, -1c, and -2, have been identified and differ in relative abundance in the liver and other various tissues. SREBP-1a is a potent activator of all SREBP-responsive genes and functions to maintain basal levels of cholesterol and fatty acid synthesis. SREBP-1c selectively activates genes involved in fatty acid synthesis, while SREBP-2 preferentially regulates genes important for cholesterol homeostasis by activating the transcription of HMG-CoA synthase, HMG-CoA reductase, LDL receptor [41].

Due to their ability to bind SREs, SREBP-2 plays an instrumental role in cholesterol homeostasis. These transcription-regulatory proteins are bound by another protein called SREBP cleavage activating proteins (SCAPs). SCAP, in turn, can bind reversibly with another endoplasmic reticulum-resident membrane protein, INSIG. SCAPs bind to SREBP-2 in the endoplasmic reticulum where a regulatory domain within SCAP responds to the level of oxysterols present in the cell. When the intracellular cholesterol and oxysterols concentrations decrease, the SREBP/SCAP complex moves to Golgi apparatus, leaving INSIG. Two proteases localized in Golgi, site-1 and -2 proteases (S1P and S2P) cleave SREBP-2 to release the transcription activation domain of SREBP-2. SREBP-2 preferentially activates transcription of target genes of LDL receptor [41]. When oxysterol levels are high, the SCAP/SREBP complex remains in the endoplasmic reticulum, preventing cleaved SREBP-2 from promoting gene expression. In addition to the up-regulation of LDLR transcription, nuclear SREBP-2 increases the transcription of PCSK9, a sterol-responsive protein that accelerates LDLR turnover in the liver, thereby limiting lipoprotein uptake. As high concentrations of cellular cholesterol suppress SREBP-2 cleavage and release from endoplasmic reticulum, PCSK9 transcription is reduced, which subsequently increases LDLR levels, helping to maintain cholesterol homeostasis [43].

7.2. Regulation of cholesterol biosynthesis

SREBPs directly activate the expression of more than 30 genes dedicated to the synthesis and uptake of cholesterol, fatty acids, triacylglycerols, and phospholipids, as well as the reduced nicotinamide adenine dinucleotide phosphate (NADPH) cofactor required to synthesize these molecules. SREBP-2–responsive genes in the cholesterol biosynthetic pathway include those for the enzymes HMG-CoA synthase, HMG-CoA reductase, farnesyl diphosphate synthase, and squalene synthase. SREBP-1c and SREBP-2 activate three genes required to generate NADPH, which is consumed at multiple stages in these lipid biosynthetic pathways [41]. High cholesterol/oxysterol levels acting on SCAP ultimately stop the maturation of SREBPs, resulting in the down regulation of key enzymes such as HMG-CoA reductase, thus, reducing the amount of cholesterol produced by the liver. To compensate the decreased cholesterol synthesis a homeostatic response in which cells increase the density of LDL receptors on their surfaces. This increases the clearance rate of LDL particles from the plasma and reduces plasma LDL cholesterol and its related health risks. The decrease in cholesterol synthesis also promotes an increase of HDL, thus, clearing even more cholesterol from the plasma.

Elevated levels of cellular cholesterol are accompanied by the increased production of oxysterols, which are specificligands of LXRs, allowing LXRs to function as cholesterol sensors [44]. LXRs respond to elevated cholesterol levels via transactivationof genes involved in sterol transport (ABCA1, ABCG1, ABCG5,and ABCG8), cholesterol efflux and HDL metabolism (ABCA1, APOE, CETP, and PLTP), and sterol catabolism(CYP7A1). Additionally, LXRs also play a central role in regulatingcellular lipid content through activation of SREBP-1c, whichis the master regulator of de novo lipogenesis [40]. In response to activation, LXRs act in a coordinated fashion to maintain cholesterol homeostasis by directing the tissue-specific expression of genes involved in sterol transport and metabolism [45]. A principal function of LXR in macrophages is to promote cholesterol removal from the cell through the induction of ABCA1, ABCG1, and apolipoprotein E. LXR also induces genes involvedin lipoprotein metabolism, including LPL, CETP, and PLTP [45].

7.3. Regulation of cholesterol absorption and secretion

At the intestine, cholesterol is absorbed into enterocytes by a mechanism involving Niemann Pick C1-like protein 1 (NPC1L1) [46]. The NPC1L1 protein is abundant on intestinal brush border membranes. It functions as a sterol transporter to mediate intestinal cholesterol absorption and counterbalances hepatobiliary cholesterol excretion [46]. NPC1L1, is not under control of a nuclear receptor LXR [47]. In the enterocyte, cholesterol is readily esterified by the action of acyl-CoA:cholesterol acyltransferase 2 (ACAT2) and released into lymph in association with chylomicrons. The ATP-binding cassette (ABC) transporter protein ABCA1 andthe ABC half-transporters, ABCG5 and ABCG8, are LXR target genesin the intestine and participate in cholesterol absorption. ABCA1 and ABCG5/8 counteract cholesterol absorption via effluxof cholesterol from the enterocyte into the gut lumen. LXR agonists exerttheir effect on cholesterol absorption through upregulationof ABCG5 and ABCG8, which is necessary for the majority of sterols secreted into bile [40, 48].

7.4. Regulation of cholesterol transport

The hepatic nuclear receptor, PPARα, exert control over many aspects of reversecholesterol transport. Hepatic synthesisof apoA-I and apoA-II, the two major apolipoproteins in discoidalHDL (HDL_2), is regulated via PPARα activation and transcriptional regulation ofRORα (NR1F1), a widely expressed nuclear receptor that is activatedby cholesterol or cholesterol sulfate ligands [49]. ABCA1, which helps in reverse transport from peripheral tissues, is PPARγ/LXR-regulated cholesterol/phospholipid transporter [50]. PLTP is activatedby both LXR and FXR whereas CETP is transactivated by LXR [40,51].

7.5. Excretion of cholesterol

Bile acids are synthesized in hepatocytes and this production is tightly controlled by the nuclear receptor transcription factors, LXR-α and LXR-β. Activation of LXRs by specific oxysterol derivatives leads to the regulation of bile acid synthesis by stimulating cholesterol 7α-hydroxylase (*CYP7A1)* transcription to convertcholesterol to bile acids. FXR, a bile acid receptor, plays a central role of lipid metabolism in liver cells. FXR may play the major roles in bileacid metabolism, reverse cholesterol transport, and protecthepatocytes against cholestasis by feedback inhibition ofbile acid synthesis by CYP7A1; stimulation of bile acid effluxfrom hepatocytes by bile salt export pump; inhibition of bile acid uptakeinto hepatocytes by Na^+-taurocholate co-transporting polypeptide; and regulation of reverse cholesteroltransport by inducing ApoCII and PLTP [40, 52].

8. Cholesterol-lowering drugs

Mainly cholesterol lowering drugs have been developed and used clinically, which includes 1) HMG-CoA reductase inhibitors, e.g., atorvastatin, fluvastatin, lovastatin, pravastatin, rosuvastatin and simvastatin, 2) bile acid sequestrants — colesevelam, cholestyramine and colestipol — and nicotinic acid (niacin), and 3) cholesterol absorption inhibitor - ezetimibe. Other available drugs are gemfibrozil, fenofibrate and clofibrate which are fibric acid derivatives primarily used for lowering high triglyceride levels

8.1. Statins – Benefits versus side effects

Statins or inhibitors of 3-hydroxy-3-methylglutaryl–coenzyme A (HMG-CoA) reductase are widely used to reduce the risk of cardiovascular events and death. Statins includes lovastatin, which is a fungal metabolite, and many synthetic derivatives, pravastatin, atorvastatin and simvastatin etc. Statins target predominantly hepatocytes and inhibit HMG-CoA reductase, the enzyme that converts HMG-CoA into mevalonic acid, a cholesterol precursor. Statins alter the conformation of the enzyme when they bind to its active site. This prevents HMG-CoA reductase from attaining a functional structure. The change in conformation at the active site makes these drugs very effective and specific [53]. Binding of statins to HMG-CoA reductase is reversible, and their affinity for the enzyme is in the nanomolar range, as compared to the natural substrate, which has micromolar affinity [54]. The inhibition of HMG-CoA reductase determines the reduction of intracellular cholesterol, inducing the activation of a protease which slices SREBPs from the endoplasmic reticulum. SREBPs are translocated into nucleus, where they increase the gene expression for LDL receptor. The reduction of cholesterol in hepatocytes leads to the increase of hepatic LDL receptors that leads to the reduction of circulating LDL and of its precursors (intermediate density - IDL and very low density- VLDL lipoproteins). All statins reduce LDL cholesterol non-linearly, dose-dependent, and after administration of a single daily dose [53]. Statins inhibit hepatic synthesis of apolipoprotein B-100, determining a reduction of the synthesis, secretion of triacylglycerols-rich lipoproteins, and an increase of receptors for apolipoproteins B/E. Statins have a modest effect on HDL increase, and no influence on lipoprotein(s) concentration. Statins can also prevent LDL oxidation by preserving the activity of the endogenous antioxidant system, like superoxide dismutase [53].

In general, the currently used statins are well tolerated and have a good safety profile [55]. Statins acting as inhibitor of HMG-CoA reductase, inhibits all the pathway in which mevalonate is a precursor such as synthesis of nonsteroid isoprenoids such as farnesylpyrophosphate (FPP), geranylgeranylpyrophosphate (GGPP), dolichol and side chain of coenzyme Q which play an essential role in cellular physiology. Coenzyme Q is a component of mitochondrial respiratory chain and a lipid-soluble antioxidant. Farnesyl- and geranylgeranyl groups are needed for protein isoprenylation and formation of small GTP-binding proteins including Ras, Rho and Rab, which are involved in signal transduction pathways. Inhibition of isoprenoid synthesis by statins decreases the activity of these proteins and modifies the respective signalling pathways; the mechanism responsible for cholesterol-independent pleiotropic effects of statins. The best recognized and most commonly reported adverse effect of statins are muscle adverse effect with muscle pain, fatigue and weakness as well as rhabdomyolysis. Rhabdomyolysis is the most severe form of statin induced myopathy, characterized by marked increase in CK activity, myoglobinemia, myoglobinuria, and myoglobin induced acute renal failure. These symptoms arising on statins are shown to be reversed with discontinuation. Coenzyme Q10 deficiency produces mitochondrial encephalomyopathy, resulting in fatigue, muscle symptoms, and cognitive problems. Gastrointestinal and neurological symptoms, psychiatric symptoms, sleep problems, glucose elevations, and a range of other symptoms are also reported on statins [56].

8.2. Ezetimibe – Benefits and side effects

Ezetimibe is the first of a new class of highly selective cholesterol absorption inhibitors. It does not inhibit cholesterol synthesis in the liver or increase bile acid excretion. It belongs to a class of lipid-lowering compounds that selectively inhibits the intestinal absorption of cholesterol and sterols. Ezetimibe's pharmacological effect is complementary to that of the statins [57]. Mechanism of action of ezetimibe involves inhibiting the absorption of cholesterol in the small intestine. Through a mechanism that is not yet fully elucidated, ezetimibe appears to block a protein transporter called Niemann-Pick C1-like 1 protein (NPC1L1) that is located at the apical membrane of the small intestine enterocytes [58]. Unlike other cholesterol-lowering agents, ezetimibe localizes and appears to act at the brush border of the small intestine and inhibits the absorption of dietary and biliary cholesterol in the small intestine, leading to a decrease in the delivery of intestinal cholesterol to the liver. This leads to a reduction of hepatic cholesterol stores and an increase in clearance of cholesterol from the blood. Ezetimibe has been demonstrated to have no significant effect on the plasma concentrations of the fat-soluble vitamins A, D, and E [57]. No published reports could be identified that assessed the potential impact of ezetimibe therapy on other traditional CVD risk factors, including blood pressure and obesity. Recent reports have raised concerns about an association between ezetimibe and an increased incidence of cancer [58]. Ezetimibe may rarely cause hepatotoxicity, severe cholestatic hepatitis, or acute autoimmune hepatitis [59].

Ezetimibe is proved to be more effective in combination with statin drugs in lowering LDL-c than monotherapy. Ezetimibe has an additive and at times synergistic effect on the reduction of LDL-C and total cholesterol (TC) concentrations when combined with statin therapy. Ezetimibe has not been associated with increased rates of myopathy or rhabdomyolysis, whether used alone or in combination with statins, although there have been some case reports of myopathy attributed to this agent. Moreover, ezetimibe has been associated with mild elevations of liver transaminases, mainly in combination with a statin. Other side effects are extremely rare. It should be noted, however, there are no long-term safety data or outcome studies for ezetimibe yet [60].

8.3. Niacin (Nicotinic acid)

Niacin is the most potent HDL increasing drug currently available and it also can efficaciously lowers triglycerides and LDL cholesterol. It is the only lipid-lowering drug that considerably lowers lipoprotein(a). Beneficial effect of niacin to reduce triglycerides and apolipoprotein-B containing lipoproteins (e.g., VLDL and LDL) are mainly through: a) decreasing fatty acid mobilization from adipose tissue triglyceride stores, and b) inhibiting hepatocyte diacylglycerol acyltransferase and triglyceride synthesis leading to increased intracellular apo B degradation and subsequent decreased secretion of VLDL and LDL particles. Niacin raises HDL by decreasing the fractional catabolic rate of HDL-apoAI without affecting the synthetic rates. Additionally, niacin selectively increases the plasma levels of lipoprotein-AI (HDL subfraction without apoAII), a cardioprotective subfraction of HDL in patients with low HDL. Recent studies indicate that niacin selectively inhibits the uptake/removal of HDL-apoAI (but not HDL-cholesterol ester) by hepatocytes, thereby increasing the capacity of retained HDL-apoAI to augment cholesterol efflux through reverse cholesterol transport pathway [61]. Niacin treatment is associated with a number of side effects, including headache, itching and gastrointestinal disturbances, but these are generally mild. The most severe of the side effects is flushing, and this is sufficiently severe to negatively affect compliance [62].

8.4. Bile acid sequestrant

Bile acid sequestrant or bile binding anion (Chloride) exchange resins that is effective in reducing total cholesterol and LDL cholesterol levels. The primary and direct action of the bile acid sequestrants is to bind to bile acids in the gut and thus interrupt the enterohepatic recirculation of bile acids [63]. Three key enzyme are affected by bile acid sequestrant, which are phosphatidic acid phosphatase, cholesterol 7-alpha-hydroxylase and HMG-CoA reductase. Activation of phosphatidic acid phosphatase promotes hepatic triglyceride synthesis, induces secretion of triglyceride-rich VLDL particles and consequently increases plasma triglyceride levels. The activation of hepatic cholesterol 7-alpha-hydroxylase promotes the conversion of intracellular cholesterol to bile acids. The decrease in intracellular cholesterol stores, in turn, increases LDL receptor expression on hepatocyte membranes and consequently, increases receptor-mediated fractional catabolism of LDL or LDL uptake by liver cells. Reduction of intracellular cholesterol may also increase the synthesis of cholesterol through activation of HMG-CoA reductase. The potential loss of the bile acid sequestrant's cholesterol-lowering efficacy can be overcome by adding HMG-CoA reductase inhibitor (statins). Finally, bile acid sequestrants promote apoprotein AI synthesis and tend to raise high-HDL cholesterol levels, primarily by increasing plasma HDL-2 concentrations. Three drugs in this class are synthetic cholestyramine, colestipol, colesevelam. The side effect profile of the bile acid sequestrants is tolerable, with most complaints related to effects on the gastrointestinal tract and the bulkiness of resins [64].

8.5. Fibrates

Fibrates are primarily effective for the treatment of hypertriglyceridemia or mixed hyperlipidemia by stimulating the peroxisomal β-oxidation pathway. Their main action is to lower plasma triglyceride levels, but they also reduce total and LDL cholesterol concentrations and induce a moderate increase in HDL cholesterol. Fibrates act by stimulating the activity of peroxisome proliferator-activated receptor (PPAR)-α, a member of the PPAR subfamily of nuclear receptors [65]. It controls the transcription of regulatory genes of fatty acids and cholesterol metabolism. It inhibits the synthesis and secretion of triglycerides by the liver and a stimulation of the degradation of triglyceride-rich lipoproteins. This increased clearance of triglycerides results from a stimulation of the expression of lipoprotein lipase and a decreased expression and concentration of apolipoprotein-CIII, an inhibitor of lipoprotein lipase activity. PPAR-α activation modifies the expression of several key genes controlling HDL cholesterol metabolism and reverse transport of cholesterol [65]. Several fibrate drugs such as ciprofibrate, bezafibrate, fenofibrate, and gemfibrozil has revolutionized lipid-lowering but research has shown the prolonged use of some of these drugs like clofibrate and ciprofibrate causes peroxisome proliferation leading to hepatomegaly and tumor formation in the liver of rodents [66].

A recent report demonstrated that between the periods 1988-1994 and 1999-2002, mean total cholesterol and mean LDL cholesterol declined in American adults. Coincidently, during this time there also was an increase in the percentage of adults receiving lipid-lowering medications. However, among adults not receiving lipid-lowering medications, trends in lipids were similar to those reported for adults overall. Among obese adults, mean total cholesterol, non–HDL cholesterol, LDL cholesterol, and geometric mean triglycerides declined between 1988 and 2010[67]. These data suggest that in addition to the increased use of lipid-lowering medications, something else must have been involved in the overall reduction of blood total cholesterol and LDL cholesterol. Although those factors, the application of natural lipid-lowering products plays a critical role and is thus described below.

9. Cholesterol-lowering natural products

9.1. Plant sterols/ stanols

Plant sterols/ stanols, naturally occurring in foods of plant origin, perform similar biological functions to cholesterol, and contain a similar chemical structure. They differ from cholesterol only in the presence of either an extra methyl or ethyl group. Absorption efficiency for plant sterols in humans is less (2-5%) than that of cholesterol (60%). The most common forms are unsaturated plant sterols β-sitosterol, campesterol, and stigmasterol and the saturated sitostanol and campestanol [68]. Plant sterols reduce the absorption of both dietary and biliary cholesterol from the intestinal tract by 30%–50% [69]. The exact mechanism is yet fully elucidated while it is generally assumed that the presence of increased quantities of plant sterols in the gut lowers the micellar solubility of cholesterol, therefore lowering the amount of cholesterol available for absorption [69]. Intake of phytosterol and stanols at an average of 2 g/day has been shown to lower low density lipoprotein cholesterol (LDL-C) by 10-15%. The effect appeared to be peaked at intakes of 2 g/d, with little additional benefit being achieved at intakes higher than 2.5 g/d. The recommended daily intake of phytosterols is 2 g/d in humans [70]. Plant sterols and their derivatives reduce plasma cholesterol levels independently from the mRNA expression of ABCG5 and ABCG8 transporters [71]. Food products such as margarine, milk, yoghurt, and cereal products enriched with plant sterols/stanols are promoted as functional foods to help lower serum cholesterol levels. Human and animal studies have shown that plant sterol and stanol esters are non-toxic [72]. There have been concerns raised over the reduced absorption of some fat soluble vitamins from the use of plant sterols. For example, plant sterols and stanols have been shown to reduce β-carotene, α-carotene, and vitamin E levels by around 25%, 10%, and 8%, respectively [72]. Used alone in the diet, or as an adjuvant to drug therapy, or in combination with other functional food components, plant sterols/stanols-enriched products are generally effective at reducing serum total and LDL-C [72], and thus the most popular natural ingredient in cholesterol-lowering product market.

9.2. Soy products

Soy foods have been consumed for centuries in Asian countries. Consumption of soy foods contribute to lower incidences of coronary heart diseases, atherosclerosis, type 2 diabetes, and decreased risk of certain types of carcinogenesis such as breast and prostate cancers [73]. Animal and human studies have also shown that consumption of soy protein or associated isoflavones has beneficial impacts such as lowering liver or blood triglyceride, total and LDL cholesterol levels, increasing HDL cholesterol and the ratio of HDL/LDL cholesterol [73, 74]. Soy protein regulates SREBP-1 expression by modulating serum insulin concentration, thus preventing the development of fatty liver [75]. Isoflavones are major soy phytoestrogens present in soy foods and Genistin, daidzin, and glycitein are the main soy isoflavones (Xiao 2008). Soy and soy bioactive components are well-tolerated and the adverse effects reported are gastrointestinal symptoms (e.g., diarrhea), followed by menstrual complaints (e.g., prolonged periods, amenorrhea) headache, dizziness, and musculoskeletal complaints [76].

9.3. Dietary fibre

Dietary fibre is one of the most studied dietary components associated with cardiovascular benefits. It is a complex of non-digestible carbohydrates and lignin that are intrinsic and intact in plants and are resistant to digestion and absorption in the small intestine. Dietary fibre can modulate body weight and promotes beneficial physiological effects such as laxation, reduction in blood cholesterol and postprandial blood glucose [77]. Traditionally, dietary fibre has been classified on the basis of its solubility in water (soluble or insoluble). Foods rich in fibre need to be chewed longer, leading to an increase in the time needed to eat and the feeling of satiety. Fibres which make up viscous solutions also delay the passage of food from the stomach to duodenum and contribute to an increase in satiety and a decrease in energy consumption [78]. In the intestine, the incorporation of fibre in food may complicate the interaction between digestive enzymes and their substrates, thus slowing down the absorption of nutrients[77]. The hypocholesterolemic action of fibre is partly mediated by a lower absorption of intestinal bile acid because the interruption of the enterohepatic bile acid circulation, thus increasing faecal bile acid loss, and its de novo synthesis in liver. The physicochemical properties of soluble fibre result in important modifications in volume, bulk and viscosity in the intestinal lumen, which will alter metabolic pathways of hepatic cholesterol and lipoprotein metabolism, also resulting in lowering of plasma LDL cholesterol [79]. Dietary fibre increases the enzymatic activity of cholesterol-7-α-hydroxylase, contributing to a higher depletion of hepatic cholesterol but increased endogenous cholesterol synthesis. However, there is an increase in the number of LDL receptors and in the recruitment of the esterified cholesterol from the circulating LDL particles. Several types of soluble dietary fibre such as pectin, glucomannan, psyllium can decrease plasma total cholesterol and LDL cholesterol. Epidemiological evidences showed a stronger association of cardiovascular protection with soluble fibre than insoluble fibre. Insoluble fibre such as that from wheat or cellulose has not been reported to have any significant effect on blood cholesterol [78]. Consumption of too much high fibre foods that have not been cooked can cause side effects of abdominal bloating and gas.

9.4. Flaxseed lignans

Flax seed is the richest source of natural lignans, with secoisolariciresinol diglucoside (SDG) being the principal lignan compound. Flaxseed or flaxseed meal have cardioprotective properties and can suppress atherosclerosis by virtue of its antioxidant properties due to the presence of flaxseed lignans. Lignan reduces serum triglycerides and LDL and raises HDL cholesterol. In addition, flaxseed oil possesses anti-inflammatory properties and reduces platelet aggregation as well [80]. Flaxseed lignans along with soy isoflavones are phytoestrogens commonly consumed in the human diet.

9.5. Polyunsaturated fatty acids and omega-3 fatty acids

An old assumption regarding fatty acids and their effects on atherosclerosis was that monounsaturated fatty acids were neutral, saturated fatty acids were bad, and polyunsaturated fatty acids were good. However, a study conducted by Scott Grundy and Fred Mattson in 1985 turned the "world of monounsaturated fatty acids" around[81]. They demonstrated that diets rich in saturated fatty acids caused a high LDL cholesterol/HDL cholesterol ratio, and that substitution of monounsaturated fatty acid for saturated fatty acids reduced LDL cholesterol but did not reduce HDL cholesterol. Consequently the LDL cholesterol/HDL cholesterol ratio was the lowest with monounsaturated fatty acids, given that polyunsaturated fatty acids reduced HDL cholesterol as well as LDL cholesterol. A similar phenomenon was observed in a 5-year study in male African green monkeys[82]. In the monkey studies, average HDL cholesterol was 50 mg/dl in the polyunsaturated fatty acids group versus 86 and 81 mg/dl in the saturated fatty acids and monounsaturated fatty acids groups, respectively. Average plasma LDL cholesterol concentrations in the polyunsaturated fatty acids and monounsaturated fatty acids-fed monkeys were 157 and 167 mg/dl, respectively (no significant difference between them) versus 257 mg/dl in the saturated fatty acids-fed animals.

The influences of dietary fatty acids on blood cholesterol profiles are also related to diet composition[83]. It is well accepted that the consumption of saturated fatty acids increases LDL cholesterol, whereas carbohydrates, monounsaturated fatty acids and polyunsaturated fatty acids do not. The effect of fatty acids on blood lipid profiles also depends on heath conditions. Among individuals who are insulin resistant, a low-fat, high-carbohydrate diet typically has an adverse effect on lipid profiles. In addition to lowering HDL cholesterol, it also increases triacylglycerols and LDL cholesterol. Consequently, a moderate fat diet in which unsaturated fatty acids replace saturated fatty acids and carbohydrates are not augmented is advised to lower LDL cholesterol[83].

Fish oil (marine n-3 fatty acids, eicosapentaenoic acid, and docosahexaenoic acid), whether from dietary sources or fish oil supplements, exhibit cardioprotective effects and reduce mortality due to cardiovascular diseases. Fish oil provides cell membrane stabilization, anti-inflammatory, antiatherogenic effects and suppression of cardiac arrhythmias[84]. Omega-3 fatty acids lower moderately the blood pressure through primarily the improvement of vascular endothelial cell function whilst a multitude of mechanisms may be involved85. Polyunsaturated fatty acids lower triacylglycerols, which has also been important in cardioprotection and the management of insulin resistance and diabetes. The effect of omega-3 fatty acids on blood cholesterol is inconsistent effect. In general, omega-3 fatty acids do not offer a benefit of directly lowering blood cholesterol. Instead, in some studies fish oil has been found to cause a small rise in LDL-cholesterol; however a change in the LDL particle size from the smaller more atherogenic form to the larger less damaging particle size have been noted85.

Health Canada has recently reconsidered the classification of food products with disease risk reduction claims or therapeutic claims in light of clarified principles for the classification of foods at the Food-Natural Health Product interface (http://www.hc-sc.gc.ca/fn-an/label-etiquet/claims-reclam/assess-evalu/sat-mono-poly-fat-gras-eng.php). Health Canada has concluded that the results of the updated literature review are consistent with the 2002 report provided by the Institute of Medicine (IOM), which forms the basis of the US and Canada dietary guidance, on the replacement of saturated fat with unsaturated fat for blood cholesterol lowering. In other words, scientific evidence exists in support of the therapeutic claim linking the replacement of saturated fat with unsaturated fat to a reduction of blood cholesterol. It is stated that the claim is relevant and generally applicable to the Canadian population as a high proportion of the Canadian population is hyperlipidemic. It is allowed now by the Health Canada's to put therapeutic claim statements such as "Replacing saturated fats with polyunsaturated and monounsaturated fats (from vegetable oils) helps lower/reduce cholesterol" in vegetable oils and foods containing vegetable oils when specific conditions for the food carrying the claim are met.

9.6. Olive oil

Olive oil can reduce LDL and raise high-density lipoprotein cholesterol and decrease lipid damage due to oxidative stress. In addition, olive oil reduces inflammatory and thrombogenic status, endothelial dysfunction, and blood pressure[86].

9.7. Green tea products

Tea catechin-especially (-)-epigallocatechin-3-gallate-inhibits the expression of soluble adhesion molecules including vascular adhesion molecule-1 and intercellular adhesion molecule-1, endothelial cell inflammatory markers, decreased oxidized LDL, and prevents the development of atherosclerosis and[87].

Certainly, there are more natural products available, for instance a number of antioxidants and phenolic compounds, to lower blood cholesterol levels. However, the big challenges that the natural products have been facing in the past years lie in their relatively lower efficacies as compared with the cholesterol-lowering drugs. The apparent advantages of natural products are their better safety profiles. In order to promote the market share of cholesterol-lowering natural products in competing with the drugs, it is critical to develop new products that can offer better efficacies than the current natural products, without losing safety or introducing increased toxic or severe side effects. Considering that the majority of the current natural products fall into the same category of cholesterol absorption inhibitor, the future direction of research and development of cholesterol-lowering products, novel distinct pathways or targets should be focused. Herewith, we will provide some brief thoughts on new approaches that we believe worth to tackle into, with a hope that the new mind in the research and development direction and focus would help to discover and develop novel natural products with significantly improved cholesterol-lowering efficacy working through distinct mechanisms than the currently available natural products, without apparent side effects.

http://dx.doi.org/10.5772/54729

10. New perspectives on the development of natural cholesterol-lowering products

Cardiovascular friendly natural products are those nutritional supplements, which can provide potential health benefits in cardiovascular diseases (CVD). Experimental, epidemiological and clinical data indicates that dietary nutrients and supplements have profound cardioprotective effects in the primary as well as secondary prevention of coronary heart disease [88]. Except for the aforementioned several cholesterol-lowering natural products, the plant alkaloid berberine has recently been introduced to the filed of lipid-lowering products. Berberine has shown a moderate or comparable cholesterol- and triacylglycerol-lowering effect in humans [89]. More importantly, recent studies have demonstrated that berberine combined with plant stanols improves cholesterol-lowering efficacy through a synergistic action on cholesterol absorption and reducing plasma triacylglycerols in animals [90], [91], with the efficacies are comparable or even better cholesterol-lowering drugs, statins. The product has been patent-protected and at the preclinical stage. Clinical trials are warranted before moving this potentially highly effective natural product to the lipid-lowering market.

10.1. Current status in the development of cholesterol-lowering products

An initial approach to control the modifiable risk factors of hyperlipidemia relies on the changes of diet, lifestyle, and other factors such as smoking. When all these fail, pharmaceutical intervention is necessary. Many of the current available drugs are those either inhibit cholesterol synthesis, or increase synthesis of bile acids and excretion. The majority of the current research focuses on lowering the "bad" LDL cholesterol, with less attention on increasing "good" HDL cholesterol. A treatment with a combination that can lower LDL cholesterol and increase HDL cholesterol would certainly provide more benefits than single approach for the treatment of hyperlipidemia, atherosclerosis and cardiovascular disease.

10.1.1. Lowering LDL cholesterol

Statins drugs, which are currently widely prescribed, lower LDL cholesterol primarily via inhibiting cholesterol biosynthesis and a secondary effect of increase LDL receptor and LDL clearance. However this family of drugs has shown several undesirable side-effects. Niacin, can also lower LDL cholesterol but not efficiently as statin but it is only one drug proved to increase HDL cholesterol with very less side effects. Therefore, a combination of niacin and statins might be superior to these drugs alone for lowering lipid levels. The scientific evidence of long-term safety and tolerability of these combination therapies are key determinants for good compliance and cardiovascular benefits.

Proprotein convertase subtilisin kexin-9 (PCSK9) is a sterol-responsive protein that accelerates LDLR turnover in the liver. When PCSK9 transcription is reduced, there will be subsequently increases LDLR levels helping to maintain cholesterol homeostasis. The transcription of PCSK9 is increased by SREBP-2, which also regulate the transcription of many other genes. Therefore, a pharmacologically specific inhibitor of PCSK9 will have atherogenic effect by increasing LDLR levels without affecting other genes regulated by SREBP-2.

10.1.2. Increasing HDL levels

Low HDL-cholesterol (HDL-C) is a strong and independent cardiovascular risk marker. Niacin is the only drug proved to increase HDLC but associated with flushing as a side-effect. Niacin-induced flushing involves both PGD_2 from mast cells and serotonin from platelets. The possibility of administering or formulating niacin together with flavonoid luteolin was recently shown to inhibit niacin flush in rats. Further investigation on inhibitors on side-effect can warrant an effective medicine for CVD[92]. Aleglitazar, a dual PPARα/γ agonist, proven has beneficial effects on both lipid and glucose parameters [93]. Activation of PPARα may increase ApoA1, apolipoprotein of HDL and increased the synthesis of LPL which hydrolyzes VLDL, IDL and LDL. PPARα agonist, with good safety profile, may have a therapeutic role in modifying cardiovascular risk factors.

10.1.3. CETP inhibition

Besides established strategies to increase HDL-C, e.g. with nicotinic acid, CETP (Cholesteryl ester transfer protein)-inhibition is a promising new therapeutic option. The failure of torcetrapib, the first CETP-inhibitor, seems to be attributed to "off-target" effects. Treatment with the newer CETP-inhibitors dalcetrapib and anacetrapib has been shown to be efficacious and safe - but their usefulness in clinical practice remains to be determined in ongoing clinical trials [94].

10.1.4. Inhibition of cannabinoid receptors

G protein-coupled cannabinoid receptor, CB-1 of the endocannabinoid system, plays a crucial role in regulating feeding pattern, lipid metabolism, and energy homeostasis. CB-1 receptors are located in the central nervous system and peripheral tissues including adipocytes, pancreas, gut, liver, and muscle. Rimonabant, a selective CB-1 antagonist drug to be developed for weight loss via increasing energy expenditure actually also increases HDL-cholesterol and triglycerides.However, the clinical efficacy and safety of these new antiobesity compounds are yet to be determined. Additional cannabinoid receptor blockers have been developed and are in testing [95].

10.1.5. Nuclear receptor modifiers

Identification of nuclear receptor LXR and FXR as regulatorof genes in bile acid and cholesterol metabolism has providedpotential new targets for screening cholesterol-lowering drugsby manipulating bile acid synthesis, transport, and absorption. Therapies targeted to LXR and FXR would be ideal for drug developmentbecause nuclear receptors are activated by natural and syntheticligands, which could be identified by high-throughput screening [96].

http://dx.doi.org/10.5772/54729

10.1.6. Acyl-coenzyme A: Cholesterol acyltransferas (ACAT) inhibitors

ACAT 1 and ACAT2 play an important role in cellular cholesterol esterification and thus modulate intestinal cholesterol absorption and hepatic lipoprotein secretion. ACAT2 is proposed to play a central role in cholesterol absorption from the intestine. ACAT1, on the other hand is widely distributed in tissues, and plays a pivotal role in cholesterol metabolism in macrophages and steroidogenic tissues. It is anticipated that inhibitors of ACAT2 activity could be developed that would decrease cholesterol absorption, whereas specific ACAT1 inhibitors could be used to reduce foam cell formation and prevent atherosclerosis. However, the results of studies have indicated that ACAT1 inhibition is not a good strategy and, in fact, could have detrimental consequence [97]. In contrast, mice lacking ACAT2 exhibited attractive metabolic findings. These include a restricted capacity to absorb cholesterol and protection against diet-induced hypercholesterolemia and gallstone formation [98, 99]. Further, ACAT2 inhibitor reduces cholesterol esters in apolipoprotein B-containing lipoproteins and protects from atherosclerosis in murine models of the disease [100]. A fundamental question remains: would ACAT2 specific inhibition in humans, either pharmacologically or with anti-sense oligonucleotides, prevent or reduce atherosclerosis? "The sole test of the validity of an idea is experiment." Until a potent and specific inhibitor of ACAT2 is tested in humans, the hypothesis remains uncertain [101].

10.2. Future perspectives of cholesterol-lowering products and their potential impact on CVD

10.2.1. Identification of new molecular targets

Target identification is an essential first step in drug development. Although cholesterol metabolism has been studied for decades and relatively well understood, the specific molecular targets that can be used for drug discovery and development are far from well-known. It is believe that with the development and use of modern molecular technology and techniques in nutritional and physiological research, more targets will be indentified and used for future drug development.

10.2.2. Application of gene silencing technology

Apart from the identification of new targets, several new approaches have been introduced or shown great potential for the development of new cholesterol-lowering products. Of them is gene-silencing technology. One technology that has generated a lot of excitement is RNA interference (RNAi) [102]. For example, clinical trials have been launched using RNA interference approaches to reduce PCSK9 expression or specific antibodies targeting and inhibiting PCSK9 interaction with the LDL receptor. They constitute very promising approaches to reducing cholesterol levels and coronary heart disease. Understanding of PCSK9 and its potential as a therapeutic target through which to reduce LDL cholesterol for prevention and treatment of coronary heart disease has been of great interest recently [103]. The administration of chemically modified small interference RNAs (siRNAs) results in silencing of a target mRNA, such as apolipoprotein B (apoB) mRNA in liver and jejunum and decreasing plasma levels of apoB protein. ApoB is a molecule involved in the metabolism of cholesterol; the concentrations of this protein in human blood samples correlate with those of cholesterol. Higher levels of both compounds are associated with an increased risk of coronary heart disease. Intravenous injections of the siRNA-cholesterol conjugates in mice resulted in a lowering of the levels of blood cholesterol comparable to that in mice in which the apoB gene had been deleted. These results demonstrate that siRNA can be delivered systemically to target the liver and suggest that RNAi has the potential to become a new therapeutic for the treatment of metabolic diseases [102].

10.2.3. Development of target-specific inhibitors or enhancers

For those molecular targets that have several different isoforms, the biggest challenge in the drug development is the specificity. A good example is ACAT inhibitors. To date, it has been demonstrated that there are two sioforms, ACAT1 and ACAT2. ACAT1 is expressed universally while ACAT2 is expressed mainly in the liver and small intestine. Both isoforms can esterify cholesterol and other sterols. However, ACAT1 primarily works on the esterification of plant sterols and other sterol products, while ACAT2 mainly converts cholesterol to its esters. Due to their different distribution and activities in the body, a universal inhibitor of both enzymes has been shown to be detrimental and recent humans trials are disappointing [104, 105]. The study of Bell et al. in 2006 breathes life back into the idea of ACAT2-specific inhibition [106]. In atherosclerosis-prone mice, ACAT2 was specifically ihibhied in the liver with antisense oligonucleotides. Biweekly intraperitoneal injections, which reduced ACAT2 expression by a remarkable 80%, decreased diet-induced hypercholesterolemia and sharply reduced cholesterol ester deposition in the aorta. The specific inhibition can be achieved from the antisense gene technology or small molecules that inhibit only ACAT2. There is no mature product in this category and lots more work needs to be done.

It has been demonstrated by numerous studies that inhibition of cholesterol absorption is associated with much less side-effects than other approaches. It remains challenge but highly promising that a potent inhibitor of cholesterol absorption would sufficiently lower blood cholesterol or keep blood cholesterol levels within the recommended healthy range. To achieve this goal, other approaches have to be take in addition to the specific inhibitor of cholesterol absorption, such as a combination of two or more products, in particular the combinations that work synergistically through one or multiple pathways of cholesterol homeostasis. Recent studies on the combination of the plant alkaloid berberine and plant sterols/stanols have shown an excellent example of this approach. The researchers have demonstrated consistently that plant sterols or stanols and berberine have a moderate effect to lower blood cholesterol levels in different animal models. However, when plant sterols/stanols were combined with berberine, a significant synergism was produced. They remarkably improved cholesterol-lowering efficacy by synergistically inhibiting cholesterol absorption [90,91].

11. Conclusions

Cardiovascular disease has long been the lead cause of mortality and morbidity in the developed countries and similar situation has arisen in recent years in the developing countries. The increased prevalence of CVD is due to the significantly improved food supply and processing and rapid shift of lifestyle from active to sedentary nature, resulting increased incidence of obesity and overweight. Although the development and clinical use of statin drugs and other cholesterol-lowering drugs has been stabilize the mortality resulted from CVD since last decade, the incidence has been stably rising. According, the control of risk factors for atherosclerosis and CVD remains critical. The primary risk factor is hypercholesterolemia. There still exists a strong demand to develop novel products, especially from distinct cholesterol metabolic pathways or molecular targets and from different new approaches as mentioned above. It is optimistic that in the near future, new cholesterol-lowering products, either drugs or natural products with higher efficacies, better specificity and better safe profiles will be developed.

Author details

Sandhya V.G. Nair and Yanwen Wang

Aquatic and Crop Resource Development, Life Sciences Branch, National Research Council Canada, Charlottetown, PE, Canada

References

[1] Mendis, S. and Banerjee, A., Equity, social determinants and public health programmes, World Health Organisation, 2010.

[2] Aje, T. O. and Miller, M. Cardiovascular disease: A global problem extending into the developing world. World J Cardiol 2009; 1: 3-10.

[3] Statistics Canada. Deaths by cause. Chapter IX: Diseases of the circulatory system (2000 to 2006). 2010.

[4] Public Health Agency of Canada. Tracking Heart Disease and Stroke in Canada. 2009.

[5] Murray, C. J. and Lopez, A. D. Mortality by cause for eight regions of the world: Global Burden of Disease Study. Lancet 1997; 349: 1269-1276.

[6] Yusuf, S., Reddy, S., Ounpuu, S. and Anand, S. Global Burden of Cardiovascular Diseases: Part I: General Considerations, the Epidemiologic Transition, Risk Factors, and Impact of Urbanization. Circulation 2001; 104: 2746-2753.

[7] Association, A. H. International Cardiovascular Disease Statistics. 2009.

[8] Zittermann, A., Schleithoff, S. S. and Koerfer, R. Putting cardiovascular disease and vitamin D insufficiency into perspective. Br J Nutr 2005; 94: 483-492.

[9] Yancy, W. S., Jr, Westman, E. C., French, P. A. and Califf, R. M. Diets and Clinical Coronary Events: The Truth Is Out There. Circulation 2003; 107: 10-16.

[10] Lakatta, E. G. Age-associated Cardiovascular Changes in Health: Impact on Cardiovascular Disease in Older Persons. Heart Failure Reviews 2002; 7: 29-49.

[11] Silander, K., Alanne, M., Kristiansson, K., Saarela, O., Ripatti, S., Auro, K., Karvanen, J., Kulathinal, S., Niemelä, M., Ellonen, P., Vartiainen, E., Jousilahti, P., Saarela, J., Kuulasmaa, K., Evans, A., Perola, M., Salomaa, V. and Peltonen, L. Gender Differences in Genetic Risk Profiles for Cardiovascular Disease. PLoS ONE 2008; 3: e3615.

[12] Jousilahti, P., Vartiainen, E., Tuomilehto, J. and Puska, P. Sex, Age, Cardiovascular Risk Factors, and Coronary Heart Disease : A Prospective Follow-Up Study of 14 786 Middle-Aged Men and Women in Finland. Circulation 1999; 99: 1165-1172.

[13] Kuhn, F. E. and Rackley, C. E. Coronary Artery Disease in Women: Risk Factors, Evaluation, Treatment, and Prevention. Arch Intern Med 1993; 153: 2626-2636.

[14] Wang, J.-G. and Staessen, J. A. Genetic polymorphisms in the renin-angiotensin system: relevance for susceptibility to cardiovascular disease. European Journal of Pharmacology 2000; 410: 289-302.

[15] Cooper, R. S. Social inequality, ethnicity and cardiovascular disease. International Journal of Epidemiology 2001; 30: S48.

[16] Onwuanyi, A. E., Abe, O., Quarshie, A., Al-Mahmoud, A., Lapu-Bula, R., Francis, C. K. and Ofili, E. Comparative frequency of angiographic coronary artery disease in African Americans and Hispanics. Ethn Dis. 2006 16: 58-63.

[17] Ludwig, D. S., Ebbeling, C. B., Pereira, M. A. and Pawlak, D. B. A Physiological Basis for Disparities in Diabetes and Heart Disease Risk among Racial and Ethnic Groups. The Journal of Nutrition 2002; 132: 2492-2493.

[18] Poirier, P., Giles, T. D., Bray, G. A., Hong, Y., Stern, J. S., Pi-Sunyer, F. X. and Eckel, R. H. Obesity and Cardiovascular Disease: Pathophysiology, Evaluation, and Effect of Weight Loss: An Update of the 1997 American Heart Association Scientific Statement on Obesity and Heart Disease From the Obesity Committee of the Council on Nutrition, Physical Activity, and Metabolism. Circulation 2006; 113: 898-918.

[19] Lavie, C. J., Milani, R. V. and Ventura, H. O. Obesity and Cardiovascular Disease: Risk Factor, Paradox, and Impact of Weight Loss. J Am Coll Cardiol 2009; 53: 1925-1932.

[20] Pocock, S. J., Shaper, A. G. and Phillips, A. N. Concentrations of high density lipoprotein cholesterol, triglycerides, and total cholesterol in ischaemic heart disease. British Medical Journal 1989; 298: 998-1002.

[21] Barr, D. P., Russ, E. M. and Eder, H. A. Protein-lipid relationships in human plasma: II. In atherosclerosis and related conditions. The American journal of medicine 1951; 11: 480-493.

[22] Morgan, J. M., Carey, C. M., Lincoff, A. and Capuzzi, D. M. The Effects of Niacin on Lipoprotein Subclass Distribution. Preventive Cardiology 2004; 7: 182-189.

[23] Kannel, W. B. Blood Pressure as a Cardiovascular Risk Factor. JAMA: The Journal of the American Medical Association 1996; 275: 1571-1576.

[24] Vasan, R. S., Massaro, J. M., Wilson, P. W. F., Seshadri, S., Wolf, P. A., Levy, D. and D'Agostino, R. B. Antecedent Blood Pressure and Risk of Cardiovascular Disease: The Framingham Heart Study. Circulation 2002; 105: 48-53.

[25] Tanasescu, M., Leitzmann, M. F., Rimm, E. B. and Hu, F. B. Physical Activity in Relation to Cardiovascular Disease and Total Mortality Among Men With Type 2 Diabetes. Circulation 2003; 107: 2435-2439.

[26] Myers, J. Exercise and Cardiovascular Health. Circulation 2003; 107: e2-5.

[27] Diabetes Mellitus: A Major Risk Factor for Cardiovascular Disease : A Joint Editorial Statement by the American Diabetes Association; the National Heart, Lung, and Blood Institute; the Juvenile Diabetes Foundation International; the National Institute of Diabetes and Digestive and Kidney Diseases; and the American Heart Association. Circulation 1999; 100: 1132-1133.

[28] Ockene, I. S. and Miller, N. H. Cigarette Smoking, Cardiovascular Disease, and Stroke : A Statement for Healthcare Professionals From the American Heart Association. Circulation 1997; 96: 3243-3247.

[29] Craig, W. Y., Palomaki, G. E. and Haddow, J. E. Cigarette smoking and serum lipid and lipoprotein concentrations: an analysis of published data. British Medical Journal 1989; 298: 784-788.

[30] Ambrose, J. A. and Barua, R. S. The pathophysiology of cigarette smoking and cardiovascular disease: An update. J Am Coll Cardiol 2004; 43: 1731-1737.

[31] Renaud, S. and de Lorgeril, M. Wine, alcohol, platelets, and the French paradox for coronary heart disease. The Lancet 1992; 339: 1523-1526.

[32] Evans, A. E., Ruidavets, J. B., McCrum, E. E., Cambou, J. P., McClean, R., Douste-Blazy, P., McMaster, D., Bingham, A., Patterson, C. C., Richard, J. L. and et al. Autres pays, autres coeurs? Dietary patterns, risk factors and ischaemic heart disease in Belfast and Toulouse. QJM 1995; 88: 469-477.

[33] Singh, R. B., Niaz, M. A., Ghosh, S., Beegom, R., Agarwal, P., Nangia, S., Moshiri, M. and Janus, E. D. Low Fat Intake and Coronary Artery Disease in a Population with Higher Prevalence of Coronary Artery Disease: The Indian Paradox. Journal of the American College of Nutrition 1998; 17: 342-350.

[34] Lusis, A. J. Atherosclerosis. Nature 2000; 407: 233-241.

[35] Ross, R. Atherosclerosis — An Inflammatory Disease. New England Journal of Medicine 1999; 340: 115-126.

[36] Witztum, J. L. and Steinberg, D. Role of oxidized low density lipoprotein in atherogenesis. The Journal of Clinical Investigation 1991; 88: 1785-1792.

[37] Badimon, L. Atherosclerosis and thrombosis: lessons from animal models. Thromb Haemost 2001; 86: 356-365.

[38] Mertens, A. and Holvoet, P. Oxidized LDL and HDL: antagonists in atherothrombosis. The FASEB Journal 2001; 15: 2073-2084.

[39] Gotto, A. M., Jr. Evolving Concepts of Dyslipidemia, Atherosclerosis, and Cardiovascular Disease: The Louis F. Bishop Lecture. J Am Coll Cardiol 2005; 46: 1219-1224.

[40] Ory, D. S. Nuclear Receptor Signaling in the Control of Cholesterol Homeostasis: Have the Orphans Found a Home? Circ Res 2004; 95: 660-670.

[41] Horton, J. D., Goldstein, J. L. and Brown, M. S. SREBPs: activators of the complete program of cholesterol and fatty acid synthesis in the liver. The Journal of Clinical Investigation 2002; 109: 1125-1131.

[42] Chawla, A., Repa, J. J., Evans, R. M. and Mangelsdorf, D. J. Nuclear Receptors and Lipid Physiology: Opening the X-Files. Science 2001; 294: 1866-1870.

[43] Dong, B., Wu, M., Li, H., Kraemer, F. B., Adeli, K., Seidah, N. G., Park, S. W. and Liu, J. Strong induction of PCSK9 gene expression through HNF1α and SREBP2: mechanism for the resistance to LDL-cholesterol lowering effect of statins in dyslipidemic hamsters. Journal of Lipid Research 2010; 51: 1486-1495.

[44] Repa, J. J., Liang, G., Ou, J., Bashmakov, Y., Lobaccaro, J.-M. A., Shimomura, I., Shan, B., Brown, M. S., Goldstein, J. L. and Mangelsdorf, D. J. Regulation of mouse sterol regulatory element-binding protein-1c gene (SREBP-1c) by oxysterol receptors, LXRα and LXRβ. Genes & Development 2000; 14: 2819-2830.

[45] Tontonoz, P. and Mangelsdorf, D. J. Liver X Receptor Signaling Pathways in Cardiovascular Disease. Molecular Endocrinology 2003; 17: 985-993.

[46] Altmann, S. W., Davis, H. R., Zhu, L.-j., Yao, X., Hoos, L. M., Tetzloff, G., Iyer, S. P. N., Maguire, M., Golovko, A., Zeng, M., Wang, L., Murgolo, N. and Graziano, M. P. Niemann-Pick C1 Like 1 Protein Is Critical for Intestinal Cholesterol Absorption. Science 2004; 303: 1201-1204.

[47] Plösch, T., Kruit, J. K., Bloks, V. W., Huijkman, N. C. A., Havinga, R., Duchateau, G. S. M. J. E., Lin, Y. and Kuipers, F. Reduction of Cholesterol Absorption by Dietary Plant Sterols and Stanols in Mice Is Independent of the Abcg5/8 Transporter. The Journal of Nutrition 2006; 136: 2135-2140.

[48] Kosters, A., Kunne, C., Looije, N., Patel, S. B., Oude Elferink, R. P. J. and Groen, A. K. The mechanism of ABCG5/ABCG8 in biliary cholesterol secretion in mice. Journal of Lipid Research 2006; 47: 1959-1966.

[49] Vu-Dac, N., Chopin-Delannoy, S., Gervois, P., Bonnelye, E., Martin, G., Fruchart, J.-C., Laudet, V. and Staels, B. The Nuclear Receptors Peroxisome Proliferator-activated Receptor α and Rev-erbα Mediate the Species-specific Regulation of Apolipoprotein A-I Expression by Fibrates. Journal of Biological Chemistry 1998; 273: 25713-25720.

[50] Oram, J. F. and Lawn, R. M. ABCA1: the gatekeeper for eliminating excess tissue cholesterol. Journal of Lipid Research 2001; 42: 1173-1179.

[51] Cao, G., Beyer, T. P., Yang, X. P., Schmidt, R. J., Zhang, Y., Bensch, W. R., Kauffman, R. F., Gao, H., Ryan, T. P., Liang, Y., Eacho, P. I. and Jiang, X.-C. Phospholipid Transfer Protein Is Regulated by Liver X Receptors in Vivo. Journal of Biological Chemistry 2002; 277: 39561-39565.

[52] Chiang, J. Y. L. Bile Acid Regulation of Gene Expression: Roles of Nuclear Hormone Receptors. Endocrine Reviews 2002; 23: 443-463.

[53] Stancu, C. and Sima, A. Statins: mechanism of action and effects. Journal of Cellular and Molecular Medicine 2001; 5: 378-387.

[54] Corsini, A., Bellosta, S., Baetta, R., Fumagalli, R., Paoletti, R. and Bernini, F. New insights into the pharmacodynamic and pharmacokinetic properties of statins. Pharmacology & Therapeutics 1999; 84: 413-428.

[55] Neuvonen, P. J., Niemi, M. and Backman, J. T. Drug interactions with lipid-lowering drugs: Mechanisms and clinical relevance. Clin Pharmacol Ther 2006; 80: 565-581.

[56] Golomb, B. A. and Evans, M. A. Statin Adverse Effects: A Review of the Literature and Evidence for a Mitochondrial Mechanism. American Journal of Cardiovascular Drugs 2008; 8: 373-418 310.2165/0129784-200808060-200800004.

[57] Patel, J., Sheehan, V. and Gurk-Turner, C. Ezetimibe (Zetia): a new type of lipid-lowering agent. Proc (Bayl Univ Med Cent). 2003 16: 354-358.

[58] Al Badarin, F. J., Kullo, I. J., Kopecky, S. L. and Thomas, R. J. Impact of Ezetimibe on Atherosclerosis: Is the Jury Still Out? Mayo Clinic Proceedings 2009; 84: 353-361.

[59] Stolk, M. F. J., Becx, M. C. J. M., Kuypers, K. C. and Seldenrijk, C. A. Severe Hepatic Side Effects of Ezetimibe. Clinical gastroenterology and hepatology : the official clinical practice journal of the American Gastroenterological Association 2006; 4: 908-911.

[60] Florentin, M., Liberopoulos, E. N. and Elisaf, M. S. Ezetimibe-associated adverse effects: what the clinician needs to know. International Journal of Clinical Practice 2008; 62: 88-96.

[61] Ganji, S. H., Kamanna, V. S. and Kashyap, M. L. Niacin and cholesterol: role in cardiovascular disease (review). The Journal of nutritional biochemistry 2003; 14: 298-305.

[62] Vosper, H. Niacin: a re-emerging pharmaceutical for the treatment of dyslipidaemia. British Journal of Pharmacology 2009; 158: 429-441.

[63] Shepherd, J. Mechanism of action of bile acid sequestrants and other lipid-lowering drugs. Cardiology 1989; 76: 65-71.

[64] Ast, M. and Frishman, W. Bile acid sequestrants. The Journal of Clinical Pharmacology 1990; 30: 99-106.

[65] Forcheron, F., Cachefo, A., Thevenon, S., Pinteur, C. and Beylot, M. Mechanisms of the Triglyceride- and Cholesterol-Lowering Effect of Fenofibrate in Hyperlipidemic Type 2 Diabetic Patients. Diabetes 2002; 51: 3486-3491.

[66] Pahan, K. Lipid-lowering drugs. Cellular and Molecular Life Sciences 2006; 63: 1165-1178.

[67] Carroll, M. D., Kit, B. K., Lacher, D. A., Shero, S. T. and Mussolino, M. E. Trends in lipids and lipoproteins in US adults, 1988-2010. JAMA 2012; 308: 1545-1554.

[68] Kochhar, S. P. Influence of processing on sterols of edible vegetable oils. Progress in Lipid Research 1983; 22: 161-188.

[69] Jones, P. H., Davidson, M. H., Stein, E. A., Bays, H. E., McKenney, J. M., Miller, E., Cain, V. A. and Blasetto, J. W. Comparison of the efficacy and safety of rosuvastatin versus atorvastatin, simvastatin, and pravastatin across doses (STELLAR* * STELLAR = Statin Therapies for Elevated Lipid Levels compared Across doses to Rosuvastatin. Trial). The American journal of cardiology 2003; 92: 152-160.

[70] Demonty, I., Ras, R. T., van der Knaap, H. C. M., Duchateau, G. S. M. J. E., Meijer, L., Zock, P. L., Geleijnse, J. M. and Trautwein, E. A. Continuous Dose-Response Relationship of the LDL-Cholesterol–Lowering Effect of Phytosterol Intake. The Journal of Nutrition 2009; 139: 271-284.

[71] Jia, X., Ebine, N., Demonty, I., Wang, Y., Beech, R., Muise, V., Fortin, M. G. and Jones, P. J. Hypocholesterolaemic effects of plant sterol analogues are independent of ABCG5 and ABCG8 transporter expressions in hamsters. Br J Nutr 2007; 98: 550-555.

[72] Patch, C., Tapsell, L., Williams, P. and Gordon, M. Plant sterols as dietary adjuvants in the reduction of cardiovascular risk: theory and evidence. Vasc Health Risk Manag 2006; 2: 157-162.

[73] Xiao, C. W. Health Effects of Soy Protein and Isoflavones in Humans. The Journal of Nutrition 2008; 138: 1244S-1249S.

[74] Wang, Y., Jones, P. J. H., Ausman, L. M. and Lichtenstein, A. H. Soy protein reduces triglyceride levels and triglyceride fatty acid fractional synthesis rate in hypercholesterolemic subjects. Atherosclerosis 2004; 173: 269-275.

[75] Ascencio, C., Torres, N., Isoard-Acosta, F., Gómez-Pérez, F. J., Hernández-Pando, R. and Tovar, A. R. Soy Protein Affects Serum Insulin and Hepatic SREBP-1 mRNA and Reduces Fatty Liver in Rats. The Journal of Nutrition 2004; 134: 522-529.

[76] Michelfelder, A. Soy: a complete source of protein. Am Fam Physician. 2009 79: 43-47.

[77] Slavin, J. L. Dietary fiber and body weight. Nutrition (Burbank, Los Angeles County, Calif.) 2005; 21: 411-418.

[78] Babio, N., Balanza, R., Basulto, J., Bulló, M. and Salas-Salvadó, J. Dietary fibre: influence on body weight, glycemic control and plasma cholesterol profile. Nutr Hosp 2010; 25: 327-340.

[79] Fernandez, M.-L. Soluble fiber and nondigestible carbohydrate effects on plasma lipids and cardiovascular risk. Current Opinion in Lipidology 2001; 12: 35-40.

[80] Peterson, J., Dwyer, J., Adlercreutz, H., Scalbert, A., Jacques, P. and McCullough, M. L. Dietary lignans: physiology and potential for cardiovascular disease risk reduction. Nutrition Reviews 2010; 68: 571-603.

[81] Mattson, F. H. and Grundy, S. M. Comparison of effects of dietary saturated, monounsaturated, and polyunsaturated fatty acids on plasma lipids and lipoproteins in man. J Lipid Res 1985; 26: 194-202.

[82] Rudel, L. L., Parks, J. S. and Sawyer, J. K. Compared with dietary monounsaturated and saturated fat, polyunsaturated fat protects African green monkeys from coronary artery atherosclerosis. Arterioscler Thromb Vasc Biol 1995; 15: 2101-2110.

[83] Baum, S. J., Kris-Etherton, P. M., Willett, W. C., Lichtenstein, A. H., Rudel, L. L., Maki, K. C., Whelan, J., Ramsden, C. E. and Block, R. C. Fatty acids in cardiovascular health and disease: a comprehensive update. J Clin Lipidol 2012; 6: 216-234.

[84] Weitz, D., Weintraub, H., Fisher, E. and Schwartzbard, A. Z. Fish oil for the treatment of cardiovascular disease. Cardiol Rev 2010; 18: 258-263.

[85] Abeywardena, M. Y. and Patten, G. S. Role of omega3 long-chain polyunsaturated fatty acids in reducing cardio-metabolic risk factors. Endocr Metab Immune Disord Drug Targets 2011; 11: 232-246.

[86] Badimon, L., Vilahur, G. and Padro, T. Nutraceuticals and Atherosclerosis: Human Trials. Cardiovascular Therapeutics 2010; 28: 202-215.

[87] Naito, Y. and Yoshikawa, T. Green Tea and Heart Health. Journal of Cardiovascular Pharmacology 2009; 54: 385-390 310.1097/FJC.1090b1013e3181b1096e1097a1091.

[88] Shukla, S. K., Gupta, S., Ojha, S. K. and Sharma, S. B. Cardiovascular friendly natural products: a promising approach in the management of CVD. Natural Product Research: Formerly Natural Product Letters 2010; 24: 873 - 898.

[89] Kong, W., Wei, J., Abidi, P., Lin, M., Inaba, S., Li, C., Wang, Y., Wang, Z., Si, S., Pan, H., Wang, S., Wu, J., Li, Z., Liu, J. and Jiang, J. D. Berberine is a novel cholesterol-lowering drug working through a unique mechanism distinct from statins. Nat Med 2004; 10: 1344-1351.

[90] Wang, Y., Jia, X., Ghanam, K., Beaurepaire, C., Zidichouski, J. and Miller, L. Berberine and plant stanols synergistically inhibit cholesterol absorption in hamsters. Atherosclerosis 2010; 209: 111-117.

[91] Jia, X., Chen, Y., Zidichouski, J., Zhang, J., Sun, C. and Wang, Y. Co-administration of berberine and plant stanols synergistically reduces plasma cholesterol in rats. Atherosclerosis 2008; 201: 101-107.

[92] Papaliodis, D., Boucher, W., Kempuraj, D., Michaelian, M., Wolfberg, A., House, M. and Theoharides, T. C. Niacin-induced "Flush" Involves Release of Prostaglandin D2 from Mast Cells and Serotonin from Platelets: Evidence from Human Cells in Vitro and an Animal Model. Journal of Pharmacology and Experimental Therapeutics 2008; 327: 665-672.

[93] Hansen, B., Tigno, X., Bénardeau, A., Meyer, M., Sebokova, E. and Mizrahi, J. Effects of aleglitazar, a balanced dual peroxisome proliferator-activated receptor α/γ agonist on glycemic and lipid parameters in a primate model of the metabolic syndrome. Cardiovasc Diabetol 2011; 10: 7.

[94] Pöss, J., Custodis, F., Werner, C., Weingärtner, O., Böhm, M. and Laufs, U. Cardiovascular Disease and Dyslipidemia: Beyond LDL. Curr Pharm Des. 2011; 17: 861-870.

[95] Pan, C., Yoo, H. J. and Ho, L. T. Perspectives of CB1 Antagonist in Treatment of Obesity: Experience of RIO-Asia. J Obes 2011; 2011: doi:10.1155/2011/957268.

[96] Chiang, J. Y. L. Bile Acid Regulation of Gene Expression: Roles of Nuclear Hormone Receptors. Endocr Rev 2002; 23: 443-463.

[97] Buhman, K. F., Accad, M. and Farese, R. V. Mammalian acyl-CoA:cholesterol acyltransferases. Biochim Biophys Acta 2000; 1529: 142-154.

[98] Buhman, K. K., Accad, M., Novak, S., Choi, R. S., Wong, J. S., Hamilton, R. L., Turley, S. and Farese, R. V., Jr. Resistance to diet-induced hypercholesterolemia and gallstone formation in ACAT2-deficient mice. Nat Med 2000; 6: 1341-1347.

[99] Repa, J. J., Buhman, K. K., Farese, R. V., Jr., Dietschy, J. M. and Turley, S. D. ACAT2 deficiency limits cholesterol absorption in the cholesterol-fed mouse: impact on hepatic cholesterol homeostasis. Hepatology 2004; 40: 1088-1097.

[100] Willner, E. L., Tow, B., Buhman, K. K., Wilson, M., Sanan, D. A., Rudel, L. L. and Farese, R. V., Jr. Deficiency of acyl CoA:cholesterol acyltransferase 2 prevents atherosclerosis in apolipoprotein E-deficient mice. Proc Natl Acad Sci U S A 2003; 100: 1262-1267.

[101] Farese, R. V., Jr. The nine lives of ACAT inhibitors. Arterioscler Thromb Vasc Biol 2006; 26: 1684-1686.

[102] Rondinone, C. M. Minireview: Ribonucleic Acid Interference for the Identification of New Targets for the Treatment of Metabolic Diseases. Endocrinology 2006; 147: 2650-2656.

[103] Abifadel, M., Pakradouni, J., Collin, M., Samson-Bouma, M.-E., Varret, M., Rabès, J.-P. and Boileau, C. Strategies for proprotein convertase subtilisin kexin 9 modulation: a perspective on recent patents. Expert Opinion on Therapeutic Patents 2010; 20: 1547-1571.

[104] Nissen, S. E., Tuzcu, E. M., Brewer, H. B., Sipahi, I., Nicholls, S. J., Ganz, P., Schoenhagen, P., Waters, D. D., Pepine, C. J., Crowe, T. D., Davidson, M. H., Deanfield, J. E., Wisniewski, L. M., Hanyok, J. J. and Kassalow, L. M. Effect of ACAT inhibition on the progression of coronary atherosclerosis. N Engl J Med 2006; 354: 1253-1263.

[105] Tardif, J. C., Gregoire, J., L'Allier, P. L., Anderson, T. J., Bertrand, O., Reeves, F., Title, L. M., Alfonso, F., Schampaert, E., Hassan, A., McLain, R., Pressler, M. L., Ibrahim, R., Lesperance, J., Blue, J., Heinonen, T. and Rodes-Cabau, J. Effects of the acyl coenzyme A:cholesterol acyltransferase inhibitor avasimibe on human atherosclerotic lesions. Circulation 2004; 110: 3372-3377.

[106] Bell, T. A., 3rd, Brown, J. M., Graham, M. J., Lemonidis, K. M., Crooke, R. M. and Rudel, L. L. Liver-specific inhibition of acyl-coenzyme a:cholesterol acyltransferase 2 with antisense oligonucleotides limits atherosclerosis development in apolipoprotein B100-only low-density lipoprotein receptor-/- mice. Arterioscler Thromb Vasc Biol 2006; 26: 1814-1820.

Chapter 8

A Glance at the Complexity of Nutrition and the Prostate: Considering Molecular Targets to Unravel the Most Recent Controversy Between Omega-3 Fatty Acids and Their Impact on Prostate Cancer Risk

Gailene Tobin, Robert Hurta and Marianna Kulka

Additional information is available at the end of the chapter

http://dx.doi.org/10.5772/55858

1. Introduction

1.1. Pathophysiology of prostate cancer

Considered part of both the male reproductive and urinary systems, the prostate gland (or prostate) is oval shaped, and is variable in size (ranging from 20 – 30 grams in adult males)[1]. The prostate gland consists of different types of cells, including gland (epithelial) cells, muscle cells and fibrous cells [2]. The overall structure of the prostate is divided in two ways: by zone, a classification more often used in pathology [2, 3] or by lobe, more often used in anatomy [2]. Prostate associated diseases usually present with urinary and sexual dysfunction and the initial symptoms related to such often necessitate diagnostic testing to indicate the presence of a certain disease state [4, 5]. Although the accuracy and use of Digital Rectal Examination (DRE) and Prostate Specific Antigen (PSA) remains controversial, these tests can be used alone, or in combination, to detect benign conditions (including benign prostatic hyperplasia (BPH) and prostatitis) or predict most forms of PCa [6, 7]. Subsequent prognosis of PCa is confirmed by prostate biopsy and involves pathological staging (Tumor/ Nodes/ Metastasis (TNM) System) and grading (Gleason Score) [8-10]. Broadly defined as the malignant growth of cells of the prostate gland, PCa occurs in many different zones of the prostate [1, 11, 12]. PCa (mostly 75%) arise in the peripheral zone, and to a lesser extent in the central and transitional zones [13]. Similar to the pattern of most epithelial cancers, cells within the prostate undergo an accumulation of genetic changes whereby the functions of cellular control are lost as the cell and tissue undergo phenotype changes from normal to prostatic intraepithelial neoplasia (PIN) [14]. This progressively leads from to an acute high-grade PIN (HGPIN) to superficial cancers, and then to invasive disease [11, 12] (See Figure 1). The most common form of PCa (around 95%) originates in the glandular/epithelial tissue, and is coined prostatic adenocarcinoma; thus, this term has emerged synonymously with PCa [13]. The residual forms of PCa are termed nonadenocarcinoma, and present as less commonly occurring cancers, but are often more aggressive. Such can be categorized as epithelial (such as squamous cell carcinoma) and nonepithelial (such as osteo- and angio-sarcoma), and also include others which rarely develop in the prostate and are derived from primary tumors of the bladder and urethra (such as transitional cell carcinoma) [13]. The diagram below gives a general overview of prostate location, the division of zones and the general progression of PCa as the cell and tissue phenotype changes from normal to A. prostatic intraepithelial neoplasia (PIN), to B. increasing and severe high-grade PIN (HGPIN), then to C. superficial cancers, and finally to D. invasive disease [11, 12, 15].

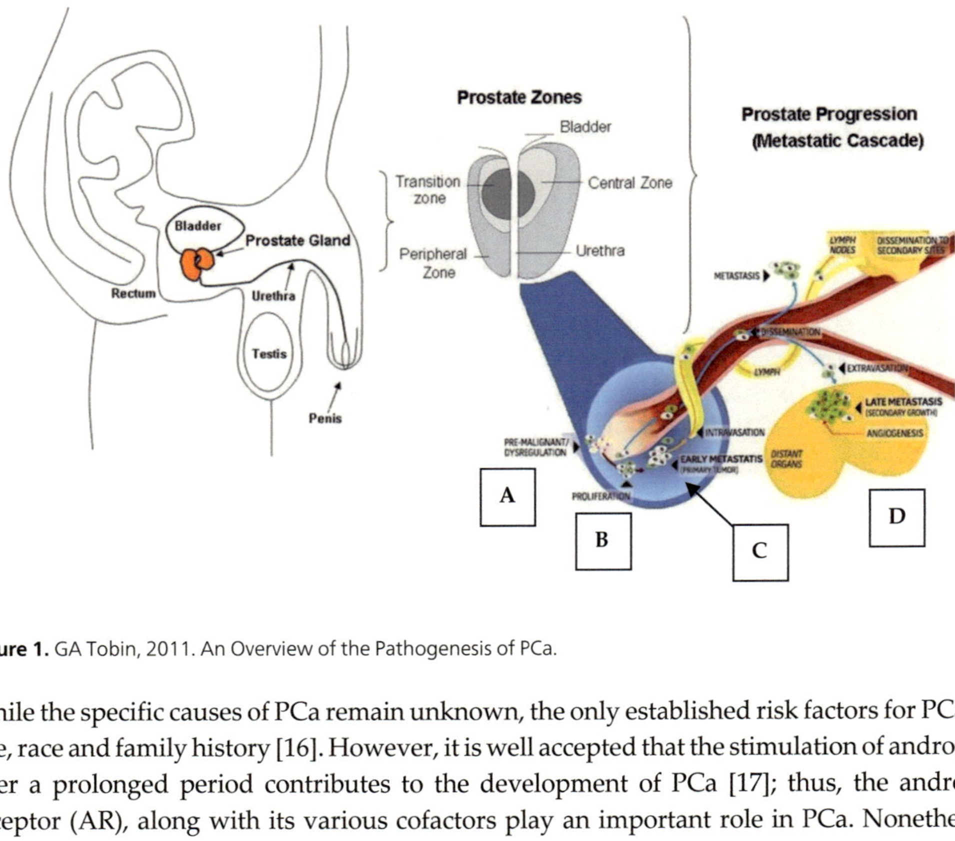

Figure 1. GA Tobin, 2011. An Overview of the Pathogenesis of PCa.

While the specific causes of PCa remain unknown, the only established risk factors for PCa are age, race and family history [16]. However, it is well accepted that the stimulation of androgens over a prolonged period contributes to the development of PCa [17]; thus, the androgen receptor (AR), along with its various cofactors play an important role in PCa. Nonetheless, progression of PCa to androgen independence (or the hormone refractory state) is one of the primary reasons for PCa-related deaths today [18]. PCa is the sixth most commonly diagnosed cancer worldwide [19]. For Canadian men, PCa is the most prevalent (based on 15 years) and frequently diagnosed non-dermatological cancer [20]. Like most other solid malignancies, PCa

http://dx.doi.org/10.5772/55858

can extend to distant organs such as the liver, lungs and brain, with an abnormally high tendency for metastasizing to the bone [21, 22]. When distant metastasis occurs, the 5 year survival rate drops to 31% [20]. Although Prostate Specific Antigen (PSA) values, TNM staging, Gleason Score, and tumor biomarkers are considered significant in their ability to predict patient outcome, alone or when incorporated into various nomogram models, there is much controversy about their accuracy. Nonetheless, treatment regimens are largely based on these combined indicators.

Standard treatments for PCa can range from watchful waiting to surgery, radiation therapy, hormone therapy, chemotherapy, and biological therapy, alone or in combination [23-26]. Additionally, in North America, a minimum of 30% of men with diagnosed prostate disease choose to use complementary and/or alternative medical (CAM) therapy [27, 28] including primarily herbal biological agents, vitamins, supplements and dietary intervention [29]. This trend is likely due to progressive research on differences in global distribution, indicating that prolonged diet and micronutrient intake intervals may possibly control whether PCa remains latent or develops into a clinically significant disease [30-34]. In particular, the role of polyunsaturated fatty acids (PUFA) has gained considerable importance in PCa in the last several years. However, the molecular basis for these observations has not been fully explained. Genetic (and epigenetic) alterations and specific signaling pathways [35] are considered important in the multi-step process of cancer [36]. Thus, dietary interventions which target signaling pathways and downstream genes known to be impacted in PCa may be a worthwhile and effective approach in developing novel therapies.

2. Endocrine and molecular biology and controls in prostate cancer

2.1. Hormones and prostate cancer

Charles Huggins introduced the phenomenon of androgen removal as a plausible means for prostate cancer treatment in men after his observation that castration in canines caused shrinkage of prostate tumors [37]. Similar to normal prostate cells, prostate cancer cells are androgen dependent at the outset with a normally functioning androgen receptor (the receptor only responds to androgen) [37]. These initial studies on the dependence of the prostate gland on androgens formed the principle behind androgen deprivation therapy. There are several avenues that can be utilized to remove androgens, and the decision to do so is largely dependent on the stage or severity of cancer. Early cancers commonly target 5alpha(α)-reductase inhibition in an effort to decrease levels of the active hormone dihydrotestosterone (DHT). In fact, in the Prostate Cancer Prevention Trial (PCPT), finasteride (a 5α-reductase inhibitor) has been reported to lower the incidence of prostate cancer in men by 25% [38]. The initial concern about finasteride causing more severe cancers was refuted. However, despite this, the FDA has published advice concerning the use of finasteride and an increased risk of high-grade PCa [39]. Interestingly, the PCPT study is the one which Brasky *et al.* used to extrapolate data for their recent findings regarding n-3 PUFA and prostate cancer [40]. AR antagonists can also be used to block both testicular and adrenally produced androgens from binding to the androgen receptor and initiating gene transcription [41]. Additionally, testicular-derived androgen production can be blocked by luteinizing hormone (LH) inhibition [42]. For more aggressive cancers, these previously mentioned methods can be used in combination blocking both androgen production and their actions [41].

Despite the fact that most prostate cancers respond well to androgen deprivation, prostate cancer cells develop survival mechanisms involving the androgen receptor that can render these treatments ineffective; this represents the progression from androgen sensitive to androgen insensitive disease. Central to this role, the AR develops abnormal signaling functions that are not seen in normal AR signaling in androgen sensitive prostate cancer progression. There are several mechanisms through which the androgen receptor can participate in androgen insensitive prostate cancer. Amplification of the AR creates a hypersensitivity to even low amounts of circulating androgens [43]. The AR can also become promiscuous; mutations of the ligand binding domain can allow for aberrant AR activation by factors other than androgens (i.e: estrogen or other steroid hormones) and increased AR activity can also occur when such mutations are found in coregulators [44]. The AR can become an outlaw receptor - receptive to transactivation, phosphorylation and activation by other signaling pathways and peptide growth factors (i.e: insulin growth factor -1 (IGF-1) in the absence of androgen [45]. Other modified functions of the AR include activation of other pro-proliferative and anti-apoptotic factors that can bypass the AR pathway, eliminating any dependence on androgens for these physiological effects. For example: bcl-2, an anti-apoptotic protein, is not expressed in normal prostate epithelium, however in the absence of AR function, bcl-2 is produced [46]. Thus, effective treatment is dependent in the ability of the AR to develop these modified survival mechanisms.

The topic of testosterone production is worthy outside the realm of AR function in androgen insensitive prostate cancer. It is well known that the testes are the main site of testosterone production. Therapies that reduce testosterone production by targeting the testes do not affect adrenal androgen synthesis which is increased in androgen insensitive prostate cancer, thus compensating for the reduced testicular androgen production. In such cases, a broad spectrum cytochrome P450 inhibitor may be recommended, although their use may introduce side effects so extensive that their utility is limited [47].

2.2. Molecular biology of prostate cancer

Hanahan and Weinberg, in 2011, summarize the unique biological capabilities of cancer [48]. The hallmarks of cancer outlined within include sustaining proliferative signaling, evading growth suppressors, resisting cell death, enabling replicative immortality, inducing angiogenesis, and activating invasion and metastasis. Interestingly, in this updated review, genomic stability and inflammation are noted as underlying these characteristics as they expedite acquisition and foster multiple functions, respectively. Additionally, two emerging hallmarks - reprogramming of energy metabolism and evading immune destruction are discussed, as well as the dimensions of tumor complexity including the ability of these acquired traits to create the tumor microenvironment [48]. We agree that the recognition of all of these concepts, alone or in combination, provide guidance in the development of new cancer treatments. The

http://dx.doi.org/10.5772/55858

paragraphs to follow are meant to provide a basic overview of some of the aforementioned concepts and their relevance in prostate cancer. While we have not specifically discussed tumor microenvironment or two of the above-mentioned emerging hallmarks and their relevance to prostate cancer in this chapter, such topics of importance subsequently emerge in broader areas of discussion.

2.2.1. *Sustaining proliferative signaling*

Although the host may provide a source of growth factors, such are not essential for the survival of cancer cells. Cancer cells can evade the requirement for exogenous growth factors in several ways, including the production of their own growth factors. Cancer cell mutations can result in constitutively active growth factors and growth factor receptor pathways. Thus the initiation of the signaling cascade occurs without the required binding of the growth factor ligand to the receptor; cell growth occurs in the absence of ligand. In this regard, mutations in both the ras family and epidermal growth factor (EGF) receptors are seen in prostate cancer [49]. Another example of such includes autocrine and/or paracrine production of IGF-1 by prostate cancer cells [50], as stromal prostate cancer cells and the adjacent epithelium produces IGF-1 and expresses IGF-1 receptor, respectively.

2.2.2. *Evading growth suppressors*

Pathway hypersensitivity can result when cancer cells over-express growth factor receptors in the presence of normal physiological levels of a growth factor. PCa cells frequently increase their expression of Human Epidermal Growth Factor Receptor (HER)2 and the androgen receptor [51]. In this way, small amounts of androgen that can direct large increases in the expression of pro-carcinogenic genes or AR regulated gene expression can even occur in the absence of androgens.

2.2.3. *Resisting cell death*

The body eliminates damaged or dysregulated cells through intrinsic mechanisms including tumor suppressor pathways responsible for the mediation of DNA repair, cell cycle arrest, apoptosis and senescence [52]. However, some of these damaged cells harbor mutations and/or have the ability to produce factors that allow them to survive. Proliferation of these cells, if not kept in check, results in tumors. The expression of Bcl-2, an anti-apoptotic protein indicates that a cell may not respond to cell death cues. Production of Bcl-2 is high in prostate cancer cells [46], rendering them resistant to apoptosis.

2.2.4. *Enabling replicative immortality*

The balance between growth and anti-growth signaling results in normal cell growth. Differentiation of cells occurs only when cells halt the growth program. Thus, rapidly proliferating (undifferentiated) cells form a mass of cells commonly referred to as a tumor. Such unimpeded growth is usually less differentiated than normal cells. Under normal conditions, transforming growth factor beta (TGFβ) is an anti-growth factor stimulating epithelial cells to a terminally differentiated state. However, this property is dysregulated in prostate cancer development [53]. As TGF-β signals through retinoblastoma (Rb) tumor suppressor gene [54], it is assumed to cause an increase in cell cycle inhibitors, such as p21. Thus, the loss of Rb in prostate cancer renders the pro-differentiation, anti-proliferation effects of TGF-β null [55].

The ability of cancer cells to replicate many more times over their natural lifespan distinguishes them from normal cells. Inherent defects in prostate cancer cells, such as losses of cell cycle inhibitors, including p21 or p27 enable this phenomenon. As with other cancer cell types, dysregulated telomere maintenance provides another explanation. The small DNA fragments at the ends of chromosomes are known as telomeres [56]. Telomere shortening to a desired length, following cell reproduction, signals a cell to stop replicating. However, cancer cells express elevated levels of telomerase, thus allowing cancer cells to replicate beyond their normal programmed number of replications by maintaining telomere length [38].

2.2.5. Inducing angiogenesis, activating invasion and metastasis

In order to expand in size, cancer cells require the support of a vasculature system. Judah Folkman's pioneering work in cancer revealed this unconditional requirement for sustained angiogenesis in cancer [57], accompanied by increased requirements for oxygen and nutrient supply, as well as waste removal; the latter is due to the ability of cancer cells to rapidly proliferate. In prostate cancer, and other cancers, vascular endothelial growth factor (VEGF) production is elevated [58]. This paracrine factor stimulates nearby endothelial cells and epithelial cells to form irregular vasculature associated with tumorigenesis. This confirms the notion that cancer cells produce factors that recruit endothelial progenitor cells and epithelial cells are capable of forming primitive vascular channels.

To further survive along the cancer cascade, and even in the presence of increased angiogenesis, cells must metastasize as the tissue of origin is capacity limiting with respect to tumor burden [57]. Metastasis of cancer cells involves degradation of the basement membrane at the site of origin and penetration to the bloodstream and/or lymph. Although few cells survive this journey through the lymph and blood stream, those that penetrate into the tissue of destination complete the metastatic cascade by invading and colonizing to secondary sites.

Cadherins, a class of membrane receptors, can undergo isoform switching (known as "cadherin switching") during normal development which allows cell types to segregate from one another. Within this family, particular cadherin members promote cell motility and invasion control via growth factor receptor signaling and pathway signaling components [59]. In tumor cells, this activity ceases resulting in aggressive tumor cells with an ability to escape the origin of the tumor and metastasize.

Therefore, the functional significance of these specific cadherins and cadherin switching provides insight into the molecular mechanism underlying tumor progression and offers an opportunity for the development of novel molecular targets for anti-cancer therapy. Integrity of the basement membrane and maintenance of epithelial integrity involves E-cadherin (epithelial calcium-dependent adhesion), a Type 1 transmembrane protein. The extracellular component of E-cadherin is responsible for homophilic interactions, while the cytoplasmic component of E-cadherin binds to beta (β-) and gamma (γ-) catenin [60]. While the loss of E-cadherin signifies the ability of a cancer cell to leave the prostate [61], it would be remiss to think that this loss alone is responsible for tumor cell invasion considering the dimensions of tumor microenvironment [48]. Aside from changes in cell-to-cell and cell-to-matrix adhesion, tumor invasion involves additional cellular events including cell migration and proteolytic degradation of the extracellular matrix (ECM), and other events which alone or in combination can affect cell signaling pathways. The initial suggestion that E-cadherin downregulation may result in the activation of specific signaling pathways triggering tumor cell invasion has been explored. Because of its dual role as a cytoplasmic cellular adhesion complex component and its fundamental role in Wnt-mediated signal transduction, β-catenin has emerged as a prime contender for activating such signaling pathways. Additionally, levels of matrix metalloproteases (MMPs) also increase in prostate cancer and degrade stromal and basement membrane components, enabling cancer cells to escape the tissue of origin [62]. Overall, such factors that allow the progression of the metastatic cascade, rather than the original tumor, are responsible for cancer death.

2.2.6. *Inflammation*

Although inflammation has been long recognized in the development of cancer [63, 64], *chronic* inflammation has emerged as one of the enabling characteristics of human cancer [48]. Chronic inflammation can be caused by numerous factors including infectious and non-infectious agents and / or other environmental aspects including hormonal changes and dietary interventions [65, 66]. Fostering multiple functions related to cancer, inflammation cuts across broad areas of study including genetics, epidemiology, molecular pathology, histopathology, immunology and animal modelling to name a few. In other words, it would be difficult to capture an association between cancer and inflammation by way of any one over-arching theory. A diverse amalgamation of evidence exist which points to the role of the inflammatory response in physiological maintenance including tissue homeostasis and the healing process involved succeeding injury or damage. Rakoff-Nahoum (2006) has provided an excellent overview of this dual role of inflammation in tumor development [52]. The inter-relationship of cancer and inflammation with respect to inflammatory cells (and their mediators) and signaling pathways involved that have been published in the past suggests that the inflammatory system can affect tumor development and inhibit the development of cancer [67-72]. The topic of inflammation in prostate carcinogenesis has been recently updated in a thorough review authored by Sfanoes and DeMarzo (2012) encompassing recent advances in prostate risk and development with respect to prostatic inflammation stimuli, immunobiology, inflammatory pathways and cytokines, proliferative inflammatory atrophy as a risk factor lesion to prostate cancer development, and the role of nutritional or other anti-inflammatory compounds [66]. While this exceptional review articulates the vast effects of inflammation in prostate cancer, we will aim to highlight evidence to date as related to some promising anti-inflammatory natural products while focusing on PUFA.

3. Promising anti-inflammatory natural products in PCa

The role of inflammation in prostate cancer etiology stems from studies accessing the relationship between intake of anti-inflammatory dietary compounds and prostate cancer risk. Epidemiological evidence associates or significantly correlates consumption of tomato [73], soy and green tea [74, 75] with decreased prostate cancer risk. Furthermore, animal studies confirm that the anti-inflammatory properties of both soy and green tea cause a decrease in prostate cancer [74, 75]. One study involving Transgenic Adenocarcinoma of the Mouse Prostate (TRAMP) mice fed a diet enriched with processed whole tomatoes reported benefits including increased survival, delayed progression from PIN to PCa cancer and a decreased incidence of poorly differentiated PCa cancer [76]. Prostate cancer cell lines treated with phytoestrogens, specifically genistein and daidzein, indicate a decrease in prostate cancer risk, however this effect seems to be linked to epigenetic modifications of DNA [77].

3.1. PUFA and prostate cancer

Interest in dietary fats and disease etiologies has emerged because of their known anti-inflammatory properties. Examples of dietary fat which are essential in a variety of mammalian biological processes and impact PCa include omega-3 (n-3) and omega-6 (n-6) PUFA [78, 79]. In published cell line and xenograft studies, n-6 PUFA (linoleic acid and arachidonic acid) typically exert a growth-promoting effect, while n-3 PUFA (EPA and DHA) have growth-inhibitory effects [80-85]. *In vitro* and animal studies suggest a trend of opposite effects for cancer development with respect to n-3 and n-6 PUFA. The n-3 PUFA, such as EPA and DHA, indicate a suppression of tumor carcinogenesis, however n-6 PUFA seems to promote tumor development. From an epidemiological perspective, evidence of an association between particular PUFA and PCa is inconsistent, with many studies reporting no association between dietary intake of n-3 or n-6 PUFA and the risk of PCa [86-92], however both pre-clinical *in vivo* and *in vitro* studies clearly indicate that there are biological mechanisms by which omega-3 PUFA can arrest growth in both PCa cells and tumors. Supplementation of n-3 PUFA in animal studies failed to produce an effect on prostate tumor growth or other markers of PCa progression and did not significantly reduce tumor growth in a PCa mouse model [93-96]. Treatment of human PCa cells with n-3 PUFA has been shown to consistently inhibit proliferation and /or increase programmed cell death, affect gene expression and deter properties of invasive human PCa in cells supporting the notion that EPA and DHA supplementation could preclude or limit the growth of prostate tumors [80, 85, 94, 97-102]. In general, and as found in a recent case-control study, while proinflammatory n-6 PUFA may present an increase in PCa risk, the anti-inflammatory properties of n-3 PUFA have been noted in their association with decreased risk [103]. Interestingly, this same study reported that mutations in the inflammation and mitogenesis related gene (COX-2), combined with low nutritional consumption of n-3 PUFA, had a higher risk of PCa; this risk was lowered with an increase in the dietary intake of n-3 PUFA [103]. Inflammatory gene expression is usually negatively associated with cancer stage and prognosis [104]. Despite these trends, a recent epidemiology study by Brasky (2011) contradicts the protective role of n-3 PUFA in PCa by reporting a positive association with

DHA for high-grade disease[40]. Specifically the findings indicate that higher blood concentrations of n-3 PUFA are associated with increased risk of high-grade prostate cancer (Gleason score 8–10), and higher concentrations of n-6 PUFA were associated with decreased risk [40]. Dr. Brasky has indicated that these findings *"turn what we know—or rather what we think we know—about diet, inflammation and the development of prostate cancer on its head and shine a light on the complexity of studying the association between nutrition and the risk of various chronic diseases* [105]." Could it be that what is deemed good and promoted for heart and brain health may be essentially harmful to the prostate? Consider the following: Data analyzed to come to this vastly different conclusion was based on a subset of more than 3200 (half of which developed PCa throughout the duration of the study) from the overall study population of 19,000 [40]. This nationwide randomized clinical trial was initiated to test the efficacy of the drug finasteride to prevent prostate cancer and considered unique as biopsy was used to confirm the absence or presence of prostate cancer in all study subjects [105]. The original intent of the study was to prove the hypothesis that n-3 PUFA would reduce and n-6 PUFA and trans-fatty acids would increase prostate cancer risk, pre-empted by two important known factors; that n-3 fatty acids originating mainly in fish and their oil supplements have anti-inflammatory properties and chronic inflammation is known to increase the risk of several cancers. All this combined with an inconsistent history of studies and the fact that the mechanisms behind the influence of n- 3 PUFA on the risk of developing high-grade PCa have not been identified, warrants further research. Nonetheless, we are presented with evidence of substantive biological activity, and thus we must explore other mechanisms, aside from inflammation, that may play a greater role in the development of certain prostate cancers. To embark upon this currently debatable journey, there are key factors concerning prostate cancer and dietary interventions that should be considered, particularly n-3 PUFA. The sections to follow are meant to generate, by example and based on the current literature, some thoughts on how to proceed in this area of research to determine the actual role of n-3 PUFA in prostate cancer.

4. Looking forward: Considerations for further research in n-3 PUFA and prostate cancer

4.1. Prostate cancer signaling pathways and n-3 PUFA

Signaling pathways and their associated molecules often have a dual role in events such as homeostasis, tissue repair, and tumorigenesis. For example, the Wnt/β-catenin pathway is critical in maintaining steady-state proliferation and tumorigenesis of tissues [106]. Numerous studies to date indicate that n-3 PUFA treatment can affect cell signaling partially through AKT (protein kinase B), mTOR (mammalian target of rapamycin) and NF-κB (nuclear factor kappa B) associated pathways [94, 95, 99, 107]. Treatment with n-3 PUFA has been indicated in the inhibition of human hepatocellular carcinoma and cholangiocarcinoma cell growth by blocking the Wnt/β-catenin pathway [108, 109], and DHA treatment has been shown to inhibit the production of β-catenin in colon cancer cells [110-112]. However, the effects of n-3 PUFA on Wnt/β-catenin signaling in PCa remain largely unknown. A single study in PCa indicates that fat-1 gene (cloned from *Caenorhabditis elegans*) that encodes for a n-3 PUFA desaturase (which converts n-6 PUFA to n-3 PUFA) expression was shown to reduce phosphorylation of glycogen synthase kinase-3β (GSK-3β), a major element in the Wnt/β-catenin pathway, resulting in subsequent down-regulation of both β-catenin and cyclin D1 thereby inhibiting PCa cell proliferation [113].

4.1.1. An introduction to Wnt/β-catenin signaling

The Wnt family constitutes 19 highly conserved glycoprotein members in mammals [114]. The most significant molecule implicated in the canonical Wnt cascade is β-catenin, a cytoplasmic protein regulated by a multi-protein destruction complex made up of Axin, adenomatous polyposis coli (APC), GSK-3β and casein kinase 1 (CK1) [115]. In the absence of Wnt signaling, the destruction complex stimulates the phosphorylation of β-catenin by GSK-3β, leading to subsequent ubiquitination and proteasomal degradation [116, 117]. Conversely, in the presence of Wnt signaling, Wnt ligand-frizzled (FZD) binding causes disheveled (DVL) protein dissociation of the β-catenin destruction complex, blocking the phosphorylation of β- catenin, and leading to β-catenin accumulation in the nucleus [116, 117]. Nuclear β-catenin functions as a transcription co-factor of the Tcf/Lef family and leads to the activation of Wnt target genes implicated in cell proliferation, differentiation and apoptosis, including c-myc, cyclin D1, Akt, MMP-7, and AR [114, 116-122].

4.1.2. Using Wnt/β-catenin signaling as a model to determine the pathogenic role of n-3 PUFA in prostate cancer

Modular in nature, the activity of the Wnt/β-catenin pathway can be modified through several points of intervention. The fundamental event in Wnt/β-catenin signaling occurs in the nucleus and is the result of stabilized β-catenin recruiting Tcf/Lef transcription factors that modulate the expression of oncogenes, such as c-myc and cyclin D1[123-128]. Abnormal expression of β-catenin has been observed in up to 71% of prostate tumor specimens [129-131], is elevated in more than 20% of advanced prostate tumors [132] and is associated with advanced stage PCa [130, 133, 134]. APC alterations alone are considered prognostic with respect to an unfavorable outcome [135] even though it varies with respect to inactivation in PCa reporting somatic loss ranging from 2– 43% [132, 136-138] and promoter hypermethylation in up to 90% of PCa [135, 139, 140]. Mutations in Axin-1 have been identified in 14% of advanced PCa, and several Axin-1 mutations and polymorphisms have been noted in PCa cell lines [138]. DVL-1, is a pathway regulator involved in Axin recruitment and inactivation, is significantly overexpressed in PCa and has also shown a positive correlation with PCa grade [141]. Pathway activators, including WNT-1, -2, -5A, and -6 have been highly overexpressed in primary PCa compared to normal prostate [142-145], and WNT-1 and -2 have been indicated as having a role in invasive PCa [143, 146]. Conversely, but also resulting in stabilized β-catenin, pathway inhibitors are commonly downregulated in PCa. Dickkopf-related protein (DKK)-1 expression is lower in PCa tissue in comparison to normal prostate tissue samples and furthermore is significantly reduced during progression to metastasis [143, 147]. Secreted frizzled-related protein (SFRP)- 1 and DKK-3 show decreased expression in prostate tumor cells [148-151]

Downregulation of SFRP-1 was also reported in PCa cell lines [152]. It is interesting to note that SFRP-4 overexpression is associated with decreased proliferation, decreased anchorage-independent growth and decreased invasiveness in a PCa cell line, and additionally predicts a good prognosis in PCa [153, 154]. WIF-1, another Wnt antagonist is downregulated at the mRNA (23%) and protein level (64%) of PCa [155]. Recently, FZD-3 inhibition by soy protein was shown to suppress the growth of PCa cell lines [156]. Similarly, FZD-5 was highly up-regulated in the prostate tissue of advanced PCa cancer patients and was downregulated by zoledronic acid in PC3 cells, but not DU145 cells [157]. Appropriate steps to determine the role of n-3 PUFA in prostate cancer may include investigating whether n-3 PUFA treatment will affect subcellular gene expression and localization of β-catenin. Beyond confirmation of the molecular mechanism(s) by which n-3 PUFA inhibits Wnt/β-catenin, subsequent experiments could target degradation of cytoplasmic β-catenin and activation of the Wnt receptor complex. Table 1 summarizes dysregulation of numerous pathway components which may be responsible for PCa tumor development/progression and as such represents potential targets for further investigation to determine n-3 PUFA/Wnt/β-catenin interactions in PCa.

4.1.3. Clinical significance of targeting the Wnt/β-catenin pathway in PCa with n-3 PUFA

Despite the noted progress of hormone-based drugs as a therapy, PCa remains as one of the primary causes of cancer deaths worldwide [20, 101]. Thus, new and improved therapeutic strategies to prevent PCa and inhibit its progression are needed. In this regard, n-3 PUFA presents tremendous opportunity as a therapeutic intervention in PCa. There is enough convincing data available to show a positive correlation between Wnt/β-catenin activation and PCa progression. It is also well established now that n-3 FAs supplementation can impact PCa development and progression *in vitro*. However, whether these effects of n-3 PUFA on PCa can occur at least in part through inhibition of Wnt/β–catenin signaling remain largely unknown. Thus, the incorporation of variations as suggested above could start by targeting nuclear interaction and progressing back through the pathway to the point of surface expression interactions of the Wnt-FRZ-LRP Receptor Complex. Furthermore, AR expression is positively correlated with an increase in cytoplasmic/nuclear β-catenin levels in epithelial cells of the prostate [175]. β-catenin interacts with AR and acts as a co-activator of AR to increase its transcriptional activity in response to androgen [17]. This leads to activation of AR target genes implicated in PCa progression. Therefore it is possible that n-3 PUFA can inhibit aberrant expression and activation of AR. As β-catenin is considered to be a ligand-dependent coactivator of AR transcription [17], the effects of n-3 PUFA on AR expression and β-catenin/ AR crosstalk is an area requiring exploration.

A series of experiments to specifically target different components of the Wnt/β-catenin pathway as noted above would be a rational approach to determining the effects of n-3 PUFA in PCa. Goss's recent textbook reviews some innovative strategies that have been utilized to antagonize signaling at various levels of the Wnt/β-catenin signaling [176]. These range from blocking β-catenin-mediated transcription to modulating the catenin destruction complex to attenuating extracellular signaling through the Wnt receptors [176]. Figure 2 illustrates the Wnt/β-catenin pathway and could serve as a model to incorporate multiple targets of interest

Pathway Component	Alteration(s)	References
A. Wnts		
Wnt-1	Increased Expression	[142]
Wnt-2	Increased Expression	[143, 146, 158]
Wnt-5A	Increased Expression	[131, 143, 158]
Wnt-6	Increased Expression	[144]
B. Secreted Wnt Antagonists		
SFRP-1	Decreased Expression	[148, 149]
SFRP-4	Decreased Expression	[153, 154]
WIF-1	Decreased Expression	[155]
DKK-3	Decreased Expression	[150-152]
DKK-1	Decreased Expression	[143, 147]
C. Wnt Receptors/coreceptors		
FZD-3	Increased Expression	[156]
FZD-5	Increased Expression	[159]
D. Pathway Regulators		
DVL-1	Increased Expression	[141]
E. Destruction Complex Components		
β-catenin	Nucleus/cytoplasm accumulation	[129-132, 134, 142, 160-163]
APC	Decreased or Loss of Expression	[132, 134-137, 139, 140, 164, 165]
GSK-3β	Increased activity	[165-170]
Axin-1	Increased Expression	[138]
F. Tcf/Lef Transcription Factor		
Tcf-4	Increased Expression	[142, 171]
F. Genes		
CyclinD1	Upregulation	[123, 124]
c-myc	Upregulation	[125-128, 172-174]

Table 1. Components of the Wnt/β–catenin Pathway Implicated in PCa: Alterations Of Primary PCa Tissues and PCa Cell Lines Compared to Normal Prostate.

to be explored in n-3 PUFA and PCa. Therefore, research focusing on targeting components of the Wnt/β-catenin pathway or other cellular pathways as a means of inhibiting PCa development and progression with a promising prospect, n-3 PUFA seems reasonable.

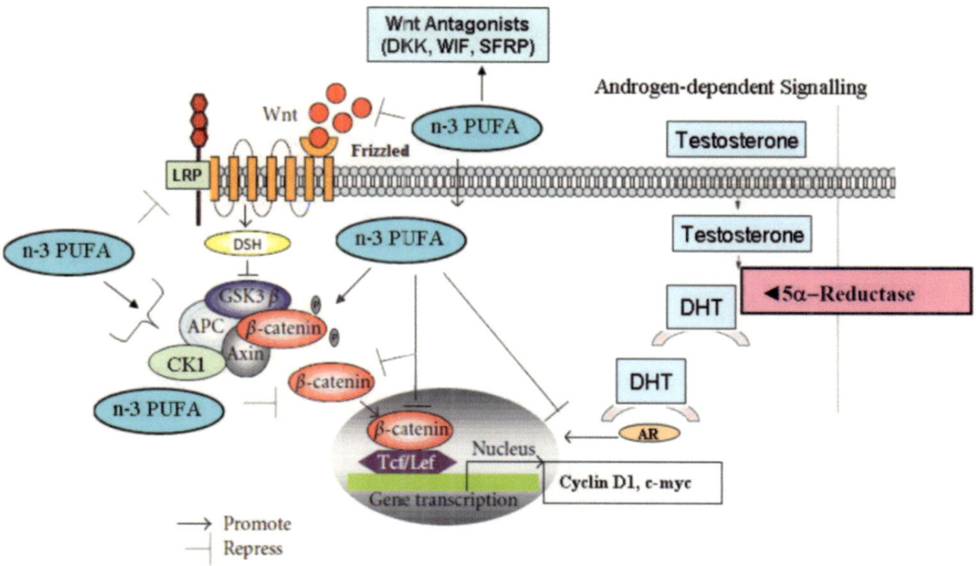

Figure 2. Tobin, GA. 2012. Adapted from articles under the Creative Commons Attribution License Copyright © 2011 Chi-Tai Yeh *et al.* [177] and from Lattouf *et al.* (Reprinted by permission from Macmillan Publishers Ltd: Nature Reviews Urology [178, 179]. Copyright © 1969). A hypothetical diagram of n-3 PUFA and n-3 PUFA/ androgen receptor induced inhibition of Wnt/β-catenin signaling pathway in PCa (directly and indirectly). When the Wnt signal is absent, a multi-complex destruction unit consisting of CK1/2, GSK3β, APC, and Axin forms the target for ubiquitination and degradation, namely a hyper-phosphorylated β-catenin. In the presence of Wnt, Fzd receptors recruit DVL to the plasma membrane to inactivate Axin. Overall, binding of Wnt ligand to a Frizzled/LRP receptor complex leads to stabilization of β-catenin. Subsequent interaction with nuclear Tcf/Lef proteins, increases the expression of genes such as cyclin D1 and c-myc. Additionally, as noted above the effects of n-3 PUFA on AR expression and β-catenin/AR crosstalk should be considered.

5. Choosing a model: *in vitro* and *in vivo* prostate cancer models and their relevance to human disease

Unpredictable pre-clinical models have been credited for the absence of effective treatments in Phase II and III trials [180, 181]. In fact, up to 70% attrition has been reported in Phase II trials; lack of efficacy accounts for about 30% of failures [180]. In the past, drug efficiency was normally assessed during the preclinical phase by xenografts of human prostate cancer cells. The limited number of cells lines that have been utilized in the past mostly include Prostate Cancer (PC)3, Lymph Node Carcinoma of the Prostate (LNCaP) and DU145 (DU-145). *In vivo* (ectopic or orthotopic xenograft models) and *in vitro* studies employing such remain at a disadvantage as these cells lack features found in chemically-induced cancers. The relevance of such models to human prostate cancer is debatable. Nonetheless, these models are valuable in initial research and preclinical assessments. While disease heterogeneity of prostate cancer continues to challenge the development of clinically relevant models, prostate cancer treatment approaches are reliant upon the development and incorporation of relevant preclinical models to confirm appropriate therapeutic targets and biomarkers. Perhaps the most significant milestone and best solution to date in providing researchers with a clinically relevant model, is the evolution of mouse models designed to intentionally inhibit or express a specific gene function by introducing foreign DNA. Over the past 15 years, these Genetically Engineered Mice (GEM) have become valuable tools in studying any combination of oncogenes expressed in specific tissues or conditionally through the tissue-specific removal of tumor suppressors [182-186]. The goal of GEM modeling is to render the best clinical and molecular characteristics of human cancer.

5.1. Prostate cancer cell lines

An exhaustive list of prostate cancer cell lines is freely available via the British Columbia Cancer Research Centre's Prostate Cancer Cell Line Database and Health Canada (website: http://capcellines.ca). This site was created to provide prostate cancer researchers with valuable information regarding cell lines to be utilized in their research. Information is available for 114 cell lines in total with information inclusive of origin, tumor forming ability in mice, doubling time (and other relevant growth factors), karyotype, as well as the status of ribonucleic acid (RNA) and protein for androgen receptor (AR), Prostate Specific Antigen (PSA), prostate-specific human kallikrein (hK2) and creatine kinase (CK). Prostate cancer xenograft models are also included as well as other relevant markers, too numerous to mention. This site conveniently includes cell lines deemed controversial in nature as well as those that have been reported as contaminated. It would seem that currently, and based on a recent search of PubMed, that the most widely used prostate cancer cell lines include PC-3, LNCaP and DU145.

Cell culture experiments provide a practical and financially viable means of investigating PCa research questions by providing preliminary and mechanistic data that justifies further research. Cell culture approaches do have limitations. In general, consider that the conditions represented in cell culture are artificial. The ideal concentrations of factors replicated to characterize the ideal environment are by no means representative of physiologic conditions. Combine this with the fact that cell culture experiments often utilize a single, clonally identical cell line of similar origin in identically constant conditions (i.e: flask culture). This is especially problematic in prostate cancer research due to the complexity of the interconnected paracrine and endocrine communications system between epithelium, stroma and endocrine organs (i.e: the pituitary) [52]. This use of a single cell type removes the ability to detect effects that a distant organ may have on the agent being tested. A co-culture *in vitro* model may prove to be a more reasonable approach. Additionally, the epithelial layer of the prostate is surrounded by a stromal layer containing fibrobasts and blood vessels, among other cell types. In cell culture models, communication of surrounding and distant tissues is not represented. In this manner, the effect of a therapeutic to surrounding and distant normal tissue is speculative. Furthermore, cell culture represents only one end of the carcinogenic spectrum as it is often conducted on transformed cells. Aside from the ability of such cells to develop various escape / survival mechanisms, this concept negates long-term exposure. Throughout a person's lifespan, exposure to agents may have varying effects prior to, during or after the transformation process to neoplastic tissue.

Choosing an appropriate cell line is largely dependent on the type of study being conducted. For example, based on the model of study represented in this chapter, the LNCaP line would be an appropriate choice to study n-3 PUFA and β-catenin as these cells are androgen sensitive, prostate-specific antigen (PSA) positive, and maintain malignant properties, even though they have low metastatic potential [187]. Furthermore, this cell line endogenously expresses β-catenin [188] and thus represents an ideal tool to elucidate the interactions of n-3PUFA/ β-catenin in PCa.

5.2. Animal models of prostate cancer

Although animal experiments are both costly and time-consuming, they are vital in the transition to Phase 1 clinical investigations. As PCa occurs naturally both in dogs and in certain strains of rats, these species represent options for animal modeling [189]. Although the dog most closely resembles human PCa characteristics [190], their use is limited and unrealistic for a variety of reasons including androgen independent tumor growth, long latency period, prohibitive costs, long gestation period, and difficulty of genetic manipulation [189]. Some strains of rats, although well characterized and capable of developing a wide range of PCa phenotypes [191], present different issues including scarcity of tumors, variability in phenotypes, long latency periods, and inability to represent metastatic disease [189]. Utilization of genetically engineered rat models for PCa will likely increase as the development of knockout rats advance [192]. In the meantime, despite anatomical differences between the murine and human prostate gland [189] and other weaknesses, mouse models have emerged as the choice for investigating the stepwise progression of PCa. Compared to earlier *in vivo* prostate cancer experiments, where rodent models were exposed to carcinogens or hormones, recent technological advances (i.e.: tissue specific promoters and conditional gene deletions) have provided multiple models for researchers to investigate genetic defects [189]. Each model has its strengths and weaknesses. For example, the transgenic mouse models of PCa that express the Simian Virus 40 (SV40) early region have a highly prognostic gene signature for cancer, however mouse prostate expressing the large probasin promoter directed by SV40-large T-antigen (LPB–Tag) is not consistent in its ability to mimic the full spectrum of PCa as it only progresses to mPIN and rarely results in progression to adenocarcinoma formation [193]. Likely the most popular mouse model, TRAMP is based on such technology and develops cancer as a result of SV40 T antigen expression resulting in many genetic defects including p53 and Rb (tumor suppressor genes) loss [54]. Because cancer is not the result of a single genetic mutation, this multi-hit effect is desirable. However, consider that certain aspects of this model may not be relevant to human disease, including viral transformation. Additionally this model does not follow the normal human prostate cancer course as it is very aggressive and progresses to advanced cancer very rapidly. Consider that it may take up to 20 years for PIN to develop, 10 or more years to advance from PIN to HGPIN and then to an early form of latent cancer, while a clinical diagnosis of PCa may occur anywhere from three to 15 years [11].

It would be reiterative to include a thorough review of mouse models utilized in prostate cancer research following the publication of such excellent work by both Valkenburg *et al.* [189] and Hensley *et al* [194]. In this section we will summarize commonly utilized transgenic mouse models; later we will discuss the reliability of mouse models to study disease effects, specifically n-3 PUFA. Table 2 summarizes the characteristics of several commonly used transgeneic mouse models.

Model	Genetic Manipulation	Characteristics	Reference
Apt121/Rbf	Fragment of SV40 Transgene to dominantly inactivate Rb	PIN at age 4 weeks and micro-invasive carcinoma at age 8 months.	[195]
PTEN (Phosphatase and tensin homologue deleted on chromosome 10)	Germline Knockout	Invasive carcinoma age 30 weeks; metastasis to lymph node and lung.	[196]
	Conditional Knockout	High grade PIN with advancement to invasive metastasis.	[194]
Hi-Myc (high Myc transgene expression)	Myc transgene Expression	PIN at age 2 weeks and invasive carcinoma at age 6-12 months with lymphovascular invasion.	[197]
LADY (LPB promoter driving the large-T antigen)	SV40 Trangene Expression	Neoplasis by age 10 weeks. Undifferentiated adenocarcinoma and invasive neuroendocrine tumors from age 5 - 9 months and metastasis to lymph node, liver and lung.	[194, 198]
Nkx3.1/Pten	Compound Deletion (Pten(+/-) Nkx3.1 (-/-))	High-grade PIN at age 6 months; invasion by age 2 months and metastasis to lymph node.	[194, 199]
TRAMP (TRansgenic Adenocarcinoma of the Mouse Prostate)	SV40 Transgene Expression	Progressive PIN at age 6 weeks. Invasive adenocarcinoma and lymph node, liver, lung and skeletal metastasis by age 6 months. Large, poorly-differentiated neuroendocrine tumors by age 16 weeks.	[182, 194]

Table 2. Common Transgenic Murine Models of Prostate Cancer

In choosing a mouse model, one must consider whether the study is aimed at treatment or prevention and the ability of a model to produce prostate phenotypes or other key features relevant to human disease. In dietary intervention studies, such as n-3 PUFA, it is important to consider whether or not models are resistant to the tumor suppressive effects of such treatments. For example, Smolinski (2011) indicates that the TRAMP model may not be ideal for studying the effects of bioactive lipids on prostate carcinogenesis. In fact, in the context of a high fat diet, including fish oil and corn oil as the primary source of lipids, the TRAMP model is reported to be resistant to the tumor suppressive effects of n-3 PUFA [200]. Thus, choosing an inappropriate mouse model may negate significant findings and lead to the conclusion that certain dietary interventions have no effect on a disease when in fact they may be responsible for disease risk or progression. When engaging in novel or controversial research such as discussed in this chapter, a rational tactic before confirming a mouse model may include the completion of a pilot study to ensure that mice are not resistant to the protective effects of n-3 PUFA and to confirm an appropriate cohort size. The goal should be to identify at least a statistically significant 15% difference in mean tumor size within an 80% confidence interval. Based on the proposed research model discussed in this chapter, the transgenic 12T-7s/Catnb $^{lox(ex3)}$/ PB*Cre4* (designated as LPB–Tag/DA β-catenin) mouse would likely be ideal and was developed recently as a model to study the expression of stabilized β-catenin in PCa and represents the full spectrum of PCa progression to invasive adenocarcinoma [169]. Additionally, this model represents AR activity and offers a reasonable study period, with an end-point of 20–22 weeks [169].

6. n-3 PUFA specific factors that make a difference: Source, purity and EPA: DHA ratio

If the general question on n-3 PUFA and PCa surrounds whether or not there is an increase or decrease in PCa cancer risk, then consideration of confounding factors for n-3 PUFA intake, including source, purity and ratio, should be addressed primarily. The foremost sources of essential fatty acids for the majority of studies are fish derived. Consider that both animal protein [201] and accumulated environmental pollutants [202] both have been linked to prostate cancer. In this regard, it is fitting that the development of n-3 PUFA as a pharmaceutical is already underway for other indications as the approval process normally removes the risk of contamination by methyl mercury, arsenic or other pollutants that are often seen in ocean or land based food sources protein [201]. Currently, there are three commercially significant formulations of pharmaceutical grade n-3 PUFAs and numerous over the counter supplements available for potential use in PCa. The noted differences between all of these formulas are purity, source and/or the ratio of EPA to DHA. Lovasa has received United States Food and Drug Administration (USFDA) approval to lower very high triglyceride levels (hypertriglyceridemia) [203]. In other major markets outside the United States, including Europe, Lovasa is known as Omacor, and can be prescribed to patients as a montherapy for hypertriglyceridemia, in combination therapy with a statin for mixed dyslipidemia, or as a secondary preventative therapeutic following myocardial infarction [204]. The expiration of GlaxoSmithKline's patent for Lovasa in September [2012] will likely increase availability of generic replacements. Such equally effective, but lower priced versions could supply markets for already proven indications as well as for subsequently approved disease indications, including for example, PCa. AMR-101, also marketed as Vascepa, received USFDA approval in July, 2012 [205]. Similar to Lovasa, this approval was based on effective treatment of hypertriglyceridemia but with the added ability to impact people with high triglycerides; the latter indication has been filed and is under review pending outcomes in clinical trials [206]. Epanova, another promising n-PUFA formula, is undergoing clinical trials for similar indications as previously mentioned for Lovasa, and USFDA approval is forthcoming [207]. Other dietary supplements, containing various amounts and ratios of n-3 PUFA which are sold over the counter in the United States and Canada would likely be based on values issued by the Institute of Medicine and National Academies as described below. Such unregulated formulary preparations do not undergo clinical trials. Studies relating to n-3 PUFA pharmaceutical preparations have focused on treating cardiovascular disease with no clinical consideration for PCa. Albeit, men diagnosed with PCa have accepted the use of such nutraceuticals and thus there is a role in ensuring that this approach constitutes safe and effective therapies. Although studies around the prescription formulas have demonstrated a very good safety and tolerability profile, the focus has been in treating cardiovascular disease and thus there has been no concern over potential adverse effects for other diseases.

Another proposed explanation for inconsistent findings in the role of n-3 PUFA in prostate cancer relates to absolute intake versus ratio of n-3 to n-6 PUFA. The latter may be more relevant for prostate cancer risk considering that the recommended dietary ratio of n-6/n-3 PUFA for health benefits are variable and range from 1:1-4:1, yet dietary intake in such studies, relative to the Western diet could contain 10 or more times the amount of n-6 compared to n-3 PUFA [208]. Also consider that in gathering and thoroughly reviewing all information toward this chapter, we were unable to find an *official* recommended daily allowance for n-3 PUFA for adults or children. In Canada and the United States, the general public and health professionals (including healthcare policy makers and public health officials) use a set of five nutrient based reference values issued by the Institute of Medicine and National Academies for a wide variety of food and dietary applications [209]. These dietary reference intakes (DRI), are inclusive of components including: estimated average requirements (EAR), recommended daily allowance (RDA), adequate intake (AI), tolerable upper intake level (UL) and an acceptable macronutrient distribution range (AMDR). Considered to be the official standard for federal agencies, these values are used to issue dietary guidance or policy directives for the health and well-being of individuals. In the absence of a DRI specific to EPA and DHA, the National Academies have recommended an AMDR of 10% for another n-3 PUFA, namely alpha-linolenic acid (ALA) to be consumed as EPA and/or DHA equating to a much lower value (about 100 mg/day) than currently recommended by many groups worldwide. For example, a number of nutritionist and physicians recommend as much as 450 milligrams of n-3 PUFA in either DHA or EPA form per day to promote a healthy diet [79, 210], a fact alone which warrants further studies to determine DRI, specifically UL. More importantly, if the effects of n-3 PUFA represent different disease specifications, then it is crucial to establish DRIs for DHA and EPA individually, and in combination. Considering the contradictory evidence that excessive DHA may be a possible cause for some types of aggressive prostate cancer, the expansion of this field of research may want to revisit the incorporation of such basic factors as the ratio of EPA to DHA as a beginning to rationalize some existing data. Altogether, in proceeding with such studies, it would be important to consider all forms of n-3 PUFA, as well as a variety of ratios and then proper incorporation of such into cell-culture media or animal models; all while considering relevant study models to reflect relevance to human disease. However, while supplementation in cell based and animal studies may produce positive results, such may not be relevant to actual human therapies.

The existing results for n-3 PUFA and prostate are contradictory, especially in the absence of consistent epidemiological data. Therefore, incorporation of n-3 PUFA related factors such as source, purity and EPA/ DHA ratios are crucial while employing *in vitro* and *in vivo* models representative of the entire PCa cascade.

7. Other considerations

7.1. Markers of tumor growth

Epidemiologic studies have shown that lower serum insulin-like growth factor (IGF)-1 levels and increased IGF binding protein-3 (IGFBP-3) levels are associated with decreased PCa risk [211]. Unlike humans, rodents do not have a PSA counterpart for monitoring prostate cancer initiation and progression, however prostatic secretory protein (PSP)-94 has been established as a serum tumor marker [212]. However, measurement of mouse serum for IGF-I, IGFBP-3 and PSP-94 can be assayed using enzyme-linked immunosorbent assay (ELISA) using mouse-specific antibodies and recombinant mouse standards (where applicable) and by methods previously described [213]. Therefore, such biomarkers could be used as indicators in both human and mouse studies in conjunction with other parameters and may be correlated with fatty acid analysis.

7.2. Fatty acid analysis: Serum blood levels of EPA and DHA

Selection of fatty acid concentration and methods of introducing fatty acids to cell cultures in such experiments are documented [214, 215]. Like most *in vitro* studies, data obtained may provide indicators of how to progress to the next levels of research. More relevant to human disease outcome, the fatty acid composition of serum (or plasma) phospholipid is an established valid biochemical marker for assessing the physiological status of various fatty acids including predictive correlations with the dietary intakes omega-3 PUFA, including EPA and DHA. [216, 217]. Serum fatty acid analysis by gas chromatography seems to be the standard for such experiments [218, 219] for both humans and animals.

8. Conclusions

As such, the features of prostate cancer, including long latency, high prevalence, significant mortality and morbidity, combined with the already accepted use of CAM, in particular n-3

PUFA presents an excellent opportunity for nutritional intervention. However, until we unravel this controversial enigma of how n-3 PUFA affects prostate cancer, much remains to be explored and examined. More research is required to support or refute the value of n-3 PUFA in prostate cancer. And thus the search continues as to how one should proceed with fatty acid intake, including supplementation, as a prophylactic or therapeutic. Currently there is not enough evidence to discount the noted beneficial effects of n-3 PUFA intake to prevent heart disease as they seem to outweigh any harm related to prostate cancer risk [40]. However, further research is required to clarify the precise mechanisms of n-3 PUFA and its role in human disease, in particular cancer. Without such, we cannot develop novel strategies for n-3 PUFA to target molecular pathways (inflammatory or other involved processes) in the prevention, development or treatment of prostate cancer or other cancers. Expansion of research in this area is warranted.

Acknowledgements

Publication costs associated with this chapter were supported by the Department of Biomedical Sciences, University of Prince Edward Island, Canada. We are grateful for their continued support.

Author details

Gailene Tobin[1], Robert Hurta[2] and Marianna Kulka[1,3]

*Address all correspondence to: Marianna.Kulka@nrc-cnrc.gc.ca

1 Department of Biomedical Sciences, University of Prince Edward Island, Charlottetown, PE, Canada

2 Department of Biology, University of Prince Edward Island, Charlottetown, PE, Canada

3 Security and Disruptive Technologies / Technologies de sécurité et de rupture, National Institute of Nanotechnology, National Research Council Canada / Conseil national de recherches, Edmonton, AB, Canada

References

[1] Wasserman NF. Benign prostatic hyperplasia: a review and ultrasound classification. Radiol Clin North Am. 2006 Sept;44(5):689-710. PubMed PMID: 17030221.

[2] Meyers RP. Structure of the Adult Prostate From a Clinician's Standpoint. Clinical Anatomy. 2000 June;13 214-15.

[3] Cohen RJ, Shannon BA, Phillips M, Moorin RE, Wheeler TM, Garrett KL. Central zone carcinoma of the prostate gland: a distinct tumor type with poor prognostic features. The Journal of Urology. 2008 May;179(5):1762-7; Discussion 7. PubMed PMID: 18343454.

[4] Anderson RU, Wise D, Sawyer T, Chan CA. Sexual dysfunction in men with chronic prostatitis/chronic pelvic pain syndrome: improvement after trigger point release and paradoxical relaxation training. The Journal of Urology. 2006 Oct;176(4 Pt 1): 1534-8; discussion 8-9. PubMed PMID: 16952676.

[5] Verhamme KM, Dieleman JP, Bleumink GS, van der Lei J, Sturkenboom MC, Artibani W, *et al*. Incidence and prevalence of lower urinary tract symptoms suggestive of benign prostatic hyperplasia in primary care--the Triumph project. European Urology. 2002 Oct;42(4):323-8. PubMed PMID: 12361895.

[6] Andriole GL, Crawford ED, Grubb RL, 3rd, Buys SS, Chia D, Church TR, *et al*. Mortality results from a randomized prostate-cancer screening trial. N Engl J Med. 2009 Mar 26;360(13):1310-9. PubMed PMID: 19297565.

[7] Boyle P, Brawley OW. Prostate cancer: current evidence weighs against population screening. CA Cancer J Clin. 2009 Jul-Aug;59(4):220-4. PubMed PMID: 19564244.

[8] Ross PL, Carroll, P. R., Small, E. J., *et al*. In Ko, A. H., Dollinger, M., & Rosenbaum, E. . Everyone's Guide to Cancer Therapy: How Cancer is Diagnosed, Treated and Managed Day to Day. (5th Edition). Prostate. 2008. pp. 789-806. .

[9] Gleason DF. Histologic grade, clinical stage, and patient age in prostate cancer. NCI Monogr. 1988 (7):15-8. PubMed PMID: 3173500.

[10] Gleason DF. Histologic grading of prostate cancer: a perspective. Hum Pathol. 1992 Mar;23(3):273-9. PubMed PMID: 1555838.

[11] Bostwick DG. Prostatic intraepithelial neoplasia (PIN): current concepts. J Cell Biochem Suppl. 1992;16H:10-9. PubMed PMID: 1289664.

[12] Kelloff GJ, Lieberman R, Steele VE, Boone CW, Lubet RA, Kopelovitch L, *et al*. Chemoprevention of prostate cancer: concepts and strategies. European Urology. 1999;35(5-6):342-50. PubMed PMID: 10325487.

[13] DeVita VH, S; Rosenberg, SA. Principles and Practise of Oncology. 2005 (7th Edition): 1419-69.

[14] Kumar NB, Cantor A, Allen K, Riccardi D, Besterman-Dahan K, Seigne J, *et al*. The specific role of isoflavones in reducing prostate cancer risk. Prostate. 2004 May 1;59(2):141-7. PubMed PMID: 15042614.

[15] Canadian Cancer Society. Canadian Cancer Encyclopedia. 2012. Available at: http://info.cancer.ca/cce-ecc/.

[16] Hsing AW, Chokkalingam AP. Prostate cancer epidemiology. Front Biosci. 2006;11:1388-413. PubMed PMID: 16368524.

[17] Narizhneva NV, Tararova ND, Ryabokon P, Shyshynova I, Prokvolit A, Komarov PG, *et al*. Small molecule screening reveals a transcription-independent pro-survival function of androgen receptor in castration-resistant prostate cancer. Cell Cycle. 2009 Dec 15;8(24):4155-67. PubMed PMID: 19946220.

[18] Canadian Cancer Society. Prostate Cancer Statistics. 2011.

[19] Ferlay J, Shin HR, Bray F, Forman D, Mathers C, Parkin DM. Estimates of worldwide burden of cancer in 2008: GLOBOCAN 2008. Int J Cancer. 2010 Dec 15;127(12): 2893-917. PubMed PMID: 21351269.

[20] Jemal A, Siegel R, Xu J, Ward E. Cancer statistics, 2010. CA Cancer J Clin. 2010 Sep-Oct;60(5):277-300. PubMed PMID: 20610543.

[21] Bubendorf L, Schopfer A, Wagner U, Sauter G, Moch H, Willi N, *et al*. Metastatic patterns of prostate cancer: an autopsy study of 1,589 patients. Hum Pathol. 2000 May; 31(5):578-83. PubMed PMID: 10836297.

[22] Lee RJ, Saylor PJ, Smith MR. Treatment and prevention of bone complications from prostate cancer. Bone. 2011 Jan;48(1):88-95. PubMed PMID: 20621630.

[23] Bray F, Moller B. Predicting the future burden of cancer. Nat Rev Cancer. 2006 Jan; 6(1):63-74. PubMed PMID: 16372017.

[24] Ferrari M. Cancer nanotechnology: opportunities and challenges. Nat Rev Cancer. 2005 Mar;5(3):161-71. PubMed PMID: 15738981.

[25] Scheinberg DA, Villa CH, Escorcia FE, McDevitt MR. Conscripts of the infinite armada: systemic cancer therapy using nanomaterials. Nat Rev Clin Oncol. 2010 May;7(5): 266-76. PubMed PMID: 20351700.

[26] Shewach DS, Kuchta RD. Introduction to cancer chemotherapeutics. Chem Rev. 2009 Jul;109(7):2859-61. PubMed PMID: 19583428.

[27] Chan JM, Gann PH, Giovannucci EL. Role of diet in prostate cancer development and progression. J Clin Oncol. 2005 Nov 10;23(32):8152-60. PubMed PMID: 16278466.

[28] Lee MM, Chang JS, Jacobs B, Wrensch MR. Complementary and alternative medicine use among men with prostate cancer in 4 ethnic populations. Am J Public Health. 2002 Oct;92(10):1606-9. PubMed PMID: 12356606.

[29] Nickel JS, D; Roehrborn,CG and Moyad, M. Nutraceuticals in Prostate Disease: The Urologist's Role. 2008. Summer (10(3):):192-206.

[30] Armstrong B, Doll R. Environmental factors and cancer incidence and mortality in different countries, with special reference to dietary practices. Int J Cancer. 1975 Apr 15;15(4):617-31. PubMed PMID: 1140864.

[31] Mononen N, Schleutker J. Polymorphisms in genes involved in androgen pathways as risk factors for prostate cancer. The Journal of Urology. 2009 Apr;181(4):1541-9. PubMed PMID: 19230916.

[32] Odedina FT, Akinremi TO, Chinegwundoh F, Roberts R, Yu D, Reams RR, *et al*. Prostate cancer disparities in Black men of African descent: a comparative literature review of prostate cancer burden among Black men in the United States, Caribbean, United Kingdom, and West Africa. Infectious Agents and Cancer. 2009;4 Suppl 1:S2. PubMed PMID: 19208207.

[33] Patel AR, Klein EA. Risk factors for prostate cancer. Nature Clinical Practice Urology. 2009 Feb;6(2):87-95. PubMed PMID: 19198622.

[34] Cheung E, Wadhera P, Dorff T, Pinski J. Diet and prostate cancer risk reduction. Expert Rev Anticancer Ther. 2008 Jan;8(1):43-50. PubMed PMID: 18095882.

[35] Lippman SM, Hong WK. Cancer prevention science and practice. Cancer Res. 2002 Sep 15;62(18):5119-25. PubMed PMID: 12234971.

[36] William WN, Jr., Heymach JV, Kim ES, Lippman SM. Molecular targets for cancer chemoprevention. Nat Rev Drug Discov. 2009 Mar;8(3):213-25. PubMed PMID: 19247304.

[37] Huggins C, Hodges CV. Studies on prostatic cancer. I. The effect of castration, of estrogen and androgen injection on serum phosphatases in metastatic carcinoma of the prostate. CA Cancer J Clin. 1972 Jul-Aug;22(4):232-40. PubMed PMID: 4625049.

[38] Redman MW, Tangen CM, Goodman PJ, Lucia MS, Coltman CA, Jr., Thompson IM. Finasteride does not increase the risk of high-grade prostate cancer: a bias-adjusted modeling approach. Cancer Prev Res (Phila). 2008 Aug;1(3):174-81. PubMed PMID: 19138953.

[39] FDA Drug Safety Communication: 5-alpha reductase inhibitors (5-ARIs) may increase the risk of a more serious form of prostate cancer. 2011. Available at: http://www.fda.gov/Drugs/DrugSafety/ucm258314.htm#sa.

[40] Brasky TM, Till C, White E, Neuhouser ML, Song X, Goodman P, *et al*. Serum phospholipid fatty acids and prostate cancer risk: results from the prostate cancer prevention trial. Am J Epidemiol. 2011 Jun 15;173(12):1429-39. PubMed PMID: 21518693.

[41] Collette L, Studer UE, Schroder FH, Denis LJ, Sylvester RJ. Why phase III trials of maximal androgen blockade versus castration in M1 prostate cancer rarely show statistically significant differences. Prostate. 2001 Jun 15;48(1):29-39. PubMed PMID: 11391684.

[42] Labrie F, Dupont A, Belanger A, St-Arnaud R, Giguere M, Lacourciere Y, *et al*. Treatment of prostate cancer with gonadotropin-releasing hormone agonists. Endocr Rev. 1986 Feb;7(1):67-74. PubMed PMID: 3514203.

[43] Visakorpi T, Hyytinen E, Koivisto P, Tanner M, Keinanen R, Palmberg C, *et al*. *In vivo* amplification of the androgen receptor gene and progression of human prostate cancer. Nat Genet. 1995 Apr;9(4):401-6. PubMed PMID: 7795646.

[44] Buchanan G, Greenberg NM, Scher HI, Harris JM, Marshall VR, Tilley WD. Collocation of androgen receptor gene mutations in prostate cancer. Clin Cancer Res. 2001 May;7(5):1273-81. PubMed PMID: 11350894.

[45] Culig Z, Hobisch A, Cronauer MV, Radmayr C, Trapman J, Hittmair A, *et al*. Androgen receptor activation in prostatic tumor cell lines by insulin-like growth factor-I, keratinocyte growth factor, and epidermal growth factor. Cancer Res. 1994 Oct 15;54(20):5474-8. PubMed PMID: 7522959.

[46] Bruckheimer EM, Brisbay S, Johnson DJ, Gingrich JR, Greenberg N, McDonnell TJ. Bcl-2 accelerates multistep prostate carcinogenesis *in vivo*. Oncogene. 2000 Nov 2;19(46):5251-8. PubMed PMID: 11077442.

[47] Trump DL, Havlin KH, Messing EM, Cummings KB, Lange PH, Jordan VC. High-dose ketoconazole in advanced hormone-refractory prostate cancer: endocrinologic and clinical effects. J Clin Oncol. 1989 Aug;7(8):1093-8. PubMed PMID: 2474059.

[48] Hanahan D, Weinberg RA. Hallmarks of cancer: the next generation. Cell. 2011. Mar 4;144(5):646-74. PubMed PMID: 21376230.

[49] de Muga S, Hernandez S, Agell L, Salido M, Juanpere N, Lorenzo M, *et al*. Molecular alterations of EGFR and PTEN in prostate cancer: association with high-grade and advanced-stage carcinomas. Mod Pathol. 2010 May;23(5):703-12. PubMed PMID: 20208477.

[50] Kawada M, Inoue H, Masuda T, Ikeda D. Insulin-like growth factor I secreted from prostate stromal cells mediates tumor-stromal cell interactions of prostate cancer. Cancer Res. 2006 Apr 15;66(8):4419-25. PubMed PMID: 16618768.

[51] Mendoza N, Phillips GL, Silva J, Schwall R, Wickramasinghe D. Inhibition of ligand-mediated HER2 activation in androgen-independent prostate cancer. Cancer Res. 2002 Oct 1;62(19):5485-8. PubMed PMID: 12359757.

[52] Rakoff-Nahoum S. Why cancer and inflammation? The Yale Journal of Biology and Medicine. 2006 Dec;79(3-4):123-30. PubMed PMID: 17940622. Pubmed Central PMCID: 1994795.

[53] Chang WY, Birch L, Woodham C, Gold LI, Prins GS. Neonatal estrogen exposure alters the transforming growth factor-beta signaling system in the developing rat prostate and blocks the transient p21(cip1/waf1) expression associated with epithelial differentiation. Endocrinology. 1999 Jun;140(6):2801-13. PubMed PMID: 10342871.

[54] Wiman KG. The retinoblastoma gene: role in cell cycle control and cell differentiation. Faseb J. 1993 Jul;7(10):841-5. PubMed PMID: 8393817.

[55] Brooks JD, Bova GS, Isaacs WB. Allelic loss of the retinoblastoma gene in primary human prostatic adenocarcinomas. Prostate. 1995 Jan;26(1):35-9. PubMed PMID: 7845865.

[56] Zhang W, Kapusta LR, Slingerland JM, Klotz LH. Telomerase activity in prostate cancer, prostatic intraepithelial neoplasia, and benign prostatic epithelium. Cancer Res. 1998 Feb 15;58(4):619-21. PubMed PMID: 9485010.

[57] Parangi S, O'Reilly M, Christofori G, Holmgren L, Grosfeld J, Folkman J, *et al*. Antiangiogenic therapy of transgenic mice impairs de novo tumor growth. Proc Natl Acad Sci U S A. 1996 Mar 5;93(5):2002-7. PubMed PMID: 8700875.

[58] Walsh K, Sriprasad S, Hopster D, Codd J, Mulvin D. Distribution of vascular endothelial growth factor (VEGF) in prostate disease. Prostate Cancer Prostatic Dis. 2002;5(2):119-22. PubMed PMID: 12497000.

[59] Wheelock MJ, Shintani Y, Maeda M, Fukumoto Y, Johnson KR. Cadherin switching. J Cell Sci. 2008 Mar 15;121(Pt 6):727-35. PubMed PMID: 18322269.

[60] Takeichi M. Morphogenetic roles of classic cadherins. Curr Opin Cell Biol. 1995 Oct; 7(5):619-27. PubMed PMID: 8573335.

[61] Tomita K, van Bokhoven A, van Leenders GJ, Ruijter ET, Jansen CF, Bussemakers MJ, *et al*. Cadherin switching in human prostate cancer progression. Cancer Res. 2000 Jul 1;60(13):3650-4. PubMed PMID: 10910081.

[62] Trudel D, Fradet Y, Meyer F, Harel F, Tetu B. Significance of MMP-2 expression in prostate cancer: an immunohistochemical study. Cancer Res. 2003 Dec 1;63(23): 8511-5. PubMed PMID: 14679018.

[63] Balkwill F, Mantovani A. Inflammation and cancer: back to Virchow? Lancet. 2001 Feb 17;357(9255):539-45. PubMed PMID: 11229684.

[64] Coussens LM, Werb Z. Inflammation and cancer. Nature. 2002 Dec 19-26;420(6917): 860-7. PubMed PMID: 12490959.

[65] De Marzo AM, Platz EA, Sutcliffe S, Xu J, Gronberg H, Drake CG, *et al*. Inflammation in prostate carcinogenesis. Nat Rev Cancer. 2007 Apr;7(4):256-69. PubMed PMID: 17384581.

[66] Sfanos KS, De Marzo AM. Prostate cancer and inflammation: the evidence. Histopathology. 2012 Jan;60(1):199-215. PubMed PMID: 22212087.

[67] Condeelis J, Pollard JW. Macrophages: obligate partners for tumor cell migration, invasion, and metastasis. Cell. 2006 Jan 27;124(2):263-6. PubMed PMID: 16439202.

[68] Egeblad M, Littlepage LE, Werb Z. The fibroblastic coconspirator in cancer progression. Cold Spring Harb Symp Quant Biol. 2005;70:383-8. PubMed PMID: 16869775.

[69] Egeblad M, Werb Z. New functions for the matrix metalloproteinases in cancer progression. Nat Rev Cancer. 2002 Mar;2(3):161-74. PubMed PMID: 11990853.

[70] Karin M. NF-kappaB as a critical link between inflammation and cancer. Cold Spring Harb Perspect Biol. 2009 Nov;1(5):141. PubMed PMID: 20066113.

[71] Wang D, Dubois RN. Prostaglandins and cancer. Gut. 2006 Jan;55(1):115-22. PubMed PMID: 16118353.

[72] Zlotnik A. Chemokines and cancer. Int J Cancer. 2006 Nov 1;119(9):2026-9. PubMed PMID: 16671092.

[73] Hadley CW, Clinton SK, Schwartz SJ. The consumption of processed tomato products enhances plasma lycopene concentrations in association with a reduced lipoprotein sensitivity to oxidative damage. J Nutr. 2003 Mar;133(3):727-32. PubMed PMID: 12612144.

[74] Hsu A, Bray TM, Ho E. Anti-inflammatory activity of soy and tea in prostate cancer prevention. Exp Biol Med (Maywood). Jun;235(6):659-67. PubMed PMID: 20511670.

[75] Hsu A, Bruno RS, Lohr CV, Taylor AW, Dashwood RH, Bray TM, *et al.* Dietary soy and tea mitigate chronic inflammation and prostate cancer via NFkappaB pathway in the Noble rat model. J Nutr Biochem. May;22(5):502-10. PubMed PMID: 20801632.

[76] Pannellini T, Iezzi M, Liberatore M, Sabatini F, Iacobelli S, Rossi C, *et al.* A dietary tomato supplement prevents prostate cancer in TRAMP mice. Cancer Prev Res (Phila). Oct;3(10):1284-91. PubMed PMID: 20716635.

[77] Vardi A, Bosviel R, Rabiau N, Adjakly M, Satih S, Dechelotte P, *et al.* Soy phytoestrogens modify DNA methylation of GSTP1, RASSF1A, EPH2 and BRCA1 promoter in prostate cancer cells. *In Vivo*. Jul-Aug;24(4):393-400. PubMed PMID: 20668305.

[78] Astorg P. Dietary N-6 and N-3 polyunsaturated fatty acids and prostate cancer risk: a review of epidemiological and experimental evidence. Cancer Causes Control. 2004 May;15(4):367-86. PubMed PMID: 15141138.

[79] Astorg P, Arnault N, Czernichow S, Noisette N, Galan P, Hercberg S. Dietary intakes and food sources of n-6 and n-3 PUFA in French adult men and women. Lipids. 2004 Jun;39(6):527-35. PubMed PMID: 15554151.

[80] Chung BH, Mitchell SH, Zhang JS, Young CY. Effects of docosahexaenoic acid and eicosapentaenoic acid on androgen-mediated cell growth and gene expression in LNCaP prostate cancer cells. Carcinogenesis. 2001 Aug;22(8):1201-6. PubMed PMID: 11470750.

[81] Karmali RA, Reichel P, Cohen LA, Terano T, Hirai A, Tamura Y, *et al*. The effects of dietary omega-3 fatty acids on the DU-145 transplantable human prostatic tumor. Anticancer Res. 1987 Nov-Dec;7(6):1173-9. PubMed PMID: 2831791.

[82] Narayanan NK, Narayanan BA, Reddy BS. A combination of docosahexaenoic acid and celecoxib prevents prostate cancer cell growth *in vitro* and is associated with modulation of nuclear factor-kappaB, and steroid hormone receptors. Int J Oncol. 2005 Mar;26(3):785-92. PubMed PMID: 15703837.

[83] Pandalai PK, Pilat MJ, Yamazaki K, Naik H, Pienta KJ. The effects of omega-3 and omega-6 fatty acids on *in vitro* prostate cancer growth. Anticancer Res. 1996 Mar-Apr;16(2):815-20. PubMed PMID: 8687134.

[84] Rose DP, Cohen LA. Effects of dietary menhaden oil and retinyl acetate on the growth of DU 145 human prostatic adenocarcinoma cells transplanted into athymic nude mice. Carcinogenesis. 1988 Apr;9(4):603-5. PubMed PMID: 3356068.

[85] Rose DP, Connolly JM. Effects of fatty acids and eicosanoid synthesis inhibitors on the growth of two human prostate cancer cell lines. Prostate. 1991;18(3):243-54. PubMed PMID: 2020620.

[86] Chavarro JE, Stampfer MJ, Li H, Campos H, Kurth T, Ma J. A prospective study of polyunsaturated fatty acid levels in blood and prostate cancer risk. Cancer Epidemiol Biomarkers Prev. 2007 Jul;16(7):1364-70. PubMed PMID: 17585059.

[87] Ghadirian P, Lacroix A, Maisonneuve P, Perret C, Drouin G, Perrault JP, *et al*. Nutritional factors and prostate cancer: a case-control study of French Canadians in Montreal, Canada. Cancer Causes Control. 1996 Jul;7(4):428-36. PubMed PMID: 8813431.

[88] Godley PA, Campbell MK, Miller C, Gallagher P, Martinson FE, Mohler JL, *et al*. Correlation between biomarkers of omega-3 fatty acid consumption and questionnaire data in African American and Caucasian United States males with and without prostatic carcinoma. Cancer Epidemiol Biomarkers Prev. 1996 Feb;5(2):115-9. PubMed PMID: 8850272.

[89] Kristal AR, Arnold KB, Neuhouser ML, Goodman P, Platz EA, Albanes D, *et al*. Diet, supplement use, and prostate cancer risk: results from the prostate cancer prevention trial. Am J Epidemiol. 2010 Sep 1;172(5):566-77. PubMed PMID: 20693267.

[90] Park SY, Wilkens LR, Henning SM, Le Marchand L, Gao K, Goodman MT, *et al*. Circulating fatty acids and prostate cancer risk in a nested case-control study: the Multiethnic Cohort. Cancer Causes Control. 2009 Mar;20(2):211-23. PubMed PMID: 18821021.

[91] Rohan TE, Howe GR, Burch JD, Jain M. Dietary factors and risk of prostate cancer: a case-control study in Ontario, Canada. Cancer Causes Control. 1995 Mar;6(2):145-54. PubMed PMID: 7749054.

[92] Terry PD, Rohan TE, Wolk A. Intakes of fish and marine fatty acids and the risks of cancers of the breast and prostate and of other hormone-related cancers: a review of

the epidemiologic evidence. Am J Clin Nutr. 2003 Mar;77(3):532-43. PubMed PMID: 12600840.

[93] Berquin IM, Min Y, Wu R, Wu J, Perry D, Cline JM, *et al*. Modulation of prostate cancer genetic risk by omega-3 and omega-6 fatty acids. The Journal of Clinical Investigation. 2007 Jul;117(7):1866-75. PubMed PMID: 17607361.

[94] Hu Y, Sun H, Owens RT, Gu Z, Wu J, Chen YQ, *et al*. Syndecan-1-dependent suppression of PDK1/Akt/bad signaling by docosahexaenoic acid induces apoptosis in prostate cancer. Neoplasia. 2011 Oct;12(10):826-36. PubMed PMID: 20927321.

[95] Kelavkar UP, Hutzley J, Dhir R, Kim P, Allen KG, McHugh K. Prostate tumor growth and recurrence can be modulated by the omega-6:omega-3 ratio in diet: athymic mouse xenograft model simulating radical prostatectomy. Neoplasia. 2006 Feb;8(2): 112-24. PubMed PMID: 16611404.

[96] Vissapragada S, Ghosh A, Ringer L, Salinas P, Brophy A, Peaceman D, *et al*. Dietary n-3 polyunsaturated fatty acids fail to reduce prostate tumorigenesis in the PB-ErbB-2 x Pten(+/-) preclinical mouse model. Cell Cycle. 2010 May;9(9):1824-9. PubMed PMID: 20404514.

[97] Aronson WJ, Barnard RJ, Freedland SJ, Henning S, Elashoff D, Jardack PM, *et al*. Growth inhibitory effect of low fat diet on prostate cancer cells: results of a prospective, randomized dietary intervention trial in men with prostate cancer. The Journal of Urology. 2010 Jan;183(1):345-50. PubMed PMID: 19914662.

[98] Bureyko T, Hurdle H, Metcalfe JB, Clandinin MT, Mazurak VC. Reduced growth and integrin expression of prostate cells cultured with lycopene, vitamin E and fish oil *in vitro*. Br J Nutr. 2009 Apr;101(7):990-7. PubMed PMID: 18718045.

[99] Cavazos DA, Price RS, Apte SS, deGraffenried LA. Docosahexaenoic acid selectively induces human prostate cancer cell sensitivity to oxidative stress through modulation of NF-kappaB. Prostate. 2011 Sep 15;71(13):1420-8. PubMed PMID: 21360560.

[100] Istfan NW, Person KS, Holick MF, Chen TC. 1alpha,25-Dihydroxyvitamin D and fish oil synergistically inhibit G1/S-phase transition in prostate cancer cells. J Steroid Biochem Mol Biol. 2007 Mar;103(3-5):726-30. PubMed PMID: 17223546.

[101] Nakajima T, Kubota N, Tsutsumi T, Oguri A, Imuta H, Jo T, *et al*. Eicosapentaenoic acid inhibits voltage-gated sodium channels and invasiveness in prostate cancer cells. Br J Pharmacol. 2009 Feb;156(3):420-31. PubMed PMID: 19154441.

[102] Yi L, Zhang QY, Mi MT, Zheng, AI. Role of Rho GTPase in inhibiting metastatic ability of human prostate cancer cell line PC-3 by omega-3 polyunsaturated fatty acid. 2007 Dec;26(12):1281-6. PubMed PMID: 18076787.

[103] Fradet V, Cheng I, Casey G, Witte JS. Dietary omega-3 fatty acids, cyclooxygenase-2 genetic variation, and aggressive prostate cancer risk. Clinical Cancer Research. 2009 Apr 1;15(7):2559-66. PubMed PMID: 19318492.

[104] Chang HY, Sneddon JB, Alizadeh AA, Sood R, West RB, Montgomery K, *et al*. Gene expression signature of fibroblast serum response predicts human cancer progression: similarities between tumors and wounds. PLoS Biol. 2004 Feb;2(2):E7. PubMed PMID: 14737219.

[105] Woodward K. A high percentage of omega-3 fatty acids in the blood is linked to an increased risk of aggressive prostate cancer. 2011. Available at: wwwfhcrc.org.

[106] Beachy PA, Karhadkar SS, Berman DM. Tissue repair and stem cell renewal in carcinogenesis. Nature. 2004 Nov 18:432(7015):324-31. PubMed PMID: 15549094.

[107] Friedrichs W, Ruparel SB, Marciniak RA, DeGraffenried L. Omega-3 fatty acid inhibition of prostate cancer progression to hormone independence is associated with suppression of mTOR signaling and androgen receptor expression. Nutrition and Cancer. 2010;63(5):771-7. PubMed PMID: 21667400.

[108] Lim K, Han C, Dai Y, Shen M, Wu T. Omega-3 polyunsaturated fatty acids inhibit hepatocellular carcinoma cell growth through blocking beta-catenin and cyclooxygenase-2. Mol Cancer Ther. 2009 Nov;8(11):3046-55. PubMed PMID: 19887546.

[109] Lim K, Han C, Xu L, Isse K, Demetris AJ, Wu T. Cyclooxygenase-2-derived prostaglandin E2 activates beta-catenin in human cholangiocarcinoma cells: evidence for inhibition of these signaling pathways by omega 3 polyunsaturated fatty acids. Cancer Res. 2008 Jan 15;68(2):553-60. PubMed PMID: 18199552.

[110] Calviello G, Resci F, Serini S, Piccioni E, Toesca A, Boninsegna A, *et al*. Docosahexaenoic acid induces proteasome-dependent degradation of beta-catenin, down-regulation of survivin and apoptosis in human colorectal cancer cells not expressing COX-2. Carcinogenesis. 2007 Jun;28(6):1202-9. PubMed PMID: 17183061.

[111] Calviello G, Serini S, Piccioni E. n-3 polyunsaturated fatty acids and the prevention of colorectal cancer: molecular mechanisms involved. Curr Med Chem. 2007;14(29): 3059-69. PubMed PMID: 18220742.

[112] Narayanan BA, Narayanan NK, Desai D, Pittman B, Reddy BS. Effects of a combination of docosahexaenoic acid and 1,4-phenylene bis(methylene) selenocyanate on cyclooxygenase 2, inducible nitric oxide synthase and beta-catenin pathways in colon cancer cells. Carcinogenesis. 2004 Dec;25(12):2443-9. PubMed PMID: 15297372.

[113] Lu Y, Nie D, Witt WT, Chen Q, Shen M, Xie H, *et al*. Expression of the fat-1 gene diminishes prostate cancer growth *in vivo* through enhancing apoptosis and inhibiting GSK-3 beta phosphorylation. Mol Cancer Ther. 2008 Oct;7(10):3203-11. PubMed PMID: 18852124.

[114] Miller JR. The Wnts. Genome Biol. 2002;3(1):REVIEWS3001. PubMed PMID: 11806834.

[115] MacDonald BT, Tamai K, He X. Wnt/beta-catenin signaling: components, mechanisms, and diseases. Dev Cell. 2009 Jul;17(1):9-26. PubMed PMID: 19619488.

[116] Clevers H. Wnt/beta-catenin signaling in development and disease. Cell. 2006 Nov 3;127(3):469-80. PubMed PMID: 17081971.

[117] Gordon MD, Nusse R. Wnt signaling: multiple pathways, multiple receptors, and multiple transcription factors. J Biol Chem. 2006 Aug 11;281(32):22429-33. PubMed PMID: 16793760.

[118] Bandapalli OR, Dihlmann S, Helwa R, Macher-Goeppinger S, Weitz J, Schirmacher P, *et al*. Transcriptional activation of the beta-catenin gene at the invasion front of colorectal liver metastases. J Pathol. 2009 Jul;218(3):370-9. PubMed PMID: 19347947.

[119] Hoppler S, Kavanagh CL. Wnt signalling: variety at the core. J Cell Sci. 2007 Feb 1;120(Pt 3):385-93. PubMed PMID: 17251379.

[120] Moon RT, Kohn AD, De Ferrari GV, Kaykas A. WNT and beta-catenin signalling: diseases and therapies. Nat Rev Genet. 2004 Sep;5(9):691-701. PubMed PMID: 15372092.

[121] Terry S, Yang X, Chen MW, Vacherot F, Buttyan R. Multifaceted interaction between the androgen and Wnt signaling pathways and the implication for prostate cancer. J Cell Biochem. 2006 Oct 1;99(2):402-10. PubMed PMID: 16741972.

[122] Tetsu O, McCormick F. Beta-catenin regulates expression of cyclin D1 in colon carcinoma cells. Nature. 1999 Apr 1;398(6726):422-6. PubMed PMID: 10201372.

[123] Comstock CE, Revelo MP, Buncher CR, Knudsen KE. Impact of differential cyclin D1 expression and localisation in prostate cancer. Br J Cancer. 2007 Mar 26;96(6):970-9. PubMed PMID: 17375037.

[124] Drobnjak M, Osman I, Scher HI, Fazzari M, Cordon-Cardo C. Overexpression of cyclin D1 is associated with metastatic prostate cancer to bone. Clinical Cancer Research. 2000 May;6(5):1891-5. PubMed PMID: 10815912.

[125] Fleming WH, Hamel A, MacDonald R, Ramsey E, Pettigrew NM, Johnston B, *et al.* Expression of the c-myc protooncogene in human prostatic carcinoma and benign prostatic hyperplasia. Cancer Res. 1986 Mar;46(3):1535-8. PubMed PMID: 2417706.

[126] Jenkins RB, Qian J, Lieber MM, Bostwick DG. Detection of c-myc oncogene amplification and chromosomal anomalies in metastatic prostatic carcinoma by fluorescence *in situ* hybridization. Cancer Res. 1997 Feb 1;57(3):524-31. PubMed PMID: 9012485.

[127] Qian J, Hirasawa K, Bostwick DG, Bergstralh EJ, Slezak JM, Anderl KL, *et al.* Loss of p53 and c-myc overrepresentation in stage T(2-3)N(1-3)M(0) prostate cancer are potential markers for cancer progression. Mod Pathol. 2002 Jan;15(1):35-44. PubMed PMID: 11796839.

[128] Sato H, Minei S, Hachiya T, Yoshida T, Takimoto Y. Fluorescence *in situ* hybridization analysis of c-myc amplification in stage TNM prostate cancer in Japanese patients. Int J Urol. 2006 Jun;13(6):761-6. PubMed PMID: 16834657.

[129] Chesire DR, Ewing CM, Sauvageot J, Bova GS, Isaacs WB. Detection and analysis of beta-catenin mutations in prostate cancer. Prostate. 2000 Dec 1;45(4):323-34. PubMed PMID: 11102958.

[130] de la Taille A, Rubin MA, Chen MW, Vacherot F, de Medina SG, Burchardt M, *et al.* Beta-catenin-related anomalies in apoptosis-resistant and hormone-refractory prostate cancer cells. Clinical Cancer Research. 2003 May;9(5):1801-7. PubMed PMID: 12738737.

[131] Yamamoto H, Oue N, Sato A, Hasegawa Y, Yamamoto H, Matsubara A, *et al.* Wnt5a signaling is involved in the aggressiveness of prostate cancer and expression of metalloproteinase. Oncogene. Apr 8;29(14):2036-46. PubMed PMID: 20101234.

[132] Gerstein AV, Almeida TA, Zhao G, Chess E, Shih Ie M, Buhler K, *et al.* APC/CTNNB1 (beta-catenin) pathway alterations in human prostate cancers. Genes Chromosomes Cancer. 2002 May;34(1):9-16. PubMed PMID: 11921277.

[133] Chesire DR, Ewing CM, Gage WR, Isaacs WB. *In vitro* evidence for complex modes of nuclear beta-catenin signaling during prostate growth and tumorigenesis. Oncogene. 2002 Apr 18;21(17):2679-94. PubMed PMID: 11965541.

[134] Yardy GW, Brewster SF. Wnt signalling and prostate cancer. Prostate Cancer Prostatic Dis. 2005;8(2):119-26. PubMed PMID: 15809669.

[135] Henrique R, Ribeiro FR, Fonseca D, Hoque MO, Carvalho AL, Costa VL, *et al.* High promoter methylation levels of APC predict poor prognosis in sextant biopsies from prostate cancer patients. Clinical Cancer Research. 2007 Oct 15;13(20):6122-9. PubMed PMID: 17947477.

[136] Brewster SF, Kemple T, MacIver AG, Astley JP, Gingell JC. The Bristol prostate cancer pilot screening study: a 3-year follow-up. Br J Urol. 1994 Nov;74(5):556-8. PubMed PMID: 7530117.

[137] Phillips SM, Barton CM, Lee SJ, Morton DG, Wallace DM, Lemoine NR, *et al.* Loss of the retinoblastoma susceptibility gene (RB1) is a frequent and early event in prostatic tumorigenesis. Br J Cancer. 1994 Dec;70(6):1252-7. PubMed PMID: 7526887.

[138] Yardy GW, Bicknell DC, Wilding JL, Bartlett S, Liu Y, Winney B, *et al.* Mutations in the AXIN1 gene in advanced prostate cancer. European Urology. 2009 Sep;56(3): 486-94. PubMed PMID: 18514389.

[139] Bastian PJ, Ellinger J, Wellmann A, Wernert N, Heukamp LC, Muller SC, *et al.* Diagnostic and prognostic information in prostate cancer with the help of a small set of hypermethylated gene loci. Clinical Cancer Research. 2005 Jun 1;11(11):4097-106. PubMed PMID: 15930345.

[140] Jeronimo C, Henrique R, Hoque MO, Mambo E, Ribeiro FR, Varzim G, *et al.* A quantitative promoter methylation profile of prostate cancer. Clinical Cancer Research. 2004 Dec 15;10(24):8472-8. PubMed PMID: 15623627.

[141] Mizutani K, Miyamoto S, Nagahata T, Konishi N, Emi M, Onda M. Upregulation and overexpression of DVL1, the human counterpart of the Drosophila dishevelled gene, in prostate cancer. Tumori. 2005 Nov-Dec;91(6):546-51. PubMed PMID: 16457155.

[142] Chen G, Shukeir N, Potti A, Sircar K, Aprikian A, Goltzman D, *et al*. Up-regulation of Wnt-1 and beta-catenin production in patients with advanced metastatic prostate carcinoma: potential pathogenetic and prognostic implications. Cancer. 2004 Sep 15;101(6):1345-56. PubMed PMID: 15316903.

[143] Hall CL, Bafico A, Dai J, Aaronson SA, Keller ET. Prostate cancer cells promote osteoblastic bone metastases through Wnts. Cancer Res. 2005 Sep 1;65(17):7554-60. PubMed PMID: 16140917.

[144] Iozzo RV, Eichstetter I, Danielson KG. Aberrant expression of the growth factor Wnt-5A in human malignancy. Cancer Res. 1995 Aug 15;55(16):3495-9. PubMed PMID: 7627953.

[145] Wang Q, Symes AJ, Kane CA, Freeman A, Nariculam J, Munson P, *et al*. A novel role for Wnt/Ca2+ signaling in actin cytoskeleton remodeling and cell motility in prostate cancer. PLoS One. 2010;5(5):e10456. PubMed PMID: 20454608.

[146] Katoh M. Differential regulation of WNT2 and WNT2B expression in human cancer. Int J Mol Med. 2001 Dec;8(6):657-60. PubMed PMID: 11712082.

[147] Hall CL, Daignault SD, Shah RB, Pienta KJ, Keller ET. Dickkopf-1 expression increases early in prostate cancer development and decreases during progression from primary tumor to metastasis. Prostate. 2008 Sep 15;68(13):1396-404. PubMed PMID: 18561248.

[148] Coutinho-Camillo CM, Salaorni S, Sarkis AS, Nagai MA. Differentially expressed genes in the prostate cancer cell line LNCaP after exposure to androgen and anti-androgen. Cancer Genet Cytogenet. 2006 Apr 15;166(2):130-8. PubMed PMID: 16631469.

[149] Kawano Y, Diez S, Uysal-Onganer P, Darrington RS, Waxman J, Kypta RM. Secreted Frizzled-related protein-1 is a negative regulator of androgen receptor activity in prostate cancer. Br J Cancer. 2009 Apr 7;100(7):1165-74. PubMed PMID: 19277043.

[150] Kawano Y, Kitaoka M, Hamada Y, Walker MM, Waxman J, Kypta RM. Regulation of prostate cell growth and morphogenesis by Dickkopf-3. Oncogene. 2006 Oct 19;25(49):6528-37. PubMed PMID: 16751809.

[151] Zenzmaier C, Untergasser G, Hermann M, Dirnhofer S, Sampson N, Berger P. Dysregulation of Dkk-3 expression in benign and malignant prostatic tissue. Prostate. 2008 Apr 1;68(5):540-7. PubMed PMID: 18247400.

[152] Lodygin D, Epanchintsev A, Menssen A, Diebold J, Hermeking H. Functional epigenomics identifies genes frequently silenced in prostate cancer. Cancer Res. 2005 May 15;65(10):4218-27. PubMed PMID: 15899813.

http://dx.doi.org/10.5772/55858

[153] Horvath LG, Henshall SM, Kench JG, Saunders DN, Lee CS, Golovsky D, *et al*. Membranous expression of secreted frizzled-related protein 4 predicts for good prognosis in localized prostate cancer and inhibits PC3 cellular proliferation *in vitro*. Clinical Cancer Research. 2004 Jan 15;10(2):615-25. PubMed PMID: 14760084.

[154] Horvath LG, Lelliott JE, Kench JG, Lee CS, Williams ED, Saunders DN, *et al*. Secreted frizzled-related protein 4 inhibits proliferation and metastatic potential in prostate cancer. Prostate. 2007 Jul 1;67(10):1081-90. PubMed PMID: 17476687.

[155] Wissmann C, Wild PJ, Kaiser S, Roepcke S, Stoehr R, Woenckhaus M, *et al*. WIF1, a component of the Wnt pathway, is down-regulated in prostate, breast, lung, and bladder cancer. J Pathol. 2003 Oct;201(2):204-12. PubMed PMID: 14517837.

[156] Liss MA, Schlicht M, Kahler A, Fitzgerald R, Thomassi T, Degueme A, *et al*. Characterization of soy-based changes in Wnt-frizzled signaling in prostate cancer. Cancer Genomics Proteomics. 2011 Sep-Oct;7(5):245-52. PubMed PMID: 20952759.

[157] Thiele S, Rauner M, Goettsch C, Rachner TD, Benad P, Fuessel S, *et al*. Expression profile of WNT molecules in prostate cancer and its regulation by aminobisphosphonates. J Cell Biochem. 2011 Jun;112(6):1593-600. PubMed PMID: 21344486.

[158] Hall CL, Kang S, MacDougald OA, Keller ET. Role of Wnts in prostate cancer bone metastases. J Cell Biochem. 2006 Mar 1;97(4):661-72. PubMed PMID: 16447163.

[159] Thiele S, Rauner M, Goettsch C, Rachner TD, Benad P, Fuessel S, *et al*. Expression profile of WNT molecules in prostate cancer and its regulation by aminobisphosphonates. J Cell Biochem. Jun;112(6):1593-600. PubMed PMID: 21344486.

[160] Bierie B, Nozawa M, Renou JP, Shillingford JM, Morgan F, Oka T, *et al*. Activation of beta-catenin in prostate epithelium induces hyperplasias and squamous transdifferentiation. Oncogene. 2003 Jun 19;22(25):3875-87. PubMed PMID: 12813461.

[161] Lu W, Tinsley HN, Keeton A, Qu Z, Piazza GA, Li Y. Suppression of Wnt/beta-catenin signaling inhibits prostate cancer cell proliferation. Eur J Pharmacol. 2009 Jan 5;602(1):8-14. PubMed PMID: 19026633.

[162] Voeller HJ, Truica CI, Gelmann EP. Beta-catenin mutations in human prostate cancer. Cancer Res. 1998 Jun 15;58(12):2520-3. PubMed PMID: 9635571.

[163] Whitaker HC, Girling J, Warren AY, Leung H, Mills IG, Neal DE. Alterations in beta-catenin expression and localization in prostate cancer. Prostate. 2008 Aug 1;68(11): 1196-205. PubMed PMID: 18459111.

[164] Bruxvoort KJ, Charbonneau HM, Giambernardi TA, Goolsby JC, Qian CN, Zylstra CR, *et al*. Inactivation of Apc in the mouse prostate causes prostate carcinoma. Cancer Res. 2007 Mar 15;67(6):2490-6. PubMed PMID: 17363566.

[165] Davies G, Jiang WG, Mason MD. The interaction between beta-catenin, GSK3beta and APC after motogen induced cell-cell dissociation, and their involvement in sig-

nal transduction pathways in prostate cancer. Int J Oncol. 2001 Apr;18(4):843-7. PubMed PMID: 11251183.

[166] Guertin DA, Stevens DM, Saitoh M, Kinkel S, Crosby K, Sheen JH, *et al*. mTOR complex 2 is required for the development of prostate cancer induced by Pten loss in mice. Cancer Cell. 2009 Feb 3;15(2):148-59. PubMed PMID: 19185849.

[167] Liao X, Zhang L, Thrasher JB, Du J, Li B. Glycogen synthase kinase-3beta suppression eliminates tumor necrosis factor-related apoptosis-inducing ligand resistance in prostate cancer. Mol Cancer Ther. 2003 Nov;2(11):1215-22. PubMed PMID: 14617795.

[168] Mazor M, Kawano Y, Zhu H, Waxman J, Kypta RM. Inhibition of glycogen synthase kinase-3 represses androgen receptor activity and prostate cancer cell growth. Oncogene. 2004 Oct 14;23(47):7882-92. PubMed PMID: 15361837.

[169] Yu X, Wang Y, DeGraff DJ, Wills ML, Matusik RJ. Wnt/beta-catenin activation promotes prostate tumor progression in a mouse model. Oncogene. 2010 Apr 21;30(16): 1868-79. PubMed PMID: 21151173.

[170] Zhu Q, Yang J, Han S, Liu J, Holzbeierlein J, Thrasher JB, *et al*. Suppression of glycogen synthase kinase 3 activity reduces tumor growth of prostate cancer *in vivo*. Prostate. 2010 Oct 28; 71(8):835-45. PubMed PMID: 21031441.

[171] Agalliu I, Suuriniemi M, Prokunina-Olsson L, Johanneson B, Collins FS, Stanford JL, *et al*. Evaluation of a variant in the transcription factor 7-like 2 (TCF7L2) gene and prostate cancer risk in a population-based study. Prostate. 2008 May 15;68(7):740-7. PubMed PMID: 18302196.

[172] Bubendorf L, Kononen J, Koivisto P, Schraml P, Moch H, Gasser TC, *et al*. Survey of gene amplifications during prostate cancer progression by high-throughout fluorescence *in situ* hybridization on tissue microarrays. Cancer Res. 1999 Feb 15;59(4):803-6. PubMed PMID: 10029066.

[173] Gurel B, Iwata T, Koh CM, Jenkins RB, Lan F, Van Dang C, *et al*. Nuclear MYC protein overexpression is an early alteration in human prostate carcinogenesis. Mod Pathol. 2008 Sep;21(9):1156-67. PubMed PMID: 18567993.

[174] Iversen PL, Arora V, Acker AJ, Mason DH, Devi GR. Efficacy of antisense morpholino oligomer targeted to c-myc in prostate cancer xenograft murine model and a Phase I safety study in humans. Clinical Cancer Research. 2003 Jul;9(7):2510-9. PubMed PMID: 12855625.

[175] Yu X, Wang Y, Jiang M, Bierie B, Roy-Burman P, Shen MM, *et al*. Activation of beta-Catenin in mouse prostate causes HGPIN and continuous prostate growth after castration. Prostate. 2009 Feb 15;69(3):249-62. PubMed PMID: 18991257.

[176] Goss, KH. and Kahn, M. Targeting the Wnt Pathway in Cancer. Springer. 2011. ISBN-10: 1441980229.

[177] Yeh CT, Yao CJ, Yan JL, Chuang SE, Lee LM, Chen CM, *et al*. Apoptotic Cell Death and Inhibition of Wnt/beta-Catenin Signaling Pathway in Human Colon Cancer Cells by an Active Fraction (HS7) from Taiwanofungus camphoratus. Evid Based Complement Alternat Med. 2011. Article ID: 750230. PubMed PMID: 21423639.

[178] Lattouf J, Srinivasan R, Pinto PA, Linehan WM, Neckers L. Mechanisms of disease: the role of heat-shock protein 90 in genitourinary malignancy. Nature Clinical Practice Urology. 2006 Nov;3(11):590-601. PubMed PMID: 17088927.

[179] Lattouf J, Srinivanasan, R. Pinto, PA. Linehan, WM and Neckers, L. Mechanisms of Disease: the role of heat-shock protein 90 in genitourinary malignancy. Nature Reviews Urology. 1969 December 31; 3(11).

[180] Booth B, Glassman R, Ma P. Oncology's trials. Nat Rev Drug Discov. 2003 Aug;2(8): 609-10. PubMed PMID: 12908467.

[181] Kola I, Landis J. Can the pharmaceutical industry reduce attrition rates? Nat Rev Drug Discov. 2004 Aug;3(8):711-5. PubMed PMID: 15286737.

[182] Greenberg NM, DeMayo F, Finegold MJ, Medina D, Tilley WD, Aspinall JO, *et al*. Prostate cancer in a transgenic mouse. Proc Natl Acad Sci U S A. 1995 Apr 11;92(8): 3439-43. PubMed PMID: 7724580.

[183] Jeet V, Russell PJ, Khatri A. Modeling prostate cancer: a perspective on transgenic mouse models. Cancer Metastasis Rev. Mar;29(1):123-42. PubMed PMID: 20143131.

[184] Mimeault M, Batra SK. Animal models relevant to human prostate carcinogenesis underlining the critical implication of prostatic stem/progenitor cells. Biochim Biophys Acta. Aug;1816(1):25-37. PubMed PMID: 21396984.

[185] Navone NM, Logothetis CJ, von Eschenbach AC, Troncoso P. Model systems of prostate cancer: uses and limitations. Cancer Metastasis Rev. 1998;17(4):361-71. PubMed PMID: 10453280.

[186] van Weerden WM, Bangma C, de Wit R. Human xenograft models as useful tools to assess the potential of novel therapeutics in prostate cancer. Br J Cancer. 2009 Jan 13;100(1):13-8. PubMed PMID: 19088719.

[187] Horoszewicz JS, Leong SS, Kawinski E, Karr JP, Rosenthal H, Chu TM, *et al*. LNCaP model of human prostatic carcinoma. Cancer Res. 1983 Apr;43(4):1809-18. PubMed PMID: 6831420.

[188] Jiang YG, Zhao JH, Luo Y, He DL, Li N, Cui XH, *et al*. Expressions of E-cadherin and beta-catenin in LNCaP and ARCaP cell lines and their significance. Zhonghua Nan Ke Xue. 2009 Oct;15(10):867-71. PubMed PMID: 20112731.

[189] Valkenburg KC, Williams BO. Mouse models of prostate cancer. Prostate cancer. 2011;2011:895238. PubMed PMID: 22111002. Pubmed Central PMCID: 3221286.

[190] Leroy BE, Northrup N. Prostate cancer in dogs: comparative and clinical aspects. Vet J. 2009 May;180(2):149-62. PubMed PMID: 18786842.

[191] Rosol TJ, Tannehill-Gregg SH, Corn S, Schneider A, McCauley LK. Animal models of bone metastasis. Cancer Treat Res. 2004;118:47-81. PubMed PMID: 15043188.

[192] Hamra FK. Gene targeting: Enter the rat. Nature. Sep 9;467(7312):161-3. PubMed PMID: 20829783.

[193] Deeb KK, Michalowska AM, Yoon CY, Krummey SM, Hoenerhoff MJ, Kavanaugh C, *et al*. Identification of an integrated SV40 T/t-antigen cancer signature in aggressive human breast, prostate, and lung carcinomas with poor prognosis. Cancer Res. 2007 Sep 1;67(17):8065-80. PubMed PMID: 17804718.

[194] Hensley PJ, Kyprianou N. Modeling prostate cancer in mice: limitations and opportunities. J Androl. 2011 Mar-Apr;33(2):133-44. PubMed PMID: 21680808.

[195] Hill R, Song Y, Cardiff RD, Van Dyke T. Heterogeneous tumor evolution initiated by loss of pRb function in a preclinical prostate cancer model. Cancer Res. 2005 Nov 15;65(22):10243-54. PubMed PMID: 16288012.

[196] Wang S, Gao J, Lei Q, Rozengurt N, Pritchard C, Jiao J, *et al*. Prostate-specific deletion of the murine Pten tumor suppressor gene leads to metastatic prostate cancer. Cancer Cell. 2003 Sep;4(3):209-21. PubMed PMID: 14522255.

[197] Ellwood-Yen K, Graeber TG, Wongvipat J, Iruela-Arispe ML, Zhang J, Matusik R, *et al*. Myc-driven murine prostate cancer shares molecular features with human prostate tumors. Cancer Cell. 2003 Sep;4(3):223-38. PubMed PMID: 14522256.

[198] Masumori N, Thomas TZ, Chaurand P, Case T, Paul M, Kasper S, *et al*. A probasin-large T antigen transgenic mouse line develops prostate adenocarcinoma and neuroendocrine carcinoma with metastatic potential. Cancer Res. 2001 Mar 1;61(5):2239-49. PubMed PMID: 11280793.

[199] Abate-Shen C, Banach-Petrosky WA, Sun X, Economides KD, Desai N, Gregg JP, *et al*. Nkx3.1; Pten mutant mice develop invasive prostate adenocarcinoma and lymph node metastases. Cancer Res. 2003 Jul 15;63(14):3886-90. PubMed PMID: 12873978.

[200] Smolinski J. Dietary Chemoprevention Studies in Preclinical Models of Prostate Cancer: Bioactive Lipids and Vitamin D. PhD Thesis. 2011. Ohio State University.

[201] Allen NE, Key TJ, Appleby PN, Travis RC, Roddam AW, Tjonneland A, *et al*. Animal foods, protein, calcium and prostate cancer risk: the European Prospective Investigation into Cancer and Nutrition. Br J Cancer. 2008 May 6;98(9):1574-81. PubMed PMID: 18382426.

[202] Multigner L, Ndong JR, Oliva A, Blanchet P. Environmental pollutants and prostate cancer: epidemiological data. Gynecol Obstet Fertil. 2008 Sep;36(9):848-56. PubMed PMID: 18693059.

[203] United States Food and Drug Administration. 2009. Available from: http://www.fda.gov/Safety/MedWatch/SafetyInformation/Safety-relatedDrugLabelingChanges/ucm155404.htm.

[204] AHP Limited. Datapharm Communication Inc.; 2008 [cited 2012]. Available from: http://www.medicines.org.uk/emc/medicine/10312/spc.

[205] Dey E, Nathan V. FDA approves Amarin's heart pill. Menon, R (editor). Reuters. 2012 July 26. Available from: http://www.reuters.com/article/2012/07/26/us-amarin-fda-vascepa-idUSBRE86P1SX20120726.

[206] Amarin Corporation. Amarin's AMR101 Phase 3 ANCHOR Trial Meets all Primary and Secondary Endpoints with Statistically Significant Reductions in Triglycerides at Both 4 Gram and 2 Gram Doses and Statistically Significant Decrease in LDL-C: Acquire Media. 2011. Available from: http://investor.amarincorp.com.

[207] Epanova® for Lowering Very High Triglycerides (EVOLVE). U.S. National Institutes of Health. 2012. Available from: http://clinicaltrials.gov/ct2/show/NCT01242527.

[208] Simopoulos AP. Evolutionary aspects of the dietary omega-6:omega-3 fatty acid ratio: medical implications. World Rev Nutr Diet. 2009;100:1-21. PubMed PMID: 19696523.

[209] Food and Nutrition Board. A Report of the Panel on Macronutrients, Subcommittees on Upper Reference Levels of Nutrients and Interpretation and Uses of Dietary Reference Intakes, Standing Committee on the Scientific Evaluation of Dietary Reference Intakes; Dietary Reference Intakes for Energy, Carbohydrate, Fiber, Fat, Fatty Acids, Cholesterol, Protein, and Amino Acids (Macronutrients). 2005. The National Academies Press, Washington, DC. Available at: http://www.nap.edu/openbook.php?record_id=10490&page=589

[210] Kris-Etherton PM, Grieger JA, Etherton TD. Dietary reference intakes for DHA and EPA. Prostaglandins, Leukotrienes and Essential Fatty Acids. 2009 81(2–3):99-104.

[211] Yu H, Rohan T. Role of the insulin-like growth factor family in cancer development and progression. J Natl Cancer Inst. 2000 Sep 20;92(18):1472-89. PubMed PMID: 10995803.

[212] Huizen IV, Wu G, Moussa M, Chin JL, Fenster A, Lacefield JC, *et al*. Establishment of a serum tumor marker for preclinical trials of mouse prostate cancer models. Clinical Cancer Research. 2005 Nov 1;11(21):7911-9. PubMed PMID: 16278416.

[213] Langdon S. Cancer Cell Culture: Methods and Protocols. 2004: 225-9. Humana Press. ISBN-10: 1588290794 ISBN-13: 978-1588290793.

[214] Schley PD, Brindley DN, Field CJ. (n-3) PUFA alter raft lipid composition and decrease epidermal growth factor receptor levels in lipid rafts of human breast cancer cells. J Nutr. 2007 Mar;137(3):548-53. PubMed PMID: 17311938.

[215] Ma DW, Ngo V, Huot PS, Kang JX. N-3 polyunsaturated fatty acids endogenously synthesized in fat-1 mice are enriched in the mammary gland. Lipids. 2006 Jan;41(1): 35-9. PubMed PMID: 16555469.

[216] Hjartaker A, Lund E, Bjerve KS. Serum phospholipid fatty acid composition and habitual intake of marine foods registered by a semi-quantitative food frequency questionnaire. Eur J Clin Nutr. 1997 Nov;51(11):736-42. PubMed PMID: 9368807.

[217] Kobayashi M, Sasaki S, Kawabata T, Hasegawa K, Akabane M, Tsugane S. Single measurement of serum phospholipid fatty acid as a biomarker of specific fatty acid intake in middle-aged Japanese men. Eur J Clin Nutr. 2001 Aug;55(8):643-50. PubMed PMID: 11477462.

[218] Chajes V, Hulten K, Van Kappel AL, Winkvist A, Kaaks R, Hallmans G, *et al.* Fatty-acid composition in serum phospholipids and risk of breast cancer: an incident case-control study in Sweden. Int J Cancer. 1999 Nov 26;83(5):585-90. PubMed PMID: 10521790.

[219] Folch J, Lees M, Sloane Stanley GH. A simple method for the isolation and purification of total lipides from animal tissues. J Biol Chem. 1957 May;226(1):497-509. PubMed PMID: 13428781.

Section 4

Bioactive Compounds in Health and Disease

Chapter 9

Mechanisms and Treatment of Photoaging and Photodamage

Marianna Kulka

Additional information is available at the end of the chapter

http://dx.doi.org/10.5772/56425

1. Introduction

Damage caused by excessive, long-term sun exposure contributes to signs of ageing and is most readily recognizable on our external surface, the skin. The damaging effects of the sun are mainly caused by ultraviolet radiation (UVR) which, on earth, consists of UVA (320 to 400 nm) and UVB (280 to 320 nm). The third type of UV radiation, UVC, also called short-wave or ionizing radiation, is absorbed by gasses in our atmosphere, does not reach the earth's surface and does not normally contribute to photodamage of skin. Ozone is one of the gases that absorbs UVC – fortunately, since UVC's ionizing effects can significantly alter cellular structures and molecules. Although UVB and UVA radiation does not have enough energy to ionize atoms, it can alter chemical bonds in molecules, thus altering their structure and functions. Skin cells are particularly susceptible to alterations mediated principally by the creation of free radicals and oxidative stress and changes in DNA structure can result in constitutive expression of protocongenes and ultimately the development of cancerous skin lesions.

Through its changes of molecular structures, UV radiation causes a series of biochemical and structural changes in skin tissues. Some of these effects, such as the induction of vitamin D production, are actually very beneficial to skin health. Niels Ryberg Finsen, a Danish physician and scientist, was one of the first to show that light can be both beneficial and detrimental to human skin and his works *Om Lysets Indvirkninger paa Huden* ("On the effects of light on the skin"), published in 1893 and *Om Anvendelse i Medicinen af koncentrerede kemiske Lysstraaler* ("The use of concentrated chemical light rays in medicine"), published in 1896 created the paradigm on which photoaging and photodamage research was based for the next fifty years. Finsen won the Nobel Prize in Physiology in 1903 for his work on phototherapy in which he showed that certain wavelengths of light (UV in particular) could treat *lupus vulgaris*, cutaneous tuberculosis. However, UV radiation can also initiate some deleterious effects that fundamentally change the structure and function of the skin and its constituent components. In fact, it has been shown that repeated, excessive sun exposure can initiate and perpetuate an inflammatory response that, given time, causes breakdown of the skin's immunological functions.

This review will focus on the effects of sun exposure on the skin microenvironment – particularly the structural proteins and immune cells that are key players in the skin's protective functions. There is sufficient evidence to suggest that photodamage is associated with a low level of chronic inflammation that ultimately breaks down the skin's structure and results in some of the manifestations of skin aging. Consequently, skin treatments that target these processes are primarily focused on rebuilding the skin's architecture and promoting its biochemical regeneration. While some treatments have been found to have some beneficial effects to the underlying cellular immune systems regulating skin inflammation and regeneration, others may, in fact, be deleterious to these processes. In this review, I will discuss some naturally-derived bioactive compounds and formulations that have been shown or are suggested to be effective at modulating the pathophysiological changes associated with photodamage and photoaging. Bioactive compounds that can address these immunological changes are uniquely poised to not only reduce the damage associated with photodamage but may ultimately improve the resiliency and protective nature of the skin surface.

2. Skin is a protective organ

2.1. The three layers of defense

Healthy human skin is an important physical barrier to the environment and protects the body from a variety of insults. It is the largest human organ and comprises approximately 15 percent of a person's body weight and covers about 1.5 to 2.0 m^2 of our surface area. Skin is mainly composed of water (70%), protein (25%) and lipids (2%) forming an effective barrier to dehydration, pathogens and mechanical insults such as abrasion. In a mechanical sense, the main function of the skin is to serve as a protective barrier to keep good things in (water, nutrients and heat) and keep bad things out (pathogens, UV radiation, toxins).

In order to understand the essential functions of the skin, it is important to review the complexity of this large organ. The skin is composed of three main layers, the uppermost epidermis, the lower dermis and the hypodermis (Fig. 1). Each of these layers is composed of a specific set of cells that perform an essential function in that layer. The epidermis contains keratinocytes, melanocytes and Langerhans cells which are critical for the structural and functional integrity of the epidermis. Keratinocytes are the major population of cells and originate in the bottom-most stem-cell pool in the stratum spinosum (Fig. 1). The epidermis itself is composed of five layers: stratum corneum, stratum lucidum, stratum granulosum, stratum spinosum and stratum basale. The uppermost layer of the skin, the keratinous stratum corneum, renews itself every 3-5 weeks and is principally composed of dead keratinocytes (see section below on keratinocytes for more detail). Keratinocytes have the capacity to

http://dx.doi.org/10.5772/56425

renew themselves every 4 weeks but this process can be increased during injury or inflammation. The underlying dermis is a vascularized, connective tissue containing nerve endings, glands and lymphatic vessels and provides structural and nutritional support to the upper epidermal cells. The dermis is, in fact, the a mucopolysaccharide matrix composed of collagen and elastin fibers. In this layer, there is a great variety of cells including mast cells, fibroblasts, macrophages and Langerhans cells all of which contribute to the immune response observed in some skin pathologies such as atopic dermatitis. These cells also maintain and regulate the essential healthy functions of skin such as repairing injury, preventing infection, regulating circulation, preventing dehydration and providing nutrition. Beneath the dermis is the superficial fascia, or hypodermis, which is comprised primarily of fat tissue.

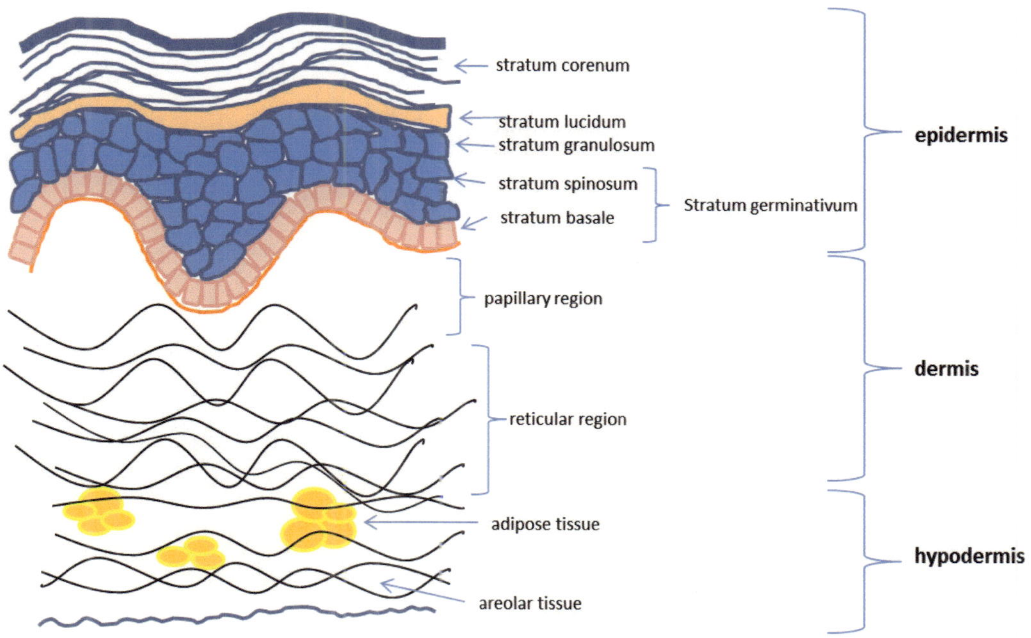

Figure 1. Structure of skin. Skin is comprised of three main layers as shown. The epidermis contains keratinocytes, melanocytes and Langerhans cells which are critical for the structural and functional integrity of the epidermis. The epidermis itself is composed of five layers: stratum corneum, stratum lucidum, stratum granulosum, stratum spinosum and stratum basale. The strata granulosum, spinosum and basale all contain keratinocytes whereas the strata corneum and lucidum have only dead keratinized cells. The underlying dermis is a vascularized, connective tissue containing nerve endings, glands and lymphatic vessels. Beneath the dermis is the superficial fascia, or hypodermis, which is comprised primarily of fat tissue.

2.2. Melanin and melanogenesis — A protective response

As a result of its optical properties, the stratum corneum scatters photons and reflects UV radiation, providing some degree of protection. However, a portion of UV radiation penetrates this uppermost layer and can potentially damage the delicate structures beneath. Melanin plays an important role in the skin's function as a protective barrier by absorbing UV radiation and thus protecting the underlying cells from DNA damage. The word melanin comes from the Greek word *melan*, meaning black. Melanin is a polymeric pigment derived from tyrosine and, in humans, it is synthesized in two main forms: the brown/black eumelanin and the cysteine-rich red/brown pheomelanin. The chemical structures of these two types of melanin are different resulting in different properties and functions (Fig. 2). Whereas eumelanin is composed of dihydroxyindole carboxylic acids, pheomelanin is a polymer of benxothiazine units. The carboxylic structure may account for pheomelanin's weak shielding capacity against ultraviolet radiation relative to eumelanin. In fact, pheomelanin has been shown to amplify UVA-induced reactive oxygen species (ROS)[1]. For this reason, pheomelanin is sometimes referred to as a UV-sensitizer and in some instances has been considered to have a weak carcinogenic effect in terms of melanoma formation.

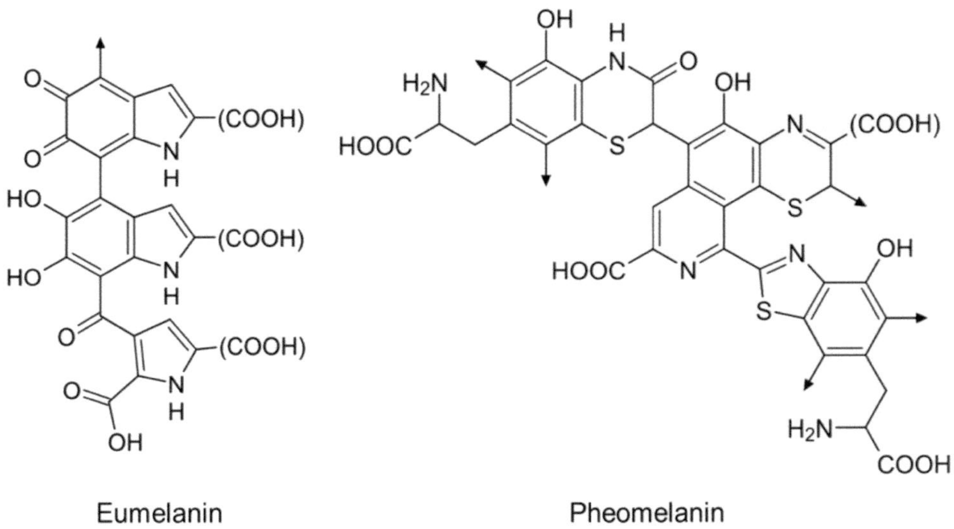

Figure 2. Chemical structure of eumelanin and pheomelanin.

Melanogenesis refers to the biochemical process by which melanin is formed. Melanocytes are the principal cell type responsible for the production and distribution of melanin in the skin. Since melanocyte differentiation and proliferation is linked very closely with their ability to produce melanin, melanogenesis is sometimes used to describe the process of melanocyte viability and reproduction. Indeed, many cosmetic products on the market that profess to alter or manipulate melanogenesis are actually cytotoxic to melanocyte and by killing healthy melanocytes they indirectly decrease the amount of melanin in the human epidermis. For example, hydroquinone (HQ), which is an U.S. Food and Drug Administration (FDA) -approved product, is used in 2 – 4 percent concentration as a skin-lightening agent but is considered to be cytotoxic to melanocytes[2]. Interestingly, some antibiotics used to treat ear infections, such as amikacin, are cytotoxic to melanocytes as well and one of its principal side-effects is ototoxicity[3].

One of the most obvious and controversial side-effects of exposing our skin to UV radiation is an increase in skin pigmentation. Certainly the issue of tanning and tanning beds has recently gained a great deal of attention because it has been shown that exposure to prolonged UV radiation (either from tanning beds or outside exposure) can cause melanoma and an effort is underway to limit the amount of time that people, especially children, spend tanning in any setting. The process of tanning is a protective mechanism and the skin's way of protecting its internal biochemical reactions from UV damage. Increased pigmentation is caused by increased production of melanin which is able to absorb some UV radiation and thus protect more sensitive biological pathways in the cell[4]. Epidemiological studies have shown that people who have high levels of constitutive pigment in their skin and are able to "tan well" are less likely to develop skin cancer[5], [6].

We still do not fully understand the precise mechanisms that initiate the malignancies associated with skin cancer and we certainly have an incomplete understanding of how photodamage and repair functions in people of different skin colors. However, mouse models and human studies have shown that albinos have a lower incidence of melanoma than their fair skinned counterparts[7] suggesting that melanin cannot just function as a protective UV-energy absorber. Recently, several groups have shown that melanin, especially pheomelanin (a yellow/red form of melanin), acts as a potent UVB photosensitizer to induce DNA damage and cause apoptosis in mouse skin. These groups believe that pheomelanin contributes to UV-induced DNA damage that is incompletely repaired. They further believe that this DNA damage maps to specific sequences of BRAF and N-RAS genes, both of which are frequently mutated in human melanoma[8], [9].

Some organic and inorganic compounds mimic the effects of melanin by absorbing or scattering UVR due to their particulate nature – often in the nanoscale. These chemicals are processed and made available as lotions, sprays, gels or other topical applications commonly known as sunscreens. There are 17 different chemicals that have been approved by the U.S. FDA as active ingredients in sunscreens. Oxybenzone (benzopehone-3) is the most widely used sunscreen chemical worldwide but other chemicals include octinoxate, avobenzone, and octyl salicylate. Some of the physical sunscreens are micro or nano-ionized to create particulate formulations capable of forming a protective UV barrier on the skin's surface. Titanium dioxide (TiO_2) are often used as a inorganic protective sunscreens in cosmetic products and to adjust their protective factor (SPF), they are often coupled with organic chemicals such as p-amino benzoic acid (PABA) which absorbs UVB but not UVA radiation. Recently, some have suggested that these nanoparticles (NP; around 200 nm) may penetrate the skin and modify the skin's immune-environment. However, several groups have shown that although nanoparticles are unable to penetrate healthy, intact human epidermis[10] they can significantly disturb cell functions through direct contact when the skin barrier is compromised[11], [12]. In fact, NP can reach the epidermal layer via hair follicles in certain circumstances such as laser-treatment[13] or inflammation[14], [15] but most compounds, although targeting the follicular region, do not permeate past the pilosebaceous region[16].

3. The production of melanin

3.1. Tyrosinase

Tyrosinase is responsible for the hydroxylation of monophenol and conversion of an *o*-diphenol to the corresponding *o*-quinone which then undergoes several modifications to become melanin (Fig. 3). Tyrosinases are ubiquitously expressed by both plants and animals, and although they may vary in structure, they all contain copper as an important cofactor. Human tyrosinase is a transmembrane protein and is sorted into specialized organelles in melanocytes called melanosomes such that melanin is ultimately synthesized and stored within these melanosomes[17]. Tyrosinase is an excellent example of convergent evolution in that although both animals and plants express tyrosinase, and although tyrosinase essentially performs the same function in all of these organisms, the structure and enzymatic requirements of these proteins are diverse. Regardless, tyrosinase regulates both the type and amount of melanin synthesized in the specialized cells that contain it. In humans, tyrosinase is encoded by the *tyr* gene which when mutated causes albinism in humans[18]. In Caucasians, tyr mutations can be identified in 56% of patients with autosomal recessive ocular albinism, characterized by reduced pigmentation of the eye[19].

3.2. Microphthalmia-Associated Transcription Factor (MITF)

Transcription of *tyr* is controlled by microphthalmia-associated transcription factor (MITF). MITF acts both as a transcription activator to promote expression of genes involved in melanogenesis within the cell cycle and as a transcriptional repressor of genes involved in invasion, making elevated MITF levels a possible biomarker for melanoma[20]. In humans, MITF regulates the expression of tyrosinase (TYR), tyrosinase-related protein-1 (TRP-1), and tyrosinase-related protein-2 (TRP-2). A complex regulatory network precisely modulates MITF expression and activation and therefore controls tyrosinase and melanogenesis. Therefore, targeting only tyrosinase or only MITF is destined to be either an ineffectual or a temporary intervention. It is likely that combination therapy that targets MITF, tyrosinase and the other regulatory pathways is more likely to produce a measurable and prolonged effect on skin pigmentation.

One of the key pathways in the stimulation of melanocytes in response to UV radiation is the adenylate cyclase pathway. UV radiation mediates the synthesis and release of alpha-melanocyte-stimulating hormone (α-MSH) which then promotes pigmentation by binding to the melanocortin 1 receptor (MC1R) on the surface of melanocytes. In people with the red-hair/fair-skin phenotype, the MC1R gene is non-signaling which leads to the increased risk for the development of melanoma. The production of cyclic adenosine monophosphate (cAMP) downstream of MC1R activates the receptors of MITF. MITF then participates in the conversion of tyrosine into melanin pigments by stimulating the transcription of melanocyte-specific genes. Therapeutic agents that are able to inhibit MITF through the down regulation of MC1R activity are likely to be particularly effective in reducing melanocyte activity.

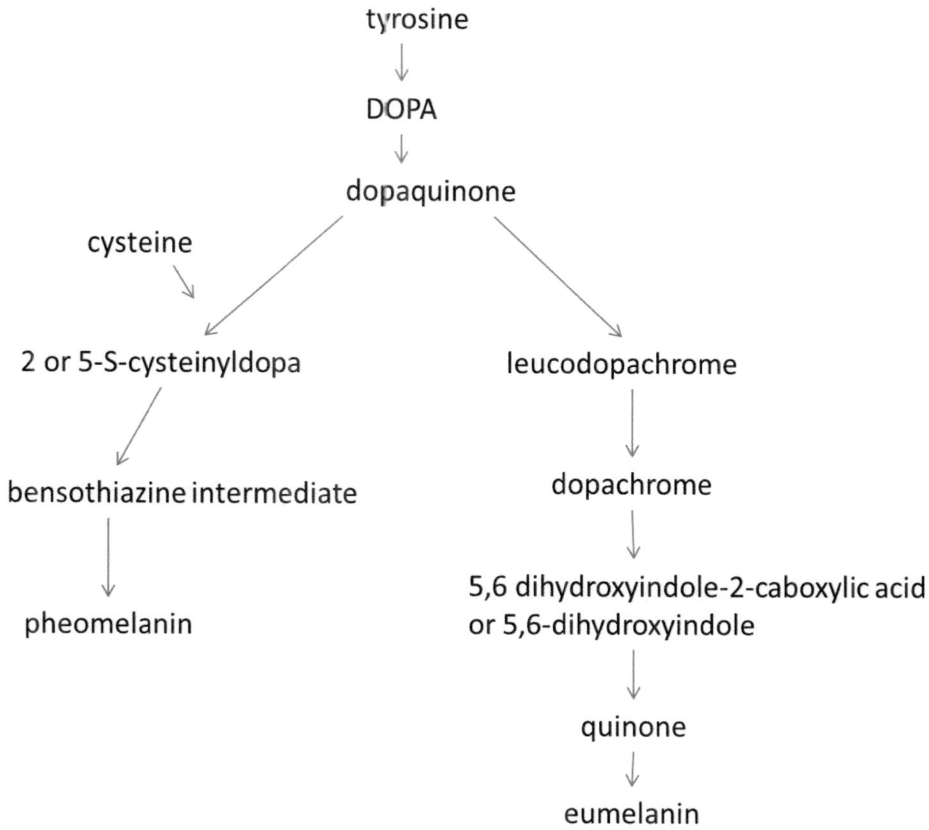

Figure 3. Melanin biosynthesis.

3.3. Keratinocytes

Keratinocytes are an important structural cell of the epidermis and comprise the majority of the cells in this layer of the skin. Throughout their life cycle, keratinocytes can take on many forms. Keratinocytes are produced by mitosis in the most basal layer of the epidermis when they begin to produce a great deal of keratin. Eventually, older keratinocytes are pushed up to the upper layers by the rapidly dividing keratinocytes beneath them until they reach the stratum granulosum where they begin to drastically change their morphological and biochemical functions. In the stratum granulosum, keratinocytes lose their organelles and acquire a flattened appearance. Due to their production of keratin, these cells become strong and their tightly bound structure makes the outermost keratinocyte layer strong and relatively impermeable.

An important role of keratinocytes is the transport of melanin through the layers of the skin. Once melanin is produced by melanocytes, the pigments are packaged into melanosomes that are subsequently translocated along the dendrites and then captured and aggregated by keratinocytes. The mechanism of transfer has long been a mystery, however a recent study summarizes the transfer mechanism in three steps: (i) the melanocyte's dendrite attaches to the surface of the keratinocyte, (ii) a portion of the melanocyte's dendrite sheds in order to deposit the melanosomes on the surface of the keratinocyte, (ii) and finally, the keratinocyte engulfs the melanosome package[21].

4. Natural ingredients that reduce pigmentation

Since a number of naturally derived bioactive molecules have been found to reduce skin pigmentation, the cosmetic industry has focused on the development of these compounds for use in their products. These compounds inhibit the production of melanin at different stages of melanogenesis. There are several compounds that specifically inhibit tyrosinase. For example, terrein, a bioactive fungal metabolite agent isolated from the *Penicilllium* species, has been shown to strongly decrease the production of tyrosinase by down-regulating MITF through dual pathways[22]. One pathway of these pathways may involve the activation of extracellular signal-regulated kinase (ERK) which has been reported to reduce melanin synthesis[23]. A second pathway recently identified may involve the ubiquitination and subsequent breakdown of tyrosinase itself[24].

Flavonoids, in particular, have received a great deal attention for their potential pigment-reducing activity because they are seen as "natural" and are associated with less side-effects than conventional medications and synthetically-designed compounds. Flavonoids are polyphenolic compounds typically found in plants. These compounds are ideal candidates for cosmetic purposes because of their potent bio-activities and low toxicity. Aloesin, a compound isolated from aloe extracts, has been shown to successfully reduce tyrosinase *in vitro* by inhibiting the hydroxylase activities[25], [26]. Resveratrol, a compound found in red wine, appears to have an affinity for tyrosinase and, by an unknown mechanism, reduces tyrosinase activity and MITF expression[27] although some studies have questioned its ability to reduce tyrosinase expression when used alone[28]. Flavonoids isolated from licorice are able to inhibit mushroom tyrosinase[29] and a skin lightening agent that uses licorice extract in its formulation (comprised of many bioactive ingredients) has been shown to reduce pigmentation in patients[30]. There are many reports of flavonoids from various sources interfering with or reducing the activity of tyrosinase, and although they all show some efficacy at reducing the biochemical pathways that lead to pigmentation, it is still unclear whether targeting these pathways in human skin would necessarily lead to reduced melanin formation *in vivo*.

Melanin formation is a complex process and there are compounds that may inhibit melanogenesis without necessarily inhibiting tyrosinase function. Anti-oxidants such as fermented rice bran and vanillic acid can reduce expression of MITF, MC1R, and associated biochemical pathways, without affecting tyrosinase activity,[31], [32] possibly due to their ability to impair peroxidase activity. Anti-oxidants, in general, may potentiate the MC1R pathway which itself is able to reduce downstream levels of hydrogen peroxide and promote nucleotide excision repair mechanisms in response to UV radiation[33]. The process of melanogenesis involves cell-to-cell communication between keratinocytes and melanosomes and compound such as niacinamide, a bioactive form of niacin (vitamin B3), has been shown to reduce pigmentation both *in vitro* and *in vivo* by downregulating the amount of melanosomes transferred to keratinocytes[34].

5. Photoaging and skin cells

5.1. Photoaging

As skin ages, a number of changes occur in the structure of the connective tissues. Healthy human dermis consists primarily of an extracellular matrix and a fibrous component formed by collagen and elastic fibers. The complex network of collagen accounts for approximately 80 percent of the dry weight of the skin and it is the component that provides the resistance to deformation. Elastic fibers comprise 2 to 4 percent of the dry weight of the skin and provide elasticity. Glycosaminoglycans (complex sugars, including hyaluronic acid) and water provide the viscous component of the deformation itself. As skin undergoes normal aging, a general reduction in the production of collagen fibers and proteins that make up the extracellular matrix contributes the formation of wrinkles and flaccid skin. Similarly an increased rate of degeneration of elastic fibers leads to the loss of elasticity.

Many of the changes that occur in skin structure as a result of aging are expressed prematurely in photodamaged skin, a phenomenon known as photoaging. Photoaging refers to the various cellular processes associated with senescence that result from photodamage. These processes are characterized by two events referred to as intrinsic (chronoaging) and extrinsic (photoaging) ageing. Leveque et al. first described the effects of chronic sun exposure on the mechanical properties of the skin and showed that long term sun exposure caused a decrease in skin extensibility and elastic recovery[35]. The skin also appeared thicker, more rigid and less susceptible to deformation. Berardesca and Maibach confirmed these findings using controlled ultraviolet (UVA) treatment and showed that even short term, low UVA and UVB exposure can impair skin elasticity and that inflammation and edema are characteristic of this process[36]. Other clinical features of photoaging include wrinkles, dyspigmentation, yellow hue, laxity, vascular ectasia, and malignancies. Adult populations in European and North American countries experience a prevalence of photoaging as high as 80 to 90 percent.

6. Photodamage and impact on skin cells

6.1. Photodamage

Photodamage refers to the damage of human skin by ultraviolet light, specifically UVA and UVB, and although the detailed mechanisms of photodamage are not fully understood, some general features have been described and are used as a standard by which topical treatments are judged. Physiological consequences of UVA radiation include thickening of the stratum corneum, epidermal hyperplasia, depletion of Langerhans cells, and dermal inflammation. Although it may seem as if these changes are random and entirely dependent upon UV exposure, photodamage is, in fact, a tightly controlled and regulated process that is facilitated by specialized skin cells. The ways in which these cells interact with each other and their extracellular matrix ultimately determines the morphological and histological consequences of light exposure in the skin. The cells and proteins involved in this process are numerous and the connections between them are complex. However, exposure of the skin to UVR initiates oxidative stress and triggers the synthesis of matrix metalloproteases (MMP) [37]. The production of MMP results in the degradation of dermal collagen and other matrix molecules thus reducing the elasticity and integrity of the skin[38].

6.2. Keratinocytes

Since keratinocytes in the upper layers of the epidermis are dead and do not underdo mitosis or metabolisis, they are relatively resistant to UVR induced damage. Younger, keratinocytes located deeper in the epidermis are much more susceptible to UVR damage and repeated UVR exposure results in accumulated DNA mutations that can lead to epidermal malignancies. Keratinocytes play a central role in elaborating innate responses that lead to inflammation and influence the generation of adaptive immune responses in skin.

Apart from the minor cellular constituents of the epidermis, specifically Langerhans cells and melanocytes, keratinocytes are the major source of cytokines. UV radiation exposure stimulates keratinocytes to secrete abundant pro-inflammatory IL-1-family proteins, IL-1α, IL-1β, IL-18, and IL-33. Normal skin contains only low levels of inactive precursor forms of IL-1β and IL-18, which require caspase 1-mediated proteolysis for their maturation and secretion. However, caspase-1 activation is not constitutive, but dependents on the UV-induced formation of an active inflammasome complex. IL-1 family cytokines can induce a secondary cascade of mediators and cytokines from keratinocytes and other cells resulting in wide range of innate processes including infiltration of inflammatory leukocytes, induction of immunosuppression, DNA repair or apoptosis. Thus, the ability of keratinocytes to produce a wide repertoire of proinflammatory cytokines can influence the immune response locally as well as systematically, and alter the host response to photodamaged cells.

6.3. Fibroblasts and langerhans cells

The most common type of cell found in the connective tissue of skin is fibroblast. They assist in producing and organizing the extracellular matrix of the dermis and also communicate with each other and other cells in the regulation of skin physiology. Dermal fibroblasts are a heterogeneous population and are identified by their location within the dermis. Fibroblasts that exist in the papillary dermis are generally in a more active state and divide at faster rates than those that exist in the reticular layer of the dermis[39]. Fibroblasts produce and secrete precursors of the extracellular matrix such as collagen, glycoproteins, and other molecules that support the structure of the skin.

http://dx.doi.org/10.5772/56425

Studies have shown that when exposed to UVA, fibroblasts proliferative activity is slowed or stopped due to morphological and functional changes. When exposed to sublethal UVA radiation does *in vitro*, researchers observed mutations in the mitochondrial DNA (mtDNA) in fibroblasts[40]. Subsequent studies have shown that the initial mutations in the mtDNA induced by UVR render the mitochondria in the fibroblasts more susceptible to ROS damage due to an increase in common deletions and a persistence of the mutations event after the termination of UVR exposure[41].

Langerhans cells are a subset of dendritic cells and are found in the epidermis of the skin. Langerhans cells play a role in the initiation and regulation of immune response by acquiring antigens in the skin and migrating to lymph nodes where immune responses are initiated. When human skin is exposed to UVR it results in a depletion of Langerhans cells and reduces the expression of immunophenotypic markers associated with antigen presentation[42]-[44]. The lack of functional Langerhans cells ultimately results in an immunosuppressive state in the skin[45] which also involves regulatory T cells and cytokine production[46].

6.4. Mast cells

It has been recognized that photoaging and normal chronological aging differ in several morphological and biological aspects, one of which is distinct alterations in elastic fibers and microvasculature. Previous studies have shown that one of the main contributors to this phenomenon is activation of immune cells in the epidermis, one of which is the mast cell. Studies comparing photo-exposed and sun-protected skin from the same individual shows that sun-exposed skin is characterized by the presence of higher numbers of infiltrating leucocytes and mast cells than is found in sun-protected skin[47]. Mast cells are cutaneous cells that contain pro-fibrotic and pro-inflammatory mediators and can contribute to skin inflammation and disease. Recent evidence has suggested that mast cells maintain tissue homeostasis and that many of the responses observed in photoaging are an attempt of the mast cell to repair damaged tissue systems. Mast cell activation can initiate or exacerbate many of the alterations associated with chronically sun-exposed skin such as massive accumulation of abnormal elastic fibers, loss of collagen, increase in glycosaminoglycans and telangiectatic vessels[47]. For example, mast cells produce fibroblast growth factors that can activate fibroblasts to produce abnormal matrix molecules. Mast cells also produce matrix-degrading enzymes and can activate the production of matrix proteinases by other skin cells such as keratinocytes. Mast cell products can recruit and activate infiltrating inflammatory cells such as neutrophils, macrophages and lymphocytes that can further damage the local tissue (see Figure 4).

Although an increased number of mast cells have been associated with photoaging, very little is known about their role in this process. The interaction between mast cells and other skin cells such as keratinocytes in photoaging is poorly understood. In fact, the precise mechanisms of mast cell activation in photodamaged skin is not known although it does not appear to be through the more common pathways such as the high affinity IgE receptor (FcεRI) or pathogen-associated pattern recognition receptors. In photoaging, mast cell acti-

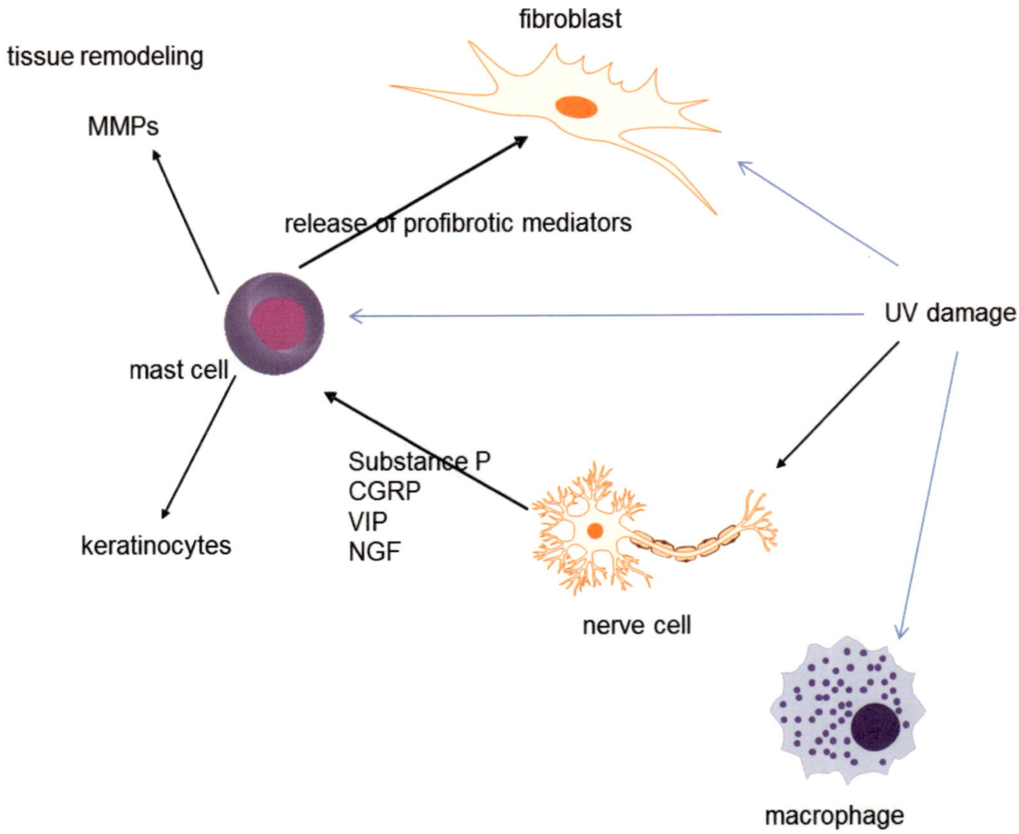

Figure 4. Role of skin cells in photoaging.

vation appears to be unique but our laboratory has shown that G protein coupled receptors (GPCR) may be responsible. Chronic exposure to UV causes sensory nerve fibers to release a series of neuropeptides including substance P (SP) and calcitonin gene-related peptide (CGRP)[48], both of which can activate mast cell degranulation and pro-inflammatory mediator release[49]. Furthermore, opiates that modify nerve function can also activate skin mast cells[50]. Interestingly, SP causes mast cells to downregulate their expression of allergen-activated receptors (FcεRI)[51] and primes them to respond to pathogen-activated (TLR) stimuli[52]. In skin that is chronically exposed to UV, mast cells may modulate a chronic inflammatory state, thus causing further damage to skin's structural integrity. Furthermore, mast cells appear to be important in the immunosuppressive environment of photodamaged skin since UVB causes a mast cell-dependent suppression of contact hypersensitivity responses[53]. This finding supports our hypothesis that human mast cells exposed to UV may undergo a phenotypic change from an allergic inflammatory effector cell to a more pathogen/structural response cell capable orchestrating structural changes in the skin. However, it is also possible that mast cell activation is a protective phenomenon and that further

http://dx.doi.org/10.5772/56425

potentiating mast cell activation in photodamaged skin may, in fact, inhibit or reverse some of the immunosuppression associated with photodamage.

6.5. Inflammation during photodamage

Traditionally, photodamage has been characterized by the mechanical damage caused to the skin's constituents – i.e. the degradation of the proteins and structures that hold the skin together and give its integrity. However, recent evidence has shown that at least some of the damage associated with UV exposure is due to the initiation of low but chronic inflammation that ultimately results in impaired cellular responses. This has some major implications because it suggests that the skin is not only losing its ability to form a physical barrier but is also losing some of its immune and regenerative abilities. Recent studies have shown that photodamage reduces immune responses by inhibiting the pathways that activate immune cells and causes changes in biochemical processes that regulate wound healing.

Using histological analysis, Bosset et al. showed that sun-exposed skin had an increase in infiltrating mononuclear cells than sun-protected skin[54]-[56]. Immunohistochemical analysis also showed an increased number of cells that one would normally associate with a Th2 inflammatory response – namely, mast cells, macrophages and CD4+ CD45RO+ T cells -- in sun-exposed dermis as well as a higher number of CD1a+ dendritic cells in sun-exposed epidermis, compared with the sun-protected samples. Although Bosset et al. found that photoaging displayed histological features of chronic skin inflammation they found a decreased expression of interleukin-1beta mRNA in sun-exposed compared with sun-protected suggesting that other pro-inflammatory mediators were mediating these effects. This hypothesis seems likely since these patients' skin looked clinically normal and would suggest an inflammatory pathology that is very different from those normally associated with acute Th2 inflammatory reactions such as atopic dermatitis or urticaria.

Inflammation is a complex process that has many different points of initiation and can be perpetuated by a diverse array of mediators. However, a study by Yan et al.[57] suggests that leukotrienes, potent lipid inflammatory mediators, may be responsible for this low but chronic inflammatory process associated with UV exposure. In their study, these investigators evaluated the protective effects of a nonsedative histamine H1-receptor antagonist, mizolastine, on UVB-exposed skin dermal fibroblasts. They found that relatively low levels of mizolastine (10 nM) inhibited UVB-induced LTB_4 production by skin fibroblasts. This decrease in LTB_4 production was associated with a down-regulation of 5-lipooxygenase (5-LO) mRNA expression and inhibition of 5-LO translocation suggesting that UV-induced leukotriene synthesis was dependent upon 5-LO expression.

The idea that chronic inflammation due to photodamage is a Th2 mediated response is possible, but some evidence suggests that it may be, in fact, a Th1 mediated event. UVB exposure of the skin results in a profound upregulation of the anti-inflammatory cytokine IL-10 and suppression of contact hypersensitivity (CHS). Furthermore, using an IL-10 transgenic mouse model (IL-10tg), Ma et al.[58] have shown that unexposed IL-10tg animals showed a diminished CHS response compared to wild-type. Yet when IL-10tg animals were exposed to UVB, the CHS response was not further suppressed, but rather was restored to the level observed in unexposed wild-type animals suggesting a normalization of the hypersensitivity response. If one believes that Th1 and Th2 responses counter-balance one another, this data would suggest that chronic inflammation associated with photodamage is mediated by a Th1 controlled inflammatory response.

7. Natural ingredients as treatments for photodamage and photodamage

7.1. Targeting the skin's immune response

Natural products that are used to treat the symptoms associated with photoaging and photodamage are designed to either stimulate new skin cell formation or inhibit the biochemical processes that cause skin damage. Sometimes, compounds are promoted as having biological activity in both of these contexts. Natural health products (NHPs) used to treat photodamaged skin are often mixtures of many different molecules and the precise mechanism of their beneficial effects are not always easy to determine from the myriad of information (anecdotal and experimental) available. However, there are a few groups of compounds that are naturally-derived and that appear to have some efficacy in at least reducing some of the biochemical manifestations of photodamage.

Botanical extracts are the most popular sources of naturally-sourced bioactives in skin health clinics. Most often, these are mixed into topical creams and applied to the epidermis. These extracts can even provide some small measure of sun protective activity (SPF) as well as reducing the biochemical and cellular consequences of photodamage described previously[59]. Topical application of green and white tea extracts, can reduce some of the detrimental immunomodulatory effects of photodamage[60]. Topical administration of Vitamin A and its analogues inhibit the expression of MMP and stimulate collagen synthesis in both photodamaged and photoprotected aged skin[61]. The list of these compounds is extensive and there are many comprehensive reviews on these compounds and their effects on human skin. However, these compounds all share the ability to modify the cellular responses in the dermis, whether through the induction of regenerative processes associated with keratinocyte renewal or inhibition of enzymes that break down the structural integrity of the skin. These compounds are all tested for their direct effect on these systems in bioassays designed to tease out the mechanisms on a single or small group of skin cells.

Some of these extracts, however, have efficacy when taken orally so their mechanisms of much more difficult to determine. For example, taking a specific *Polypodium leucotomos* extract (Fernblock, *Cantabria Farmaceutica*) 7.5 mg/kg daily for two doses before UVA treatment can modestly reduce erythema, edema, and signs of epidermal damage and may decrease subsequent hyperpigmentation in some patients[62]. In fact, it has been suggested that a diet rich in green tea polyphenols, grape seed proanthocyanidins and silymarin may act as chemopreventative agents to protect skin from photocarcinogenesis[63]. Taking what we know about the skin immune system and the possible molecular targets of these compounds we can hypothesize that this process may involve the induction of interleukin-12 (IL-12), DNA repair mechanisms, protection of Langerhans cell depletion and stimulation of cytotoxic T cells. However, many questions remain. How much of these chemoprotective agents must we eat and how often? Are some people (i.e. different skin tones) better protected by these dietary compounds than others? What are the best sources of these compounds in our diet? These are all relevant questions that are difficult to answer experimentally.

In addition to prophylactic treatments to alleviate the symptoms of photoaging, there is a strong market for compounds that can either stop or delay the sigs of photoaging. Anti-aging products are used to reduce the various cellular processes associated with senescence – both intrinsic (chronoaging) and extrinsic (photoaging) ageing. Younger individuals seek to prevent or reduce the manifestations of the extrinsic aging process which is responsible for approximately 80 percent of facial aging. Older individuals are often concerned with preventing or reversing the signs of both intrinsic and extrinsic aging processes. As such, treatments used to prevent photoaging target the underlying inflammatory and molecular responses associated with damage of skin integrity. Treatments used to reverse or stop the appearance of photoaging often target the biomechanical properties of skin.

There are numerous compounds currently on the market and in development and it is beyond the scope of this chapter to cover all of them. However, alpha hydroxy acids serve as excellent example to illustrate their effects on the skin microenvironment. AHA include glycolic, citric, lactic, malic, tartaric and lactic acids and are used extensively to promote skin rejuvenation and renewal. They are sometimes marketed as "fruit acids" because citric acid is found in citric fruits, malic acid is present in apples and tartaric acid is sometimes isolated from grapes. However, other foods also contain these acids (sugarcane contains glycolic acid and sour milk contains lactic acid). AHA work mainly by exfoliating the stratum corneum thus improving the smoothness and texture of skin. Although the exact mechanism of this effect is unknown, it is believed that AHA inhibit the enzymes that form ionic sulfate and phosphate bonds in the stratum corneum[64]. In the dermis, AHA induce desquamation and promoting cell renewal as well as stimulate collagen synthesis and induce dermal thickness[65].

AHA peels have recently been recognized as important adjunctive therapy in a variety of conditions including photodamage, actinic damage, melasma, hyperpigmentation disorders, acne, and rosacea. Since AHA are considered to have a reasonable level of safety and efficacy in a variety of skin types, they have been used extensively in the cosmetic industry as well[66]. Although their exact mechanism of action is unknown, it has been suggested that AHA improve skin pathological disorders by thinning the stratum corneum, promoting epidermolysis, dispersing basal layer melanin, and increasing collagen synthesis within the dermis[67]. Specifically in patients with photodamaged skin, AHA peels and topical products are often combined with retinoids and other antioxidants to reduce the thickness of the stratum corneum and smooth out the skin's surface. It has been suggested that AHA may help increase the skin's barrier function, making it more resilient to chemical damage[68].

A new class of hydroxy acids called polyhydroxy acids (PHAs), have similar effects as AHA but irritate the skin the same way as classical AHAs. PHAs cam be used on clinically sensitive skin, including rosacea and atopic dermatitis, and are compatible with cosmetic procedures[69]. Compared to AHA, PHA formulations are more moisturizing and can enhance stratum corneum barrier function. PHAs such as gluconolactone or lactobionic acid may be used in combination with other products, ingredients, or procedures such as laser and microdermabrasion to provide additional benefits to therapy or to enhance the therapeutic effect. PHAs used in combination with retinyl acetate (pro-vitamin A) in a cream base can have some anti-aging skin benefits such as skin smoothing and plumping although it is unclear if these also involve biochemical or immunomodulatory effects. In some formulations, PHA and hydroquinone together have demonstrated some superficial improvement in morphological changes associated with photoaging and have resulted in a decrease in skin pigmentation.

8. Conclusions

The skin is a complex and dynamic organ that is constantly bombarded with environmental trauma including UV radiation. UV light can cause major and often irreversible changes in the skin including damage to the three layers of skin. In the context of this constantly changing and sometimes harsh environment, the skin must maintain homeostasis and protect a delicate network of biochemical and physiological systems. There are a number of processes that are designed to protect the skin from photodamage, including the stratum corneum, melanin and underlying immunological processes to control inflammation. However, it is becoming increasingly clear that, over time, the skin's protective mechanisms can become overwhelmed by the damage caused by UV radiation, resulting in irreversible structural damage, chronic inflammation and, in some cases, photocarcinogenesis. Understanding the role that the microenvironment plays in this complex process is important to developing innovative new strategies for its treatment and possibly reversal.

Author details

Marianna Kulka*

National Research Council, Canada

References

[1] Wakamatsu K, Nakanishi Y, Miyazaki N, Kolbe L, Ito S. UVA-induced oxidative degradation of melanins: fission of indole moiety in eumelanin and conversion to benzothiazole moiety in pheomelanin. Pigment cell & melanoma research 2012; 25(4): 434-45.

[2] Curto EV, Kwong C, Hermersdorfer H, et al. Inhibitors of mammalian melanocyte tyrosinase: in vitro comparisons of alkyl esters of gentisic acid with other putative inhibitors. Biochemical pharmacology 1999; 57(6): 663-72.

[3] Wrzesniok D, Beberok A, Otreba M, Buszman E. Modulation of melanogenesis and antioxidant defense system in melanocytes by amikacin. Toxicology in vitro : an international journal published in association with BIBRA 2013; 27(3): 1102-8.

[4] Tadokoro T, Yamaguchi Y, Batzer J, et al. Mechanisms of skin tanning in different racial/ethnic groups in response to ultraviolet radiation. The Journal of investigative dermatology 2005; 124(6): 1326-32.

[5] Aalborg J, Morelli JG, Mokrohisky ST, et al. Tanning and increased nevus development in very-light-skinned children without red hair. Archives of dermatology 2009; 145(9): 989-96.

[6] Langholz B, Richardson J, Rappaport E, Waisman J, Cockburn M, Mack T. Skin characteristics and risk of superficial spreading and nodular melanoma (United States). Cancer causes & control : CCC 2000; 11(8): 741-50.

[7] Mitra D, Luo X, Morgan A, et al. An ultraviolet-radiation-independent pathway to melanoma carcinogenesis in the red hair/fair skin background. Nature 2012; 491(7424): 449-53.

[8] Gibney GT, Smalley KS. An unholy alliance: cooperation between BRAF and NF1 in melanoma development and BRAF inhibitor resistance. Cancer discovery 2013; 3(3): 260-3.

[9] Nagore E, Hacker E, Martorell-Calatayud A, et al. Prevalence of BRAF and NRAS mutations in fast-growing melanomas. Pigment cell & melanoma research 2013; 26(3): 429-31.

[10] Kuntsche J, Bunjes H, Fahr A, et al. Interaction of lipid nanoparticles with human epidermis and an organotypic cell culture model. International journal of pharmaceutics 2008; 354(1-2): 180-95.

[11] Kiss B, Biro T, Czifra G, et al. Investigation of micronized titanium dioxide penetration in human skin xenografts and its effect on cellular functions of human skin-derived cells. Experimental dermatology 2008; 17(8): 659-67.

[12] Larese FF, D'Agostin F, Crosera M, et al. Human skin penetration of silver nanoparticles through intact and damaged skin. Toxicology 2009; 255(1-2): 33-7.

[13] Lee WR, Shen SC, Al-Suwayeh SA, Yang HH, Li YC, Fang JY. Skin permeation of small-molecule drugs, macromolecules, and nanoparticles mediated by a fractional carbon dioxide laser: the role of hair follicles. Pharmaceutical research 2013; 30(3): 792-802.

[14] Abdel-Mottaleb MM, Moulari B, Beduneau A, Pellequer Y, Lamprecht A. Surface-charge-dependent nanoparticles accumulation in inflamed skin. Journal of pharmaceutical sciences 2012; 101(11): 4231-9.

[15] Abdel-Mottaleb MM, Moulari B, Beduneau A, Pellequer Y, Lamprecht A. Nanoparticles enhance therapeutic outcome in inflamed skin therapy. European journal of pharmaceutics and biopharmaceutics : official journal of Arbeitsgemeinschaft fur Pharmazeutische Verfahrenstechnik eV 2012; 82(1): 151-7.

[16] Chourasia R, Jain SK. Drug targeting through pilosebaceous route. Current drug targets 2009; 10(10): 950-67.

[17] Seiji M, Fitzpatrick TB. The reciprocal relationship between melanization and tyrosinase activity in melanosomes (melanin granules). Journal of biochemistry 1961; 49: 700-6.

[18] Kinnear PE, Jay B, Witkop CJ, Jr. Albinism. Survey of ophthalmology 1985; 30(2): 75-101.

[19] Hutton SM, Spritz RA. A comprehensive genetic study of autosomal recessive ocular albinism in Caucasian patients. Investigative ophthalmology & visual science 2008; 49(3): 868-72.

[20] Koludrovic D, Davidson I. MITF, the Janus transcription factor of melanoma. Future oncology 2013; 9(2): 235-44.

[21] Wu XS, Masedunskas A, Weigert R, Copeland NG, Jenkins NA, Hammer JA. Melanoregulin regulates a shedding mechanism that drives melanosome transfer from melanocytes to keratinocytes. Proceedings of the National Academy of Sciences of the United States of America 2012; 109(31): E2101-9.

[22] Park SH, Kim DS, Kim WG, et al. Terrein: a new melanogenesis inhibitor and its mechanism. Cellular and molecular life sciences : CMLS 2004; 61(22): 2878-85.

[23] Kim HE, Ishihara A, Lee SG. The effects of Caffeoylserotonin on inhibition of melanogenesis through the downregulation of MITF via the reduction of intracellular cAMP and acceleration of ERK activation in B16 murine melanoma cells. BMB reports 2012; 45(12): 724-9.

[24] Park SH, Kim DS, Lee HK, et al. Long-term suppression of tyrosinase by terrein via tyrosinase degradation and its decreased expression. Experimental dermatology 2009; 18(6): 562-6.

[25] Jones K, Hughes J, Hong M, Jia Q, Orndorff S. Modulation of melanogenesis by aloesin: a competitive inhibitor of tyrosinase. Pigment cell research / sponsored by the European Society for Pigment Cell Research and the International Pigment Cell Society 2002; 15(5): 335-40.

[26] Gillbro JM, Olsson MJ. The melanogenesis and mechanisms of skin-lightening agents--existing and new approaches. International journal of cosmetic science 2011; 33(3): 210-21.

[27] Solano F, Briganti S, Picardo M, Ghanem G. Hypopigmenting agents: an updated review on biological, chemical and clinical aspects. Pigment cell research / sponsored by the European Society for Pigment Cell Research and the International Pigment Cell Society 2006; 19(6): 550-71.

[28] Kim SY, Park KC, Kwon SB, Kim DS. Hypopigmentary effects of 4-n-butylresorcinol and resveratrol in combination. Die Pharmazie 2012; 67(6): 542-6.

[29] Fu B, Li H, Wang X, Lee FS, Cui S. Isolation and identification of flavonoids in licorice and a study of their inhibitory effects on tyrosinase. Journal of agricultural and food chemistry 2005; 53(19): 7408-14.

[30] Makino ET, Mehta RC, Banga A, Jain P, Sigler ML, Sonti S. Evaluation of a hydroquinone-free skin brightening product using in vitro inhibition of melanogenesis and clinical reduction of ultraviolet-induced hyperpigmentation. Journal of drugs in dermatology : JDD 2013; 12(3): s16.

[31] Chou TH, Ding HY, Hung WJ, Liang CH. Antioxidative characteristics and inhibition of alpha-melanocyte-stimulating hormone-stimulated melanogenesis of vanillin and vanillic acid from Origanum vulgare. Experimental dermatology 2010; 19(8): 742-50.

[32] Chung SY, Seo YK, Park JM, et al. Fermented rice bran downregulates MITF expression and leads to inhibition of alpha-MSH-induced melanogenesis in B16F1 melanoma. Bioscience, biotechnology, and biochemistry 2009; 73(8): 1704-10.

[33] Abdel-Malek ZA, Knittel J, Kadekaro AL, Swope VB, Starner R. The melanocortin 1 receptor and the UV response of human melanocytes--a shift in paradigm. Photochemistry and photobiology 2008; 84(2): 501-8.

[34] Hakozaki T, Minwalla L, Zhuang J, et al. The effect of niacinamide on reducing cutaneous pigmentation and suppression of melanosome transfer. The British journal of dermatology 2002; 147(1): 20-31.

[35] Leveque JL, Poelman MC, Legall F, de Rigal J. New experimental approach to measure the skin-reflected light. Application to cutaneous erythema and blanching. Dermatologica 1985; 170(1): 12-6.

[36] Berardesca E, Farage M, Maibach H. Sensitive skin: an overview. International journal of cosmetic science 2013; 35(1): 2-8.

[37] Fisher GJ, Datta SC, Talwar HS, et al. Molecular basis of sun-induced premature skin ageing and retinoid antagonism. Nature 1996; 379(6563): 335-9.

[38] Szendroi M, Meimon G, Bakala H, et al. On the presence of a metalloprotease in human skin fibroblasts that degrades the human skin elastic fiber system. The Journal of investigative dermatology 1984; 83(3): 224-9.

[39] Sorrell JM, Caplan AI. Fibroblast heterogeneity: more than skin deep. Journal of cell science 2004; 117(Pt 5): 667-75.

[40] Berneburg M, Grether-Beck S, Kurten V, et al. Singlet oxygen mediates the UVA-induced generation of the photoaging-associated mitochondrial common deletion. The Journal of biological chemistry 1999; 274(22): 15345-9.

[41] Gremmel T, Wild S, Schuller W, et al. Six genes associated with the clinical phenotypes of individuals with deficient and proficient DNA repair. Translational oncogenomics 2008; 3: 1-13.

[42] Aberer W, Schuler G, Stingl G, Honigsmann H, Wolff K. Ultraviolet light depletes surface markers of Langerhans cells. The Journal of investigative dermatology 1981; 76(3): 202-10.

[43] Stingl G, Gazze-Stingl LA, Aberer W, Wolff K. Antigen presentation by murine epidermal langerhans cells and its alteration by ultraviolet B light. Journal of immunology 1981; 127(4): 1707-13.

[44] Aberer W, Leibl H. Effect of UVB radiation on the biosynthesis of HLA-DR antigens. Archives of dermatological research 1987; 279(5): 321-6.

[45] Schwarz A, Noordegraaf M, Maeda A, Torii K, Clausen BE, Schwarz T. Langerhans cells are required for UVR-induced immunosuppression. The Journal of investigative dermatology 2010; 130(5): 1419-27.

[46] Schwarz T, Schwarz A. Molecular mechanisms of ultraviolet radiation-induced immunosuppression. European journal of cell biology 2011; 90(6-7): 560-4.

[47] Lavker RM. Structural alterations in exposed and unexposed aged skin. The Journal of investigative dermatology 1979; 73(1): 59-66.

[48] Eschenfelder CC, Benrath J, Zimmermann M, Gillardon F. Involvement of substance P in ultraviolet irradiation-induced inflammation in rat skin. The European journal of neuroscience 1995; 7(7): 1520-6.

[49] Kulka M, Sheen CH, Tancowny BP, Grammer LC, Schleimer RP. Neuropeptides activate human mast cell degranulation and chemokine production. Immunology 2008; 123(3): 398-410.

[50] Sheen CH, Schleimer RP, Kulka M. Codeine induces human mast cell chemokine and cytokine production: involvement of G-protein activation. Allergy 2007; 62(5): 532-8.

[51] McCary C, Tancowny BP, Catalli A, et al. Substance P downregulates expression of the high affinity IgE receptor (FcepsilonRI) by human mast cells. Journal of neuroimmunology 2010; 220(1-2): 17-24.

[52] Tancowny BP, Karpov V, Schleimer RP, Kulka M. Substance P primes lipoteichoic acid- and Pam3CysSerLys4-mediated activation of human mast cells by up-regulating Toll-like receptor 2. Immunology 2010; 131(2): 220-30.

[53] Hart PH, Grimbaldeston MA, Swift GJ, Jaksic A, Noonan FP, Finlay-Jones JJ. Dermal mast cells determine susceptibility to ultraviolet B-induced systemic suppression of contact hypersensitivity responses in mice. The Journal of experimental medicine 1998; 187(12): 2045-53.

[54] Bosset S, Barre P, Chalon A, et al. Skin ageing: clinical and histopathologic study of permanent and reducible wrinkles. European journal of dermatology : EJD 2002; 12(3): 247-52.

[55] Bosset S, Bonnet-Duquennoy M, Barre P, et al. Photoageing shows histological features of chronic skin inflammation without clinical and molecular abnormalities. The British journal of dermatology 2003; 149(4): 826-35.

[56] Bosset S, Bonnet-Duquennoy M, Barre P, et al. Decreased expression of keratinocyte beta1 integrins in chronically sun-exposed skin in vivo. The British journal of dermatology 2003; 148(4): 770-8.

[57] Yan Y, Wang B, Zuo YG, Qu T. Inhibitory effects of mizolastine on ultraviolet B-induced leukotriene B4 production and 5-lipoxygenase expression in normal human dermal fibroblasts in vitro. Photochemistry and photobiology 2006; 82(3): 665-9.

[58] Ma LJ, Guzman EA, DeGuzman A, et al. Unexpected effects of UVB in IL-10 transgenic mice: normalization of contact hypersensitivity response. Archives of dermatological research 2006; 297(9): 417-20.

[59] Matsui MS, Hsia A, Miller JD, et al. Non-sunscreen photoprotection: antioxidants add value to a sunscreen. The journal of investigative dermatology Symposium proceedings / the Society for Investigative Dermatology, Inc [and] European Society for Dermatological Research 2009; 14(1): 56-9.

[60] Camouse MM, Domingo DS, Swain FR, et al. Topical application of green and white tea extracts provides protection from solar-simulated ultraviolet light in human skin. Experimental dermatology 2009; 18(6): 522-6.

[61] Offord EA, Gautier JC, Avanti O, et al. Photoprotective potential of lycopene, beta-carotene, vitamin E, vitamin C and carnosic acid in UVA-irradiated human skin fibroblasts. Free radical biology & medicine 2002; 32(12): 1293-303.

[62] Middelkamp-Hup MA, Pathak MA, Parrado C, et al. Oral Polypodium leucotomos extract decreases ultraviolet-induced damage of human skin. Journal of the American Academy of Dermatology 2004; 51(6): 910-8.

[63] Katiyar SK. UV-induced immune suppression and photocarcinogenesis: chemoprevention by dietary botanical agents. Cancer letters 2007; 255(1): 1-11.

[64] Berardesca E, Distante F, Vignoli GP, Oresajo C, Green B. Alpha hydroxyacids modulate stratum corneum barrier function. The British journal of dermatology 1997; 137(6): 934-8.

[65] Inan S, Oztukcan S, Vatansever S, et al. Histopathological and ultrastructural effects of glycolic acid on rat skin. Acta histochemica 2006; 108(1): 37-47.

[66] Van Scott EJ, Yu RJ. Alpha hydroxy acids: procedures for use in clinical practice. Cutis; cutaneous medicine for the practitioner 1989; 43(3): 222-8.

[67] Fartasch M, Teal J, Menon GK. Mode of action of glycolic acid on human stratum corneum: ultrastructural and functional evaluation of the epidermal barrier. Archives of dermatological research 1997; 289(7): 404-9.

[68] Rawlings AV, Davies A, Carlomusto M, et al. Effect of lactic acid isomers on keratinocyte ceramide synthesis, stratum corneum lipid levels and stratum corneum barrier function. Archives of dermatological research 1996; 288(7): 383-90.

[69] Grimes PE, Green BA, Wildnauer RH, Edison BL. The use of polyhydroxy acids (PHAs) in photoaged skin. Cutis; cutaneous medicine for the practitioner 2004; 73(2 Suppl): 3-13.

Chapter 10

Asthma in the 21st Century — Unexpected Applications of Ancient Treatments

Priyanka Pundir, Xiaofeng Wang and
Marianna Kulka

Additional information is available at the end of the chapter

http://dx.doi.org/10.5772/56428

1. Introduction

Asthma comes from the Greek word for "panting" and has been described as a pathological condition for centuries. It is a chronic inflammatory disorder of the airways in which many immunological cells play a role, including mast cells and eosinophils. In susceptible individuals, this inflammation causes symptoms which are usually associated with widespread variable airflow obstruction that is often reversible, either spontaneously or with treatment, and causes an associated airway hyperresponsiveness (AHR) to a variety of stimuli. The clinical features of asthma include dyspnea, wheezing and coughing.

During the last forty years there has been an increased understanding of the wide spectrum of this disease and as a result a number of effective treatments have been developed. Despite these advances, however, the mortality continues to increase and approximately 500 Canadians and 3500 Americans die each year from asthma. It remains a major cause of morbidity, as the leading cause of school absenteeism and the third leading cause of work absenteeism. The prevalence of asthma in North America has been on a constant rise over the last 25 years and it is estimated that currently over 3 million Canadians and 25 million Americans suffer from asthma. Worldwide the prevalence rates of asthma are rising on average by 50% each decade and developing a better understanding of the risk factors associated with this trend is critical. These may be broadly classified as either host genetic factors or environmental factors (Table 1).

One of the marked risk factors of asthma associated with the westernized lifestyle is our changing diet and/or nutritional status. It has been hypothesized that the significant change in our diet plays a dominant role in the etiology of asthma. Seaton *et al.* have proposed that

Genetic Factors	Environmental Factors
Atopy Gender Genetic predisposition Race/ethnicity	Smoking Allergens Occupational sensitizers Respiratory infections Parasitic infections Perinatal risk factors Diet and nutrition

Table 1. Risk factors associated with asthma

asthma prevalence has increased in UK because of an alteration in diet associated with industrialization [1]. This has lead to a substantial decline in the consumption of fresh fruits, green vegetables, fish and red meat, and as a result decrease in pulmonary antioxidant defences and an increase in susceptibility to inhaled irritants and allergens [1]. These foods are the main sources of antioxidants, substances that protect cells against the effects of free radicals generated during oxidative stress.

Oxidative stress is important in the pathophysiology of asthma [2] and development of AHR [3]. A large number of epidemiologic studies have reported the protective effects of dietary antioxidants such as micronutrients vitamin A, C, and E, polyphenol, and carotenoids against the development of asthma and decline of lung function. In a study on American children higher levels of antioxidants beta-carotene and Vitamin C, along with antioxidant trace mineral selenium is associated with a lower risk of asthma [4]. Dietary vitamin C intake is positively associated with 1 Second Forced Expiratory Volume (FEV_1) in children and adults [5-8] but less frequently with asthma or wheeze in children and adults [4, 9-11]. Dietary vitamin E intake is positively associated with ventilatory function [5, 6, 12] but negatively associated with asthma and wheeze in children [13], adult-onset wheeze [11] and the likelihood of atopic sensitization in adults [14]. Fresh fruits intake is inversely associated with wheeze [15] and chronic lung disease onset [16] and is positively associated with FEV_1 [17]. Total fruit and vegetable intake is inversely related to asthma prevalence [18] but not to FEV_1 [19] or airway obstruction [20]. Vegetables may protect against chronic bronchitis, asthma [21], and wheeze [22]. Moreover, dietary polyphenols intake are associated with lower disease risk with beneficial clinical outcomes attributed to both the antioxidants and anti-inflammatory properties of polyphenols [23]. Polyphenols consist of a large group of natural antioxidants extracted from plants and flavonoids comprise the most studied group.

In addition to antioxidants, intake of fats, particularly the changing composition of polyunsaturated fatty acids (PUFA) in westernized diets, has been implicated in the etiology of asthma. There has been a reduced intake of saturated fat accompanied by an increase in n-6 PUFA consumption, particularly linoleic acid and arachidonic acid. In addition, there has been a decrease in consumption of n-3 PUFA such as eicosapentaenoic acid (EPA) and docosahexaenoic acid (DHA). Thus, it has been postulated that the increased ratio of n-6:n-3 PUFA in diets of industrialized countries may also contributed to the increased asthma incidence.

Ancient Egyptian papyrus writings contain prescriptions for asthma that include several herbs suggesting that naturally occurring bioactive compounds may been used to effectively treat asthma. This chapter summarizes the current knowledge on the effects of dietary compounds and nutrients on allergy and asthma, with a focus on the mechanisms involved, wherever possible.

2. Pathogenesis of asthma

Airway inflammation in asthma is a complex process involving the interactions between immunological mediators produced by inflammatory cells such as mast cells, eosinophils, basophils, neutrophils, dendritic cells and lymphocytes [24]. This inflammation leads to structural and architectural changes in the airways of asthmatic patients including collagen and fibronectin deposition, wall thickening, subepithelial fibrosis and hypertrophy, goblet and airway smooth muscle cell hyperplasia, and angiogenesis, all of which collectively contribute to the phenomenon known as airway remodeling [25].

Allergic inflammation is often classified into four phases [26]:

a. Induction of allergic reaction involving antigen uptake, processing and presentation (Figure 1),

b. Early-phase asthmatic reaction (EAR, Figure 2),

c. Late-phase asthmatic reactions (LAR, Figure 3), and

d. Chronic allergic inflammation (Figure 4)

3. Common molecular targets used in current asthma therapy

Inspite of the advances made in the field of asthma treatments, some patients remain less responsive to conventional therapies than others. Current treatment strategy includes the combinations of bronchodilators, particularly short or long acting β_2-adrenergic agonists (SABA, LABA), and inhaled and oral corticosteroids. The current approach to the management of asthma includes the addition of drugs in a stepwise fashion based on the severity of symptoms, however the stronger drugs include more severe side effects. The treatment aims to reverse airflow obstruction and reduces asthma exacerbations thus improving quality of life. However, long-term use of high dose inhaled corticosteroids therapy may lead to detrimental effects, such as cataracts [46], osteoporosis in elderly patients [47], and stunting of growth in children [48]. Moreover, the combination therapy may not modify the disease progression and are not curative.

The limited efficacy and side effects associated with conventional treatments has lead to the introduction of nutraceuticals as a "safer"alternative therapy and for those whom symptoms

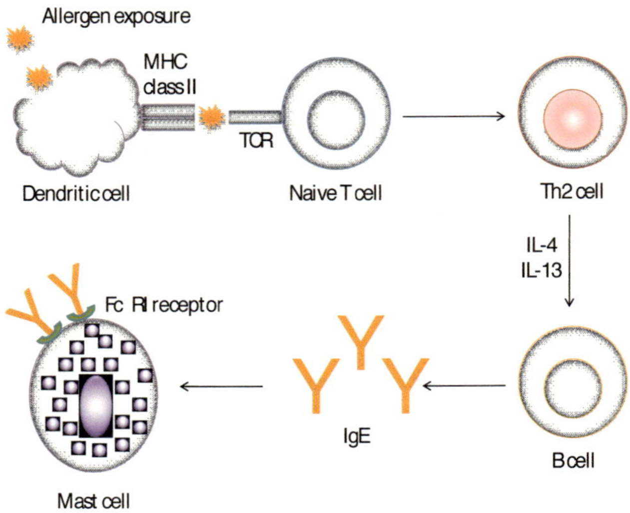

Figure 1. AHR and bronchial inflammation starts with the inhalation of an allergen. The allergen enters tissues through disrupted epithelium. It is then captured by antigen-presenting cells (APCs), usually dendritic cells (DCs), but also alveolar macrophages and B cells [27]. Allergen-loaded DCs migrate to regional lymph nodes where they present peptides to naïve T cells [28]. Presentation of processed allergen in the form of peptide fragments on MHC class II molecules to naïve T cells signals activation and clonal expansion of T cells [27]. In the presence of interleukin (IL)-4, naïve T cells acquire the characteristic of T helper 2 (Th2) cells [29]. Activated Th2 cells secrete greater amounts of IL-4 and IL-13 which triggers the isotype switch to immunoglobulin (Ig)E synthesis [29, 30]. IgE produced by B cells diffuses locally, enters the blood and is then distributed systematically. Allergen-specific or non-specific IgE binds to the high-affinity receptor for IgE (FcεRI) on the surface of tissue-resident mast cells and peripheral blood basophils, thereby sensitizing them to future allergen exposures [30].

are not improved with current therapies. Nutraceuticals is a very general term which encompasses many classifications of food products and derivatives that have the potential to either prevent or treat pathological conditions in humans or animals. For example, micronutrients such as vitamins and minerals and non-nutritive components of plant products such as polyphenols have some anti-inflammatory activity and have been used to supplement some foods to improve their health benefits. Table 3 summarizes some of the major nutraceuticals used to treat allergy and asthma currently.

The following sections discuss the current knowledge on the effects of nutraceuticals on inflammation associated with asthma with a focus on the cellular and molecular mechanism involved.

3.1. Anti-mediator agents

Anti-mediator agents are a group of drugs that antagonize the release of granule-associated preformed mediators, lipid mediators, cytokines, chemokines, and growth factors released by allergen-activated inflammatory cells. Several important groups of specific inhibitors against many of these inhibitors have been developed.

http://dx.doi.org/10.5772/56428

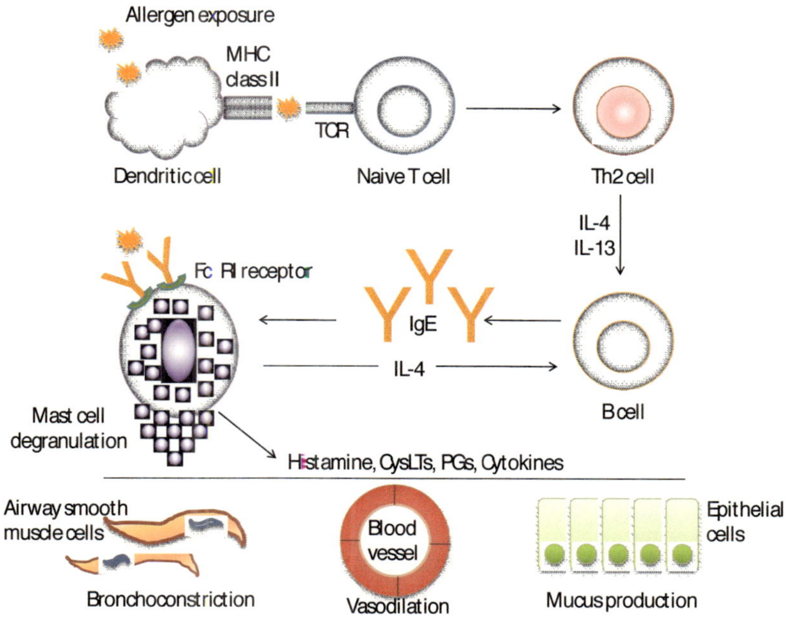

Figure 2. The EAR occurs within 30 min of allergen exposure and is principally initiated by mast cell and basophil activation [26]. Mast cells are widely distributed throughout the human respiratory tract and are found in large numbers in the walls of the alveoli and airways [31]. Asthmatics have allergen-specific IgE bound to the FcεRI receptors on mast cell surface. Upon cross-linking of adjacent IgE molecules by allergen, aggregation of FcεRI triggers a complex intracellular signaling process [32]. Activated mast cells release a diverse array of biologically active mediators: preformed granule-associated mediators, lipid-derived mediators, and *de novo* synthesized cytokines, chemokines, growth factors and other biologically active molecules (Table 2) [33]. The release of mast cell-derived mediators contributes to acute signs and symptoms associated with EAR that may range from mild rhinitis to anaphylactic shock. These mediators induce vasodilation, contraction of the bronchial smooth muscle (producing airflow obstruction and wheezing) and increased mucus secretion (exacerbating airflow obstruction in the lower airways) [26].

3.1.1. Lipid mediator blockers

Montelukast is a current FDA approved drug used in asthma treatment and serves a prototypical drug for Lipid Mediator Blocking class of drugs. Its mechanism of actions works through the blocking of the CysLT receptor for leukotriene D_4 which reduces bronchoconstriction and inflammation. Zileuton, a related drug in the same class, is a 5-lipoxygenase inhibitor which blocks the synthesis of cysLTs and leukotriene B_4. These drugs while not natural products serve as a models in the search for nutraceuticals whom may share same or related mechanism of action and therefore may prove useful in asthma management. Antagonists of the prostaglandin D_2 receptors DP1 and CRTH2 reduce inflammation in a murine model of asthma, possibly by inhibiting prostaglandin synthesis [49, 50]. Antagonist of the leukotriene B_4 receptor BLT1 (R05101576) prevents airway inflammation and AHR in animal models and non-human primates [51]. Quercetin and luteolin, flavonoids found in fruits, vegetables and wine, inhibit the release of leukotrienes and PGD2 from human cultured mast cells [52]. Table 4 summarizes phytochemicals that act on pathways related to the synthesis of lipid mediators in allergic inflammation.

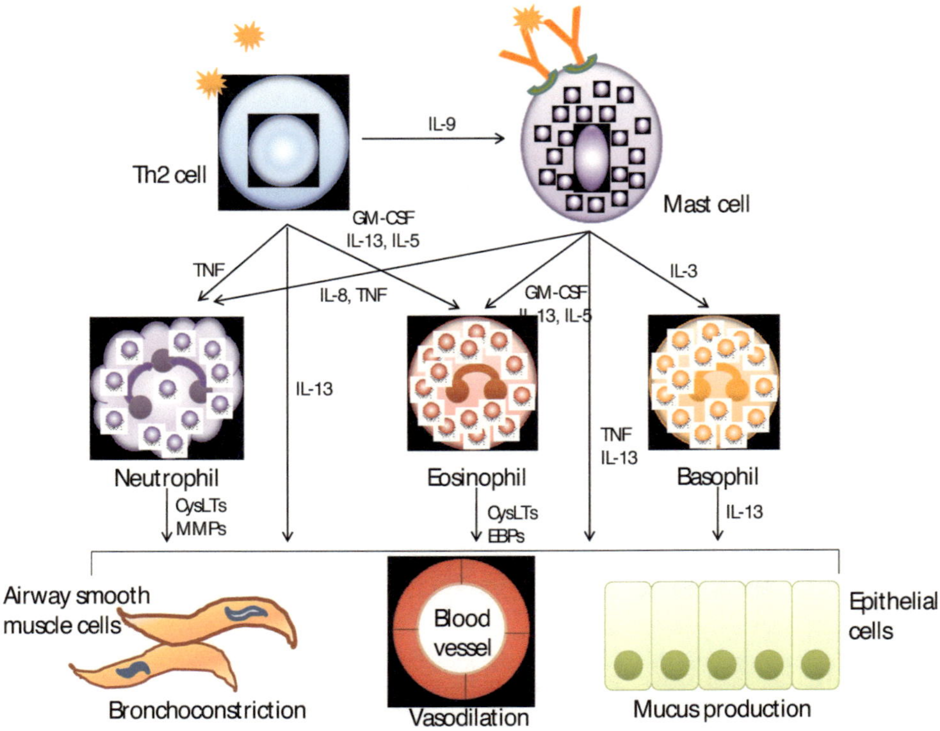

Figure 3. The LAR typically develops 2-6 hr following allergen challenge, often peaks after 6-9 hr, and has a more severe and prolonged phase. In general, allergen activated mast cells release various *de novo* synthesized cytokines, chemokines and growth factors, which are released more slowly than granule-associated mediators [34]. Thus, LAR is sustained by *de novo* synthesized mast cell-derived mediators which recruit inflammatory cells to the airways several hours after allergen challenge. These recruited cells include effector cells, such as eosinophils, basophils, neutrophils, macrophages, T cells, and DCs [34, 35]. These inflammatory cells are activated when they reach the airway and produce a vast array of inflammatory mediators that act on specific receptors and exacerbate airway inflammation and airway remodeling. Eosinophils are the central effector cells in the LAR [36], and are present not only in the airway wall [37] but are also found in large numbers in the sputum and bronchoalveolar lavage fluid (BALF) [38]. Eosinophils are a rich source of granule basic proteins (EBP), such as major basic proteins (MBP), eosinophil cationic protein (ECP), eosinophil peroxidase (EPO), and eosinophil-derived neurotoxin (EDN), and can also generate lipid-mediators (prostaglandins and cysteinyl leukotrienes), cytokines (such as TNF, TGF-β, IL-4 and IL-13) and chemokines [39]. These eosinophil-derived products promote some of the pathophysiological hallmarks of asthma such as AHR [40]. The activation of peripheral blood neutrophils during allergen challenge results in their intravascular migration, adhesion to the endothelium, and migration to the site of inflammation and can be responsible for significant damage. Nocturnal asthma is associated with high levels of neutrophils, which correlate with the severity of the disease [41]. Furthermore, in a small number of patients who died of sudden-onset asthma, the predominant cell type in the sputum is the neutrophils, not eosinophils [42]. Neutrophils also predominate more frequently in the sputum of patients with acute exacerbations of asthma, mostly associated with respiratory tract infection [43]. T cells are not only important during the induction phase, but play also a very important role during ongoing inflammation. Th2 cells and their cytokines are crucial for promoting acute hypersensitivity responses, and for maintaining the state of chronic and relapsing eosinophil-predominant inflammation that is characteristic of chronic allergic inflammation. Elevated levels of $CD4^+$ T cells are observed in the bronchial mucosa of biopsy samples, BALF and sputum from patients with asthma [44]. In a majority of studies, T cells found in asthmatic patients express cytokines or transcription factors characteristic of Th2 cells, especially IL-4, IL-5, IL-9 and IL-13 [45].

http://dx.doi.org/10.5772/56428

Class of Product	Examples	Biological Effects
Preformed Mediators	Histamine, heparin	Increase vascular permeability, smooth muscle contraction
Enzymes	Tryptase, chymase, cathepsin G, carboxypeptidase	Remodel tissue matrix
Cytokines	IL-4, IL-13	Stimulate Th2 cell response
	IL-3, IL-5, GM-CSF	Promote eosinophil production and activation
	Tumor necrosis factor (TNF)	Promotes inflammation and cytokine release by immune cells
Chemokines	CCL2, CCL3, CCL4, CXCL1, CXCL2, CXCL3, CXCL10	Attract monocytes, macrophages and neutrophils
Lipid Mediators	Prostaglandin D_2, E2 Leukotriene B4, C4	Cause smooth muscle contraction, increase vascular permeability, stimulate mucus secretion
	Platelet-activating factor	Attracts leukocytes, amplifies production of lipid mediators, activates neutrophils, eosinophils and platelets

Table 2. Mast cell-derived proinflammatory mediators

Antioxidants		
Vitamin A	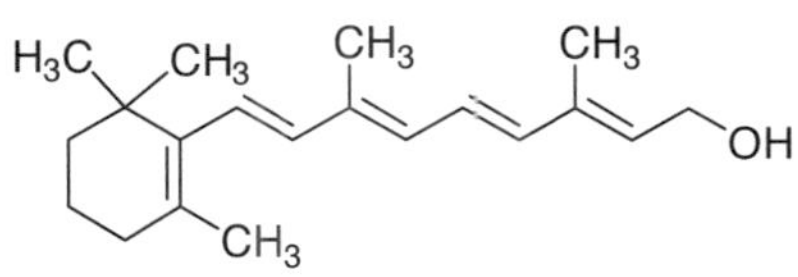	Vitamin A (retinoid) occurs in many foods, including carrots, broccoli, sweet potato, butter, spinach, pumpkin, and liver, cod liver oil. The form found in colorful fruits and vegetables is called provitamin A carotenoid.
Vitamin C	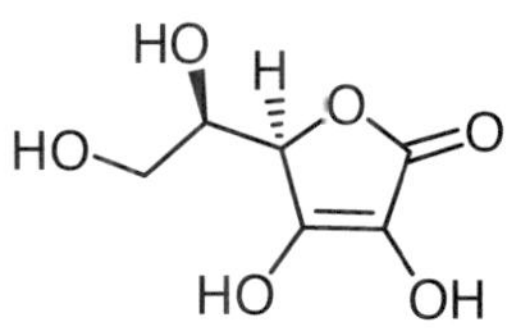	Vitamin C (ascorbic acid) is an essential nutrient for humans as it protects the body against oxidative stress and is a necessary in collagen synthesis. Fruits (kakadu plum, camu camu, rose hip, indian gooseberry, blackcurrant, orange, tangerine, and guava) and vegetables (green and red chilli pepper, red pepper, broccoli, Brussels sprout, spinach, and cabbage) are good sources of Vitamin C.
Vitamin E	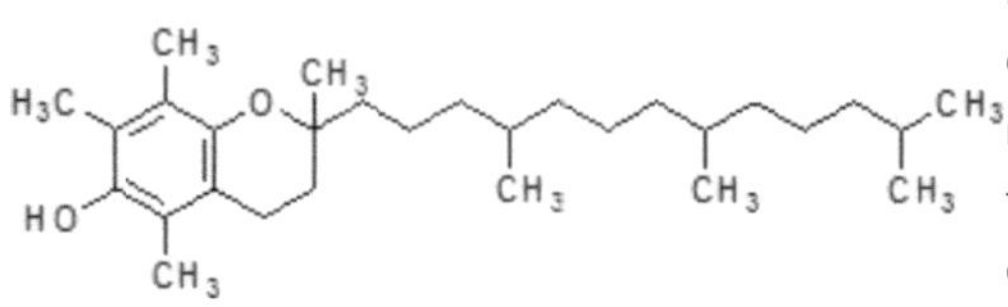	Vitamin E is a fat-soluble vitamin that exists in eight different forms. It consists of a group of substances belonging to two closely related families, the tocopherols and tocotrienols, with each existing in a number of isomeric forms (α, β, γ, and δ). α-tocopherol is the most active form of Vitamin E in humans and is considered the major

Antioxidants		
		membrane-bound antioxidant employed by cells. Its main antioxidant function is protection against lipid peroxidation. There is an interaction between Vitamin E and other nutrients, particularly selenium and vitamin C in the antioxidant role. Vitamin E is found in fruits (tomato, mango, and papaya), green leafy vegetables (lettuce, spinach, turnip, and beet), nuts and nut oils (almonds and hazelnuts), vegetable oils (wheat germ oil, sunflower oil, and safflower oil), meat, and poultry.
Vitamin D	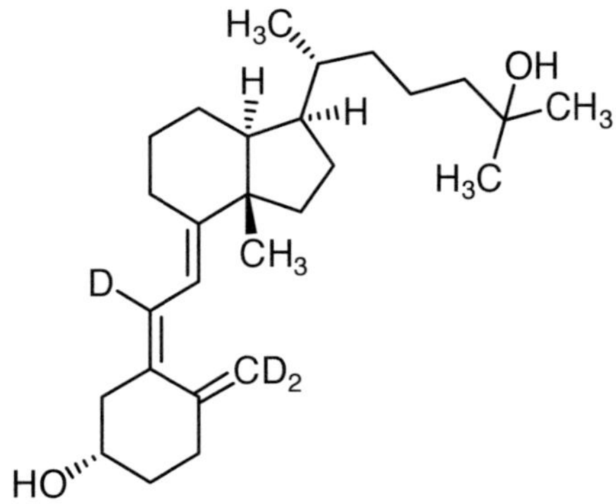	
Flavonoids	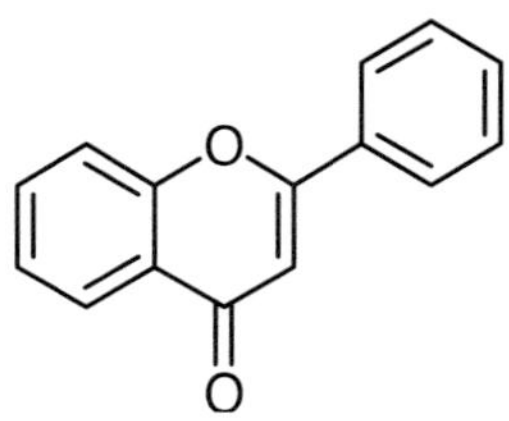 Flavones 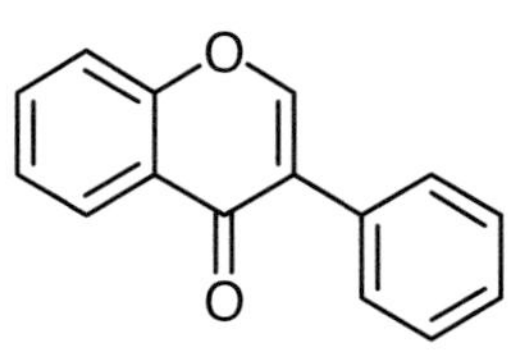 Isoflavones	Flavonoids constitute the most important single group of polyphenols of low molecular weight polyphenolic secondary plant metabolites, with more than 8,000 compounds described. They are found in fruits, vegetables, nuts, seeds, stems, flowers, roots, tea, wine, and coffee and are common substances in our daily diet. Their structure is a heterocyclic hydrocarbon, chromane, and substitution of its ring C in position 2 or 3 with a phenyl group (B-ring) results in flavans or isoflavans. An oxo-group in position 4 leads to flavanones and isoflavanones. The presence of a double bond between C2 and C3 provides flavones and isoflavones. An additional double bond in between C1 and C2 makes these compounds colourful anthocyanidins. Based on their structure, flavonoids are categorized into eight groups:

http://dx.doi.org/10.5772/56428

Antioxidants		
	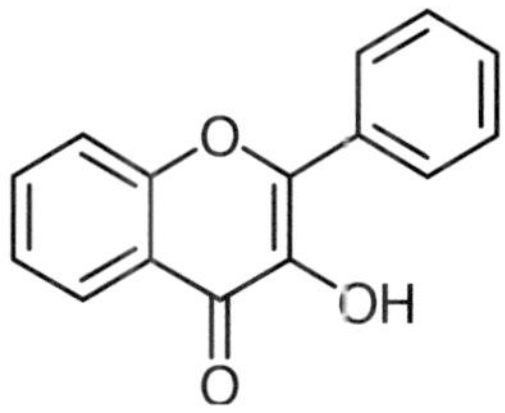 Flavonols	flavans, flavanones, isoflavanones, flavones, isoflavones, anthocyanidins, chalcones, and flavonolignans (Table 11].
Resveratrol	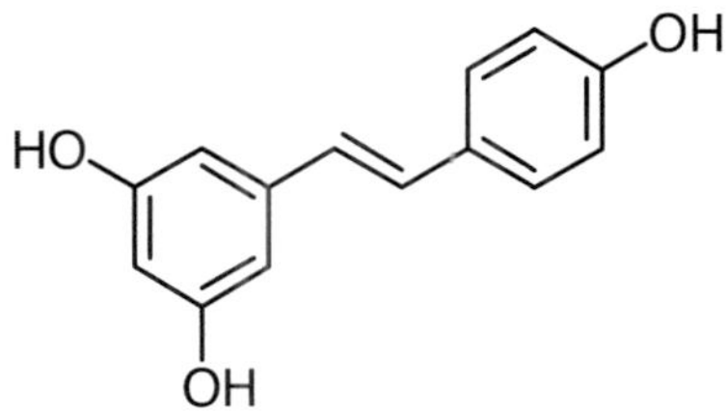	Resveratrol is a stilbenoid, a type of natural phenol, and a phytoalexin produced naturally by several plants when under attack by pathogens such as bacteria or fungi. Resveratrol is found in the skin of red grapes and in other fruits. It is sold as a nutritional supplement derived primarily from Japanese knotweed.
Selenium		Selenium is derived from both vegetable and animal products, particularly seafood, liver, and cereals. As a member of the sulfur family of elements, it shares several chemical properties with sulfur, including valence states and the ability to form covalent bonds with carbon. It is unique among antioxidants in that it exerts its biological effects through direct incorporation into proteins (selenoproteins) as the amino acid selenocysteine. Some selenoproteins that have been characterized as important antioxidant enzymes include GPX-1, GPX-4, thioredoxin reductase-1 and thioredoxin reductase-2, and selenoprotein P. The selenium-dependent enzyme, GPX recycles glutathione, reducing lipid peroxidation by catalyzing the reduction of peroxides, including hydrogen peroxide.
Avenanthramide	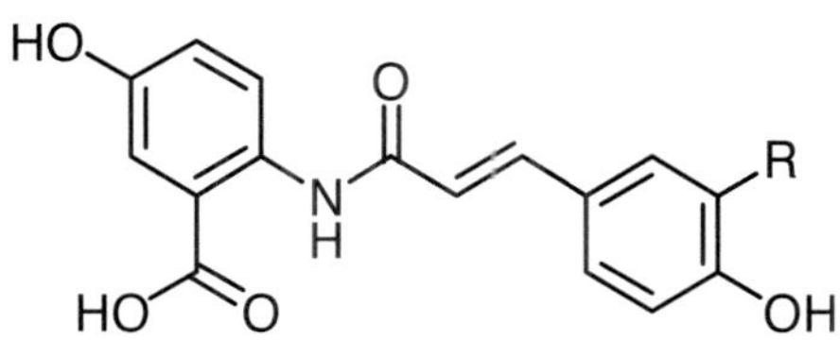	Oats contain unique, low-molecular-weight, soluble phenolic compounds called avenanthramides (Avns), which are not present in other cereal grains. These compounds are antipathogens (phytoalexins), which are produced by the plant in response to exposure to pathogens

Antioxidants		
		such as fungi. Avns are conjugates of a phenylpropanoid with anthranilic acid or 5-hydroxy anthranilic acid. More than 20 different forms of Avns are present when extracted from oats, and the three major forms are A, B, and C.

Table 3. Some of the dietary nutraceuticals indicated in asthma prevention.

Phytochemicals Flavonoids	Target/Function
4,3',5'-trihydroxystilbene	Inhibits Cyclooxygenase 1
4,3'-dihydoxy-5'methoxystilbene	inhibits Cyclooxygenase 1
4-hydoxy-3'5'-dimethoxystilbene	Inhibits Cyclooxygenase 1
Acacetin	Inhibits Cyclooxygenase 1
Andanthoflavone	Inhibits 12-Lipoxygenase, 15-Lipoxygenase
Apigenin	Inhibits Cyclooxygenase 2, 12-Lipoxygenase, 15-Lipoxygenase
Artonin E	Inhibits Cyclooxygenase 1, 5-Lipoxygenase, 12-Lipoxygenase, 15-Lipoxygenase
Baicalein	Inhibits Cyclooxygenase 1, Cyclooxygenase 2, 5-Lipoxygenase, 12-Lipoxygenase, 15-Lipoxygenase
Bicalin	Inhibits Cyclooxygenase 1, Cyclooxygenase 2
Buddledin A	Inhibits Cyclooxygenase 1
Chrysin	Inhibits Cyclooxygenase 1, 5-Lipoxygenase
Chrysol	Inhibits 5-Lipoxygenase
Cirsiliol	Inhibits 5-Lipoxygenase, 12-Lipoxygenase
Daidzein	Inhibits Cyclooxygenase 2
Epicatechin	Inhibits 5-Lipoxygenase
Epigallocatechin	Inhibits 5-Lipoxygenase
Fisetin	Inhibits Phospholipase A2, 5-Lipoxygenase, 12-Lipoxygenase, 15-Lipoxygenase
Flavone	Inhibits 5-Lipoxygenase
Gambogenic acid	Inhibits Cyclooxygenase 2
Genistein	Inhibits Cyclooxygenase 2

Ginkgetin	Inhibits 5-Lipoxygenase
Glycitein	Inhibits Cyclooxygenase 2
Isoliquiritigenin	Inhibits Cyclooxygenase 1, Cyclooxygenase 2
Kampferol	Inhibits Phospholipase A2
Kaempferol	Inhibits 5-Lipoxygenase
Kenusanone A	Inhibits 5-Lipoxygenase
Kisetin	Inhibits Phospholipase A2
Kuraridin	Inhibits Cyclooxygenase 1, 5-Lipoxygenase
Kurarinone	Inhibits Cyclooxygenase 1, 5-Lipoxygenase
Kuwanon C	Inhibits 5-Lipoxygenase, 12-Lipoxygenase
Luteolin	Inhibits 5-Lipoxygenase, 15-Lipoxygenase
Morelloflavone	Inhibits Phospholipase A2
Morusin	Inhibits Cyclooxygenase 1, 12-Lipoxygenase
Mosuin	Inhibits 15-Lipoxygenase
Myricetin	Inhibits 5-Lipoxygenase
Narigenin	Inhibits Phospholipase A2, 5-Lipoxygenase
Oroxidin	Inhibits 5-Lipoxygenase
Pedalitin	Inhibits 5-Lipoxygenase
Quercetin	Inhibits Cyclooxygenase 1, Cyclooxygenase 2, 5-Lipoxygenase, 12-Lipoxygenase
Resveratrol	Inhibits Cyclooxygenase 1, Cyclooxygenase 2, 5-Lipoxygenase
Rhamnetin	Inhibits 5-Lipoxygenase
Sanggenon B	Inhibits Cyclooxygenase 1, 5-Lipoxygenase
Sanggenon D	Inhibits 5-Lipoxygenase
Scutellarein	Inhibits Phospholipase A2
Silibinin	Inhibits 5-Lipoxygenase
Sophoflavanone A	Inhibits Cyclooxygenase 1
Sophoflavanone G	Inhibits Cyclooxygenase 1, 5-Lipoxygenase, 12-Lipoxygenase
Tectorigenin	Inhibits Cyclooxygenase 2
Wogonin	Inhibits Cyclooxygenase 2
Polyphenols	
Anisic acid	Inhibits Phospholipase A2
Caffeic acid	Inhibits 5-Lipoxygenase
Catechin	Inhibits Cyclooxygenase 1, 5-Lipoxygenase

Curcumin	Inhibits Phospholipase A2, Cyclooxygenase 1, Cyclooxygenase 2, 5-Lipoxygenase
Diphyllin acetapioside	Inhibits 5-Lipoxygenase
EGCG	Inhibits Cyclooxygenase 2
Eugenol	Inhibits 5-Lipoxygenase
Gingerol	Inhibits 5-Lipoxygenase
Ginkgetin	Inhibits Phospholipase A2, 5-Lipoxygenase
Hydroxytyrosol	Inhibits 5-Lipoxygenase
Hyperforin	Inhibits 5-Lipoxygenase
Medicarpin	Inhibits 5-Lipoxygenase
Ohenethyl ferulate	Inhibits Cyclooxygenase 2
Onosmins A and B	Inhibits 5-Lipoxygenase
Panaxynol	Inhibits 5-Lipoxygenase
Phenethyl ferulate	Inhibits 5-Lipoxygenase
Quercetagetin-7-O-beta-O-glucoside	Inhibits 5-Lipoxygenase
Rosmarinic acid	Inhibits 5-Lipoxygenase
Rosmarinic acid methylester	Inhibits 5-Lipoxygenase
Rosmarol	Inhibits Cyclooxygenase 20
n-3 PUFA	Inhibits Cyclooxygenase 2 and 5-Lipoxygenase

Table 4. Phytochemical inhibitors of lipid mediators

3.1.2. Cytokines blockers

Cytokines exhibit pleiotropy and have overlapping functions in the pathogenesis of asthma, making them a major target for new asthma therapies. Allergic inflammation is driven by an imbalance between Th1 and Th2 cytokines, favoring the Th2 arm of the immune response and inhibition of Th2 cytokines IL-4, IL-5 and IL-13 prevents asthma progression in animal models. Anti-IL-4 administration in mice prevents development of acute and chronic allergic inflammation [53], therefore, natural products that specifically target cytokines or their receptors have the potential to be effective asthma treatments.

Our current pharmacological approach include the use humanized monoclonal antibodies against specific cytokine or receptor targets. This class of drugs, known as the biologics, has been approved for use in treatment of cancer, autoimmune and inflammatory diseases. Omalizumab is a drug currently approved for the management of asthma and is antibody targeting IgE. While not specifically a cytokine blocker it functions through the same mechanism of action. These drugs while very effective carry the risk of unforeseen side effects and under current production treatment costs remain very high ranging upwards from $15,000 to 60,000 per annum. Others examples including humanized IL-4-specific antibodies that block

IL-4 receptor α that are under clinical trial [54]. Neutralizing antibodies against IL-5 (Mepolizumab and Reslizumab) and IL-5 receptor α (MEDI-563) remarkably inhibits IL-5 related pathways resulting in reduction of asthma exacerbations [55]. Tralokinumab, an anti-IL-13 monoclonal antibody, prevents the development of asthmatic phenotype, both in murine model as well asthmatic patients [56]. Suplatast tosilate inhibits IL-4 and IL-5 production from T cells and reduces AHR in asthmatic patients.

Some of the phytochemicals and potential treatments indicated against cytokines function are listed in Table 5. These products if proved to be effective, could be cost effective alternatives and being natural products have the potential to have less side effects.

Phytochemicals **Anti-oxidants**	**Target/Function and Effective Concentration(s)**	**References**
Vitamin A	Inhibits release of Th2 cytokines IL-4, IL-5 and IL-13 *in vitro* as well as *in vivo*. Suppresses production of IP-10, IL-6, TNF, GM-CSF and IFN-γ.	
Vitamin C	Effect on Th1/Th2 balance controversial.	
Vitamin E	Inhibits IL-1β, IL-6 and TNF response of human monocytes in asthmatic patients. Suppresses IL-4 levels in lungs of experimental allergic mice.	
Flavonoids		
Apigenin	Reduces airway inflammation by down-regulating Th2 cytokines IL-4 and IL-13. Suppresses the expression of Th2 cytokines (IL-4, IL-13 and IL-5) in human basophils. Inhibits production of TNF, IL-6 and GM-CSF in HMC-1 cells.	[57, 58]
Baicalein	Decreases inflammatory cytokines such as TNF and IL-6 in allergic inflammation. Inhibits production of IL-6 in activated human mast cells, and GM-CSF from human cultured mast cells.	[52, 59]
Bicalin	Reduces TNF and IL-6 levels in plasma and BALF in cigarette smoke-induced COPD rat model.	[60]
Chrysin	Downregulates IL-4 and IL-13 expression and production in allergen-sensitized mice. Inhibits TNF, IL-1β, IL-4 and IL-6 expression in RBL-2H3 and HMC-1 cells.	[61]
Chrysol	Inhibits IL-4 production in antigen-stimulated RBL-2H3 cells.	[62]
Daidzein	Mast cell stabilizer inhibits Th2 cytokines production.	
Fisetin	Inhibits IL-13 production in RBL-2H3 cells, and TNF, IL-6, IL-4 and IL-1β production in HMC-1 cells. Suppresses the expression of Th2 cytokines (IL-4, IL-13 and IL-5)in human basophils. Attenuates LPS-induced TNF, IL-6 and IL-10 release in leukocytes of patients with COPD.	[57, 63-65]
Genistein	Inhibits TNF production in PBMCs from asthmatic patients.	
Ginkgetin	Inhibits TNF expression in activated macrophages.	

Phytochemicals Anti-oxidants	Target/Function and Effective Concentration(s)	References
Isoliquiritigenin	Inhibits the release of TNF and IL-6 in activated inflammatory cells.	
Kaempferol	Impairs Th2 cytokines production (IL-5 and IL-13) in OVA-sensitized mice. Suppresses the release of IL-4 and TNF in RBL-2H3 cells and macrophages. Inhibits IgE-mediated TNF and IL-6 release in hCBMCs.	
Kuraridin	Suppresses expression of TNF and IL-1β in LPS-stimulated macrophages (40 μM).	[66]
Kurarinone	Suppresses expression of TNF and IL-1β in LPS-stimulated macrophages (40 μM).	[66]
Luteolin	Reduces the levels of TNF and IL-1β in LPS-stimulated macrophages (8 & 16 μM). Inhibits induction of TNF, IL-6 and GM-CSF in HMC-1 cells (10 & 50 μM). Inhibits Th2 cytokines (IL-4, IL-5 and IL-13) expression in murine asthma model (50 & 100 mg/kg body wt.). Inhibits myelin basic protein-induced IL-6, TGF-β1, and TNF release in hCBMCs (10 & 100 μM). Decreases TNF (IC_{50} 7.9±4.6 μM) and IL-1β (IC_{50} 5.1±0.4 μM) in PBMCs. Reduces IL-4 and IL-5 levels in BALF of murine asthma model (0.1 mg/kg body wt.). Inhibits antigen-IgE-mediated TNF (IC_{50} 5.8 μM) and IL-4 (IC_{50} 3.7 μM) production in RBL-2H3 cells.	[57, 67-73]
Morin	Inhibits IgE-mediated TNF and IL-6 release in hCBMCs (10 & 100 μM). Inhibits TNF secretion in LPS-activated macrophages.	[74, 75]
Myricetin	Inhibits TNF (30 μM) and IL-6 (30 μM) production in HMC-1 cells. Inhibits IgE-mediated TNF (10 & 100 μM) and IL-6 (1, 10 & 100 μM) release from hCBMCs.	[75, 76]
Naringenin	Suppresses Th2 cytokines production from CD4 T cells (0.8 mg/kg body wt.). Reduces IL-4 (25, 50 & 100 mg/kg body wt.) and IL-13 (50 & 100 mg/kg body wt.) levels in BALF of murine asthma model. Suppresses LPS-induced IL-1β (10, 25 & 50 μg/mL), IL-6 (5, 10, 25 & 50 μg/mL), and TNF (25 & 50 μg/mL) production in macrophages and human whole-blood samples.	[77-79]
Pedalitin	Inhibits TNF and IL-12 production in LPS-activated macrophages (40 μM).	[80]
Quercetin	Inhibits IgE-mediated TNF (10 & 100 μM) and IL-6 (1, 10 & 100 μM) release from hCBMCs.	[75]
Resveratrol	Inhibits increase in Th2 cytokines (IL-4 and IL-5) in plasma and BALF in asthmatic mouse model (30 mg/kg body wt.). Inhibits TNF induced GM-CSF and VEGF release in HASM cells. Inhibits PMA- and A23187-induced TNF and IL-6 release in HMC-1 cells. Decreases production of IL-1β in lung tissue of mice with LPS-induced acute lung injury (1	[68, 81-86]

Phytochemicals Anti-oxidants	Target/Function and Effective Concentration(s)	References
	mg/kg body wt.). Attenuates C5a-induced TNF, IL-1β and IL-6 production in mouse model (10 mg/kg body wt.).	
Scutellarein	Inhibits TNF and IL-12 production in LPS-activated macrophages (40 μM).	[80]
Silibinin	Polarizes Th1/Th2 balance towards Th1 by increasing IFN-γ (200 & 400 mg/kg body wt.) and decreasing IL-4 levels (200 & 400 mg/kg body wt.) in asthmatic mouse model.	[87]
Polyphenols		
Caffeic acid	Inhibits increase in TNF and Th2 cytokines (IL-4 and IL-5) in BALF in asthmatic mouse model (10 mg/kg body wt. IP). Inhibits IL-10 expression in allergic patients' DCs (10 μM). Suppresses TNF and IL-6 levels in asthmatic patients (13% solution).	[88-90]
Curcumin	Attenuates the expression of IL-4 and IL-5 in BALF in asthmatic mouse model (20 mg/kg body wt.). Inhibits release of IL-10, TNF and IL-1β in HDM-activated eosinophils and bronchial epithelial cells (10 μM). Inhibits IL-5, GM-CSF and IL-4 production in lymphocytes from bronchial asthmatics (10 μM). Inhibits TNF secretion in activated HMC-1 cells (10 & 100 μM/L). Inhibits tryptase-induced IL-6 release in eosinophils (25 μM).	[91-95]
EGCG	Reduces TNF in BALF in asthmatic guinea pigs (25 mg/kg body wt. SC). Inhibits TNF and IL-6 production in HMC-1 cells (100 μM). Attenuates production of TNF in lungs of mice with LPS-induced acute lung injury (10 mg/kg body wt. IP).	[96-99]
Eugenol	Inhibits IL-1β, TNF and IL-6 release in macrophages.	[100, 101]
Gallic acid	Inhibits TNF and IL-6 in HMC-1 cells (10 μM).	[102]
Gingerol	Inhibits IL-1β and IL-12 release in peritoneal macrophages 100 ng/mL)	[103]
Hydroxytyrosol	Inhibits LPS-induced TNF production in THP-1 cells (25, 50 & 100 μM). Reduces TNF levels in LPS-treated mice.	[104, 105]
Rosmarinic acid	Reduces IL-4, IL-5 and IL-13 expression in lung of HDM-sensitized asthmatic mouse model (1.5 mg/day PO). Attenuates IL-1β, IL-6, and TNF increase in spleen and nasal mucosa of asthmatic mouse model (4 mg/kg body wt.). Inhibits IL-4 and IFN-γ release from $CD4^+$ T cells (1 & 5 μM). Inhibits diesel exhaust particles-induced IL-1β expression in mice lung (4.6 μg/kg body wt.).	[106-110]
Terpenes		
Celastrol	Reduced mRNA expression of IL-5, IL-5, IL-13, TNF, and IFN-γ in BAL cells and lung tissue of asthmatic mouse model.	

Phytochemicals Anti-oxidants	Target/Function and Effective Concentration(s)	References
Costunolide	Inhibits production of TNF, IL-1β and IL-6 by LPS-stimulated macrophages (0.1, 0.5 & 1 μM).	[111, 112]
Helenalin	Inhibits TNF and IL-6 secretion by ASMCs (1 μM).	[113]
n-3 PUFA	EPA and DHA Lower BALF concentration of pro-inflammatory cytokines IL-1α, IL-2, IL-5, IL-9, IL-13, G-CSF and RANTES. EPA (120 μM) suppress TNF and IL-1β expression and production in LPS-stimulated alveolar macrophages from asthmatic patients	Ref?

Table 5. Phytochemical inhibitors of proinflammatory cytokines

3.1.3. Chemokines and chemokine receptors blockers

Chemokines (CC) and their receptors (CCR) play a crucial role in the recruitment of inflammatory cells into the airways and development of asthma. CC-chemokine receptor 3 CCR3, CCR4, and CRTH2 antagonists are being targets currently being evaluated for the treatment of asthma. A study found that treatment of asthmatic mice with an anti-CCR3 monoclonal antibody inhibits allergen-induced eosinophilia and $CD34^+$ progenitor cell infiltration into the lung, which is accompanied by reduced AHR [114, 115]. RS-1748, a CCR4 antagonist, inhibits OVA-induced airway inflammation in guinea pigs [116]. The number of CCR4-expressing Th2 cells is increased in the airways of asthmatic patients which can be blocked by a selective CCR4 antagonist [117], and therefore could be an effective therapy for asthma. Ramatroban and closely related TM30089 are antagonists for CRTH2, a chemokine receptor expressed on Th2 cells. They have been shown to attenuate allergen-induced EAR and LAR in animal models of asthma [118, 119]. Some of the phytochemicals indicated against chemokines function are listed in Table 6.

Phytochemicals Flavonoids	Target/Function and Effective Concentration(s)	References
Apigenin	Suppresses the production of MDC and IP-10 in THP-1 cells (10^{-6} and 10^{-5} M). Inhibits release of LPS-induced MCP-1 in J774.2 macrophages (10 & 30 μM). Inhibits production of IL-8 in HMC-1 cells.	[58, 120, 121]
Baicalein	Inhibits IL-8 and MCP-1 release in activated human mast cells. Inhibits eotaxin production in human dermal fibroblasts (10 μg/mL).	[59, 122]
Baicalin	Reduces IL-8 levels in plasma and BALF in cigarette smoke-induced COPD rat model. Inhibits eotaxin production in human dermal fibroblasts (10 μg/mL).	[60, 122]

http://dx.doi.org/10.5772/56428

Phytochemicals Flavonoids	Target/Function and Effective Concentration(s)	References
Chrysin	Inhibits TNF-induced IL-8 expression in HEK 293 cells (20, 40 & 80 μM).	[123]
Chrysol	Inhibits MCP-1 production in antigen-stimulated RBL-2H3.	[62]
Fisetin	Inhibits TNF-induced IL-8 expression in HEK 293 (20, 40 & 80 μM). Inhibits IL-8 production in HMC-1 cells.	[65, 123]
Genistein	Blocks HDM-induced IL-8 release in human lung epithelial cells (50 μM). Inhibits IL-8 release in TNF-stimulated human keratinocytes (60 μM). Inhibits chemokine-stimulated eosinophil adherence (10^{-7}, 10^{-6} and 10^{-5} M).	[124-126]
Isoliquiritigenin	Inhibits eotaxin-1 secretion in human fetal lung fibroblasts (IC_{50} 0.92±0.05 μg/mL).	[127]
Kaempferol	Suppresses LPS-induced production of MDC, IP-10 and IL-8 in THP-1. Inhibits MCP-1 production in antigen-stimulated RBL-2H3 and J774.2 macrophages (10 & 30 μM). Inhibits TNF-induced IL-8 expression in HEK 293 (20, 40 & 80 μM).	[62, 123, 128, 129]
Kuraridin	Suppresses expression of MCP-1 in LPS-stimulated macrophages (40 μM).	[66]
Kurarinone	Inhibits MCP-1-induced chemotaxis of THP-1 cells (IC_{50} 19.2 μg/mL). Suppresses expression of MCP-1 in LPS-stimulated macrophages (40 μM).	[130]
Luteolin	Inhibits TNF-induced expression of MCP-1 (10, 20 & 30 μM) and CXCL-1 (20 & 30 μM) expression in keratinocytes. Inhibits induction of IL-8 in activated HMC-1 cells (50 μM) and hCBMCs.	[70, 131, 132]
Morin	Inhibits IL-8 production in antigen-stimulated hCBMCs (100 μM).	[75]
Myricetin	Inhibits IL-8 production in antigen-stimulated hCBMCs (100 μM).	[75]
Naringenin	Decreases secretion of PMA-induced IL-8 in HL-60 cells (20 μM). Suppresses LPS-induced IL-8 production by macrophages and human whole-blood samples (25 & 50 μg/mL). Inhibits expression of RANTES and eotaxin-1 in BALF and lungs in asthmatic mouse model (50 & 100 mg/kg body wt.).	[78, 79, 133]
Quercetin	Decreases production of IL-8 (3 & 30 μM) and MCP-1 (10^{-4}, 10^{-5} and 10^{-6} M) in activated HMC-1 and IL-8 in human bronchial epithelial cells (0.1, 10 & 25 μM).	[134-136]
Resveratrol	Decreases production of MIP-1α in lung tissue of mice with LPS-induced acute lung injury (10 mg/kg body wt.). Reduces TNF-induced IL-8 release in HASMCs in COPD. Inhibits IFNγ-induced production of IP-10 and MIG in macrophages and HMC-1 cells.	[68, 82, 83, 85, 86, 137]

Phytochemicals Flavonoids	**Target/Function and Effective Concentration(s)**	**References**
	Inhibits IL-8 production in THP-1 cells (0.1, 1, 10 & 100 μg/mL). Attenuates C5a-induced MIP-1α production in mouse model (1 mg/kg body wt.).	
Tectorigenin	Inhibits MCP-1 expression in endothelial cells.	[138]
Wogonin	Suppresses mite antigen-induced TARC expression in human keratinocytes (250 ng/mL).	[139]
Polyphenols		
Caffeic acid	Decreases IL-8 release in chitinase-activated human airway epithelial cells (1 μM). Inhibits production of eotaxin in human lung fibroblast cells (1, 10 & 100 μM). Inhibits IP-10 expression in allergic patients' DCs (10 μM). Decreases expression of CXCR4 receptor on CD4 T cells (20 μg/mL). Suppresses IL-8 levels in asthmatic patients (13% soln.).	[89, 90, 140-143]
Curcumin	Inhibits tryptase-induced IL-8 release in eosinophils (25 μM).	
EGCG	Inhibits IL-8 release in TNF-stimulated human keratinocytes (0.5, 1, 5 & 10 μM). Reduces airway inflammation in asthmatic mouse model by binding to chemokines CXCL9, CXCL10 and CXCL11 (10 & 100 μM). Decreases MCP-1 and CCR2 expression on THP-1 cells (100 μM). Attenuates production of MIP-2 in lungs of mice with LPS-induced acute lung injury. Reduces expression of MCP-1 and IL-8 in HMC-1 cells (100 μM). Inhibits neutrophil migration by suppression of CINC-1 production (15, 50 & 150 μg/mL). Downregulates cigarette smoke-induced IL-8 release from bronchial epithelial cells.	[97, 99, 125, 144-147]
Gallic acid	Inhibits production of IL-8 and TARC (5 & 10 μg/mL) in neutrophils and keratinocytes respectively. Inhibits eotaxin and RANTES in pleural lavage fluid of allergen-challenged mouse model (100 mg/kg body wt.). Inhibits IL-8 release in HMC-1 cells (10 μM).	[148-150]
Rosmarinic acid	Inhibits LPS-induced production of MCP-1 and MIP-1α in bone-marrow derived DCs (100 μM). Reduces diesel exhaust particles-induced MIP-1α, MCP-1 and KC expression in mice lung (4.6 μg/kg body wt.). Inhibits expression of eotaxin in lungs of mite antigen-sensitized mice (1.5 mg/kg body wt. PO). Inhibits expression of CCL11 and CCR3 genes induced by TNF in human dermal fibroblast cells.	[102, 107, 110, 151]
Helenalin	Inhibits eotaxin and RANTES secretion in ASMCs (1 μM).	[113]

Table 6. Phytochemical inhibitors of chemokines

http://dx.doi.org/10.5772/56428

3.1.4. Miscellaneous: IgE, histamine, enzymes

The activation of mast cells involves the cross-linking of IgE bound to the $F_C\varepsilon RI$ surface receptor. Activation is measured in the laboratory by the release of the Beta-hexosaminidase enzyme (β-hex) from cytosolic granules into the interstitial fluid. The following compounds (Table 7) have been found to be inhibitors of β-Hex release in vitro and have to potential to be inhibitor of IgE-antigen activation.

Phytochemicals	IC_{50}	References
Anti-oxidants		
Vitamin A/carotenoid	?	[152]
Flavonoids		
Apigenin	4.5 μM	[153]
Baicalein	17 μM	[153]
Chrysin	?	[62]
Daidzein	?	[83]
Fisetin	3 μM	[73]
Genistein	28.5 μg/mL	[83]
Ginkgetin	6.52 μM	[154]
Glycitein	28.5 μg/ml	[83]
Isoliquiritigenin	24 μM	[155]
Kaempferol	7.5 μM	[62]
Luteolin	3 μM	[73]
Morin	51 μM	[153]
Myricetin	6.7 μM	[153]
Naringenin	29 μM	[156]
Quercetin	3 μM	[73]
Resveratrol	14 μM	[157]
Sophoflavanone G	20 μM	[158]
Tectorigenin	0.193 mM	[159]
Polyphenols		
Caffeic acid	?	[160]
Curcumin	5.3 μM	[161]
EGCG	?	[162]
Ginkgetin	?	

	Phytochemicals	IC_{50}	References
	Medicarpin	>100 μM	[155]
	Rosmarinic acid	?	[160]
Terpenes			
	Celastrol	?	[163]
	Costunolide	34 μM	[164]

Table 7. Phytochemical inhibitors of beta-hexosaminidase enzyme

3.2. Inhibitors of intracellular signaling pathways

The previous section focused on compounds that affected the function of extracellular, cell surface/receptor and cell to cell interactions. The following group of compounds affect the intercellular functions of the cells particular the components of cell signalling pathways.

3.2.1. Protein kinase inhibitor

Protein kinases have a key role in the expression and activation of inflammatory mediators implicated in airway inflammation. Enhanced activation of p38 mitogen-activated protein kinase (MAPK), c-Jun N-terminal kinase (JNK), spleen tyrosine kinase (Syk), and phosphoinositol 3-kinase (PI3K) signaling pathways have all been proposed to have a role in the pathogenesis of asthma.

p38 MAPK is involved in the airway inflammation and remodeling. A selective synthetic p38 MAPK inhibitor SB2439063 reduces synthesis of Th2 cytokines [54] and thus has a potential application in asthma treatment. Inhaled p38 MAPK antisense oligonucleotide attenuates asthma in OVA-sensitized and –challenged mice [165]. The natural product limonene inhibits eosinophil migration in p38 MAPK dependent manner and was investigation in an *in vitro* bronchial asthma model [166].

JNK activity is increased in corticosteroid-resistant asthma and SP600125, a JNK inhibitor, reduces cytokines expression and inflammatory cells accumulation in BALF of asthmatic animal models. Celastrol, a natural compound, modulates the expression of JNK in asthma [167]. It supresses allergen-induced mouse asthma by decreasing expression of MAP kinases, ERK and JNK [168].

Syk is a protein kinase involved in signal transduction in many inflammatory cells, and its aberrant regulation is associated with asthma, thus is considered an interesting target for asthma therapies. BAY 61-3606, a synthetic Syk inhibitor, inhibits inflammatory mediator release from mast cells, basophils, eosinophils, and monocytes, and reduces allergic asthma in rats [169]. Eupatilin, a biological extract, inhibits Syk and blocks downstream signaling pathways in mast cell from guinea pig lung tissues, leading to inhibition of mediator release [170]. Thus, Syk inhibitors may have use clinically as a treatment for asthma.

The PI3K pathway plays a major role in the pathogenesis of asthma by promoting eosinophil and neutrophil recruitment and degranulation [171]. Sorbus commixta water extract, an anti-inflammatory medicinal plant, remarkably blocks PI3K activity in antigen-activated macrophages, suggesting the usefulness of PI3K inhibitors in asthma [172].

3.2.2. Transcription factor inhibitors

The increased expression of various inflammatory proteins seen in asthma is the result of enhanced gene transcription, since many of the genes are not expressed in normal cells but are selectively induced during inflammation. Changes in gene transcription are under the control of transcription factors which therefore play a key role in the pathogenesis of asthma.

Transcription factors such as nuclear factor-κB (NF-κB), GATA-3, signal transducers and activators of transcription protein (STAT)s, nuclear factor of activated T cells (NFAT), and peroxisome proliferator-activated receptors (PPAR) have been implicated in asthma and therefore represent therapeutic targets.

NF-κB is induced by many factors involved in asthmatic inflammation and is implicated in glucocorticoid-resistant asthma. Inhibition of IκB (inhibitor of NF-κB) by small molecule inhibitors suppresses inflammatory responses in mast cell [173], OVA-induced rat model of airway inflammation [174], and macrophages from BALF of asthmatic patients. A number of herbal preparations (i.e. andrographolide and narigenin) have been demonstrated to inhibit airway inflammation and AHR by inhibiting NF-κB activity in OVA-induced murine asthma [78, 175]. Many inhibitors of NF-κB have been identified belonging to the Flavonoids, Polyphenols and Terpenoids classes of compounds as well as n-3 PUFA (see Table 8).

Flavonoid	Polyphenols	Terpenoids	PUFA
Apigenin	CAPE	Parthenolide	n-3 PUFA
Capsaicin	Curcumin	Costunolide	
Fisetin	Epigallocatechin-3-gallate	Helenalin	
Kuraridin	Gallic acid	Celastrol	
Kurarinone	Gingerol	Celaphanol A	
Luteolin	Rosmarinic acid	Kamebanin	
Myrecitin		Kamebacetal A	
Naringenin		Excisanin A	
Quercetin		Orbiculin	
Resveratrol			

Table 8. Naturally occurring NF-κB inhibitors

GATA-3 is a critical transcription factor that is specifically expressed by Th2 cells and is involved in their differentiation [176]. GATA-3 has been indicated in the development of airway eosinophilia and expression is increased in atopic asthma [177] and therefore is an obvious target for inhibition. Direct inhibition by using a specific antisense oligonucleotide or interference RNA promises a novel approach for asthma treatment [178]. Polyphenols, such as apigenin and quercetin, ameliorate asthma symptoms, and suppress the translocation of GATA-3 in the cytosol of lung tissue of OVA-sensitized and -challenged mice [179].

NFAT transcription factor is mostly involved in the production of Th2 cytokines through its interaction with GATA-3 and activator protein-1 (AP-1) [180]. Immunosupressive drugs cyclosporin A and FK506 block NFAT activation [181]. The use of peptides known as inhibitors of NFAT-calcineurin association (INCA) represents an alternative asthma treatment strategy [182].

PPARs are transcription factors belonging to the nuclear receptor superfamily activated by PUFA derivatives, oxidized fatty acids and phospholipids. PPARγ activation might exhibit anti-inflammatory properties in different inflammatory processes. In a murine model of asthma, treatment with PPARγ ligand ciglitazone significantly reduces AHR and lung inflammation [183]. PPARα and PPARγ ligands also decreases allergen-induced AHR, lung inflammation as well as serum IgE levels in different asthma models [184]. Popular anti-asthmatic Traditional Chinese Medicine San-ao Decoction (SAD), comprising *Herba Ephedrae, Radix et Rhizoma Glycyrrhizae* and *Seneb Armeniacae Amarum*, has a significant effect on PPARγ activation [185].

3.3. Inhibitors of oxidative stress

Oxidative stress plays a critical role in the development of asthmatic conditions. Oxidative stress and its by-products drive a Th2-dependent immune response. A number of antioxidants have been explored for their anti-inflammatory and anti-asthmatic properties, and a number of natural products have emerged as promising candidates. Resveratrol, a component of red wine, possesses anti-inflammatory and antioxidant properties. It inhibits inflammatory cytokines release in patients with chronic obstructive pulmonary diseases (COPD) [186] and may be beneficial in asthma. Several other biological compounds such as *Sanguisorba offcinalis* [187], aqueous extract from the root of *Platycodi Radix* [188], stem and bark of *Ulmus davidiana* [189], and *Alpinia katsumadai* seed extracts [190] attenuate oxidative stress and asthmatic activity in OVA-induced murine asthma. The flavonoids and polyphenols are the main groups of compounds that display anti-oxidative properties as listed in table 9.

Phytochemicals	Function and effective concentration(s)	References
Flavonoids		
Apigenin	Suppresses LPS-induced NO production in RAW264.7 macrophages	[191]
Baicalein	Inhibits LPS-induced NO production and iNOS expression in RAW264.7 macrophages	[192]
Chrysin	Inhibits NO production (IC_{50} 7.50±1.84 μM) in LPS-activated RAW264.7 macrophages	[74]
Fisetin	Inhibits TNF-induced ROS production in HEK cells	[123]

http://dx.doi.org/10.5772/56428

Phytochemicals	Function and effective concentration(s)	References
Kaempferol	Inhibits NO production (IC_{50} 9.83±1.55 μM) in LPS-activated RAW264.7 macrophages	[74]
Kuraridin	Inhibits ROS, NO production (20 & 40 μM) and iNOS gene expression (40 μM) in LPS-activated RAW264.7 macrophages.	[66]
Kurarinone	Inhibits ROS, NO production (40 μM) and iNOS gene expression (40 μM) in LPS-activated RAW264.7 macrophages.	[66]
Luteolin	Inhibits NO production (4, 8 & 16 μM) in LPS-activated RAW264.7 macrophages.	[67]
Morin	Inhibits NO production (IC_{50} 44.86±1.05 μM) in LPS-activated RAW264.7 macrophages	[74]
Naringenin	Inhibits lung iNOS expression in allergen-induced mouse asthma model	[78]
Quercetin	Inhibits NO production (IC_{50} 36.9±1.24 μM) in LPS-activated RAW264.7 macrophages	[74]
Resveratrol	Inhibits NO production in mice with acute lung injury (1 mg/kg body wt.).	[85]
Polyphenols		
Caffeic acid	Reduces ROS levels in BALF of OVA-sensitized and –challenged mice (10 mg/kg body wt. IP).	[88]
Curcumin	Reduces iNOS expression in lung tissue of OVA-sensitized asthmatic mice.	[91]
EGCG	Reduces NOS activity in lungs of OVA-sensitized asthmatic guinea pigs.	[96]
Hydroxytyrosol	Inhibits NO_2 production as well as iNOS expression in THP-1 cells (50 & 100 μM)	[104]
Rosmarinic acid	Inhibits formation of ROS and RNS in activates macrophages	[193]
Helenalin	Inhibits iNOS expression in LPS-stimulated macrophages (10 μM)	[137]
n-3 PUFA	Decreases exhaled NO from asthma patients challenged with mite allergen	[194]

Table 9. Phytochemical inhibitors of oxidative stress

4. Experimental models of asthma

Understanding respiratory sensitization mechanisms is the first step to designing therapeutic agents that may relieve patients of their asthma symptoms. A number of *in vitro* and *in vivo* experimental models are able to reproduce one or more features of allergic response and have been studied for a few decades. Animal models of asthma are the best characterized in terms of the inflammatory and remodeling processes. The use of gene knockout and transgenic animals and the therapeutic administration of antibodies or pharmacological antagonists/ inhibitors have helped to identify a range of pre-clinical targets for subsequent evaluation in humans. Small animal models of asthma, using mice, rats and guinea pigs, are most commonly used. Most of these models are based on active sensitization to an allergen such as OVA via the airways. *In vitro* model systems using inflammatory cells and airway-related cell types are widely used in studies on immuno-biological mechanisms of asthma. A more detailed description of the most commonly used models of asthma can be found in Table 10.

In Vivo Model	**Route(s) of Administration**	**Primary Effects**
OVA-induced allergic asthma	Intranasal or aerosol challenge, intrathoracic inoculation, intradermal challenge	Increased serum IgE levels, histological changes in airways including cellular infiltration, mediator release, AHR, and remodeling.
LPS lung inflammation model	Intranasal	Leukocytes (mainly neutrophils) recruitment to lung within 4 hr of LPS treatment.
House dust mite exposure	Intraperitoneal sensitization followed by inhalational challenge	Increased serum IgE levels, histological changes in airways including cellular infiltration, mediator release, AHR, and remodeling.
Infection by Aspergillus fumigatus	Intraperitoneal sensitization followed by inhalational challenge	Increased serum IgE levels, histological changes in airways including cellular infiltration, mediator release, AHR, and remodeling.
Ragweed allergen exposure	Intraperitoneal sensitization followed by inhalational challenge	Airway inflammation and AHR.
Infection with Ascaris suum	Subcutaneous and intratracheal sensitization, aerosol challenge	Bronchoconstriction, AHR and cellular infiltration.
In Vitro Cell Model	**Cell Type**	**Primary Response(s)**
Mast cells:		
Human mast cells	$CD34^{+}$-derived primary mast cells, cord blood mast cells, skin mast cells, lung mast cells, LAD2, LUVA , HMC-1, RBL-2H3	Release of proinflammatory mediators such as histamine, tryptase, chymase, cytokines, chemokines, leukotrienes, and prostaglandins.
Rodent mast cells	Bone marrow-derived mast cells, peritoneal mast cells	Release of proinflammatory mediators such as histamine, tryptase, chymase, cytokines, chemokines, leukotrienes, and prostaglandins.
Eosinophils	Primary cells, EoL-1, AML14.3D10	Release of proinflammatory mediators such as ECP, EPO, EDN, MBP, cytokines, and chemokines.

In Vivo Model	Route(s) of Administration	Primary Effects
Bronchial epithelial cells	Primary cells, NHBE, BEAS-2B	Release of proinflammatory mediators such as cytokines and chemokines. Morphological changes.
Alveolar epithelial cells	Primary cells, A549	Release of proinflammatory mediators such as cytokines and chemokines. Morphological changes.
Monocytes/ Macrophages	Primary cells, Mono-Mac-6, THP-1, RAW 264.7	Release of proinflammatory mediators such as cytokines, chemokines, leukotrienes, prostaglandins, ROS, and RNS.
Dendritic cells	Primary cells, U-937, CD34-DC, Mo-DC, KG-1, MUTZ-3	Release of proinflammatory mediators such as cytokines and chemokines.

Table 10. *In vivo* and *in vitro* models for asthma studies

5. Evidence for the association between diet and asthma

5.1. Antioxidants

The airways are continuously exposed to oxidants, either generated endogenously by various metabolic reactions (e.g. from mitochondrial respiration or released from phagocytes) or derived from exogenous sources (e.g. air pollutants and cigarette smoke). Allergen-activated inflammatory cells from asthmatic patients produce more ROS than from healthy individuals. In addition, several inflammatory mediators including histamine, lipid mediators, cytokines, chemokines, ECP, and EPO are potential stimuli for ROS production in the airways, leading to asthma exacerbation.

Deficiency of endogenous antioxidant defenses has been reported in asthma [195]. Since a diet rich in vitamin A or carotenoids, vitamin C vitamin E, and flavonoids, has been associated with a decreased prevalence of asthma, understanding the relationship between dietary antioxidants and asthma-associated inflammatory responses has been a recent focus.

5.1.1. Vitamin A and carotenoids

A systemic review and meta-analysis by Allen *et al.* has shown that dietary vitamin A intake is significantly lower in asthmatic patients than in healthy subjects [196]. Asthmatic children have a lower serum vitamin A concentration than healthy controls [197]. Supplementation of the diet with lycopene, a carotene found in tomatoes and carrots, has a protective effect against asthma development in a murine model [198].

All-trans retinoic acid (ARTA), a derivative of vitamin A, inhibits airway inflammation in asthmatic rats. ARTA inhibits total cell counts and the proportion of inflammatory cells in BALF, suppresses the expression of NF-κB and intercellular adhering molecule-1 (ICAM-1), and increases the expression of iκB [199]. Retinoid acid also downregulates the expression of Th1 and Th2 chemokines in monocytes, including macrophage-derived chemokine and IP-10, which are all important in the inflammatory process [200]. Airway smooth muscle cell migration, which contributes to the airway remodeling in chronic asthma is also inhibited by ARTA [201]. However, excessive intake of vitamin A exacerbates pulmonary hyperresponsiveness in murine asthma model, suggesting that excessive vitamin A may increase the risk and severity of asthma [202].

Mechanistically, vitamin A may regulate bronchial hyperreactivity by altering the function and abundance of the muscarinic M(2) receptors in bronchial tissue [203]. Moreover, carotenoids may regulate activation of a variety of transcription factors. Treatment of cells exposed to oxidative stress with β-carotene suppresses oxidative stress-induced activation of NF-κB and production of IL-6, TNF, and inflammatory cytokines. Carotenoids may influence the process of apoptosis in healthy cells. While the pro-apoptotic protein Bax is downregulated after induction of external stimuli, β-carotene is able to increase expression of the anti-apoptotic protein Bcl-2 in normal cells. In addition, β-carotene exhibits a pro-apoptotic effect in colon and leukemic cancer cells, and this effect occurs by a redox-dependent mechanism linked with NF-κB activity. These dual roles of vitamin A, including carotenoids, on apoptosis provide the capability of carotenoids as an effective anti-inflammatory agent in various diseases.

5.1.2. Vitamin C

Many observational studies have reported associations between reduced dietary/blood vitamin C levels and reduced lung functions. Asthmatic children undergoing an exacerbation have significant lower serum levels of vitamin C [204]. There is a positive correlation between serum vitamin C levels and asthma development in children (OR=0.72 per mg/dl, 95% CI=0.55, 0.95) [10]. Furthermore, asthma patients have significantly lower vitamin C level in both the cellular and fluid-phase fraction in induced sputum [205]. Higher maternal intake of citrus fruits rich in vitamin C during pregnancy is significantly associated with a reduced risk of allergic inflammation in the offspring [206]. Administration of vitamin C in OVA-challenged mice decreases AHR, influx of inflammatory cells in BALF and attenuates lung inflammation [207]. Similarly, high dose vitamin C supplementation significantly reduces eosinophilic infiltration in BALF and increases the Th1/Th2 cytokine secretion ratio; thus, skewing the Th1/Th2 balance toward non-allergic Th1 immune response in asthmatic mice [208].

A randomized, placebo controlled, double-blinded crossover trial has shown that vitamin C supplementation (1500 mg/day) attenuates asthma symptoms. Moreover, exhaled nitric oxide, urinary leukotriene C_4, D_4, E_4 and 9α, 1β-prostaglandin F_2 after exercise are downregulated [209]. On the contrary, there are also studies showing no significant effect of vitamin C supplementation on asthma symptoms. For example, in a randomized, placebo-controlled, double-blind parallel group trial three hundred asthma patients provided with 1 g/day vitamin C or placebo for 6 weeks do not show any improvements of asthma symptoms [210], therefore, there is insufficient evidence from randomised-controlled trials to support the use of vitamin C for asthma treatment [211].

As its mechanism of action, vitamin C may regulate factors that can influence gene expression, apoptosis, and other cellular functions indicated in inflammation. In fact, vitamin C protects against cell death triggered by various stimuli, and major proportion of this protection is associated with its antioxidant ability [212]. Vitamin C inhibits the AP-1 activation by regulating MAPK-ERK pathway [213]. Treatment of cells exposed to UV-B irradiation with vitamin C results in a 50% decrease in JNK phosphorylation, which activates AP-1, therewith inhibiting the JNK/AP-1 signaling pathways [214]. At present, however, evidence from randomized controlled trials is insufficient to recommend a specific role for vitamin C in the treatment of asthma due to variable study design and generally poor reporting system.

5.1.3. Vitamin E

The body of evidence from multiple studies suggests that a positive association between asthma outcomes and vitamin E intake or serum vitamin E levels. Asthmatic children have significantly lower serum levels of vitamin E than non-asthmatic children [204, 215]. A longitudinal birth cohort study has explored association between maternal plasma vitamin E, fetus and fetal lungs growth, and childhood asthma. The findings have shown that maternal vitamin E status has a positive effect on the growth of fetus and fetal lungs during early pregnancy and better asthma outcomes during childhood [216]. Moreover, high maternal vitamin E intake during pregnancy also reduces the risk of infantile wheeze [206]. Vitamin E intake is higher in control subjects than in asthma patients [217]. However there is no relationship found between serum vitamin E level and asthma [4, 218]. On the other hand, administration of vitamin E for 6 weeks does not have an effect on asthma features and serum immunoglobulin levels in adults [219].

Role of Vitamin E has been investigated in animal models of allergic asthma. Administration of Vitamin E to allergen-challenged mice reduces mitochondrial dysfunction, Th2 cytokines production, allergen-specific IgE, and expression of lipid mediators in lung leading to alleviation of asthmatic features [220]. Expression of IL-5 mRNA and protein in lung, and plasma IgE level are reduced after OVA sensitization and challenge compared to wild type mice in vitamin E transfer protein knockout mice [221]. Moreover, dietary supplementation with vitamin E affords variable degree of protection against ozone-induced enhanced airway response in allergen-sensitized guinea pigs [222]. However, oral α-tocopherol has no protective effect on lung response in rat model of allergic asthma. There is no improvement in OVA-induced AHR, the inflammatory cell infiltrate and histological changes [223]. The observed opposite effects of vitamin E could be associated with the study design in an animal model of asthma. The effect of vitamin E deserves further evaluation.

Vitamin E may induce immunological effects via modulation of the functional activity of T cells and enhancing the phagocytic activity of peripheral granulocytes [224]. A derivative γ-tocopherol appears to be a more potent anti-inflammatory agent than α-tocopherol. It decreases systemic oxidative stress, cytokine release from monocytes in asthmatic patients, and inhibits monocyte response to LPS and LPS-induced degradation of IκB and JNK activation [225]. There is a contradictory study demonstrating that γ-tocopherol elevates inflammation and ablates the anti-inflammatory benefit of the α-tocopherol by regulation of endothelial cell signals during leukocyte recruitment in experimental asthma [226]. Dietary tocopherols are taken up from the intestine and transported via the lymph to the blood and then to the liver.

In the liver, α-tocopherol is transferred to plasma lipoproteins, resulting in retention of γ-tocopherol in tissues at 10% that of α-tocopherol. On interpreting these two contradictory results, one should consider their serum levels with caution since low plasma level of γ-tocopherol (1.2–7.0 μM) may act as prooxidant, while higher level of γ-tocopherol (19.5 μM at 8 days) exerts antioxidative and anti-inflammatory effects.

5.1.4. Vitamin D

Over the past several years, the role of vitamin D in immunomodulation has been studied and shown to have a significant impact on innate and adaptive immunity to infections, including the pathophysiology of allergic asthma. It has been proposed that the increase in allergy and asthma is a consequence of widespread vitamin D insufficiency which appears to be frequent in industrialized countries, reflecting the insufficient intake of diet-sourced vitamin D.

The serum vitamin D level is associated with asthma in children as well as adults. A randomized, placebo controlled clinical study with 1024 children suffering from mild-to-moderate persistent asthma has shown that Vitamin D deficiency ias associated with a higher rate of severe asthma [227]. There is a significant positive correlation between forced vital capacity percent predicted and serum vitamin D level children with asthma. Moreover, 91.6% of these asthmatic children are not sufficient in serum vitamin D level [228]. Low level of vitamin D in serum are also associated with increased hyperresponsiveness and reduced glucocorticoid response in adults with asthma [229]. These studies have indicated that the low serum vitamin D level is related to reduced lung function and higher risk of asthma. Reduced the risk of asthma exacerbation triggered by acute respiratory tract infection is observed in a vitamin D supplementation [230]. Higher consumption of vitamin D during pregnancy may reduce the risk of childhood wheeze and asthma.

One possible mechanism of vitamin D's protective effect against asthma can be that it inhibits the maturation process of dendritic cells by suppressing the expression of costimulatory molecules HLA-DR, CD86, CD80, the maturation marker CD83, and IL-12 which are important for the recruitment of Th1 cells [231]. Vitamin D also upregulates the expression of IL-10 receptor in dendritic cells, which is an anti-inflammatory cytokine. In addition, it can promote the production of FoxP3 positive and IL-10 positive regulatory T cells, and induce the release of IL-10, TGF-β and CTLA-4 [232]. Furthermore, it may reverse steroid-resistance in asthmatic patients through induction of IL-10 secreting T-regulatory cells [233], and vitamin D has been shown to regulate expression of many genes in ASM cells, including genes previously implicated in asthma predisposition and pathogenesis [234].

5.2. Flavonoids

Flavonoids interfere with oxidation of lipids and other molecules and this strong antioxidative property makes them protective against airway diseases linked to oxidative stress. In fact, several epidemiologic studies suggest the beneficial effects of flavonoids on asthma. A population-based case-control study has shown that apple consumption and red wine intake are inversely associated with asthma prevalence or severity, perhaps due to a protective effect of flavonoids [18]. Moreover, a 30-year longitudinal epidemiological study has reported that the incidence of asthma is lower in populations with higher intake of flavonoids [235].

Flavonoid Subclass	Dietary Flavonoids	Some Common Food Sources
Anthocyanidins	Cyanidin, Delphinidin, Malvidin, Pelargonidin, Peonidin, Petunidin	Red, blue, and purple berries; red and purple grapes; red wine
Flavanols	Monomers (Catechins): Catechin, Epicatechin, Epigallocatechin Epicatechin gallate, Epigallocatechin gallate Dimers and Polymers: Theaflavins, Thearubigins, Proanthocyanidins	**Catechins:** Teas (particularly green and white), chocolate, grapes, berries, apples **Theaflavins, Thearubigins:** Teas (particularly black and oolong) **Proanthocyanidins:** Chocolate, apples, berries, red grapes, red wine
Flavanones	Hesperetin, Naringenin, Eriodictyol	Citrus fruits and juices, e.g., oranges, grapefruits, lemons
Flavonols	Quercetin, Kaempferol, Myricetin, Isorhamnetin	Widely distributed: yellow onions, scallions, kale, broccoli, apples, berries, teas
Flavones	Apigenin, Luteolin	Parsley, thyme, celery, hot peppers
Isoflavones	Daidzein, Genistein, Glycitein	Soybeans, soy foods, legumes

Table 11. Common dietary flavanoids.

Beyond antioxidative effects, flavonoids inhibit the release of histamine and other preformed granule associated mediators by inhibiting the activation of basophils and mast cells [66]. Flavonoids inhibit synthesis of IL-4, IL-13, and CD40 ligand but initiate generation of new phospholipid-derived mediators. One of the well-characterized flavonoids, quercetin, inhibits eosinophilic secretion of Charcot-Leyden crystal protein and ECP in a concentration-dependent manner. Very recently, Li *et al.* demonstrated that apigenin exhibits an anti-inflammatory activity in a murine asthma model and can switch the immune response to allergens toward the Th1 profile. These findings suggest that flavonoids are anti-allergenic and anti-inflammatory agents effective in treating/preventing asthma.

Vascular changes are one of the major components of asthmatic pathogenesis. These changes include an increase in vascular permeability, vascular dilation/engorgement, and vasculogenesis/angiogenesis. Flavonoids and their related compounds have been shown to modulate expression of HIF-1, VEGF, matrix metalloproteinases (MMPs), and epidermal growth factor receptor but also inhibit NF-κB, PI3K/Akt, and ERK1/2 signaling pathways [236]. These observations suggest that flavonoids as well as their related compounds inhibit certain steps of angiogenesis including cell migration, microcapillary tube formation, and MMP expression.

Many flavonoids have been tested for their anti-asthma effect. Quercetin decreases the eosinophil recruitment, reduces IL-5 and IL-4 levels, and inhibits NF-κB activation in BALF in OVA-induced mouse model [237]. It also regulates Th1/Th2 balance by enhancing IFN-γ and decreasing IL-4 levels in mouse asthma model [179]. Naringenin alleviates airway inflammation and reactivity by decreasing serum total IgE level and IL-4, IL-13 level in BALF and inhibiting NF-κB activity [78]. Licorice is a Traditional Chinese Medicine, which contain many flavonoids. Flavonoids extracted from licorice attenuates LPS-induced acute pulmonary inflammation by inhibiting inflammatory cells infiltration and inflammatory mediator release [238]. Neutrophils, macrophages and lymphocytes accumulation in BALF, lung TNF and IL-1β mRNA expression and lung myeloperoxidase activity are reduced; whereas BALF superoxide dismutase activity is increased [238]. Flavonoids from red algae decrease eosinophil infiltration, levels of TNF, IL-4 and IL-5 in BALF, airway luminal narrowing, AHR and level of allergen-specific IgE in the serum [239]. A complex mixture of bioflavonoids derived from purple passion fruit peel extract supplemented to asthma patients in a randomized, placebo-controlled, double-blinded trial alleviates asthma clinical symptoms, including FVC and FEV1 [240].

5.3. Resveratrol

Resveratrol scavenges intracellular ROS by inducing and stabilizing antioxidant enzymes such as catalase, SOD, and glutathione peroxidase hemoxygenase. In addition to its reducing properties, resveratrol has been shown to attenuate inflammation via inhibition of prostaglandin production [241] and to decrease the phosphorylation of ERK1/2, COX-2 activity, and activity of various transcription factors including NF-κB, STAT3, HIF-1α, and β-catenin [236]. Resveratrol also inhibits protein kinases (e.g. src, PI3K, JNK, and Akt) and the production of inflammatory mediators (e.g. IFN-γ, TNF, COX-2, iNOS, CRP and various interleukins). Recent studies have reported that resveratrol activates sirtuin1 (SIRT1) which is modulates apoptosis and has been shown to increase longevity in some experimental systems [242]. SIRT1 modulates poly (ADP-ribose) polymerase-1 (PARP-1) activity upon DNA damage. Activation of SIRT1 by resveratrol leads to a decrease in PARP-1 activity and promotes cell survival, which can attenuate the inflammatory reaction. We investigated the effects of resveratrol on human mast cell activation in comparison to the anti-allergic drug tranilast. The results show that resveratrol inhibits mast cell degranulation, cytokine, chemokine and leukotriene release, and is more efficacious than tranilast [316].

Resveratrol is able to modulate innate immune response by inhibiting expression of costimulatory molecules (CD80 and CD86) and major histocompatibility complex classes I and II in bone marrow-derived dendritic cells and inhibit angiogenesis pathway that is mediated through expression of MMPs, VEGF, cathepsin D, ICAM-1, and E-selectin [236]. These findings suggest that resveratrol can be a very attractive compound for preventing/treating asthma since this compound displays multiple therapeutic effects, showing antioxidative, anti-inflammatory, immune modulating, and vascular protective property.

Resveratrol has been shown to inhibit the airway inflammation and hyperresponsiveness in OVA-induced mouse asthma by reducing eosinophil/neutrophils infiltration, the levels of IL-4 and IL-5 in plasma and BALF [81]. It can modulate Th1/Th2 balance, polarization of naive $CD4^+$ T cells to the Th2 phenotype, and the expression of Th2 regulatory transcription factor, GATA-3 [81]. It also inhibits cytokine release in vitro by alveolar macrophages from patients with COPD, including IL-8 and GM-CSF [186].

5.4. Selenium

Selenium is an important molecule in both innate and adaptive immune responses. It stabilizes activated platelets by inhibiting platelet aggregation and secretion of adenine nucleotide, thus possibly blocking the release of acrachidonic acid from platelet membrane [243]. In asthma, platelets participate by acting as inflammatory cells, by releasing mediators, spasmogens and/or by interacting with other inflammatory cell types [168]. Selenium affects the expression of endothelial cell adhesion molecules, E-selectin, P-selectin, ICAM-1, VCAM-1, and ELAM-1, which are crucial in the inflammatory process for recruitment of inflammatory cells into the target tissue [244].

Some studies have reported that asthma patients have lower selenium level in platelets and serum compared to healthy controls [245, 246]. While others studies have found no relationship between serum selenium level and asthma in Japanese and Europe populations [247, 248]. Selenium supplementation studies in mouse OVA-induced asthma models have shown that selenium has some protective effects on asthma-associated inflammation. Mice with decreased and increased levels of selenium intake show lower cytokine levels, airway inflammatory cell infiltration, serum anti-OVA IgE, airway hyperreactivity, and phosphorylated STAT-6 levels in the lung compared to medium selenium intake [249]. Selenium supplementation does not show any clinical benefit in adult asthma patients [250].

Despite the data showing positive effects of selenium on some of the pathologies associated with asthma, there are still some conflicting findings of selenium supplementation in animal and human studies. Thus the issue regarding selenium is not conclusive.

5.5. Avenanthramides

Avenanthramides (Avns) are extracted from oats and those synthetically prepared exhibit potent antioxidant properties *in vitro* and *in vivo*. The antioxidant activity of Avns is 10–30 times greater than that of oats' other phenolic antioxidants such as vanillin and caffeic acid. Avn-C, one of the three major Avns of oats, often comprises about one-third of the total concentration of Avns in oat grain (although the relative proportion of Avns is highly variable), it has the highest antioxidant activity *in vitro*. By far, these Avns constitute the major phenolic antioxidants present in the oat kernel. The antioxidant activity of Avn-enriched extract of oats has been investigated in laboratory animals. Supplementing the diet of rats at 100 mg/kg diet (providing about 20 mg Avns/kg body weight) has been reported to increase superoxide dismutase (SOD) activity in skeletal muscle, liver, and kidneys, and to enhance glutathione peroxidase activity in heart and skeletal muscles [251]. Supplementation at 200 mg/kg diet, which provides about 40 mg Avns/kg body weight in rats, attenuated the exercise-induced production of ROS [251].

In addition to demonstrating antioxidant activity, Avn compounds may also interact with cellular components, through their interactions with the molecular and signaling pathways that govern cellular responses during inflammation. Using the human aortic endothelial cell (HAEC) culture system, the potentially beneficial health effects of oat Avns was found to be mediated via modulation of the cellular and molecular processes that are known to play an important role in the inflammation of arteries and the development of atherosclerosis [251]. They have been shown to inhibit vascular endothelial cell expression of adhesion molecules, including ICAM-1, VCAM-1, and E-selectin. Suppression of these adhesion molecules resulted in inhibition of monocyte adhesion to HAEC monolayers and reduced production of several inflammatory cytokines and chemokines, including IL-6, IL-8, and MCP-1, the inflammatory components involved in fatty streak formation in arteries. The production of proinflammatory cytokines, chemokines, and adhesion molecules by endothelial cells has been shown to be regulated by redox-sensitive signal transduction involving nuclear transcription factor NF-κB. The above-observed effects of Avns on HAEC and other cells are reported to be mediated through inhibition of NF-κB. More recently, dihydroavenanthramide (DHAv), a synthetic analog of Avn, has been shown to protect pancreatic β-cells from damage via inhibition of NF-κB. In a series of experiments, Guo *et al.* determined that suppression of the expression of NF-κB activity by Avns is mediated via inhibition of the phosphorylation of IKK and iκB, and by suppression of proteasome activity in endothelial cells [252]. A study by Sur *et al.* demonstrated anti-inflammatory activity of Avns in skin, inhibiting the degradation of IκB-α in human keratinocytes which correlates with decreased activation of NF-κB and subsequent reduction in IL-8 release [253]. Topical application mitigates skin inflammation in murine model of contact hypersensitivity and neurogenic inflammation and reduces pruritogen-induced scratching in murine itch model [253]. Taken together these observations suggest that Avns are potent anti-inflammatory agents with a potential application in asthma treatment.

5.6. Herbal preparations

Herbs have been used to treat airway diseases including asthma for thousands years in many nations, especially in Asian and African countries. In recent decades, some Chinese, Japanese, Indian, and African herbs have been tested for their anti-asthmatic effects.

5.6.1. Boswellia serrata

Boswellia serrata, Indian frankincense, is commonly found in many regions of the world, such as South Asia, Northern Africa, and Middle East. Traditional medicine using extract made from sap, has long been used to treat inflammatory diseases [204]. These extracts contain resin, amino acids, phenols, terpenes, polysaccharides [205] and β-boswellic acid the major active anti-inflammatory component [206].

Extract of Boswellia Serrata or β-boswellic acid has been reported to inhibit hypersensitivity reactions by regulating both the humoral and cellular immune systems They decrease primary antibody synthesis, inhibit polymorphonuclear leukocyte proliferation and infiltration, enhance the phagocytotic function of macrophages, and suppress the classical and alternate complement pathways [254, 255] and suppress the inflammation process, one of the critical pathological features in asthma. It has been shown that β-boswellic acid inhibits the production of proinflammatory cytokines, including TNF, IL-1, IL-2, IL-6, IL-12 and IFN-γ by suppressing the activation of NF-κB [256]. It also inhibits histamine release from mast cells challenged with G protein stimulator c48/80 in a dose-dependent manner [257]. β-boswellic acid can down-regulate the synthesis of prostaglandins by inhibiting COX-1 in intact human platelets [258].

The synthesis of 5-hydroxyeicosatetraenoic acid (5-HETE) and leukotriene B_4 from rat peritoneal polymorphonuclear leukocytes, which contribute to bronchoconstriction, and increased vascular permeability, are reduced by Boswellia Serrata extract as a result of 5-LO inhibition [259]. These results suggest that Boswellia Serrata might be effective in controlling the inflammation process and contraction of airway smooth muscle in asthmatic condition by inhibiting enzymes required for production of proinflammatory mediators and bronchoconstrictor.

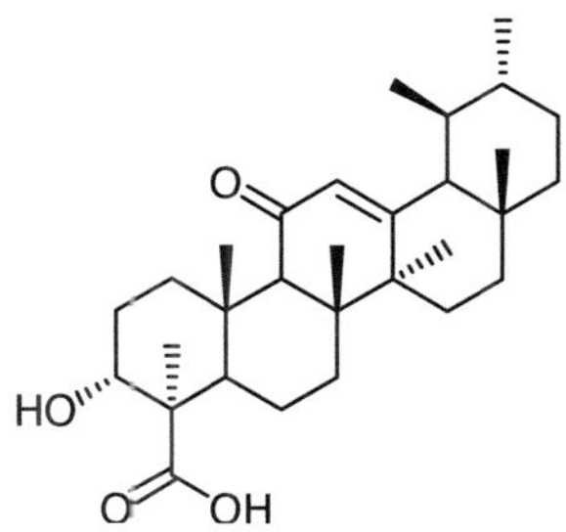

Boswellia serrata

Preliminary clinical investigation has shown Boswellia Serrata's potential therapeutic effect on asthma. In a double-blind, placebo-controlled clinical study [260], 40 patients took 300 mg of extract daily for six weeks, while a control group received a lactose placebo for the same period of time. Lung and immune functions were recorded, including dyspnoea, rhonchi, frequency of attacks, FEV1, FVC, peak expiratory flow rate (PEFR), eosinophil count and erythrocyte sedimentation rate. In the treatment group 70% of patients and 27% in the control group showed improvement in terms of recorded physical symptoms and signs. These results suggest that Boswellia Serrata extract has potential benefit for asthma patients, although the age for control and treatment group was not perfectly matched. However, there is not enough evidence to draw a conclusion on the potential use of Boswellia Serrata for treating asthma in human.

5.6.2. Bromelain

Bromelain is an extract from the pineapple stem, Ananas comosus, containing a mixture of cysteine proteases, peroxidase, acid phosphatase, protease inhibitors, and calcium, with cysteine proteases being the main functional components [214].

Bromelain modulates immune responses both *in vitro* and *in vivo*. In *vitro*, it downregulates mRNA expression of IL-2, IL-4, and IFN-γ in T cells induced by phorbol myristate acetate (PMA), with the mechanism thought to be the inhibitionof p21ras and subsequent ERK-2 [261, 262]. In a study using peripheral blood mononuclear cells (PBMC), Bromelain decreases the expression of migration/activation related cell surface markers on leukocyte by proteolysis, including CD14, CD16, CD21, CD25, CD44, CD45RA, CD62L [263]. In addition, it can dose-dependently reduce CD25 expression in anti-CD3 antibody-stimulated $CD4^+$ T cells, which is upregulated when T cells are activated in inflammation, autoimmunity and allergy [264].

These results indicate that Bromelain may regulate inflammatory process by interfering the migration and activation of immune cells, primarily T cells. *In vivo*, Bromelain may inhibit IgG production and decrease IL-2 gene transcription in spleen, and significantly reduce blood $CD4^+$ T cell count [262]. In addition, it downregulates IFN-γ mRNA expression in spleen [265]. These results indicate that Bromelain has regulatory effects on the adaptive immunity, principally by targeting T cell responses.

Bromelain administration via intraperitoneal injection alleviates some of the features of airway inflammation in the OVA-induced murine asthma model. It reduces the total numbers of leukocytes, eosinophils, $CD4^+$ and $CD8^+$ T cells in BALF, and decreases IL-13 concentration, which is a critical mediator for AHR in asthma [266]. In separate study, oral supplementation has been shown to suppress airway methacholine sensitivity, decrease IL-13 level, and eosinophils, $CD19^+$ B cells and $CD8^+$ T cells counts in BAL [267]. These results suggest that Bromelain modulates airway reactivity by altering the presence of leukocytes in airway, which is consistent with the *in vitro* results mentioned above. However, there is no clinical report available on the use of Bromelain against asthma so far.

5.6.3. Butterbur (Petasites hybridus)

Butterbur is a member of the perennial sunflower family found in Europe and northern Asia. The ancient Greeks used butterbur roots to treat airway diseases and alleviate bronchial spasms [268].

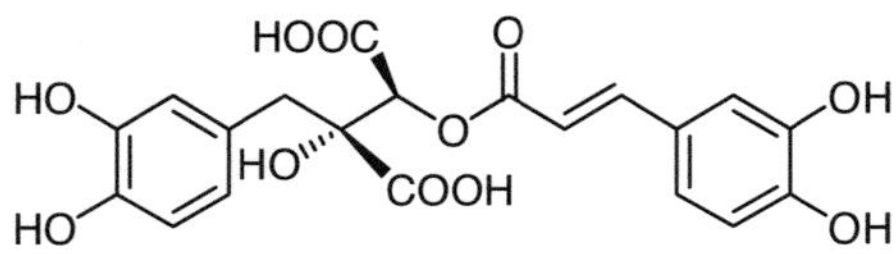

Fukinolic acid

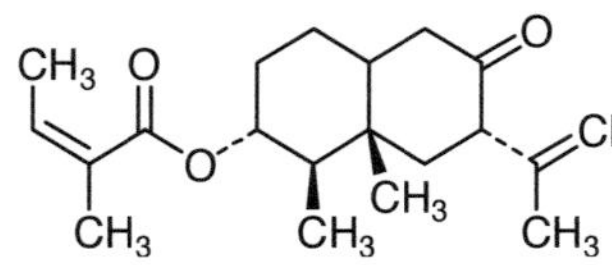

Petasin

Extract from the flower bud, leaves and root have been shown to inhibit β-hexosaminidase release, leukotriene C4/D4/E4 synthesis, and TNF production from IgE-sensitized RBL-2H3 cell [223]. A group of Japanese researchers reported that Japanese butterbur contains multiple active compounds including two eremophilane-type sesquiterpenes, six polyphenolic compounds, and two triterpene glycosides [223], and based on its inhibitory activity on mast cell degranulation, fukinolic acid is believed to be the most active component [269]. Another active component petasin, can reduce leukotriene and ECP production from eosinophils activated

http://dx.doi.org/10.5772/56428

by platelet-activating factor (PAF) or C5a via suppression of cytosolic phospholipase A2 (cPLA2) activity, decreasing intracellular calcium concentration and inhibiting 5-LO translocation from the cytosol to nuclear membrane [270]. Pepsin inhibits leukotriene production from macrophages [271] and suppresses bronchial constriction induced by histamine, carbachol, KCl and leukotriene D_4 in isolated guinea pig trachea [272]. In the OVA murine model, butterbur extract given intranasally together with antigen challenge has been shown to inhibit airway inflammation induced by OVA and hyperresponsiveness to aerosolized methacholine, reduce eosinophil count and decrease Th2 cytokine production including IL-4, IL-5 and RANTES in BALF [227]. These results suggest that Butterbur may have inhibitory effects on proinflammatory mediator release from a broad range of immune cells.

In 2003, a prescription-based Butterbur extract was approved in Switzerland for the treatment of seasonal allergic rhinitis and in response some researchers have tested Butterbur extract for the treatment of asthma. Ziolo *et al* conducted an open clinical study on its effects on bronchial reactivity in asthma patients. Provided orally in a single dose for three time periods patients show significant improvement on FEV1, especially subjects those in longer treatment group[273]. In another randomized, double-blind, placebo-controlled clinical study, results have shown that the signs of asthma are significantly suppressed by Butterbur treatment including FEV1, exhaled NO, serum ECP and peripheral blood eosinophil count, suggesting Butterbur reduces some of the inflammatory markers associated with allergic respiratory inflammation [274], However, some long term adverse side effects have ben reported including abdominal pain, flatulence, and sneezing in pediatric patients and hair loss, cough, dyspnea, and severe depression for adult patients [230]. More studies with larger sample size are needed for the evaluation of Butterbur's clinical use on asthma.

5.6.4. Curcumin

Curcumin is a yellow polyphenol compound, extracted from the rhizomes of *Curcuma longa* [231]. In ancient time, curcumin containing turmeric plants were widely used to treat swelling and wounds in Southern Asia [275].

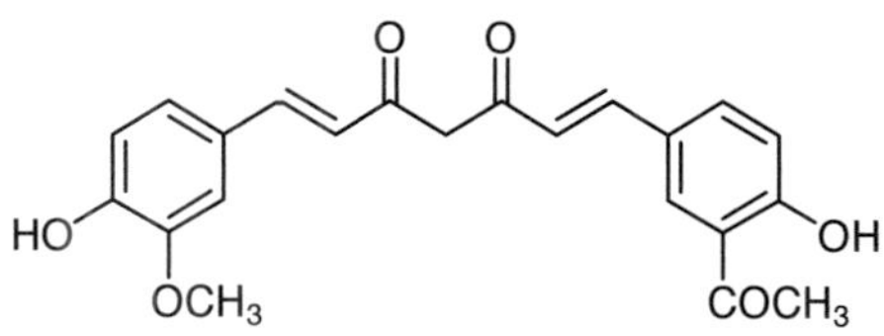

Curcumin

Many pharmacological effects of curcumin have been reported, including antioxidative, anti-inflammatory and antimicrobial activities [276]. In terms of its antioxidative effects, curcumin is thought to be more potent than vitamin E [277] with the mechanism including downregulation of NO production, scavenging free radicals, and inducing heme oxygenase-1 to repair the oxidative damage caused by free radicals [278-280]. Curcumin can inhibit the production of proinflammatory cytokines such as IL-1β and IL-8, suppress inducible iNOS and NO production, and modulate steroid activity. It's effect on steroid activity may be the result of inhibition of NF-κB through blocking IKK activity [281-284].

During allergic inflammation, curcumin may modulate both early and late phase responses by altering Th2 responses. In a murine latex-induced allergy model, characterized by an increased serum total IgE and latex specific IgG_1, elevated peripheral blood eosinophils count, and enhanced lung tissue IL-4, IL-5 and IL-13, intragastric curcumin administration reduces lung inflammation. Protein expression of costimulatory molecules CD80, CD86, and OX40-Ligand, and RNA expression of MMP-9, ornithine aminotransferase (OAT), and thymic stromal lymphopoietin (TSLP) in antigen-presenting cells are all decreased. These results suggest that curcumin may disrupt antigen presentation, so that has potential therapeutic value on allergen triggered airway inflammation [285].

Curcumin has been shown to have anti-asthmatic effects in both *in vivo* and *in vitro* studies. In OVA-induced asthma model in guinea pigs, curcumin treatment during OVA sensitization or following antigen challenge shows significant protective effects through attenuation of bronchial constriction and hyperreactivity [286]. This indicates curcumin has both preventive and therapeutic effects on asthma. In another study in an OVA-induced murine asthma model, curcumin's anti-asthmatic function is attributed to the suppression of iNOS and subsequent NO production, inhibition of inflammatory cytokine synthesis and downregulation of eosinophil recruitment to airway [91]. *In vitro,* curcumin supplementation inhibits IgE/antigen activation of mast cells through the principal activation pathway mediated by FcεRI directly inhibiting Syk kinase phosphorylation, which is critical for the propagation of signaling cascade. Subsequently, the phosphorylation of MAP kinases including p38, ERK 1/2 and JNK are supressed, which are crucial for gene transcription and production of proinflammatory cytokines [287]. In addition, curcumin inhibits HDM-induced lymphocyte proliferation and production of IL-2, IL-4, IL-5, and GM-CSF by lymphocytes from asthma patients [246]. These results indicate that curcumin may attenuate asthma symptom by inhibiting production of cytokines related to eosinophil function and IgE synthesis, and suppressing IgE-mediated reactions and hyperreactivity.

5.6.5. Licorice root (Glycyrrhiza glabra)

Licorice root has been widely used around the world to treat cough since ancient time [247]. It contains the active compounds including glycyrrhizin, glycyrrhetinic acid, flavonoids, isoflavonoids, and chalcones [248]. Glycyrrhizin and glycyrrhetinic acid are considered to be the main active components [249] and are potent inhibitors of cortisol metabolism, due to their steroid like structures inhibiting the key steroid metabolic enzymes, delta 4-5-reductase, 11 beta-hydroxysteroid dehydrogenase and 20-hydroxysteroid dehydrogenase [250, 251]. Therefore, the benefits and side effects of steroid are both expected to be enhanced in the presence of glycyrrhetinic acid and glycyrrhizin.

http://dx.doi.org/10.5772/56428

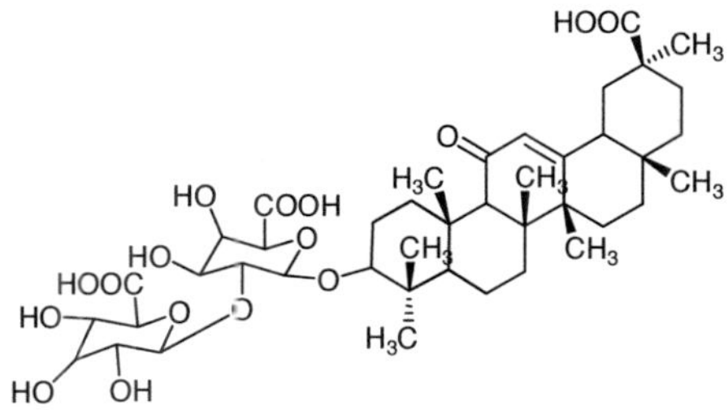

Glycyrrhizin

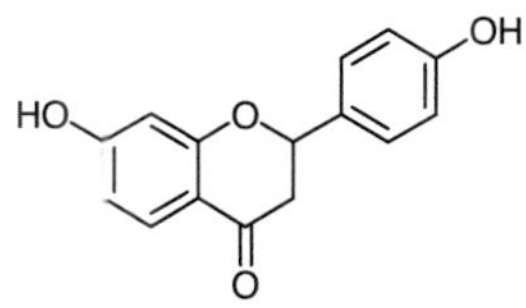

Liquiritige

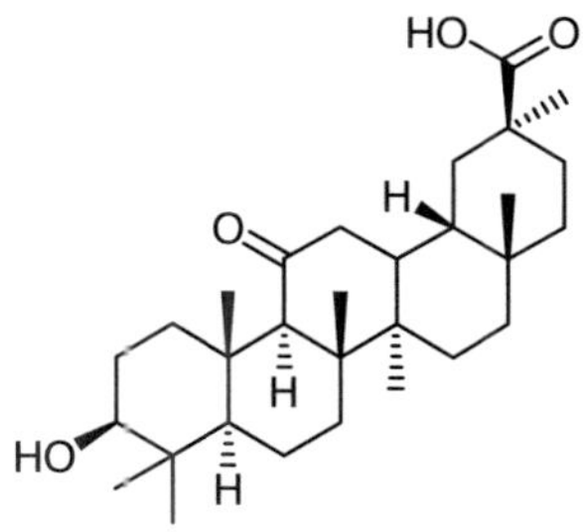

Glycyrrhetinic acid

The anti-inflammatory effect of glycyrrhizin during virus infection has been well documented [288-290] and may alleviate allergic inflammation as well. In a contact skin hypersensitivity mouse model, glycyrrhizin and its metabolite 18 β-glycyrrhetinic acid-3-O-β-D-glucuronide show protective effects in terms of reduced passive cutaneous anaphylaxis and inflammation, with glycyrrhizin being more potent than 18 β-glycyrrhetinic acid-3-O-β-D-glucuronide [291]. In an OVA-induced murine asthma model, glycyrrhizin provided orally alleviates airway constriction and hyperreactivity, pulmonary inflammation. In BAL, IFNγ level is increased, while IL-4, IL-5 levels and eosinophil count are decreased. It also reduces OVA-specific IgE levels and upregulates total IgG_{2a} in serum as well [292]. These results indicate that glycyrrhizin interfere the production of IgE by decreasing the IgE-stimulating cytokines.

The effects of glycyrrhetinic acid and liquiritigenin (a flavonoid of licorice root) on asthma have been tested both *in vivo* and *in vitro*. *In vitro*, glycyrrhetinic acid and liquiritigenin inhibits β-hexosaminidase release from RBL-2H3 cells induced by IgE/DNP, and from rat peritoneal mast cells challenged with c48/80. *In vivo*, they can suppress c48/80 induced passive cutaneous anaphylactic reaction in mice. In OVA-induced murine asthma model, glycyrrhetinic acid but not liquiritigenin reduces the level of IgE in serum [293]. Flavonoids extracted from licorice root quench LPS-induced pulmonary inflammation by inhibiting the recruitment of neutrophils, macrophages and lymphocytes in BALF, and suppressing the mRNA expression of TNF and IL-1β in LPS-challenged lung tissue in mice [238]. The reported side effects of licorice root includes headache, hypertension, hypokalemia, premature birth, muscle weakness, and increase body weight, which were attributed to its function on inhibiting the steroid metabolism [294].

5.6.6. Modified Mai-Men-Dong-Tang

Mai-Men-Dong-Tang is an old Chinese herb formula commonly used for treating lung diseases, which contains Ophiopogon, Ginseng, Pinellia, Licorice, Jujube, and Oryza [260]. It is reported to increase the cough threshold to inhaled capsaicin in asthmatic patients. Also, the eosinophil count in peripheral blood, sputum eosinophil ratio, and serum eosinophil cationic protein level are significantly decreased, especially in patients with severe airway inflammation [261], which suggests that Mai-Men-Dong-Tang may alleviate asthma-related cough by inhibiting eosinophil function.

Modified Mai-Men-Dong-Tang (mMMDT) contains five herbs, Ophiopogon, American ginseng, Pinellia, Licorice root, and Lantern tridax [262]. The efficacy and safety of this formula to persistent, mild to moderate asthma has been evaluated in a double-blind, randomized clinical study of 100 patients with mild to moderate asthma. After 4 months, improvements in FEV1 and symptom scores has been reported in mMMDT treatment groups with decreased serum IgE and no drug-related adverse effects seen in terms of blood test, and liver, kidney functions [295]. Modified Mai-Men-Dong-Tang is a potential effective herb formula in treatment of childhood asthma for long time use. However, recommendation cannot be made because of small sample size used in the study.

5.6.7. Ding-Chuan-Tang

Ding-Chuan-Tang (DCT) is a traditional Chinese herb formula used for the treatment of cough, wheezing, and chest tightness, developed about four hundred years ago during the Ming dynasty. This formula contains nine herbs including *Radix glycyrrhizae, Tuber pinellia, Gingko bilboae, Herba ephedrae, Flos tussilaginis farfarae, Cortex mori albae radicis, Fructus perilla frutescens, Semen pruni armeniacae, Radix scutellariae baicalensis* [263]. In OVA-induced pig asthma model, DCT given orally to animals 30 min before antigen challenge inhibits the antigen induced immediate asthmatic responses. If it is given together with sensitization, immediate and late asthmatic responses are all suppressed. In addition, DCT relaxes trachea contracted with carbachol. The effects are attributed to decreased eosinophil infiltration to airway [263].

Randomized double-blind, placebo-controlled study to assess the effect of DCT on airway hyperreactivity in children with mild to moderate persistent asthma has shown that the FEV1 is significantly increased in DCT group (196%, p=0.034), but not in placebo control group. Compared to placebo control group, total clinical/medication score shows improvement in the DCT group (p=0.004). No side effects have been reported [296]. These results suggest that DCT might be effective in treating asthma in children. Larger sample size and wider population are required in further investigations.

5.6.8. STA-1 and STA-2

STA is a combination of mMMDT and another Chinese herb formula Liu-Wei-Di-Huang-Wan (LWDHW), which is also used by Chinese as an anti-cough agent. LWDHW contains six herbs including *Rehmannia* root, *Alisma* rhizome, *Dioscorea* rhizome, *Poria, Hoelen, Moutan* root bark, *Shanzhu yu*. The formula for STA-1 and 2 are the same while the only difference being in the preparation of LWDHW is different [265]. In a mouse asthma model induced by intraperitoneally administrated dermatophagoides pteronyssinus group 5 allergen (Der p 5), oral STA-1 treatment during sensitization suppresses Der p 5-specific IgE production from animals in response to inhaled Der p 5 challenge. In addition, eosinophil and neutrophil airway infiltration, and airway hyperreactivity are all significantly reduced in STA-1 group compared to control animals [266]. The efficacy and side effects of STA-1 and STA-2 on childhood asthma treatment have been evaluated in a randomized, double-blind, placebo-controlled study. The herbs and placebo provided to pediatric patients with mild to moderate asthma reduces symptom scores, serum steroid concentration, total IgE, and allergen-specific IgE levels and improves FEV1 in the STA-1 group. STA-2 does not show protective effects. No severe side effects were reported [297]. These results indicate that STA-1 might be a valuable formula for childhood asthma, especially subjects induced by dust mite antigen. However, there is not enough evidence to draw a concrete conclusion. It is worthwhile to evaluate their potential use as immunotherapy as well.

5.6.9. Anti-Asthma Herbal Medicine Intervention (ASHMI)

ASHMI is a relatively new formula developed by a group of Chinese researchers and physicians, which is an extract from three herbs: *Radix glycyrrhizaen prednisone, Radix sophorae flavescentis*, and *Ganoderma* [267]. In OVA-induced asthma, oral ASHMI treatment before and during OVA sensitization and challenge reduces AHR represented by time-integrated change in peak airway pressure. Eosinophil infiltration in BALF, lung inflammation, OVA-specific IgE production, and level of IL-4, IL-5, and IL-13 in lung and splenocyte cultures are significantly lower in ASHMI treated mice, whereas IFN-γ production is increased [267, 268]. A 6-week treatment of ASHMI beginning 24 hr after the first OVA challenge in mice reduces early phase response by decreasing histamine, leukotriene C, and OVA-specific IgE levels, and suppresses late phase responses by decreasing eosinophil count and Th2 cytokines in BALF. In addition, it relieves contraction of murine tracheal rings by increasing the production of PGI_2 [269]. These results suggest that ASHMI inhibits asthmatic inflammation and airway muscle contraction, primarily by inhibiting Th2 cell function and might be suitable for treating antigen-induced asthma in both young and old subjects.

In clinical trial, ASHMI has been shown to improve lung function indicated by increased FEV1 and peak expiratory flow. Clinical symptom scores, use of β2-bronchodilators, serum IgE level, serum IL-5, IL-13 concentrations are all reduced, and some effects are even better than prednisone. During the study no adverse effect were recorded [298]. These results indicate the effectiveness of ASHMI on treating asthma in both young and old adult patients. More adequately powered investigations are needed to evaluate ASHMI's effect on asthma.

5.7. n-3 polyunsaturated fatty acids

PUFA are a group of fatty acids with more than two carbon-carbon double bonds. There are three types of PUFA, n-3, n-6 and n-9, with their names based on the position of first double band from methyl end in their chemical structures. Currently, many studies have focused on n-3 and n-6 PUFA because EPA (20:4 n-3), Dihomo-γ-Linolenic acid (DGLA, 20:3 n-6) and Arachidonic acid (AA, 20:4 n-6) in cell membrane can be metabolized and become eicosanoid precursors, which are important modulatory autocrine molecules. Eicosanoids include prostaglandins, leukotrienes, thromboxanes, resolvins, lipoxins, are signal molecules that exert complex effects on health. They can modulate inflammation, fever, blood pressure, the immune system, etc. Eicosanoids can be made by oxidation of twenty carbon n-3 (EPA) and n-6 (DGLA, AA) PUFA. Eicosanoids from AA are proinflammatory, while those from EPA and DGLA are less so. There is competition between n-3 PUFA and n-6 PUFA in oxidation in terms of cyclooxygenase and lipoxygenase, which are critical enzymes for eicosanoid generation. AA is the predominant n-6 PUFA in body. In general, n-3 and n-6 are hypothesized to be beneficial and detrimental respectively [299, 300]. Fish, fish oil, krill, mussel and seal oil are natural sources of n-3 PUFA.

The major n-3 PUFA are listed in Table 12. In mammals, including humans, n-3 PUFA cannot be synthesized *de novo*. Therefore they must be absorbed through the diet or produced from α-Linolenic acid (ALA), which is an essential fatty acid. Among them, the health beneficial effects of EPA and DHA (22:6 n-3) are well documented in a broad range of health and disease conditions. The consumption of EPA and DHA are associated with lower risk of cancer, hyperlipidemia, and cardiovascular disease, high blood pressure, and neurodegenerative diseases [301-304]. Their regulating function on immune system was also well known and are involved in activation of immune cells like of T cells, B cells, mast cells and basophils [305, 306].

In recent decade, the relationship between n-3 PUFA and inflammatory diseases has been investigated in many studies. In a study conducted in rheumatoid arthritis patients, significant improvement in symptoms have been reported after 3 month fish oil supplementation in terms of tender joint count and duration of morning stiffness [307]. Besides reduction in the production of proinflammatory eicosanoids by competition with n-6 PUFA, n-3 PUFA has been found to be effective in inhibiting the synthesis of proinflammatory cytokines. In *fat-1* transgenic mice, which have a much lower n-6:n-3 PUFA in tissues because they are genetically modified to possess the ability to convert n-6 PUFA to n-3 PUFA, serum proinflammatory cytokines, including TNF, IL-1β, and IL-6 are lower. [280]. DHA and ALA also reduce the mRNA expression of IL-1β, IL-6 in a cerulein-induced pancreatitis model. They inhibit the activation of AP-1, suppress DNA fragmentation and decrease mRNA expression of apoptotic genes including p53, Bax and apoptosis-inducing factor in hydrogen peroxide-treated pancreatic acinar cells [308]. A randomized, double-blind human study has confirmed their suppressing effect on production of proinflammatory cytokines [309]. It has been shown that n-3 fatty acids

Common name	Lipid name	Chemical name	Formula/MW	Structure
(HTA)	C16:3 (*n*−3)	all-cis-7,10,13-hexadecatrienoic acid	$C_{16}H_{26}O_2$/250.376	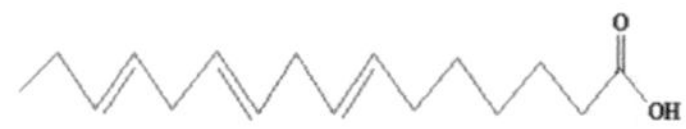
α-Linolenic acid (ALA)	C18:3 (*n*−3)	all-cis-9,12,15-octadecatrienoic acid	$C_{18}H_{30}O_2$/278.430	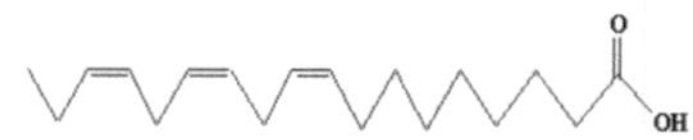
α -Parinaric acid	C18:4 (*n*−3)	all-cis-9,11,13,15-octadecatetraenoic acid	$C_{18}H_{28}O_2$/276.414	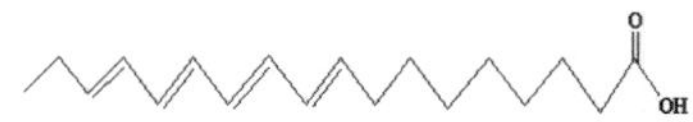
Stearidonic acid (SDA)	C18:4 (*n* −3)	all-cis-6,9,12,15-octadecatetraenoic acid	$C_{18}H_{28}O_2$/276.414	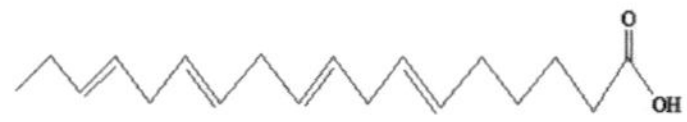
(ETE)	C20:3 (*n*−3)	all-cis-11,14,17-eicosatrienoic acid	$C_{20}H_{34}O_2$/306.483	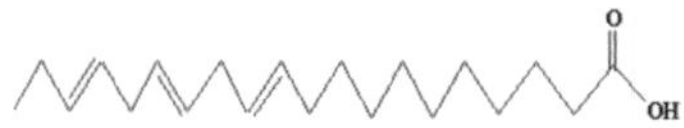
(ETA)	C20:4 (*n*−3)	all-cis-8,11,14,17-eicosatetraenoic acid	$C_{20}H_{32}O_2$/304.467	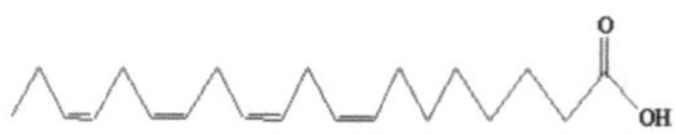
(EPA)	C20:5 (*n*−3)	all-cis-5,8,11,14,17-eicosapentaenoic acid	$C_{20}H_{30}O_2$/302.451	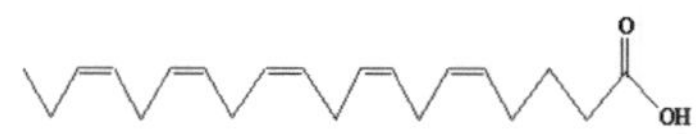
(DPA)	C22:5 (*n*−3)	all-cis-7,10,13,16,19-docosapentaenoic acid	$C_{22}H_{34}O_2$/330.504	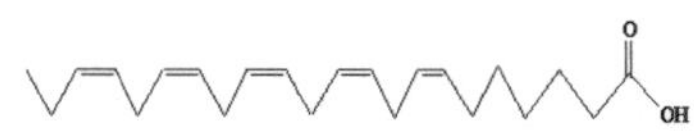
(DHA)	C22:6 (*n*−3)	all-cis-4,7,10,13,16,19-docosahexaenoic acid	$C_{22}H_{32}O_2$/328.488	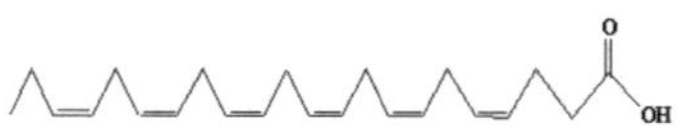

Table 12. The common name, lipid name and chemical name of major n-3 PUFA

can alleviate inflammatory process by modulating cell signalling pathways in immune cells, such as T cell receptor pathway and cytokine receptor pathways. [310-312]

There have been a number of clinical studies that have shown n-3 PUFA's potentially protective effects on asthma, especially on childhood patients. There is a positive association between the n-6:n-3 PUFA in diet and risk for asthma [313]. A randomized, double-blind, placebo-controlled 3-year study on effect of n-3 PUFA supplementation on asthma has found that high n-3 PUFA diet intervention significantly reducesd the prevalence of cough in atopic children, suggesting that n-3 PUFA may be effective in preventing the development of asthma in early childhood [314]. In a cohort study on the relations between fish/cod oil intake and asthma, results have shown that adults with low fish intake frequency (less than weekly) have increased risk to have asthma [315]. Another randomized double-blind study with 5-weeks n-3 PUFA supplementation has reported a significant decrease in exhaled NO from asthma patients challenged with mite allergen. Serum eosinophils count and ECP, and the production of CysLTs from isolated leukocyte stimulated with mite antigen are also reduced [194]. Overall, n-3 PUFA might be a promising remedy agents for allergic diseases like asthma but the mechanism remains to be elucidated.

6. Conclusion

The prevalence of asthma is becoming the mortality and morbidity pandemic of the 21st century. The cost of in quality of patient's lives and economic burden of treatment is continuing to grow at pace unmatched in our current health system. It is impossible to enter public classroom now without seeing a young sufferer of this condition and any trip to the emergency department will show how dangerous this disease can be. As the incidence and severity of the disease continues to rise, medical research is continuing to search new treatment strategies. While many treatments currently exists those reserve for the severest of conditions carry their own inherent risk which may match the severity of disease itself. It is for these reasons alone that health care professionals are now examining the traits of our ancestors in time when this epidemic was less severe to determine if their medicines and practices hold the answer for the next treatment strategy. By combining the scientific knowledge at the molecular and clinical level and the resources of past it might hold the answer to breathless pandemic of the 21st century.

Acknowledgements

The authors are thankful to Dr. Clayton Macdonald for his assiatance with the manuscript preparation. This work is supported by the National Research Council Canada. Priyanka Pundir is the recipient of Innovation PEI Graduate Student Fellowship.

Author details

Priyanka Pundir[1,2], Xiaofeng Wang[1,2] and Marianna Kulka[3]

1 National Research Council Canada, Charlottetown, PE, Canada

2 Department of Biomedical Sciences, Atlantic Veterinary College, University of Prince Edward Island, Charlottetown, PE, Canada

3 National Research Council Canada, Edmonton, AB, Canada

References

[1] Seaton A, Godden DJ, Brown K. Increase in asthma: a more toxic environment or a more susceptible population? Thorax. 1994;49(2):171-4. Epub 1994/02/01.

[2] Wood LG, Gibson PG, Garg ML. Biomarkers of lipid peroxidation, airway inflammation and asthma. Eur Respir J. 2003;21(1):177-86. Epub 2003/02/07.

[3] Katsumata U, Miura M, Ichinose M, Kimura K, Takahashi T, Inoue H, et al. Oxygen radicals produce airway constriction and hyperresponsiveness in anesthetized cats. The American review of respiratory disease. 1990;141(5 Pt 1):1158-61. Epub 1990/05/01.

[4] Rubin RN, Navon L, Cassano PA. Relationship of serum antioxidants to asthma prevalence in youth. Am J Respir Crit Care Med. 2004;169(3):393-8.

[5] Gilliland FD, Berhane KT, Li YF, Gauderman WJ, McConnell R, Peters J. Children's lung function and antioxidant vitamin, fruit, juice, and vegetable intake. Am J Epidemiol. 2003;158(6):576-84. Epub 2003/09/11.

[6] Hu G, Cassano PA. Antioxidant nutrients and pulmonary function: the Third National Health and Nutrition Examination Survey (NHANES III). Am J Epidemiol. 2000;151(10):975-81. Epub 2000/06/15.

[7] Britton JR, Pavord ID, Richards KA, Knox AJ, Wisniewski AF, Lewis SA, et al. Dietary antioxidant vitamin intake and lung function in the general population. Am J Respir Crit Care Med. 1995;151(5):1383-7. Epub 1995/05/01.

[8] Schwartz J, Weiss ST. Relationship between dietary vitamin C intake and pulmonary function in the First National Health and Nutrition Examination Survey (NHANES I). The American journal of clinical nutrition. 1994;59(1):110-4. Epub 1994/01/01.

[9] Soutar A, Seaton A, Brown K. Bronchial reactivity and dietary antioxidants. Thorax. 1997;52(2):166-70. Epub 1997/02/01.

[10] Harik-Khan RI, Muller DC, Wise RA. Serum vitamin levels and the risk of asthma in children. Am J Epidemiol. 2004;159(4):351-7.

[11] Bodner C, Godden D, Brown K, Little J, Ross S, Seaton A. Antioxidant intake and adult-onset wheeze: a case-control study. Aberdeen WHEASE Study Group. Eur Respir J. 1999;13(1):22-30. Epub 2000/06/03.

[12] Butland BK, Fehily AM, Elwood PC. Diet, lung function, and lung function decline in a cohort of 2512 middle aged men. Thorax. 2000;55(2):102-8. Epub 2000/01/20.

[13] Hijazi N, Abalkhail B, Seaton A. Diet and childhood asthma in a society in transition: a study in urban and rural Saudi Arabia. Thorax. 2000;55(9):775-9. Epub 2000/08/19.

[14] Fogarty A, Lewis S, Weiss S, Britton J. Dietary vitamin E, IgE concentrations, and atopy. Lancet. 2000;356(9241):1573-4. Epub 2000/11/15.

[15] Butland BK, Strachan DP, Anderson HR. Fresh fruit intake and asthma symptoms in young British adults: confounding or effect modification by smoking? Eur Respir J. 1999;13(4):744-50. Epub 1999/06/11.

[16] Miedema I, Feskens EJ, Heederik D, Kromhout D. Dietary determinants of long-term incidence of chronic nonspecific lung diseases. The Zutphen Study. Am J Epidemiol. 1993;138(1):37-45. Epub 1993/07/01.

[17] Carey IM, Strachan DP, Cook DG. Effects of changes in fresh fruit consumption on ventilatory function in healthy British adults. Am J Respir Crit Care Med. 1998;158(3):728-33. Epub 1998/09/10.

[18] Shaheen SO, Sterne JA, Thompson RL, Songhurst CE, Margetts BM, Burney PG. Dietary antioxidants and asthma in adults: population-based case-control study. Am J Respir Crit Care Med. 2001;164(10 Pt 1):1823-8. Epub 2001/12/06.

[19] Dow L, Tracey M, Villar A, Coggon D, Margetts BM, Campbell MJ, et al. Does dietary intake of vitamins C and E influence lung function in older people? Am J Respir Crit Care Med. 1996;154(5):1401-4. Epub 1996/11/01.

[20] Morabia A, Sorenson A, Kumanyika SK, Abbey H, Cohen BH, Chee E. Vitamin A, cigarette smoking, and airway obstruction. The American review of respiratory disease. 1989;140(5):1312-6. Epub 1989/11/01.

[21] La Vecchia C, Decarli A, Pagano R. Vegetable consumption and risk of chronic disease. Epidemiology. 1998;9(2):208-10. Epub 1998/03/21.

[22] Ellwood P, Asher MI, Bjorksten B, Burr M, Pearce N, Robertson CF. Diet and asthma, allergic rhinoconjunctivitis and atopic eczema symptom prevalence: an ecological analysis of the International Study of Asthma and Allergies in Childhood (ISAAC) data. ISAAC Phase One Study Group. Eur Respir J. 2001;17(3):436-43. Epub 2001/06/19.

[23] Arts IC, Hollman PC. Polyphenols and disease risk in epidemiologic studies. The American journal of clinical nutrition. 2005;81(1 Suppl):317S-25S. Epub 2005/01/11.

[24] Barrett NA, Austen KF. Innate cells and T helper 2 cell immunity in airway inflammation. Immunity. 2009;31(3):425-37.

[25] Halwani R, Al-Muhsen S, Hamid Q. Airway remodeling in asthma. Curr Opin Pharmacol.10(3):236-45.

[26] Galli SJ, Tsai M, Piliponsky AM. The development of allergic inflammation. Nature. 2008;454(7203):445-54. Epub 2008/07/25.

[27] Holt PG. Antigen presentation in the lung. Am J Respir Crit Care Med. 2000;162(4 Pt 2):S151-6.

[28] Willart MA, Hammad H. Alarming dendritic cells for allergic sensitization. Allergol Int.59(2):95-103.

[29] Robinson DS. The role of the T cell in asthma. J Allergy Clin Immunol.126(6):1081-91; quiz 92-3.

[30] Holgate ST. Pathogenesis of asthma. Clin Exp Allergy. 2008;38(6):872-97.

[31] Fox B, Bull TB, Guz A. Mast cells in the human alveolar wall: an electronmicroscopic study. J Clin Pathol. 1981;34(12):1333-42.

[32] Rivera J, Fierro NA, Olivera A, Suzuki R. New insights on mast cell activation via the high affinity receptor for IgE. Adv Immunol. 2008;98:85-120.

[33] Pundir P, Kulka M. The role of G protein-coupled receptors in mast cell activation by antimicrobial peptides: is there a connection? Immunol Cell Biol.88(6):632-40.

[34] Pradalier A. Late-phase reaction in asthma: basic mechanisms. Int Arch Allergy Immunol. 1993;101(3):322-5.

[35] Bradding P, Holgate ST. Immunopathology and human mast cell cytokines. Crit Rev Oncol Hematol. 1999;31(2):119-33.

[36] Leckie MJ, ten Brinke A, Khan J, Diamant Z, O'Connor BJ, Walls CM, et al. Effects of an interleukin-5 blocking monoclonal antibody on eosinophils, airway hyper-responsiveness, and the late asthmatic response. Lancet. 2000;356(9248):2144-8.

[37] Larsen GL, Wilson MC, Clark RA, Behrens BL. The inflammatory reaction in the airways in an animal model of the late asthmatic response. Fed Proc. 1987;46(1):105-12.

[38] De Monchy JG, Kauffman HF, Venge P, Koeter GH, Jansen HM, Sluiter HJ, et al. Bronchoalveolar eosinophilia during allergen-induced late asthmatic reactions. Am Rev Respir Dis. 1985;131(3):373-6.

[39] Kariyawasam HH, Robinson DS. The eosinophil: the cell and its weapons, the cytokines, its locations. Semin Respir Crit Care Med. 2006;27(2):117-27.

[40] Panettieri RA, Tan EM, Ciocca V, Luttmann MA, Leonard TB, Hay DW. Effects of LTD4 on human airway smooth muscle cell proliferation, matrix expression, and contraction In vitro: differential sensitivity to cysteinyl leukotriene receptor antagonists. Am J Respir Cell Mol Biol. 1998;19(3):453-61.

[41] Laitinen LA, Laitinen A, Haahtela T, Vilkka V, Spur BW, Lee TH. Leukotriene E4 and granulocytic infiltration into asthmatic airways. Lancet. 1993;341(8851):989-90. Epub 1993/04/17.

[42] Sur S, Crotty TB, Kephart GM, Hyma BA, Colby TV, Reed CE, et al. Sudden-onset fatal asthma. A distinct entity with few eosinophils and relatively more neutrophils in the airway submucosa? The American review of respiratory disease. 1993;148(3): 713-9. Epub 1993/09/01.

[43] Fahy JV, Kim KW, Liu J, Boushey HA. Prominent neutrophilic inflammation in sputum from subjects with asthma exacerbation. J Allergy Clin Immunol. 1995;95(4): 843-52. Epub 1995/04/01.

[44] Hamzaoui A, Hamzaoui K, Salah H, Chabbou A. Lymphocytes apoptosis in patients with acute exacerbation of asthma. Mediators of inflammation. 1999;8(4-5):237-43. Epub 2000/03/07.

[45] Robinson D, Hamid Q, Bentley A, Ying S, Kay AB, Durham SR. Activation of CD4+ T cells, increased TH2-type cytokine mRNA expression, and eosinophil recruitment in bronchoalveolar lavage after allergen inhalation challenge in patients with atopic asthma. J Allergy Clin Immunol. 1993;92(2):313-24. Epub 1993/08/01.

[46] Cumming RG, Mitchell P, Leeder SR. Use of inhaled corticosteroids and the risk of cataracts. The New England journal of medicine. 1997;337(1):8-14. Epub 1997/07/03.

[47] van Staa TP, Leufkens HG, Cooper C. Use of inhaled corticosteroids and risk of fractures. Journal of bone and mineral research : the official journal of the American Society for Bone and Mineral Research. 2001;16(3):581-8. Epub 2001/03/30.

[48] Guilbert TW, Morgan WJ, Zeiger RS, Mauger DT, Boehmer SJ, Szefler SJ, et al. Long-term inhaled corticosteroids in preschool children at high risk for asthma. The New England journal of medicine. 2006;354(19):1985-97. Epub 2006/05/12.

[49] Lou HQ, Ying YF, Hu Y. [CRTH2 antagonist ameliorates airway inflammation in rats with asthma]. Zhejiang Da Xue Xue Bao Yi Xue Ban.39(1):64-70.

[50] Lukacs NW, Berlin AA, Franz-Bacon K, Sasik R, Sprague LJ, Ly TW, et al. CRTH2 antagonism significantly ameliorates airway hyperreactivity and downregulates inflammation-induced genes in a mouse model of airway inflammation. Am J Physiol Lung Cell Mol Physiol. 2008;295(5):L767-79.

[51] Hicks A, Goodnow R, Jr., Cavallo G, Tannu SA, Ventre JD, Lavelle D, et al. Effects of LTB4 receptor antagonism on pulmonary inflammation in rodents and non-human primates. Prostaglandins Other Lipid Mediat.92(1-4):33-43.

[52] Kimata M, Shichijo M, Miura T, Serizawa I, Inagaki N, Nagai H. Effects of luteolin, quercetin and baicalein on immunoglobulin E-mediated mediator release from human cultured mast cells. Clin Exp Allergy. 2000;30(4):501-8.

[53] Siegle JS, Hansbro N, Dong C, Angkasekwinai P, Foster PS, Kumar RK. Blocking induction of T helper type 2 responses prevents development of disease in a model of childhood asthma. Clin Exp Immunol.

[54] Caramori G, Groneberg D, Ito K, Casolari P, Adcock IM, Papi A. New drugs targeting Th2 lymphocytes in asthma. J Occup Med Toxicol. 2008;3 Suppl 1:S6. Epub 2008/03/05.

[55] Rosenwasser LJ, Rothenberg ME. IL-5 pathway inhibition in the treatment of asthma and Churg-Strauss syndrome. J Allergy Clin Immunol.125(6):1245-6.

[56] Walsh GM. Tralokinumab, an anti-IL-13 mAb for the potential treatment of asthma and COPD. Curr Opin Investig Drugs.11(11):1305-12.

[57] Hirano T, Higa S, Arimitsu J, Naka T, Shima Y, Ohshima S, et al. Flavonoids such as luteolin, fisetin and apigenin are inhibitors of interleukin-4 and interleukin-13 production by activated human basophils. Int Arch Allergy Immunol. 2004;134(2): 135-40.

[58] Kang OH, Lee JH, Kwon DY. Apigenin inhibits release of inflammatory mediators by blocking the NF-kappaB activation pathways in the HMC-1 cells. Immunopharmacol Immunotoxicol.

[59] Hsieh CJ, Hall K, Ha T, Li C, Krishnaswamy G, Chi DS. Baicalein inhibits IL-1beta- and TNF-alpha-induced inflammatory cytokine production from human mast cells via regulation of the NF-kappaB pathway. Clin Mol Allergy. 2007;5:5.

[60] Lixuan Z, Jingcheng D, Wenqin Y, Jianhua H, Baojun L, Xiaotao F. Baicalin attenuates inflammation by inhibiting NF-kappaB activation in cigarette smoke induced inflammatory models. Pulm Pharmacol Ther.23(5):411-9.

[61] Bae Y, Lee S, Kim SH. Chrysin suppresses mast cell-mediated allergic inflammation: Involvement of calcium, caspase-1 and nuclear factor-kappaB. Toxicol Appl Pharmacol.254(1):56-64.

[62] Nakamura R, Nakamura R, Watanabe K, Oka K, Ohta S, Mishima S, et al. Effects of propolis from different areas on mast cell degranulation and identification of the effective components in propolis. Int Immunopharmacol.10(9):1107-12.

[63] Higa S, Hirano T, Kotani M, Matsumoto M, Fujita A, Suemura M, et al. Fisetin, a flavonol, inhibits TH2-type cytokine production by activated human basophils. J Allergy Clin Immunol. 2003;111(6):1299-306.

[64] Weseler AR, Geraets L, Moonen HJ, Manders RJ, van Loon LJ, Pennings HJ, et al. Poly (ADP-ribose) polymerase-1-inhibiting flavonoids attenuate cytokine release in blood from male patients with chronic obstructive pulmonary disease or type 2 diabetes. J Nutr. 2009;139(5):952-7.

[65] Park HH, Lee S, Oh JM, Lee MS, Yoon KH, Park BH, et al. Anti-inflammatory activity of fisetin in human mast cells (HMC-1). Pharmacol Res. 2007;55(1):31-7.

[66] Han JM, Jin YY, Kim HY, Park KH, Lee WS, Jeong TS. Lavandulyl flavonoids from Sophora flavescens suppress lipopolysaccharide-induced activation of nuclear factor-kappaB and mitogen-activated protein kinases in RAW264.7 cells. Biol Pharm Bull. 33(6):1019-23.

[67] Park CM, Jin KS, Lee YW, Song YS. Luteolin and chicoric acid synergistically inhibited inflammatory responses via inactivation of PI3K-Akt pathway and impairment of

NF-kappaB translocation in LPS stimulated RAW 264.7 cells. Eur J Pharmacol. 660(2-3):454-9.

[68] Kang OH, Jang HJ, Chae HS, Oh YC, Choi JG, Lee YS, et al. Anti-inflammatory mechanisms of resveratrol in activated HMC-1 cells: pivotal roles of NF-kappaB and MAPK. Pharmacol Res. 2009;59(5):330-7.

[69] Jin M, Yang JH, Lee E, Lu Y, Kwon S, Son KH, et al. Antiasthmatic activity of luteolin-7-O-glucoside from Ailanthus altissima through the downregulation of T helper 2 cytokine expression and inhibition of prostaglandin E2 production in an ovalbumin-induced asthma model. Biol Pharm Bull. 2009;32(9):1500-3.

[70] Kempuraj D, Tagen M, Iliopoulou BP, Clemons A, Vasiadi M, Boucher W, et al. Luteolin inhibits myelin basic protein-induced human mast cell activation and mast cell-dependent stimulation of Jurkat T cells. Br J Pharmacol. 2008;155(7):1076-84.

[71] Hougee S, Sanders A, Faber J, Graus YM, van den Berg WB, Garssen J, et al. Decreased pro-inflammatory cytokine production by LPS-stimulated PBMC upon in vitro incubation with the flavonoids apigenin, luteolin or chrysin, due to selective elimination of monocytes/macrophages. Biochem Pharmacol. 2005;69(2):241-8.

[72] Das M, Ram A, Ghosh B. Luteolin alleviates bronchoconstriction and airway hyperreactivity in ovalbumin sensitized mice. Inflamm Res. 2003;52(3):101-6.

[73] Mastuda H, Morikawa T, Ueda K, Managi H, Yoshikawa M. Structural requirements of flavonoids for inhibition of antigen-Induced degranulation, TNF-alpha and IL-4 production from RBL-2H3 cells. Bioorg Med Chem. 2002;10(10):3123-8.

[74] Harasstani OA, Moin S, Tham CL, Liew CY, Ismail N, Rajajendram R, et al. Flavonoid combinations cause synergistic inhibition of proinflammatory mediator secretion from lipopolysaccharide-induced RAW 264.7 cells. Inflamm Res.59(9):711-21.

[75] Kempuraj D, Madhappan B, Christodoulou S, Boucher W, Cao J, Papadopoulou N, et al. Flavonols inhibit proinflammatory mediator release, intracellular calcium ion levels and protein kinase C theta phosphorylation in human mast cells. Br J Pharmacol. 2005;145(7):934-44.

[76] Park HH, Lee S, Son HY, Park SB, Kim MS, Choi EJ, et al. Flavonoids inhibit histamine release and expression of proinflammatory cytokines in mast cells. Arch Pharm Res. 2008;31(10):1303-11.

[77] Iwamura C, Shinoda K, Yoshimura M, Watanabe Y, Obata A, Nakayama T. Naringenin chalcone suppresses allergic asthma by inhibiting the type-2 function of CD4 T cells. Allergol Int.59(1):67-73.

[78] Shi Y, Dai J, Liu H, Li RR, Sun PL, Du Q, et al. Naringenin inhibits allergen-induced airway inflammation and airway responsiveness and inhibits NF-kappaB activity in a murine model of asthma. Can J Physiol Pharmacol. 2009;87(9):729-35.

[79] Bodet C, La VD, Epifano F, Grenier D. Naringenin has anti-inflammatory properties in macrophage and ex vivo human whole-blood models. J Periodontal Res. 2008;43(4):400-7.

[80] Rao YK, Fang SH, Hsieh SC, Yeh TH, Tzeng YM. The constituents of Anisomeles indica and their anti-inflammatory activities. J Ethnopharmacol. 2009;121(2):292-6.

[81] Lee M, Kim S, Kwon OK, Oh SR, Lee HK, Ahn K. Anti-inflammatory and anti-asthmatic effects of resveratrol, a polyphenolic stilbene, in a mouse model of allergic asthma. Int Immunopharmacol. 2009;9(4):418-24.

[82] Knobloch J, Sibbing B, Jungck D, Lin Y, Urban K, Stoelben E, et al. Resveratrol impairs the release of steroid-resistant inflammatory cytokines from human airway smooth muscle cells in chronic obstructive pulmonary disease. J Pharmacol Exp Ther.335(3):788-98.

[83] Oh YC, Kang OH, Choi JG, Chae HS, Lee YS, Brice OO, et al. Anti-inflammatory effect of resveratrol by inhibition of IL-8 production in LPS-induced THP-1 cells. Am J Chin Med. 2009;37(6):1203-14.

[84] Bereswill S, Munoz M, Fischer A, Plickert R, Haag LM, Otto B, et al. Anti-inflammatory effects of resveratrol, curcumin and simvastatin in acute small intestinal inflammation. PLoS One.5(12):e15099.

[85] Cao Q, Jing C, Tang X, Yin Y, Han X, Wu W. Protective effect of resveratrol on acute lung injury induced by lipopolysaccharide in mice. Anat Rec (Hoboken).294(3): 527-32.

[86] Issuree PD, Pushparaj PN, Pervaiz S, Melendez AJ. Resveratrol attenuates C5a-induced inflammatory responses in vitro and in vivo by inhibiting phospholipase D and sphingosine kinase activities. Faseb J. 2009;23(8):2412-24.

[87] Kuo FH, Jan TR. Silibinin attenuates antigen-specific IgE production through the modulation of Th1/Th2 balance in ovalbumin-sensitized BALB/c mice. Phytomedicine. 2009;16(2-3):271-6.

[88] Jung WK, Lee DY, Choi YH, Yea SS, Choi I, Park SG, et al. Caffeic acid phenethyl ester attenuates allergic airway inflammation and hyperresponsiveness in murine model of ovalbumin-induced asthma. Life Sci. 2008;82(13-14):797-805.

[89] Wang LC, Lin YL, Liang YC, Yang YH, Lee JH, Yu HH, et al. The effect of caffeic acid phenethyl ester on the functions of human monocyte-derived dendritic cells. BMC Immunol. 2009;10:39.

[90] Khayyal MT, el-Ghazaly MA, el-Khatib AS, Hatem AM, de Vries PJ, el-Shafei S, et al. A clinical pharmacological study of the potential beneficial effects of a propolis food product as an adjuvant in asthmatic patients. Fundam Clin Pharmacol. 2003;17(1): 93-102.

[91] Moon DO, Kim MO, Lee HJ, Choi YH, Park YM, Heo MS, et al. Curcumin attenuates ovalbumin-induced airway inflammation by regulating nitric oxide. Biochem Biophys Res Commun. 2008;375(2):275-9.

[92] Wong CK, Li ML, Wang CB, Ip WK, Tian YP, Lam CW. House dust mite allergen Der p 1 elevates the release of inflammatory cytokines and expression of adhesion molecules in co-culture of human eosinophils and bronchial epithelial cells. Int Immunol. 2006;18(8):1327-35.

[93] Kobayashi T, Hashimoto S, Horie T. Curcumin inhibition of Dermatophagoides farinea-induced interleukin-5 (IL-5) and granulocyte macrophage-colony stimulating factor (GM-CSF) production by lymphocytes from bronchial asthmatics. Biochem Pharmacol. 1997;54(7):819-24.

[94] Baek OS, Kang OH, Choi YA, Choi SC, Kim TH, Nah YH, et al. Curcumin inhibits protease-activated receptor-2 and -4-mediated mast cell activation. Clin Chim Acta. 2003;338(1-2):135-41.

[95] Temkin V, Kantor B, Weg V, Hartman ML, Levi-Schaffer F. Tryptase activates the mitogen-activated protein kinase/activator protein-1 pathway in human peripheral blood eosinophils, causing cytokine production and release. J Immunol. 2002;169(5): 2662-9.

[96] Bani D, Giannini L, Ciampa A, Masini E, Suzuki Y, Menegazzi M, et al. Epigallocatechin-3-gallate reduces allergen-induced asthma-like reaction in sensitized guinea pigs. J Pharmacol Exp Ther. 2006;317(3):1002-11.

[97] Shin HY, Kim SH, Jeong HJ, Kim SY, Shin TY, Um JY, et al. Epigallocatechin-3-gallate inhibits secretion of TNF-alpha, IL-6 and IL-8 through the attenuation of ERK and NF-kappaB in HMC-1 cells. Int Arch Allergy Immunol. 2007;142(4):335-44.

[98] Syed DN, Afaq F, Kweon MH, Hadi N, Bhatia N, Spiegelman VS, et al. Green tea polyphenol EGCG suppresses cigarette smoke condensate-induced NF-kappaB activation in normal human bronchial epithelial cells. Oncogene. 2007;26(5):673-82.

[99] Bae HB, Li M, Kim JP, Kim SJ, Jeong CW, Lee HG, et al. The effect of epigallocatechin gallate on lipopolysaccharide-induced acute lung injury in a murine model. Inflammation.33(2):82-91.

[100] Rodrigues TG, Fernandes A, Jr., Sousa JP, Bastos JK, Sforcin JM. In vitro and in vivo effects of clove on pro-inflammatory cytokines production by macrophages. Nat Prod Res. 2009;23(4):319-26.

[101] Adhami VM, Malik A, Zaman N, Sarfaraz S, Siddiqui IA, Syed DN, et al. Combined inhibitory effects of green tea polyphenols and selective cyclooxygenase-2 inhibitors on the growth of human prostate cancer cells both in vitro and in vivo. Clin Cancer Res. 2007;13(5):1611-9.

[102] Kim SH, Jun CD, Suk K, Choi BJ, Lim H, Park S, et al. Gallic acid inhibits histamine release and pro-inflammatory cytokine production in mast cells. Toxicol Sci. 2006;91(1):123-31.

[103] Tripathi S, Maier KG, Bruch D, Kittur DS. Effect of 6-gingerol on pro-inflammatory cytokine production and costimulatory molecule expression in murine peritoneal macrophages. J Surg Res. 2007;138(2):209-13.

[104] Zhang X, Cao J, Zhong L. Hydroxytyrosol inhibits pro-inflammatory cytokines, iNOS, and COX-2 expression in human monocytic cells. Naunyn Schmiedebergs Arch Pharmacol. 2009;379(6):581-6.

[105] Bitler CM, Viale TM, Damaj B, Crea R. Hydrolyzed olive vegetation water in mice has anti-inflammatory activity. J Nutr. 2005;135(6):1475-9.

[106] Inoue K, Takano H, Shiga A, Fujita Y, Makino H, Yanagisawa R, et al. Effects of volatile constituents of a rosemary extract on allergic airway inflammation related to house dust mite allergen in mice. Int J Mol Med. 2005;16(2):315-9.

[107] Sanbongi C, Takano H, Osakabe N, Sasa N, Natsume M, Yanagisawa R, et al. Rosmarinic acid in perilla extract inhibits allergic inflammation induced by mite allergen, in a mouse model. Clin Exp Allergy. 2004;34(6):971-7.

[108] Oh HA, Park CS, Ahn HJ, Park YS, Kim HM. Effect of Perilla frutescens var. acuta Kudo and rosmarinic acid on allergic inflammatory reactions. Exp Biol Med (Maywood).236(1):99-106.

[109] Jang AH, Kim TH, Kim GD, Kim JE, Kim HJ, Kim SS, et al. Rosmarinic acid attenuates 2,4-dinitrofluorobenzene-induced atopic dermatitis in NC/Nga mice. Int Immunopharmacol.

[110] Inoue K, Takano H, Shiga A, Fujita Y, Makino H, Yanagisawa R, et al. Effects of volatile constituents of rosemary extract on lung inflammation induced by diesel exhaust particles. Basic Clin Pharmacol Toxicol. 2006;99(1):52-7.

[111] Pae HO, Jeong GS, Kim HS, Woo WH, Rhew HY, Kim HS, et al. Costunolide inhibits production of tumor necrosis factor-alpha and interleukin-6 by inducing heme oxygenase-1 in RAW264.7 macrophages. Inflamm Res. 2007;56(12):520-6.

[112] Kang JS, Yoon YD, Lee KH, Park SK, Kim HM. Costunolide inhibits interleukin-1beta expression by down-regulation of AP-1 and MAPK activity in LPS-stimulated RAW 264.7 cells. Biochem Biophys Res Commun. 2004;313(1):171-7.

[113] Seidel P, Merfort I, Hughes JM, Oliver BG, Tamm M, Roth M. Dimethylfumarate inhibits NF-{kappa}B function at multiple levels to limit airway smooth muscle cell cytokine secretion. Am J Physiol Lung Cell Mol Physiol. 2009;297(2):L326-39.

[114] Ben S, Li X, Xu F, Xu W, Li W, Wu Z, et al. Treatment with anti-CC chemokine receptor 3 monoclonal antibody or dexamethasone inhibits the migration and differentia-

tion of bone marrow CD34 progenitor cells in an allergic mouse model. Allergy. 2008;63(9):1164-76.

[115] Das AM, Vaddi KG, Solomon KA, Krauthauser C, Jiang X, McIntyre KW, et al. Selective inhibition of eosinophil influx into the lung by small molecule CC chemokine receptor 3 antagonists in mouse models of allergic inflammation. J Pharmacol Exp Ther. 2006;318(1):411-7.

[116] Nakagami Y, Kawase Y, Yonekubo K, Nosaka E, Etori M, Takahashi S, et al. RS-1748, a novel CC chemokine receptor 4 antagonist, inhibits ovalbumin-induced airway inflammation in guinea pigs. Biol Pharm Bull.33(6):1067-9.

[117] Vijayanand P, Durkin K, Hartmann G, Morjaria J, Seumois G, Staples KJ, et al. Chemokine receptor 4 plays a key role in T cell recruitment into the airways of asthmatic patients. J Immunol.184(8):4568-74.

[118] Sugimoto H, Shichijo M, Iino T, Manabe Y, Watanabe A, Shimazaki M, et al. An orally bioavailable small molecule antagonist of CRTH2, ramatroban (BAY u3405), inhibits prostaglandin D2-induced eosinophil migration in vitro. J Pharmacol Exp Ther. 2003;305(1):347-52.

[119] Uller L, Mathiesen JM, Alenmyr L, Korsgren M, Ulven T, Hogberg T, et al. Antagonism of the prostaglandin D2 receptor CRTH2 attenuates asthma pathology in mouse eosinophilic airway inflammation. Respir Res. 2007;8:16.

[120] Huang CH, Kuo PL, Hsu YL, Chang TT, Tseng HI, Chu YT, et al. The natural flavonoid apigenin suppresses Th1- and Th2-related chemokine production by human monocyte THP-1 cells through mitogen-activated protein kinase pathways. J Med Food.13(2):391-8.

[121] Kowalski J, Samojedny A, Paul M, Pietsz G. [Apigenin inhibits release and gene expression of monocyte chemoattractant protein 1 (MCP-1) in J774.2 macrophages]. Wiad Lek. 2006;59(9-10):634-8. Hamujacy wplyw apigeniny na wydzielanie i ekspresji genu bialka chemotaktycznego monocytow (MCP-1) w hodowli makrofagow linii J774.2.

[122] Nakajima T, Imanishi M, Yamamoto K, Cyong JC, Hirai K. Inhibitory effect of baicalein, a flavonoid in Scutellaria Root, on eotaxin production by human dermal fibroblasts. Planta Med. 2001;67(2):132-5.

[123] Lee S, Kim YJ, Kwon S, Lee Y, Choi SY, Park J, et al. Inhibitory effects of flavonoids on TNF-alpha-induced IL-8 gene expression in HEK 293 cells. BMB Rep. 2009;42(5): 265-70.

[124] Sohn MH, Lee KE, Kim KW, Kim ES, Park JY, Kim KE. Calcium-calmodulin mediates house dust mite-induced ERK activation and IL-8 production in human respiratory epithelial cells. Respiration. 2007;74(4):447-53.

[125] Trompezinski S, Denis A, Schmitt D, Viac J. Comparative effects of polyphenols from green tea (EGCG) and soybean (genistein) on VEGF and IL-8 release from normal hu-

man keratinocytes stimulated with the proinflammatory cytokine TNFalpha. Arch Dermatol Res. 2003;295(3):112-6.

[126] Saito N, Yamada Y, Sannohe S, Honda K, Adachi T, Kayaba H, et al. Possible involvement of C-C chemokines in functional augmentation of adhesion molecules in asthmatic patients. Lung. 2002;180(5):251-63.

[127] Jayaprakasam B, Doddaga S, Wang R, Holmes D, Goldfarb J, Li XM. Licorice flavonoids inhibit eotaxin-1 secretion by human fetal lung fibroblasts in vitro. J Agric Food Chem. 2009;57(3):820-5.

[128] Huang CH, Jan RL, Kuo CH, Chu YT, Wang WL, Lee MS, et al. Natural Flavone Kaempferol Suppresses Chemokines Expression in Human Monocyte THP-1 Cells through MAPK Pathways. J Food Sci.75(8):H254-H9.

[129] Kowalski J, Samojedny A, Paul M, Pietsz G, Wilczok T. Effect of kaempferol on the production and gene expression of monocyte chemoattractant protein-1 in J774.2 macrophages. Pharmacol Rep. 2005;57(1):107-12.

[130] Lee SW, Lee HS, Nam JY, Kwon OE, Baek JA, Chang JS, et al. Kurarinone isolated from Sophora flavescens Ait inhibited MCP-1-induced chemotaxis. J Ethnopharmacol. 2005;97(3):515-9.

[131] Funakoshi-Tago M, Nakamura K, Tago K, Mashino T, Kasahara T. Anti-inflammatory activity of structurally related flavonoids, Apigenin, Luteolin and Fisetin. Int Immunopharmacol.

[132] Kang OH, Choi JG, Lee JH, Kwon DY. Luteolin isolated from the flowers of Lonicera japonica suppresses inflammatory mediator release by blocking NF-kappaB and MAPKs activation pathways in HMC-1 cells. Molecules.15(1):385-98.

[133] Yeh SL, Wang HM, Chen PY, Wu TC. Interactions of beta-carotene and flavonoids on the secretion of pro-inflammatory mediators in an in vitro system. Chem Biol Interact. 2009;179(2-3):386-93.

[134] Min YD, Choi CH, Bark H, Son HY, Park HH, Lee S, et al. Quercetin inhibits expression of inflammatory cytokines through attenuation of NF-kappaB and p38 MAPK in HMC-1 human mast cell line. Inflamm Res. 2007;56(5):210-5.

[135] Castellani ML, Kempuraj D, Frydas S, Theoharides TC, Simeonidou I, Conti P, et al. Inhibitory effect of quercetin on tryptase and MCP-1 chemokine release, and histidine decarboxylase mRNA transcription by human mast cell-1 cell line. Neuroimmunomodulation. 2006;13(3):179-86.

[136] Nanua S, Zick SM, Andrade JE, Sajjan US, Burgess JR, Lukacs NW, et al. Quercetin blocks airway epithelial cell chemokine expression. Am J Respir Cell Mol Biol. 2006;35(5):602-10.

[137] Chung EY, Roh E, Kwak JA, Lee HS, Lee SH, Lee CK, et al. alpha-Viniferin suppresses the signal transducer and activation of transcription-1 (STAT-1)-inducible inflam-

matory genes in interferon-gamma-stimulated macrophages. J Pharmacol Sci.112(4): 405-14.

[138] Wang J, Zhang Y, Yang C, Hou M, Wang F, Wang G, et al. [Effect of tectorigenin on MCP-1 and ICAM-1 mRNA expression in injured vascular endothelial cells]. Zhongguo Zhong Yao Za Zhi.35(15):2001-3.

[139] Lee BS, Shim SM, Heo J, Pae HO, Seo BY, Han SY, et al. Wogonin suppresses TARC expression induced by mite antigen via heme oxygenase 1 in human keratinocytes. Suppressive effect of wogonin on mite antigen-induced TARC expression. J Dermatol Sci. 2007;46(1):31-40.

[140] Hong JY, Lee KE, Kim KW, Sohn MH, Kim KE. Chitinase induce the release of IL-8 in human airway epithelial cells, via Ca2+-dependent PKC and ERK pathways. Scand J Immunol.72(1):15-21.

[141] Liao YR, Hsu JY, Chu JJ, Fu LS. Caffeic acid phenethyl ester suppresses the induction of eotaxin in human lung fibroblast cells. J Asthma.47(3):233-7.

[142] Han KH, Hong KH, Ko J, Rhee KS, Hong MK, Kim JJ, et al. Lysophosphatidylcholine up-regulates CXCR4 chemokine receptor expression in human CD4 T cells. J Leukoc Biol. 2004;76(1):195-202.

[143] Lin YT, Hsu JY, Chen CJ, Chu JJ, Fu LS. Caffeic acid phenethyl ester suppresses eotaxin secretion and nuclear p-STAT6 in human lung fibroblast cells. J Microbiol Immunol Infect.

[144] Qin S, Alcorn JF, Craigo JK, Tjoeng C, Tarwater PM, Kolls JK, et al. Epigallocatechin-3-gallate reduces airway inflammation in mice through binding to proinflammatory chemokines and inhibiting inflammatory cell recruitment. J Immunol.186(6): 3693-700.

[145] Melgarejo E, Medina MA, Sanchez-Jimenez F, Urdiales JL. Epigallocatechin gallate reduces human monocyte mobility and adhesion in vitro. Br J Pharmacol. 2009;158(7):1705-12.

[146] Melgarejo E, Medina MA, Sanchez-Jimenez F, Botana LM, Dominguez M, Escribano L, et al. (-)-Epigallocatechin-3-gallate interferes with mast cell adhesiveness, migration and its potential to recruit monocytes. Cell Mol Life Sci. 2007;64(19-20):2690-701.

[147] Takano K, Nakaima K, Nitta M, Shibata F, Nakagawa H. Inhibitory effect of (-)-epigallocatechin 3-gallate, a polyphenol of green tea, on neutrophil chemotaxis in vitro and in vivo. J Agric Food Chem. 2004;52(14):4571-6.

[148] Kiss AK, Filipek A, Czerwinska M, Naruszewicz M. Oenothera paradoxa defatted seeds extract and its bioactive component penta-O-galloyl-beta-D-glucose decreased production of reactive oxygen species and inhibited release of leukotriene B4, interleukin-8, elastase, and myeloperoxidase in human neutrophils. J Agric Food Chem. 58(18):9960-6.

[149] Ju SM, Song HY, Lee SJ, Seo WY, Sin DH, Goh AR, et al. Suppression of thymus- and activation-regulated chemokine (TARC/CCL17) production by 1,2,3,4,6-penta-O-galloyl-beta-D-glucose via blockade of NF-kappaB and STAT1 activation in the HaCaT cells. Biochem Biophys Res Commun. 2009;387(1):115-20.

[150] Cavalher-Machado SC, Rosas EC, Brito Fde A, Heringe AP, de Oliveira RR, Kaplan MA, et al. The anti-allergic activity of the acetate fraction of Schinus terebinthifolius leaves in IgE induced mice paw edema and pleurisy. Int Immunopharmacol. 2008;8(11):1552-60.

[151] Kim HK, Lee JJ, Lee JS, Park YM, Yoon TR. Rosmarinic acid down-regulates the LPS-induced production of monocyte chemoattractant protein-1 (MCP-1) and macrophage inflammatory protein-1alpha (MIP-1alpha) via the MAPK pathway in bone-marrow derived dendritic cells. Mol Cells. 2008;26(6):583-9.

[152] Sakai S, Sugawara T, Matsubara K, Hirata T. Inhibitory effect of carotenoids on the degranulation of mast cells via suppression of antigen-induced aggregation of high affinity IgE receptors. J Biol Chem. 2009;284(41):28172-9.

[153] Cheong H, Ryu SY, Oak MH, Cheon SH, Yoo GS, Kim KM. Studies of structure activity relationship of flavonoids for the anti-allergic actions. Arch Pharm Res. 1998;21(4):478-80.

[154] Son JK, Son MJ, Lee E, Moon TC, Son KH, Kim CH, et al. Ginkgetin, a Biflavone from Ginko biloba leaves, inhibits cyclooxygenases-2 and 5-lipoxygenase in mouse bone marrow-derived mast cells. Biol Pharm Bull. 2005;28(12):2181-4.

[155] Xu F, Matsuda H, Hata H, Sugawara K, Nakamura S, Yoshikawa M. Structures of new flavonoids and benzofuran-type stilbene and degranulation inhibitors of rat basophilic leukemia cells from the Brazilian herbal medicine Cissus sicyoides. Chem Pharm Bull (Tokyo). 2009;57(10):1089-95.

[156] Park SH, Park EK, Kim DH. Passive cutaneous anaphylaxis-inhibitory activity of flavanones from Citrus unshiu and Poncirus trifoliata. Planta Med. 2005;71(1):24-7.

[157] Cheong H, Ryu SY, Kim KM. Anti-allergic action of resveratrol and related hydroxystilbenes. Planta Med. 1999;65(3):266-8.

[158] Quan W, Lee HJ, Kim CY, Noh CW, Um BH, Oak MH, et al. Anti-allergic prenylated flavonoids from the roots of Sophora flavescens. Planta Med. 2008;74(2):168-70.

[159] Park EK, Shin YW, Lee HU, Lee CS, Kim DH. Passive cutaneous anaphylaxis-inhibitory action of tectorigenin, a metabolite of tectoridin by intestinal microflora. Biol Pharm Bull. 2004;27(7):1099-102.

[160] Ito H, Miyazaki T, Ono M, Sakurai H. Antiallergic activities of rabdosiin and its related compounds: chemical and biochemical evaluations. Bioorg Med Chem. 1998;6(7):1051-6.

[161] Matsuda H, Tewtrakul S, Morikawa T, Nakamura A, Yoshikawa M. Anti-allergic principles from Thai zedoary: structural requirements of curcuminoids for inhibition of degranulation and effect on the release of TNF-alpha and IL-4 in RBL-2H3 cells. Bioorg Med Chem. 2004;12(22):5891-8.

[162] Nishikawa H, Wakano K, Kitani S. Inhibition of NADPH oxidase subunits translocation by tea catechin EGCG in mast cell. Biochem Biophys Res Commun. 2007;362(2): 504-9.

[163] Kim Y, Kim K, Lee H, Han S, Lee YS, Choe J, et al. Celastrol binds to ERK and inhibits FcepsilonRI signaling to exert an anti-allergic effect. Eur J Pharmacol. 2009;612(1-3):131-42.

[164] Kim TJ, Nam KW, Kim B, Lee SJ, Oh KB, Kim KH, et al. Inhibitory Effects of Costunolide Isolated from Laurus nobilis on IgE-induced Degranulation of Mast Cell-like RBL-2H3 Cells and the Growth of Y16 pro-B Cells. Phytother Res.

[165] Duan W, Chan JH, McKay K, Crosby JR, Choo HH, Leung BP, et al. Inhaled p38alpha mitogen-activated protein kinase antisense oligonucleotide attenuates asthma in mice. Am J Respir Crit Care Med. 2005;171(6):571-8. Epub 2004/11/24.

[166] Hirota R, Roger NN, Nakamura H, Song HS, Sawamura M, Suganuma N. Anti-inflammatory effects of limonene from yuzu (Citrus junos Tanaka) essential oil on eosinophils. J Food Sci.75(3):H87-92.

[167] Kannaiyan R, Shanmugam MK, Sethi G. Molecular targets of celastrol derived from Thunder of God Vine: potential role in the treatment of inflammatory disorders and cancer. Cancer Lett.303(1):9-20.

[168] Kim DY, Park JW, Jeoung D, Ro JY. Celastrol suppresses allergen-induced airway inflammation in a mouse allergic asthma model. Eur J Pharmacol. 2009;612(1-3):98-105. Epub 2009/04/10.

[169] Adcock IM, Caramori G, Chung KF. New targets for drug development in asthma. Lancet. 2008;372(9643):1073-87. Epub 2008/09/23.

[170] Kim JY, Kwon EY, Lee YS, Kim WB, Ro JY. Eupatilin blocks mediator release via tyrosine kinase inhibition in activated guinea pig lung mast cells. Journal of toxicology and environmental health Part A. 2005;68(23-24):2063-80. Epub 2005/12/06.

[171] Kampe M, Lampinen M, Stolt I, Janson C, Stalenheim G, Carlson M. PI3-kinase regulates eosinophil and neutrophil degranulation in patients with allergic rhinitis and allergic asthma irrespective of allergen challenge model. Inflammation.35(1):230-9.

[172] Yu T, Lee YJ, Jang HJ, Kim AR, Hong S, Kim TW, et al. Anti-inflammatory activity of Sorbus commixta water extract and its molecular inhibitory mechanism. J Ethnopharmacol.134(2):493-500.

[173] Wen D, Nong Y, Morgan JG, Gangurde P, Bielecki A, Dasilva J, et al. A selective small molecule IkappaB Kinase beta inhibitor blocks nuclear factor kappaB-mediated

inflammatory responses in human fibroblast-like synoviocytes, chondrocytes, and mast cells. J Pharmacol Exp Ther. 2006;317(3):989-1001. Epub 2006/03/10.

[174] Ziegelbauer K, Gantner F, Lukacs NW, Berlin A, Fuchikami K, Niki T, et al. A selective novel low-molecular-weight inhibitor of IkappaB kinase-beta (IKK-beta) prevents pulmonary inflammation and shows broad anti-inflammatory activity. Br J Pharmacol. 2005;145(2):178-92. Epub 2005/03/09.

[175] Li J, Luo L, Wang X, Liao B, Li G. Inhibition of NF-kappaB expression and allergen-induced airway inflammation in a mouse allergic asthma model by andrographolide. Cell Mol Immunol. 2009;6(5):381-5.

[176] Zhang DH, Cohn L, Ray P, Bottomly K, Ray A. Transcription factor GATA-3 is differentially expressed in murine Th1 and Th2 cells and controls Th2-specific expression of the interleukin-5 gene. J Biol Chem. 1997;272(34):21597-603. Epub 1997/08/22.

[177] Nakamura Y, Ghaffar O, Olivenstein R, Taha RA, Soussi-Gounni A, Zhang DH, et al. Gene expression of the GATA-3 transcription factor is increased in atopic asthma. J Allergy Clin Immunol. 1999;103(2 Pt 1):215-22. Epub 1999/02/09.

[178] Popescu FD, Popescu F. A review of antisense therapeutic interventions for molecular biological targets in asthma. Biologics : targets & therapy. 2007;1(3):271-83. Epub 2007/09/01.

[179] Park HJ, Lee CM, Jung ID, Lee JS, Jeong YI, Chang JH, et al. Quercetin regulates Th1/Th2 balance in a murine model of asthma. Int Immunopharmacol. 2009;9(3): 261-7.

[180] Macian F, Lopez-Rodriguez C, Rao A. Partners in transcription: NFAT and AP-1. Oncogene. 2001;20(19):2476-89. Epub 2001/06/13.

[181] Martinez-Martinez S, Redondo JM. Inhibitors of the calcineurin/NFAT pathway. Current medicinal chemistry. 2004;11(8):997-1007. Epub 2004/04/14.

[182] Roehrl MH, Kang S, Aramburu J, Wagner G, Rao A, Hogan PG. Selective inhibition of calcineurin-NFAT signaling by blocking protein-protein interaction with small organic molecules. Proceedings of the National Academy of Sciences of the United States of America. 2004;101(20):7554-9. Epub 2004/05/08.

[183] Honda K, Marquillies P, Capron M, Dombrowicz D. Peroxisome proliferator-activated receptor gamma is expressed in airways and inhibits features of airway remodeling in a mouse asthma model. J Allergy Clin Immunol. 2004;113(5):882-8. Epub 2004/05/08.

[184] Belvisi MG, Mitchell JA. Targeting PPAR receptors in the airway for the treatment of inflammatory lung disease. Br J Pharmacol. 2009;158(4):994-1003. Epub 2009/08/26.

[185] Zhou L, Tang YP, Gao L, Fan XS, Liu CM, Wu DK. Separation, characterization and dose-effect relationship of the PPARgamma-activating bio-active constituents in the

Chinese herb formulation 'San-Ao decoction'. Molecules. 2009;14(10):3942-51. Epub 2009/11/20.

[186] Culpitt SV, Rogers DF, Fenwick PS, Shah P, De Matos C, Russell RE, et al. Inhibition by red wine extract, resveratrol, of cytokine release by alveolar macrophages in COPD. Thorax. 2003;58(11):942-6. Epub 2003/10/31.

[187] Lee NH, Lee MY, Lee JA, Jung DY, Seo CS, Kim JH, et al. Anti-asthmatic effect of Sanguisorba officinalis L. and potential role of heme oxygenase-1 in an ovalbumin-induced murine asthma model. Int J Mol Med. 2010;26(2):201-8. Epub 2010/07/03.

[188] Choi JH, Hwang YP, Lee HS, Jeong HG. Inhibitory effect of Platycodi Radix on ovalbumin-induced airway inflammation in a murine model of asthma. Food Chem Toxicol. 2009;47(6):1272-9. Epub 2009/03/07.

[189] Lee MY, Seo CS, Ha H, Jung D, Lee H, Lee NH, et al. Protective effects of Ulmus davidiana var. japonica against OVA-induced murine asthma model via upregulation of heme oxygenase-1. J Ethnopharmacol. 2010;130(1):61-9. Epub 2010/04/28.

[190] Lee MY, Lee NH, Seo CS, Lee JA, Jung D, Kim JH, et al. Alpinia katsumadai seed extract attenuate oxidative stress and asthmatic activity in a mouse model of allergic asthma. Food Chem Toxicol. 2010;48(6):1746-52. Epub 2010/04/14.

[191] Lee JH, Zhou HY, Cho SY, Kim YS, Lee YS, Jeong CS. Anti-inflammatory mechanisms of apigenin: inhibition of cyclooxygenase-2 expression, adhesion of monocytes to human umbilical vein endothelial cells, and expression of cellular adhesion molecules. Arch Pharm Res. 2007;30(10):1318-27.

[192] Lin HY, Juan SH, Shen SC, Hsu FL, Chen YC. Inhibition of lipopolysaccharide-induced nitric oxide production by flavonoids in RAW264.7 macrophages involves heme oxygenase-1. Biochem Pharmacol. 2003;66(9):1821-32.

[193] Qiao S, Li W, Tsubouchi R, Haneda M, Murakami K, Takeuchi F, et al. Rosmarinic acid inhibits the formation of reactive oxygen and nitrogen species in RAW264.7 macrophages. Free Radic Res. 2005;39(9):995-1003.

[194] Schubert R, Kitz R, Beermann C, Rose MA, Lieb A, Sommerer PC, et al. Effect of n-3 polyunsaturated fatty acids in asthma after low-dose allergen challenge. Int Arch Allergy Immunol. 2009;148(4):321-9.

[195] Riedl MA, Nel AE. Importance of oxidative stress in the pathogenesis and treatment of asthma. Current opinion in allergy and clinical immunology. 2008;8(1):49-56. Epub 2008/01/12.

[196] Allen S, Britton JR, Leonardi-Bee JA. Association between antioxidant vitamins and asthma outcome measures: systematic review and meta-analysis. Thorax. 2009;64(7): 610-9.

[197] Al Senaidy AM. Serum vitamin A and beta-carotene levels in children with asthma. J Asthma. 2009;46(7):699-702.

[198] Hazlewood LC, Wood LG, Hansbro PM, Foster PS. Dietary lycopene supplementation suppresses Th2 responses and lung eosinophilia in a mouse model of allergic asthma. J Nutr Biochem.22(1):95-100.

[199] Fang H, Jin H, Wang H. Effect of all-trans retinoic acid on airway inflammation in asthmatic rats and its mechanism. J Huazhong Univ Sci Technolog Med Sci. 2004;24(3):229-32.

[200] Tsai YC, Chang HW, Chang TT, Lee MS, Chu YT, Hung CH. Effects of all-trans retinoic acid on Th1- and Th2-related chemokines production in monocytes. Inflammation. 2008;31(6):428-33.

[201] Day RM, Lee YH, Park AM, Suzuki YJ. Retinoic acid inhibits airway smooth muscle cell migration. Am J Respir Cell Mol Biol. 2006;34(6):695-703.

[202] Schuster GU, Kenyon NJ, Stephensen CB. Vitamin A deficiency decreases and high dietary vitamin A increases disease severity in the mouse model of asthma. J Immunol. 2008;180(3):1834-42.

[203] McGowan SE, Smith J, Holmes AJ, Smith LA, Businga TR, Madsen MT, et al. Vitamin A deficiency promotes bronchial hyperreactivity in rats by altering muscarinic M(2) receptor function. Am J Physiol Lung Cell Mol Physiol. 2002;282(5):L1031-9.

[204] Al-Abdulla NO, Al Naama LM, Hassan MK. Antioxidant status in acute asthmatic attack in children. J Pak Med Assoc.60(12):1023-7.

[205] Kongerud J, Crissman K, Hatch G, Alexis N. Ascorbic acid is decreased in induced sputum of mild asthmatics. Inhal Toxicol. 2003;15(2):101-9.

[206] Miyake Y, Sasaki S, Tanaka K, Hirota Y. Consumption of vegetables, fruit, and antioxidants during pregnancy and wheeze and eczema in infants. Allergy.65(6):758-65.

[207] Jeong YJ, Kim JH, Kang JS, Lee WJ, Hwang YI. Mega-dose vitamin C attenuated lung inflammation in mouse asthma model. Anat Cell Biol.43(4):294-302.

[208] Chang HH, Chen CS, Lin JY. High dose vitamin C supplementation increases the Th1/Th2 cytokine secretion ratio, but decreases eosinophilic infiltration in bronchoalveolar lavage fluid of ovalbumin-sensitized and challenged mice. J Agric Food Chem. 2009;57(21):10471-6.

[209] Tecklenburg SL, Mickleborough TD, Fly AD, Bai Y, Stager JM. Ascorbic acid supplementation attenuates exercise-induced bronchoconstriction in patients with asthma. Respir Med. 2007;101(8):1770-8.

[210] Fogarty A, Lewis SA, Scrivener SL, Antoniak M, Pacey S, Pringle M, et al. Oral magnesium and vitamin C supplements in asthma: a parallel group randomized placebo-controlled trial. Clin Exp Allergy. 2003;33(10):1355-9.

[211] Kaur B, Rowe BH, Arnold E. Vitamin C supplementation for asthma. Cochrane Database Syst Rev. 2009(1):CD000993.

[212] Guaiquil VH, Vera JC, Golde DW. Mechanism of vitamin C inhibition of cell death induced by oxidative stress in glutathione-depleted HL-60 cells. J Biol Chem. 2001;276(44):40955-61. Epub 2001/09/05.

[213] Benkoussa M, Brand C, Delmotte MH, Formstecher P, Lefebvre P. Retinoic acid receptors inhibit AP1 activation by regulating extracellular signal-regulated kinase and CBP recruitment to an AP1-responsive promoter. Molecular and cellular biology. 2002;22(13):4522-34. Epub 2002/06/08.

[214] Meves A, Stock SN, Beyerle A, Pittelkow MR, Peus D. Vitamin C derivative ascorbyl palmitate promotes ultraviolet-B-induced lipid peroxidation and cytotoxicity in keratinocytes. The Journal of investigative dermatology. 2002;119(5):1103-8. Epub 2002/11/26.

[215] Bakkeheim E, Mowinckel P, Carlsen KH, Burney P, Carlsen KC. Altered oxidative state in schoolchildren with asthma and allergic rhinitis. Pediatr Allergy Immunol. 22(2):178-85.

[216] Turner SW, Campbell D, Smith N, Craig LC, McNeill G, Forbes SH, et al. Associations between fetal size, maternal {alpha}-tocopherol and childhood asthma. Thorax. 65(5):391-7.

[217] de Luis DA, Armentia A, Aller R, Asensio A, Sedano E, Izaola O, et al. Dietary intake in patients with asthma: a case control study. Nutrition. 2005;21(3):320-4.

[218] Misso NL, Brooks-Wildhaber J, Ray S, Vally H, Thompson PJ. Plasma concentrations of dietary and nondietary antioxidants are low in severe asthma. Eur Respir J. 2005;26(2):257-64.

[219] Pearson PJ, Lewis SA, Britton J, Fogarty A. Vitamin E supplements in asthma: a parallel group randomised placebo controlled trial. Thorax. 2004;59(8):652-6.

[220] Mabalirajan U, Aich J, Leishangthem GD, Sharma SK, Dinda AK, Ghosh B. Effects of vitamin E on mitochondrial dysfunction and asthma features in an experimental allergic murine model. J Appl Physiol. 2009;107(4):1285-92.

[221] Lim Y, Vasu VT, Valacchi G, Leonard S, Aung HH, Schock BC, et al. Severe vitamin E deficiency modulates airway allergic inflammatory responses in the murine asthma model. Free Radic Res. 2008;42(4):387-96.

[222] Chhabra SK, Yasir A, Chaudhry K, Shah B. Effect of ozone on response to ovalbumin & its modulation by vitamins C & E in sensitized guinea pigs. Indian J Med Res. 132:87-93.

[223] Suchankova J, Voprsalova M, Kottova M, Semecky V, Visnovsky P. Effects of oral alpha-tocopherol on lung response in rat model of allergic asthma. Respirology. 2006;11(4):414-21.

[224] Grabarczyk M, Podstawka U, Kopec-Szlezak J. [Protection of human peripheral blood leukocytes with vitamin E and C from toxic effects of fenarimol in vitro]. Acta haematologica Polonica. 1991;22(1):136-44. Epub 1991/01/01. Oslanianie leukocytow ludzkiej krwi obwodowej za pomoca witamin E i C przed skutkami toksycznego dzialania fenarimolu in vitro.

[225] Wiser J, Alexis NE, Jiang Q, Wu W, Robinette C, Roubey R, et al. In vivo gamma-tocopherol supplementation decreases systemic oxidative stress and cytokine responses of human monocytes in normal and asthmatic subjects. Free radical biology & medicine. 2008;45(1):40-9. Epub 2008/04/15.

[226] Berdnikovs S, Abdala-Valencia H, McCary C, Somand M, Cole R, Garcia A, et al. Isoforms of vitamin E have opposing immunoregulatory functions during inflammation by regulating leukocyte recruitment. J Immunol. 2009;182(7):4395-405. Epub 2009/03/21.

[227] Brehm JM, Schuemann B, Fuhlbrigge AL, Hollis BW, Strunk RC, Zeiger RS, et al. Serum vitamin D levels and severe asthma exacerbations in the Childhood Asthma Management Program study. J Allergy Clin Immunol.126(1):52-8 e5.

[228] Chinellato I, Piazza M, Sandri M, Peroni D, Piacentini G, Boner AL. Vitamin D serum levels and markers of asthma control in Italian children. J Pediatr.158(3):437-41.

[229] Sutherland ER, Goleva E, Jackson LP, Stevens AD, Leung DY. Vitamin D levels, lung function, and steroid response in adult asthma. Am J Respir Crit Care Med.181(7): 699-704.

[230] Majak P, Olszowiec-Chlebna M, Smejda K, Stelmach I. Vitamin D supplementation in children may prevent asthma exacerbation triggered by acute respiratory infection. J Allergy Clin Immunol.127(5):1294-6.

[231] Penna G, Adorini L. 1 Alpha,25-dihydroxyvitamin D3 inhibits differentiation, maturation, activation, and survival of dendritic cells leading to impaired alloreactive T cell activation. J Immunol. 2000;164(5):2405-11. Epub 2000/02/29.

[232] Chambers ES, Hawrylowicz CM. The impact of vitamin D on regulatory T cells. Curr Allergy Asthma Rep.11(1):29-36.

[233] Xystrakis E, Kusumakar S, Boswell S, Peek E, Urry Z, Richards DF, et al. Reversing the defective induction of IL-10-secreting regulatory T cells in glucocorticoid-resistant asthma patients. The Journal of clinical investigation. 2006;116(1):146-55. Epub 2005/12/13.

[234] Damera G, Fogle HW, Lim P, Goncharova EA, Zhao H, Banerjee A, et al. Vitamin D inhibits growth of human airway smooth muscle cells through growth factor-in-

duced phosphorylation of retinoblastoma protein and checkpoint kinase 1. Br J Pharmacol. 2009;158(6):1429-41. Epub 2009/10/10.

[235] Knekt P, Kumpulainen J, Jarvinen R, Rissanen H, Heliovaara M, Reunanen A, et al. Flavonoid intake and risk of chronic diseases. The American journal of clinical nutrition. 2002;76(3):560-8. Epub 2002/08/29.

[236] Aggarwal BB, Shishodia S. Molecular targets of dietary agents for prevention and therapy of cancer. Biochem Pharmacol. 2006;71(10):1397-421. Epub 2006/03/28.

[237] Rogerio AP, Dora CL, Andrade EL, Chaves JS, Silva LF, Lemos-Senna E, et al. Anti-inflammatory effect of quercetin-loaded microemulsion in the airways allergic inflammatory model in mice. Pharmacol Res.61(4):288-97.

[238] Xie YC, Dong XW, Wu XM, Yan XF, Xie QM. Inhibitory effects of flavonoids extracted from licorice on lipopolysaccharide-induced acute pulmonary inflammation in mice. Int Immunopharmacol. 2009;9(2):194-200.

[239] Jung WK, Choi I, Oh S, Park SG, Seo SK, Lee SW, et al. Anti-asthmatic effect of marine red alga (Laurencia undulata) polyphenolic extracts in a murine model of asthma. Food Chem Toxicol. 2009;47(2):293-7.

[240] Watson RR, Zibadi S, Rafatpanah H, Jabbari F, Ghasemi R, Ghafari J, et al. Oral administration of the purple passion fruit peel extract reduces wheeze and cough and improves shortness of breath in adults with asthma. Nutr Res. 2008;28(3):166-71.

[241] Candelario-Jalil E, de Oliveira AC, Graf S, Bhatia HS, Hull M, Munoz E, et al. Resveratrol potently reduces prostaglandin E2 production and free radical formation in lipopolysaccharide-activated primary rat microglia. Journal of neuroinflammation. 2007;4:25. Epub 2007/10/12.

[242] Lagouge M, Argmann C, Gerhart-Hines Z, Meziane H, Lerin C, Daussin F, et al. Resveratrol improves mitochondrial function and protects against metabolic disease by activating SIRT1 and PGC-1alpha. Cell. 2006;127(6):1109-22. Epub 2006/11/23.

[243] Zbikowska HM, Wachowicz B, Krajewski T. Selenium compounds inhibit the biological activity of blood platelets. Platelets. 1999;10(2-3):185-90. Epub 2006/06/28.

[244] Horvathova M, Jahnova E, Gazdik F. Effect of selenium supplementation in asthmatic subjects on the expression of endothelial cell adhesion molecules in culture. Biological trace element research. 1999;69(1):15-26. Epub 1999/06/26.

[245] Guo CH, Liu PJ, Hsia S, Chuang CJ, Chen PC. Role of certain trace minerals in oxidative stress, inflammation, CD4/CD8 lymphocyte ratios and lung function in asthmatic patients. Ann Clin Biochem.48(Pt 4):344-51.

[246] Hassan AM. Selenium status in patients with aspirin-induced asthma. Ann Clin Biochem. 2008;45(Pt 5):508-12.

[247] Urushidate S, Matsuzaka M, Okubo N, Iwasaki H, Hasebe T, Tsuya R, et al. Association between concentration of trace elements in serum and bronchial asthma among Japanese general population. J Trace Elem Med Biol.24(4):236-42.

[248] Burney P, Potts J, Makowska J, Kowalski M, Phillips J, Gnatiuc L, et al. A case-control study of the relation between plasma selenium and asthma in European populations: a GAL2EN project. Allergy. 2008;63(7):865-71.

[249] Hoffmann PR, Jourdan-Le Saux C, Hoffmann FW, Chang PS, Bollt O, He Q, et al. A role for dietary selenium and selenoproteins in allergic airway inflammation. J Immunol. 2007;179(5):3258-67.

[250] Shaheen SO, Newson RB, Rayman MP, Wong AP, Tumilty MK, Phillips JM, et al. Randomised, double blind, placebo-controlled trial of selenium supplementation in adult asthma. Thorax. 2007;62(6):483-90.

[251] Nie L, Wise ML, Peterson DM, Meydani M. Avenanthramide, a polyphenol from oats, inhibits vascular smooth muscle cell proliferation and enhances nitric oxide production. Atherosclerosis. 2006;186(2):260-6. Epub 2005/09/06.

[252] Guo W, Wise ML, Collins FW, Meydani M. Avenanthramides, polyphenols from oats, inhibit IL-1beta-induced NF-kappaB activation in endothelial cells. Free radical biology & medicine. 2008;44(3):415-29. Epub 2007/12/08.

[253] Sur R, Nigam A, Grote D, Liebel F, Southall MD. Avenanthramides, polyphenols from oats, exhibit anti-inflammatory and anti-itch activity. Arch Dermatol Res. 2008;300(10):569-74. Epub 2008/05/08.

[254] Ammon HP. Modulation of the immune system by Boswellia serrata extracts and boswellic acids. Phytomedicine.17(11):862-7.

[255] Khajuria A, Gupta A, Suden P, Singh S, Malik F, Singh J, et al. Immunomodulatory activity of biopolymeric fraction BOS 2000 from Boswellia serrata. Phytother Res. 2008;22(3):340-8.

[256] Gayathri B, Manjula N, Vinaykumar KS, Lakshmi BS, Balakrishnan A. Pure compound from Boswellia serrata extract exhibits anti-inflammatory property in human PBMCs and mouse macrophages through inhibition of TNFalpha, IL-1beta, NO and MAP kinases. Int Immunopharmacol. 2007;7(4):473-82.

[257] Pungle P, Banavalikar M, Suthar A, Biyani M, Mengi S. Immunomodulatory activity of boswellic acids of Boswellia serrata Roxb. Indian J Exp Biol. 2003;41(12):1460-2.

[258] Siemoneit U, Hofmann B, Kather N, Lamkemeyer T, Madlung J, Franke L, et al. Identification and functional analysis of cyclooxygenase-1 as a molecular target of boswellic acids. Biochem Pharmacol. 2008;75(2):503-13.

[259] Ammon HP, Mack T, Singh GB, Safayhi H. Inhibition of leukotriene B4 formation in rat peritoneal neutrophils by an ethanolic extract of the gum resin exudate of Boswellia serrata. Planta Med. 1991;57(3):203-7.

[260] Gupta I, Gupta V, Parihar A, Gupta S, Ludtke R, Safayhi H, et al. Effects of Boswellia serrata gum resin in patients with bronchial asthma: results of a double-blind, placebo-controlled, 6-week clinical study. Eur J Med Res. 1998;3(11):511-4.

[261] Mynott TL, Ladhams A, Scarmato P, Engwerda CR. Bromelain, from pineapple stems, proteolytically blocks activation of extracellular regulated kinase-2 in T cells. J Immunol. 1999;163(5):2568-75.

[262] Engwerda CR, Andrew D, Ladhams A, Mynott TL. Bromelain modulates T cell and B cell immune responses in vitro and in vivo. Cell Immunol. 2001;210(1):66-75.

[263] Hale LP, Greer PK, Sempowski GD. Bromelain treatment alters leukocyte expression of cell surface molecules involved in cellular adhesion and activation. Clin Immunol. 2002;104(2):183-90.

[264] Secor ER, Jr., Singh A, Guernsey LA, McNamara JT, Zhan L, Maulik N, et al. Bromelain treatment reduces CD25 expression on activated CD4+ T cells in vitro. Int Immunopharmacol. 2009;9(3):340-6.

[265] Manhart N, Akomeah R, Bergmeister H, Spittler A, Ploner M, Roth E. Administration of proteolytic enzymes bromelain and trypsin diminish the number of CD4+ cells and the interferon-gamma response in Peyer's patches and spleen in endotoxemic balb/c mice. Cell Immunol. 2002;215(2):113-9.

[266] Secor ER, Jr., Carson WFt, Cloutier MM, Guernsey LA, Schramm CM, Wu CA, et al. Bromelain exerts anti-inflammatory effects in an ovalbumin-induced murine model of allergic airway disease. Cell Immunol. 2005;237(1):68-75.

[267] Secor ER, Carson WF, Singh A, Pensa M, Guernsey LA, Schramm CM, et al. Oral Bromelain Attenuates Inflammation in an Ovalbumin-induced Murine Model of Asthma. Evid Based Complement Alternat Med. 2008;5(1):61-9.

[268] Szelenyi I, Brune K. Herbal remedies for asthma treatment: between myth and reality. Drugs Today (Barc). 2002;38(4):265-303.

[269] Shimoda H, Tanaka J, Yamada E, Morikawa T, Kasajima N, Yoshikawa M. Anti type I allergic property of Japanese butterbur extract and its mast cell degranulation inhibitory ingredients. J Agric Food Chem. 2006;54(8):2915-20.

[270] Thomet OA, Wiesmann UN, Blaser K, Simon HU. Differential inhibition of inflammatory effector functions by petasin, isopetasin and neopetasin in human eosinophils. Clin Exp Allergy. 2001;31(8):1310-20.

[271] Bickel D, Roder T, Bestmann HJ, Brune K. Identification and characterization of inhibitors of peptido-leukotriene-synthesis from Petasites hybridus. Planta Med. 1994;60(4):318-22.

[272] Ko WC, Lei CB, Lin YL, Chen CF. Relaxant effects of petasins in isolated guinea pig trachea and their structure-activity relationships. Planta Med. 2000;66(7):650-2.

[273] Ziolo G, Samochowiec L. Study on clinical properties and mechanisms of action of Petasites in bronchial asthma and chronic obstructive bronchitis. Pharm Acta Helv. 1998;72(6):378-80.

[274] Lee DK, Haggart K, Robb FM, Lipworth BJ. Butterbur, a herbal remedy, confers complementary anti-inflammatory activity in asthmatic patients receiving inhaled corticosteroids. Clin Exp Allergy. 2004;34(1):110-4.

[275] Esatbeyoglu T, Huebbe P, Ernst IM, Chin D, Wagner AE, Rimbach G. Curcumin--from molecule to biological function. Angew Chem Int Ed Engl.51(22):5308-32.

[276] Aggarwal BB, Harikumar KB. Potential therapeutic effects of curcumin, the anti-inflammatory agent, against neurodegenerative, cardiovascular, pulmonary, metabolic, autoimmune and neoplastic diseases. Int J Biochem Cell Biol. 2009;41(1):40-59.

[277] Reddy AC, Lokesh BR. Studies on spice principles as antioxidants in the inhibition of lipid peroxidation of rat liver microsomes. Mol Cell Biochem. 1992;111(1-2):117-24.

[278] Dikshit M, Rastogi L, Shukla R, Srimal RC. Prevention of ischaemia-induced biochemical changes by curcumin & quinidine in the cat heart. Indian J Med Res. 1995;101:31-5.

[279] Motterlini R, Foresti R, Bassi R, Green CJ. Curcumin, an antioxidant and anti-inflammatory agent, induces heme oxygenase-1 and protects endothelial cells against oxidative stress. Free Radic Biol Med. 2000;28(8):1303-12.

[280] Brouet I, Ohshima H. Curcumin, an anti-tumour promoter and anti-inflammatory agent, inhibits induction of nitric oxide synthase in activated macrophages. Biochem Biophys Res Commun. 1995;206(2):533-40.

[281] Pan MH, Lin-Shiau SY, Ho CT, Lin JH, Lin JK. Suppression of lipopolysaccharide-induced nuclear factor-kappaB activity by theaflavin-3,3'-digallate from black tea and other polyphenols through down-regulation of IkappaB kinase activity in macrophages. Biochem Pharmacol. 2000;59(4):357-67.

[282] Onoda M, Inano H. Effect of curcumin on the production of nitric oxide by cultured rat mammary gland. Nitric Oxide. 2000;4(5):505-15.

[283] Literat A, Su F, Norwicki M, Durand M, Ramanathan R, Jones CA, et al. Regulation of pro-inflammatory cytokine expression by curcumin in hyaline membrane disease (HMD). Life Sci. 2001;70(3):253-67.

[284] Biswas S, Rahman I. Modulation of steroid activity in chronic inflammation: a novel anti-inflammatory role for curcumin. Mol Nutr Food Res. 2008;52(9):987-94.

[285] Kurup VP, Barrios CS, Raju R, Johnson BD, Levy MB, Fink JN. Immune response modulation by curcumin in a latex allergy model. Clin Mol Allergy. 2007;5:1.

[286] Ram A, Das M, Ghosh B. Curcumin attenuates allergen-induced airway hyperresponsiveness in sensitized guinea pigs. Biol Pharm Bull. 2003;26(7):1021-4.

[287] Lee JH, Kim JW, Ko NY, Mun SH, Her E, Kim BK, et al. Curcumin, a constituent of curry, suppresses IgE-mediated allergic response and mast cell activation at the level of Syk. J Allergy Clin Immunol. 2008;121(5):1225-31.

[288] Sato H, Goto W, Yamamura J, Kurokawa M, Kageyama S, Takahara T, et al. Therapeutic basis of glycyrrhizin on chronic hepatitis B. Antiviral Res. 1996;30(2-3):171-7.

[289] van Rossum TG, Vulto AG, de Man RA, Brouwer JT, Schalm SW. Review article: glycyrrhizin as a potential treatment for chronic hepatitis C. Aliment Pharmacol Ther. 1998;12(3):199-205.

[290] Sekizawa T, Yanagi K, Itoyama Y. Glycyrrhizin increases survival of mice with herpes simplex encephalitis. Acta Virol. 2001;45(1):51-4.

[291] Park HY, Park SH, Yoon HK, Han MJ, Kim DH. Anti-allergic activity of 18beta-glycyrrhetinic acid-3-O-beta-D-glucuronide. Arch Pharm Res. 2004;27(1):57-60.

[292] Ram A, Mabalirajan U, Das M, Bhattacharya I, Dinda AK, Gangal SV, et al. Glycyrrhizin alleviates experimental allergic asthma in mice. Int Immunopharmacol. 2006;6(9):1468-77.

[293] Shin YW, Bae EA, Lee B, Lee SH, Kim JA, Kim YS, et al. In vitro and in vivo antiallergic effects of Glycyrrhiza glabra and its components. Planta Med. 2007;73(3):257-61.

[294] Asl MN, Hosseinzadeh H. Review of pharmacological effects of Glycyrrhiza sp. and its bioactive compounds. Phytother Res. 2008;22(6):709-24.

[295] Hsu CH, Lu CM, Chang TT. Efficacy and safety of modified Mai-Men-Dong-Tang for treatment of allergic asthma. Pediatr Allergy Immunol. 2005;16(1):76-81.

[296] Chan CK, Kuo ML, Shen JJ, See LC, Chang HH, Huang JL. Ding Chuan Tang, a Chinese herb decoction, could improve airway hyper-responsiveness in stabilized asthmatic children: a randomized, double-blind clinical trial. Pediatr Allergy Immunol. 2006;17(5):316-22.

[297] Chang TT, Huang CC, Hsu CH. Clinical evaluation of the Chinese herbal medicine formula STA-1 in the treatment of allergic asthma. Phytother Res. 2006;20(5):342-7.

[298] Wen MC, Wei CH, Hu ZQ, Srivastava K, Ko J, Xi ST, et al. Efficacy and tolerability of anti-asthma herbal medicine intervention in adult patients with moderate-severe allergic asthma. J Allergy Clin Immunol. 2005;116(3):517-24.

[299] Calder PC. n-3 polyunsaturated fatty acids, inflammation, and inflammatory diseases. Am J Clin Nutr. 2006;83(6 Suppl):1505S-19S.

[300] Tapiero H, Ba GN, Couvreur P, Tew KD. Polyunsaturated fatty acids (PUFA) and eicosanoids in human health and pathologies. Biomed Pharmacother. 2002;56(5): 215-22.

[301] Morris MC, Sacks F, Rosner B. Does fish oil lower blood pressure? A meta-analysis of controlled trials. Circulation. 1993;88(2):523-33.

[302] Davidson MH, Stein EA, Bays HE, Maki KC, Doyle RT, Shalwitz RA, et al. Efficacy and tolerability of adding prescription omega-3 fatty acids 4 g/d to simvastatin 40 mg/d in hypertriglyceridemic patients: an 8-week, randomized, double-blind, placebo-controlled study. Clin Ther. 2007;29(7):1354-67.

[303] Bucher HC, Hengstler P, Schindler C, Meier G. N-3 polyunsaturated fatty acids in coronary heart disease: a meta-analysis of randomized controlled trials. Am J Med. 2002;112(4):298-304.

[304] Iso H, Rexrode KM, Stampfer MJ, Manson JE, Colditz GA, Speizer FE, et al. Intake of fish and omega-3 fatty acids and risk of stroke in women. Jama. 2001;285(3):304-12.

[305] Yaqoob P. Fatty acids as gatekeepers of immune cell regulation. Trends Immunol. 2003;24(12):639-45.

[306] Yaqoob P. Mechanisms underlying the immunomodulatory effects of n-3 PUFA. Proc Nutr Soc.69(3):311-5.

[307] Fortin PR, Lew RA, Liang MH, Wright EA, Beckett LA, Chalmers TC, et al. Validation of a meta-analysis: the effects of fish oil in rheumatoid arthritis. J Clin Epidemiol. 1995;48(11):1379-90.

[308] Park KS, Lim JW, Kim H. Inhibitory mechanism of omega-3 fatty acids in pancreatic inflammation and apoptosis. Ann N Y Acad Sci. 2009;1171:421-7.

[309] Tartibian B, Maleki BH, Abbasi A. Omega-3 fatty acids supplementation attenuates inflammatory markers after eccentric exercise in untrained men. Clin J Sport Med. 21(2):131-7.

[310] Mingam R, Moranis A, Bluthe RM, De Smedt-Peyrusse V, Kelley KW, Guesnet P, et al. Uncoupling of interleukin-6 from its signalling pathway by dietary n-3-polyunsaturated fatty acid deprivation alters sickness behaviour in mice. Eur J Neurosci. 2008;28(9):1877-86.

[311] McMurray DN, Jolly CA, Chapkin RS. Effects of dietary n-3 fatty acids on T cell activation and T cell receptor-mediated signaling in a murine model. J Infect Dis. 2000;182 Suppl 1:S103-7.

[312] Gorjao R, Hirabara SM, de Lima TM, Cury-Boaventura MF, Curi R. Regulation of interleukin-2 signaling by fatty acids in human lymphocytes. J Lipid Res. 2007;48(9): 2009-19.

[313] Oddy WH, de Klerk NH, Kendall GE, Mihrshahi S, Peat JK. Ratio of omega-6 to omega-3 fatty acids and childhood asthma. J Asthma. 2004;41(3):319-26.

[314] Peat JK, Mihrshahi S, Kemp AS, Marks GB, Tovey ER, Webb K, et al. Three-year outcomes of dietary fatty acid modification and house dust mite reduction in the Childhood Asthma Prevention Study. J Allergy Clin Immunol. 2004;114(4):807-13.

[315] Laerum BN, Wentzel-Larsen T, Gulsvik A, Omenaas E, Gislason T, Janson C, et al. Relationship of fish and cod oil intake with adult asthma. Clin Exp Allergy. 2007;37(11):1616-23.

[316] Catalli A, MacDonald C, Pundir P, Kulka M. Inhibitory effects of resveratrol on human mast cell degranulation, cytokine, chemokine and leukotriene release. Open J Immunol. (2):187-194. doi:10.4236/oji.2012.24022

Chapter 11

Plant Based Natural Products and Breast Cancer: Considering Multi-Faceted Disease Aspects, Past Successes, and Promising Future Interventions

Gailene Tobin, Ruwani Kalupahana and
Marianna Kulka

Additional information is available at the end of the chapter

http://dx.doi.org/10.5772/55794

1. Introduction

1.1. Dealing with the burden

World-wide, approximately 410,000 of the estimated 1 million females diagnosed annually with breast cancer will die from the disease [1]. According to Canadian Cancer Statistics, breast cancer continues to be the most commonly diagnosed cancer among Canadian women over the age of 20 (excluding non-melanoma skin cancer) and is the second leading cause of cancer deaths [2]. In 2012, it was estimated that 22,700 Canadian women would be diagnosed with breast cancer and 5,200 would succumb to the disease [2]. Furthermore, the recently published Prince Edward Island (PEI) Cancer Trends Report outlining cancer cases diagnosed from 1980 to 2009 indicates that in PEI, breast cancer is the most commonly diagnosed cancer in women [3]. While the overall incidence rate of breast cancer has increased marginally (0.5% per annum) and mortality rates have stabilized since 1992, the long-term survival in PEI women is significantly lower than the Canadian rate [3]. In summary, breast cancer continues to be a world-wide issue requiring attention. Increased awareness and advanced screening, resulting in early detection, is attributed to the increased incidence of the disease and such factors have led to a high percentage (approximately 95%) of all breast cancer patients being initially diagnosed with curable disease [4]. However, 30-40% of patients diagnosed with curable breast cancer succumb to disease reoccurrence [5]. Although increased diagnosis and advances in the treatment of breast cancer are clearly contributing factors in disease progression, eradication of residual malignancies and metastatic tumors via a systemic approach is considered the key for success in treating cancer and increasing cancer patient survival [6]. There is an urgent need to explore agents that will be effective in preventing and treating metastasis of breast tumors.

1.2. The biology of breast cancer

In general, cancer occurs when a normal cell accumulates genetic and/or epigenetic changes caused by the activation or amplification of oncogenes and/or the mutation or loss of tumor suppressor function, resulting in the ability to proliferate indefinitely [7]. While these specific alterations lead to the transformation of the normal cell and partly determine the characterization of the tumor, the cell of origin and tumor (micro-) environment are also considered important factors contributing to tumor cell establishment, progression and therapeutic resistance [8].

2. Clinical characteristics and classification of breast cancer

2.1. Classifying breast cancer

Breast cancer classifications are largely explained by differences in tumor characteristics as determined by tumor appearance, histology, tumor marker expression (immunohistochemistry) or receptor status, and gene expression profiles. Alone, or in combination, these aspects can influence treatment, response and prognosis.

2.1.1. Histology

Breast cancer represents many different histologies, however the majority (estimated to be more than 85%) of breast cancers are collectively derived from the epithelium lining in the ducts or lobes, and are classified as mammary ductal or lobular carcinoma [9]. Furthermore, this classification can be defined as *in situ* (meaning the proliferation of cancer cells within the epithelial tissue without invasion of the surrounding tissue) or *invasive* whereby the surrounding tissue is affected [9]. Included in the histological description of breast cancer is the status of invasion to the perineural and/or lymphovascular space and the presence of such is associated with more aggressive disease [10].

2.1.2. Grade

Tumor grade is determined by comparing differentiation in normal and cancerous breast tissues. Normal cells in the breast become differentiated and acquire specific shapes and forms that reflect their function as part of the mammary system [9]. When cell division becomes uncontrolled, differentiation is lost. Breast cancers are either well differentiated (low grade), moderately differentiated (intermediate grade), or poorly differentiated (high grade) [9]. This progressive loss of features seen in normal breast cells is indicative of disease progression and poorly differentiated or high grade cancers have a worse prognosis than others [11].

http://dx.doi.org/10.5772/55794

2.1.3. *Stage*

Between 1943 and 1952, Pierre Denoix devised the TNM staging systems for all solid tumors to classify the progression of cancer [12]; the acronym can be explained by the fact that this model utilizes the size and extension of the primary tumor (T), its spread to the lymph nodes (N), and the presence of metastases (M). Although it is not utilized for all cancers (i.e.: brain and spinal cord cancer), the TNM system has progressed to the 7th textbook edition (TNM Classification of Malignant Tumors) [12] and remains the major system by which breast cancer is staged. An increase in stage number is based on larger tumor size, nodal spread (in particular, the sentinel node*) and metastasis and is positively correlated with a worse prognosis [13, 14].

* Certain cancers spread in a predictable manner, from the site of origin to nearby lymph nodes (lymph glands) and then to other parts of the body. The very first draining lymph node is termed the "sentinel node" and is important in the sentinel lymph node biopsy (SLNB) technique utilized to stage the spread of certain types of cancer. The absence of cancer within the sentinel lymph node indicates that there is a high likelihood that the cancer has not spread to any other area of the body. Lymph node metastasis is considered one of the most important predictive signs in breast cancer, and thus can serve to guide the surgeon/oncologist to the appropriate therapy.

2.2. Receptor status and gene expression profiles

Recent progress in molecular technologies has led to distinct breast cancer categories and five distinct tumor types and a normal breast-like group have been identified to date based on gene expression profiling [15], as summarized in Table 1.

Molecular Sub-type based on Gene Expression Profiling	Receptor Status based on Immunohistochemistry	Reference
Luminal A	ER+ve and/or PR+ve, Her2–ve, any CK5/6/Her1	[15-17]
Luminal B	ER+ve and/or PR+ve, Her2+ve, any CK5/6/Her1	[15-17]
Basal-like (triple –ive)	ER–ve, PR–ve, Her2–ve, CK5,6+ve and/or Her1+	[18]
Her-2+over-expressing (ERBB2)	ER–ve, PR–ve, Her2+ve, any CK5/6/Her1	[19]
Normal Breast –like	"unclassified" (negative for all 5 markers), displays putative-initiating stem cell phenotype	[20, 21]
"claudin-low" group	"unclassified" (negative for all 5 markers), displays putative-initiating stem cell phenotype, Often triple negative, displays low expression of cell-cell junction proteins and e-cadherin, frequently infiltration with lymphocytes	[20, 22]

Positive (+ve), negative (–ve), estrogen receptor (ER), progesterone receptor (PR), human epidermal growth factor receptors (EGFR) 1 and 2 (Her 1 and 2) and cytokeratin 5, 6 (CK5,6).

Table 1. Distinct Molecular Tumor Categories of Breast Cancer and their Receptor Status

However, most investigators use the presence (+) or absence (-) of immunohistochemical (IHS) markers or receptor combinations that are expressed by neoplastic cells. In this manner, distinct tumor categories to-date are identified by the expression of estrogen receptors (ER), progesterone receptors (PR), human epidermal growth factor receptors (EGFR) 1 and 2 (Her 1 and 2) and cytokeratin 5, 6 (CK5,6) [15-19, 23-25]. Generally, molecular sub-types correspond to IHC receptor status [26]. These subtypes are of great clinical and research importance as they are utilized to administer and target therapeutic regimes based on predictions of response. Furthermore, these subtypes have been shown to display a wide variety of responses to different treatments [27-30] and are associated with other clinical outcomes, such as patient relapse and overall survival. The most favorable outcomes are noted for the luminal A subtype, which are hormone sensitive [31]. The Her2+ and basal subtypes are noted as more aggressive and have fewer therapeutic options [31-33]. The normal-like and claudin-low are unclassified (negative for all major receptors), and associated with poor prognosis [20-22, 30, 34]. Several small studies support the concept that molecular subtype and tumor receptor status may change during ordinary disease progression and a major study completed by MacFarlane *et al.* in 2008 revealed that 21% of relapsed tumors had changes in either ER/PR or HER2 receptor status [35]. This significant proportion led the author to suggest that biopsies of relapsed/ metastatic breast cancers should be performed routinely. This also should be an important consideration in research. In summary, treatment options considered effective in primary stage cancer may no longer be optimal in later stages of the disease, including relapses and metastasis as determined by the current classification scheme.

2.3. Other classification approaches

Other breast cancer classification approaches are also used to assist in both prognostic and treatment decisions. These include computer models that are based on a combination of several factors and offer individual survival predictions and calculations of treatment benefits [36]. For example, patients undergoing systemic adjuvant therapy can determine optimal treatment through the commercially available computer model *Adjuvant* which has been successfully validated in several cohorts, including the United States and Canada [36, 37]. Other useful classification tools utilized for breast cancer treatment choices include prognostic assessments (such as USC/Van Nuys prognostic index (VNPI)) and general comorbidity assessments [38, 39]. Also consider the case of familial breast cancer (genetic classification) whereby a patient may opt to undergo preventative measures such as mastectomy. Additionally, immunohistochemistry testing, other than those mentioned earlier, continue to prove favorable as prognostic markers across various molecular subtypes [40]. For example, in human breast cancer epithelial cell proliferation is considered a significant prognostic marker [41] and could possibly be used as a prediction tool to measure different hormone treatment related risks [42]. Therefore, the immunohistochemical marker, Ki67 (a nuclear protein expressed by cells in all active phases of the cycle except for quiescent or resting cells) is utilized frequently to evaluate proliferation [43]. Such labeling indicates a significant association with higher carcinoma grade, clinical response to endocrine therapy, higher risk of relapse, and worse survival in patients with early breast cancer [44].

3. Cell of origin

While scientists have predicted that specific breast cancer types may arise from different types of progenitor cells, it has been difficult to identify the cells of origin, and the topic remains controversial to date. Breast tumors represent a heterogeneous collection of cell populations with different biological properties [45]. Shared molecular features have made it difficult to distinguish the cell populations of breast cancer tumors and only recently have researchers been able to differentiate stem cells from other progenitor cells. Within this context, tumor evolution has been explained by two main theories. The traditional clonal evolution model is based on the premise that all tumor cells have the capacity to undergo self-renewal which is an indication of their potential to undergo tumor progression and drug resistance [46, 47]. The Cancer Stem Cell (CSC) theory emphasizes the ability of only a minor population of tumorigenic cells capable of self-renewal and differentiation [20, 48] and this specific sub-set of CSC's gives rise to new tumors which are phenotypically identical to the original tumors [49]. CSC's are believed to be a small population of cells with dysregulated self–renewal properties capable of continuous self-renewal and differentiation and responsible for tumor existence treatment resistance and relapse. Existence of CSC's in various types of tumours, including breast cancer [50],[51] has been identified. ALDH (aldehyde dehydrogenase)-1 is a marker of normal and malignant human mammary stem cells [52], and these cells can also be isolated using the cell surface markers epithelial-specific antigen (ESA), CD44 and the absence of the expression of CD24 [53]. When transformed cells undergo epithelial-mesenchymal transition (EMT), they have been noted to gain properties of stem cells [54]. Although evidence supporting the CSC model was initially obtained from acute myeloid leukemia [55], successive studies maintain that solid tumors, including breast cancer tumors, are also driven and sustained by CSCs [50].

Regardless of origin, an abundance of research has clearly confirmed the existence of cancer stem cells (CSCs) or tumor-initiating cells (TICs) in a variety of human cancers [55-58], including breast cancer [50]. Nonetheless, most of the therapeutic approaches available, inclusive of chemotherapy and radiation, lack the ability to effectively kill these populations [59-62]. This may explain the lack of progress in eliminating cancerous tumors and preventing metastasis and may help to rationalize therapeutic resistance; therefore, the CSC or TIC population has become a target for cancer prevention and therapy [63]. A general consensus exists in the literature that breast cancer re-occurrence is assumed to be caused by a sub-population of tumor initiating cells possessing stem cell attributes of a tumor as well as resistance to chemotherapy, radiation and other forms of treatment [64-66]. Of great interest is the role of CSC's in tumor relapse and resistance to therapy and recent articles suggesting that such resistance can be overcome.

4. Breast cancer progression models

The combined research efforts of various scientific disciplines have resulted in the development of a disease progression model for breast cancer (See Figure 1) and include a continuum of lesions through to invasive carcinoma and eventually metastatic disease [30, 48, 67, 68]. For decades, it was thought that metastatic dissemination occurred as a final step in cancer and was the responsibility of genetic changes of malignant cells in the primary tumor [69]. In 2008, Husemann *et al*, used transgenic mice to show systemic dissemination (specifically to lungs and bone marrow) of mammary tissue derived premalignant cells prior to the emergence of mammary tumors [70]. Additionally, this research reported that systemic dissemination of tumor cells can occur in pre-invasive stages of tumor progression as observed in female patients with ductal carcinoma *in situ*. A complementary accumulation of evidence supports the evolution of an early dissemination model, where malignant cells outside the primary lesion can also migrate to distal sites (such as lung and bone marrow) and cause tumors via various genetic programs [54, 71, 72]. Such a model is inclusive to "self-seeding", the term coined when cancer cells not only seeds regional (lymph nodes) and distant sites but also fuel the growth of the original tumor itself [73].

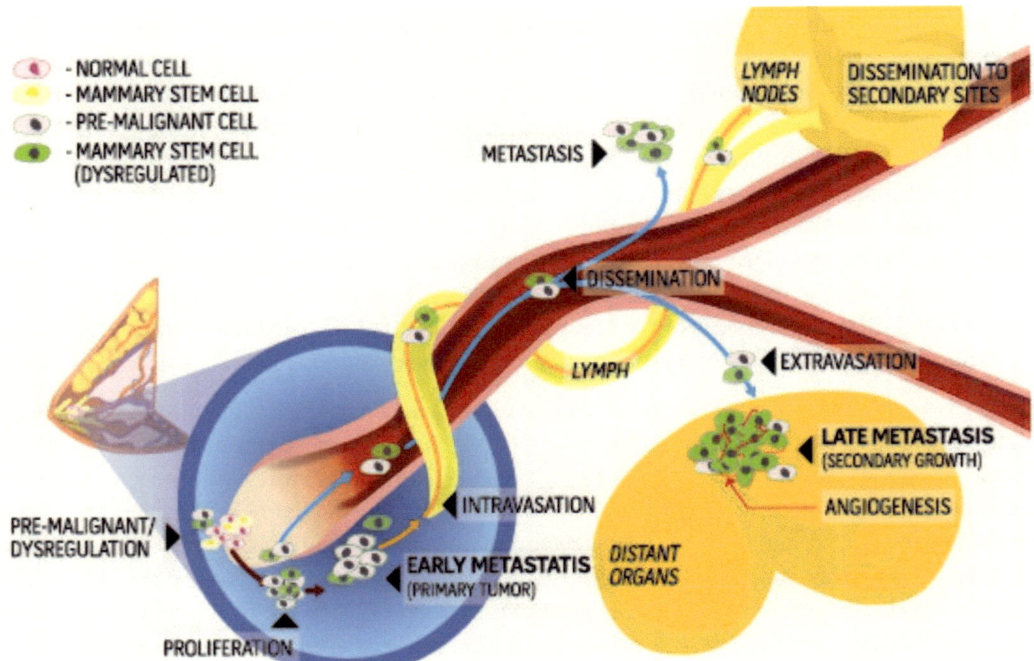

Figure 1. (Tobin, GA, 2011) Physiological Aspects of Disease Progression in Breast Cancer: The development of breast cancer has been proposed as a multi-step process. The most deadly aspect of breast cancer is metastasis and involves a cascade of reactions. Although the molecular mechanisms underlying this process are not fully understood, any disruption along the cascade could arrest disease progression.

Thus, breast cancer is not a single disease, but rather an assortment of diseases with diverse characteristics and clinical outcomes which will likely always require a variety and/or combination of treatments or alternatively, a broad spectrum application. Combine this with the fact that, despite major advances in our understanding of the biology of cancer, further research is required to improve our understanding of tumor establishment, progression and dissemination - the principal cause of mortality. Then, our goal in breast cancer research

http://dx.doi.org/10.5772/55794

regarding treatment would be to identify novel therapies and maximize, based on our current understanding of the disease, the use of such in preventing and treating as many aspects of the disease as possible.

5. Molecular and endocrine controls

5.1. BRCA and other gene expression signatures associated with increased risk of breast cancer

Less time, low cost and new sequencing technologies are all accomplishments that yield impact on molecular biomedical research. Recently, for example, such advances (combined with some prospective epidemiology studies) have allowed researchers to compare the DNA from healthy breast tissue, initial tumor cells and then cells obtained nine years later when the breast cancer had metastasized [74]. The 32 DNA mutations reported in the metastasized cells are a prime example of how technological advances can serve to provide us with ample data regarding gene expression that may offer insights into the progression of breast cancer disease. However, consider that gene expression profiling / signatures of primary breast tumors can only be used as a predictor of susceptibility or disease progression in breast cancer, particularly metastasis. Currently, it is not possible to accurately predict the risk of metastasis or prevent it. As a result, more than ½ of the patients treated with adjuvant chemotherapy are needlessly exposed to harmful side effects [5]. This presents another compelling reason to further study drug targets that are specific to, and have potential for, treatment in metastatic breast cancer.

Nonetheless, based on current knowledge, and aside from the many identified factors that could impact the risk of developing breast cancer (including personal and environmental), genetic mutations in critical cancer genes (both tumor suppressor and oncogenes) have been identified for their increased or associated risk with breast cancer [75]. Of the many that have been reported throughout the history of cancer genetics, Table 2 below captures those that stand out principally for their research and/or clinical significance in relation to breast cancer and summarizes major function, encoded proteins and known disease associations or risk factors. Such genetic aberrations are acquired over a person's lifetime; or less commonly, are inherited. While it is estimated that only 5% to 10% of breast cancers are hereditary, some gene variations are associated with both hereditary and somatic mutations [75]. The tumor suppressor genes *BRCA1* and *BRCA2* are the major genes related to hereditary breast cancer [76], and mutations in these and other *BRCA* genes in women are associated with a 60-80% risk of developing breast cancer throughout their life span [77]. Other genes with inherited alterations, including *CDH1, PTEN, TP53, CHEK 2*, and *ATM* have been noted to increase or are associated with the risk of developing breast cancer [78]. Most notably, the latter three have presented the strongest evidence related to the risk of developing breast cancer [79]. Somatic mutations mostly reference *ERBB2/HER2(neu)* in breast cancer, however *TP53* genes and others have been associated with some cases of breast cancer in this manner [80]. It is noteworthy that not all people who inherit mutations in these genes will develop cancer.

Gene	Major Function: Associated Proteins	Risk Factor	Ref.
BRCA1 (BReast CAncer gene one)	Encodes breast cancer type 1 susceptibility protein; responsible for DNA repair, transcriptional regulation and cell cycle check point control.	Strong evidence indicating a 60 – 80% risk of developing breast cancer for people with mutations.	[81 - 86]
BRCA2 (BReast CAncer gene two)	Encodes BRCA2 susceptibility protein involved in the repair of chromosomal damage, especially in the error-free repair of DNA double strand breaks. As with BRCA1, indicates a high degree of risk.	Reduced levels of the BRCA2 protein may cause Fanconi anemia. Patients with such are prone to several types of cancers, including reproductive system associated tumors.	[87] [88]
ATM (Ataxia telangiectasia mutation)	Encodes protein with a phosphatidylinositol 3-kinase (PI3K)–like domain which plays a central role in the complex processes that repair DNA double-strand breaks. Also involved in regulation of cell cycle progression and the maintenance of genomic stability.	Confers susceptibility and linked to an modest increase (up to 2 times) of breast cancer.	[89-93]
p53 (TP53) (Tumor Protein p53)	Encodes p53 protein and regulates cell cycle, preventing tumor growth.	Causes Li-Fraumeni syndrome: results in higher-than-average-risk of breast cancer and several other cancers.	[94-96]
CHEK2 (Checkpoint kinase 2)	Encodes a serine/threonine-protein kinase which plays a critical role in DNA damage signaling pathways. Phosphorylates and regulates the functions of p53 and BRCA1.	Causes Li-Fraumeni syndrome. Can double breast cancer risk.	[97-99]
PTEN (Phosphatase and tensin homolog)	Encodes phosphatase and tensin homolog protein, namely phosphatidylinositol-3,4,5-trisphosphate 3-phosphatase, which is involved in the regulation of the cell cycle.	Causes Cowden syndrome which presents a higher risk of both benign and cancerous tumors in the breast, digestive tract, thyroid, uterus, and ovaries.	[100, 101]
CDH1 (Cadherin 1 Gene) or E-cadherin (epithelial cadherin)	Encodes E-cadherin protein. Down-regulation decreases the strength of cellular adhesion, increases cellular motility; allowing cell invasion.	Increased risk of breast cancer, particularly invasive lobular breast cancer.	[102-104]
** ERBB2, (HER2/neu), or VEGF	Encodes a transmembrane receptor with constitutive tyrosine-kinase activity.	Amplification occurs in 15-30% of human breast cancers.	[34] [80]

** ERBB2 (erythroblastosis oncogene B), HER2/neu (Human Epidermal growth factor Receptor2, neu: derived from a rodent (neu)ral tumor), VEGF (vascular endothelial growth factor).

Table 2. Familiar Genetic Mutations, Encoding Proteins and their Major Functions in Relation to the Associated and Increased Risk of Developing Breast Cancer.

Those listed in Table 2, as mentioned, represent familiar genes associated with breast cancer. However, others genes that are applicable in breast cancer progression will be reviewed in terms of their associated cell signaling pathways. Considering the profound implications that the CSC theory has for cancer chemoprevention and therapy, combined with our interest in plant based molecules, we will also examine gene function in the context of opportunities for natural product compounds in CSC self-renewal.

5.2. Endocrine controls

Over the years, and more notably since the discovery of suitable breast cancer cell lines and animal models, the symbiotic relationship between lab research and clinical investigations have advanced our knowledge of endocrine action. Breast cancer is influenced and highly regulated by several sex and growth hormones (including estrogens, androgens, progesterone, prolactin and insulin-like growth factors) and each of the sub-types and gene expression patterns of breast cancer are characterized by both unique and specific endocrine controls [105]. Particularly, estrogens and progesterone have received the greatest attention likely because of their involvement in normal and neoplastic mammary tissue and the scale of their associated risk estimation for breast cancer. Research into the role of androgens has likely been a consideration in breast cancer research as androgens are necessary precursors to all endogenous estrogens. The role of prolactin in the pathogenesis of breast cancer remains unclear given the scarcity of studies to date. Similarly, although well studied, the role of Insulin-like growth factor (IGF) in breast cancer is inconsistent.

There are challenges in defining the role of progesterone in breast cancer and the role of progesterone receptor (PR) action in breast cancer remains divisive. In breast cancer, progesterone has biphasic effects (both proliferative and inhibitory) on breast cancer cell lines grown *in vitro* [106, 107]. Depending upon cellular context and/or the presence of secondary agents, there may be a role for progesterone as a priming agent with growth promoting activity [106].

While progesterone is found as a single hormone, the major endogenous estrogens in females include estrone (E1), estradiol (E2), and estriol (E3) and are primarily produced during menopause, in non-pregnant and pregnant females, respectively [108]. A variety of synthetic (xenoestrogens) and natural substances have been identified that also possess estrogenic activity including those derived from plant products (phytoestrogens) and fungi (mycoestrogens) [108]. The actions of estrogens are mediated by their respective receptors binding to specific DNA sequences to activate the transcription of estrogen receptor (ER)-regulated genes, including direct target genes [109]. Approximately 80% of breast cancers demonstrate expression of PR and/or ER [110]. Once established, these breast cancers which are classified as either hormone-sensitive or hormone-receptor-positive cancers are reliant on hormones to grow. Thus, treatment includes the suppression of hormone production in the body for these specific breast cancers. Therefore, this section will provide an overview of estrogens, their past indications in the treatment of breast cancer and their potential role in relation to naturally occurring dietary compounds.

5.2.1. The role of estrogens and breast cancer

The link involving estrogen and breast cancer can be traced back to as early as 1896 when a surgeon in England reported an improvement in condition in three young female breast cancer patients after the removal of their ovaries [111]. Since estrogen had not yet been discovered, the surgeon had unknowingly removed the source of estrogen that promotes the survival and division of cancer cells [111]. Since that time, a lot of evidence has shown that interactions between estrogens and their receptors influence the pathogenesis of breast cancer. Estrogen promotes proliferative effects on cultured human breast cancer cells [112]. Estradiol affects breast cancer risk by controlling the mitotic rate of breast epithelial cells and high levels of estradiol in post-menopausal women are also known to increase the risk of breast cancer [113]. Estradiol has also been shown to increase breast cancer risk via its metabolite, catechol estrogen 4-hydroxyestradiol, causing direct DNA damage through the formation of free radicals [114]. Estradiol has also been shown to modulate breast cancer cell apoptosis [115]. ER is a major determinant of the cellular response of estrogen and has been indicated in breast cancer promotion [116, 117]. The binding of estrogen to the ER modulates the transcription of a series of genes, including those coding for proliferation.

The close relationship between the etiology of breast cancer and exposure to estrogen warrants examination of key variables that may affect estrogen homeostasis, in particular those exhibiting anti-estrogen activity. Because of their impact on the primary and metastatic aspects of disease, anti-hormonal drugs are the mainstay breast cancer treatment. The goal in treating hormone receptor +ve breast cancers is to utilize drugs which suppress production of estrogen in the body. Estrogens in naturally occurring dietary compounds such as soy are used as an alternative to hormone therapy because of their anti-proliferative effects. This practice, in breast cancer treatment, is widely known as hormonal therapy, or anti-estrogen therapy, but is not representative of the term hormone replacement therapy [118].

6. *In vitro* and *in vivo* breast cancer models and their relevance to human disease

In 2007, Vargo-Gogola and Rosen summarized appropriately, within their title, the challenge of modelling breast cancer; "One size does not fit all"[31]. Considering the heterogeneity nature of this disease, these researchers rather addressed the reasonable question of the most powerful way to investigate breast cancer with respect to cell lines and animal models. We agree with their conclusion that an integrated and multi-systems approach is the strongest way to model this disease. Here, we briefly discuss the most commonly utilized *in vivo* and *in vitro* models and their relevance in human breast cancer.

6.1. Mammary carcinoma cell lines

Our current knowledge of breast cancer is mainly based on *in vivo* and *in vitro* studies completed with breast cancer cell (BCC) lines. The first BCC line, namely BT-20, was established in 1958 [119] and since then the number of permanent lines sustained are relatively low despite continuous research in breast cancer [120]. In fact, the number of commercially available BCC lines (ranging from 70 – 80 based on ATCC and similar commercial suppliers) represent mostly cell lines that were established more than 25 years ago. It has been suggested that this inefficiency in producing new and improved lines is likely due to technical difficulties in extracting viable tumor cells from their neighboring stroma [120]. In the past, it has been estimated that more than two-thirds of all scientific abstracts related to studies on mentioned BCC lines include the MCF-7, T-47D, and MDA-MB-231 lines [120]. Although no single cell line is entirely representative of human breast cancer, cell lines have been widely used. As a result, we have a greater understanding of breast cancer biology. Additionally, these cell lines have advanced the ability of pre-clinical models to predict pharmaceutical activity and therapeutic applications for further study. Despite this, the use of cell lines for application in human disease is limited. The single most significant question, considering the devastating effects or outcomes of metastasis, is the issue of whether these cell lines are representative of metastatic conditions, or contain tumor initiating subpopulations. There are studies to indicate distinctions between tumor and non-tumor initiating populations at the cellular and molecular level [31, 121]. Research indicates that the two luminal subsets (A and B) evident in tumors are not apparent in the cell lines, and the basal-like cell lines are actually representative of two distinctive clusters (A and B) that are not apparent in analyses of primary tumors [16]. The differences in cell culture may be due to the absence of stromal or physiological interactions and/or signaling [122] [123]. However, there is evidence that cell lines may be derived from subpopulations of tumor cells that are selected because they grow well. For example, it has been noted that differences between the genome aberration patterns for the basal-like and luminal clusters in the cell line system don't match differences in these subtypes in primary tumors. Furthermore, the highly invasive Basal B cells carry the distinctive phenotype associated with the subpopulation of tumorigenic stem cells identified in breast cancer [50, 124]. Also, one must consider the issue of variants of the same cell lines and the phenotypic changes that can occur due to environmental exposures, rate of passage and age of cells.

Perhaps the most highly debated topic regarding the use of breast cancer cell lines revolves around the MDA-MB-435 cell line, and by extension MDA-MB-435S (ATCC® HTB-129™) and derivatives. Spontaneously metastatic and originally designated as Basal B and being derived from a breast carcinoma, the MDA-MB-435 cell line has subsequently been questioned because of recent evidence indicating that it might originate from melanoma or may have been cross-contaminated with the M14 melanoma cell line [125-130]. While some researchers continue to use this cell line as a breast cancer mouse model [131] and conclude that this cell line is in fact breast cancer cells [132], others insist that the MDA-MB-425 cell line is a melanoma cell line and renders its use as improper in breast cancer studies [133]. Later in the chapter, we will describe some research that has been conducted using MDA-MB435 cell lines and/or its derivatives as breast cancer models in research involving natural, despite this controversy. This may not be all bad news for natural product researchers. On the bright side, natural product therapies indicated in the controversial cells line MDA-MB-435 and its derivatives then point toward activity in melanoma as opposed to breast cancer.

Nonetheless, there is clearly a need for new cell lines that are representative of all the known sub-types of breast cancer. Currently, researchers have the option of using a group (or panel) of subtype cell lines to increase power in their research, as proposed by Neve [2006] [129]. To date, and based on our knowledge, there has been no evidence of a male breast cancer derived cell line. With the incidence of male breast cancer rising [2], relevant models require further development.

Cell lines are easy to culture, inexpensive in comparison to animal models, and provide an unlimited source of homogenous material to work with. Comparisons between researcher and studies are usually fairly consistent and reproducible. A limitation of cell cultures is their inability to measure tumor-stromal cell interactions, however the growth of cell lines for transplantation allows for such *in vivo*.

6.2. Animal models

Animal models have allowed researchers to gain much insight into the disease progression, in particular metastasis. In addition to advancing the concept of metastasis [134, 135], our knowledge of the biological function of genes and signaling pathways has progressed as a result of the vast amount of information generated from animal models. Experimental systems based on mouse models that are currently used to study breast cancer can be categorized as tumor transplantation and genetically engineered mice (GEM) – often termed as transgenic. Here we will focus on commonly utilized models within each of these categories and discuss some of the advantages and limitations of each in relation to human breast cancer disease relevance.

6.2.1. Transgenic or (GEM) models

Different GEM breast cancer models are useful for studying distinct signaling interactions and for testing therapies that target pathways involved. Genomic deletion of tumor suppressor genes or the transgenic insertion of oncogenes allow these mice to be a relevant tool to investigate the spontaneous initiation of breast tumors in each step of metastasis [136]. Specific to breast cancer, the expression of oncogenes in explicit breast regions are restricted via a mammary gland specific promoter [136]. MMTV (mouse mammary tumor virus) or WAP (Whey Acidic Protein) promoter control the expression of oncogenes (i.e: PyMT, ErbB2, Wnt1, or Ras) in transgenic mice and initiate mammary gland tumors which lead to metastasis in various organs [137]. The MMTV-PyMT transgenic mouse model represents hyperplasia, adenoma, and early or late carcinoma as seen in human cancer stages. In breast cancer, this model demonstrates short latency tumor development specific to the mammary gland with a high incidence pulmonary metastasis [138]. The deletion of mammary epithelial cell-specific tumor suppressor genes results in similar conditions observed in human cancer patients, including spontaneous tumors, bone metastasis, loss of estrogen receptor (ER) expression, and hormone-responsiveness [139, 140]. Crossing GEM mice with other transgenic mice has allowed researchers to investigate the role of genes and signaling pathways in tumorigenesis and metastasis. While tumor progression was delayed in MMTV-PyMT or MMTV-ErbB2/neu mice crossed into an Akt or PTP1B-deleted genetic background [141, 142], increased metastasis was observed in the MMTV-PyMT mouse in a CD44_/_ background; the later indicates the importance of receptors and other secreted factors in epithelial–stromal interactions or overall tumor environment [139]. In this regard, much insight has been gained through the use of GEM models to indicate the role of both innate and adaptive immune responses in the progression of breast cancer. For example, pulmonary metastasis is notably diminished via the selective loss of the interleukin (IL-) 4 cytokine in PyMT/IL-4_/_ mice through inhibition of IL-4 mediated EGFR signaling of mammary tumors [143]. The understanding of such interactions are important if we consider that tumor-associated immune cells release numerous growth factors, including cytokines, chemokines, and enzymes that promote tumor growth, angiogenesis, and metastasis, and thus are associated with poor prognosis [136]. Inducible GEM mouse models (those capable of expression or repression of certain genes) have advanced knowledge with respect to the association of multiple genetic mutations of oncogenes in relation to tumor establishment and maintenance [144]. There are several drawbacks to consider in the use of GEM models. There are inherent differences in mouse and human, for example: BRCA1 and p53 are on the same chromosome in mice, but not in humans [136, 144]. Technical discrepancies, depending on methods used to generate the model and the interpretation of results can present varying outcomes. Also, temporal and spatial tumor development and metastasis differ depending on the mouse strain used. For example the percentage of ER/progesterone receptor (PR)+ve tumors in Wap-Cre/Trp53_/_ mice are high while MMTV-Cre/Trp53_/_ mice report a low incidence of such [145]. The molecular profile of mammary tumors from GEM models represent the subtypes of human breast cancers, including those included in Table 1, however no single model to date is representative of all expression patterns and characteristics of human cancer.

6.2.2. Tumor transplantation model

Syngeneic transplantation refers to the transfer of cancer cells from one mouse into another with identical genetic background [146] and such models are used to establish organ specific metastasis [147]. The 4T1 breast cancer tumor model (a syngeneic mouse model) is considered excellent for testing experimental cell-based immunotherapy strategies and is comparable with stage IV human breast cancer [148]. The injection of 4T1 cells, originally derived from a spontaneous mouse mammary tumor are injected into the mammary fat pad of a syngeneic animal and the rapid proliferation of cells forms tumors and eventually metastasizes to the lungs, liver, bone and brain [146, 147, 149]. Furthermore, this model has been refined through the development of 4T1 cell lines to employ varying degrees of metastasis that are location specific and representative of distinct gene expression signatures [150]. Xenograft transplantation encompasses the use of human cancer cells into immuno-compromised mice via intravenous, intraperitoneal or subcutaneous injection, orthptopically or ectopically [136, 151]. First discovered in 1962, nude mice have been commonly used for xenotransplantation because they lack a thymus and are unable to mount most types of immune responses, including rejection of allografts and xenografts [152]. Severe Combined Immunodeficiency (SCID) mice present with impaired ability to make T or B lymphocytes and are used as model organisms for research into transplantation strategies as they cannot reject tumors and transplants [153]. In general, rodents with immunological defects are typically resistant to growth of mammary carcinomas, and despite improvements these approaches have yielded low percentage of successful breast tumor engraftment compared to other types of cancers

[154]. Recent mouse models have contributed significantly to the understanding of breast cancer, however further research into suitable animal models will be required to advance development of new therapies for breast cancer. The growth and metastasis of human breast cancer cell lines *in vivo* allows the measurement of gene function relative to disease progression and has provided much insight into the use of investigational drugs intended interrupt or interfere with tumor growth [155].

Table 3 provides an overview of the defining characteristics of established breast cancer cell lines (mouse and human) commonly used in both *in vitro* and transplantation models.

Cell line	Species	ER Status	PR Status	Metastasis Location	Ref.
4T1	Mouse	+	+	Lymph node, blood, liver, lung, brain, bone	[149]
BT-474	Human	+	+	Bone	[156]
FII3	Mouse	+	+	Lung	[157, 158]
MCF-7	Human	+	+	Lymph node, lymphatic vessel	[159, 160, 161]
MDA-MB-231	Human	–	–	Lung, liver, brain and bone	[162, 163]
MDA-MB-435	Human	–	–	Lung	[164]
MDA-MB-453	Human	–	–	Bone	[165]
SUM1315	Human	–	–	Lung, bone	[166, 167]
SUM149	Human	–	–	Lung	[167]
T47D	Human	+	+	Lymph node, lymphatic vessel	[168]

Table 3. Breast Cancer Cell Lines for *in vitro* and transplantation models

It is unlikely that any one transplantation model will ever replicate the complexity of the whole cancer process; however studies to date demonstrate that xenographs are relevant in human breast cancer. Treatment with Herceptin was shown to improve the anti-tumor activity of paclitaxel and doxorubicin against HER2/neu-overexpressing human breast cancer xenografts leading to consecutive favorable clinical trials [169, 170]. Davis *et al.* [2004] reported the effective inhibition of tumor growth and metastasis in an orthotopic xenograft model by the use of combination therapy of paclitaxel and neutralizing antibodies targeting vascular endothelial growth factor receptor 2 (VEGFR2] [171]. The results of this research likely led to the development of bevacizumab, a humanized monoclonal antibody that targets vascular endothelial growth factor A (VEGF-A) [172]. Although, bevacizumab was removed as a breast cancer indication by the FDA [173], this is yet another example of how transplantation models lead to further development in the clinic. While these are merely a few cases for breast cancer and the use of xenograft studies, the information obtained from such has been translated into successful clinical trials for a variety of cancers [174-178]. Furthermore, useful information has been gained from transplantation models with respect to toxicity and in the identification of predictive biomarkers.

http://dx.doi.org/10.5772/55794

In spite of these successes, the xenograft model presents disadvantages in its ability to predict clinical response to therapy. Most animal tumors do not accurately model clinical metastatic disease. The use of immuno-compromised mice prevents an immune rejection response which is fundamentally different from the human system where the immune response promotes primary growth of tumor cells and their migration to secondary organs [136, 179]. Most xenograph models do not metastasize at the common sites of human breast cancer (such as lymph nodes, liver, bone and brain) as they prefer to colonize in the lungs [5]. However, improved models that have been created to represent human breast cancer metastasis from a primary orthotopic site to human bone, such as initially published in 2005 by Kuperwasser *et al* [167]. Consider that some xenograph models which utilize subcutaneous injection of tumor cells into the flank and mammary fat pad are not as representative of clinical disease as those that use orthotopic transplantation of cells into the mammary gland. Inherent discrepancies in the background of mice and humans should be considered, and this is of particular importance in predicting side effects for cancer therapy targets [180]. Additionally, the area of metastasis can change depending on the cells line utilized or methods of inoculation [167]; thus, there are considerable technical issues. One could overcome such restrictions by use of clinical isolates. However the utility of primary xerographs is inefficient; access is limited, results are restricted by sample size and thus, studies to date indicate only some degree of success [181]. Current research with aims to generate partial human immune systems or intact populations of human cells in mice systems may also overcome such limitations. We must consider that despite all advances to date, animals do not represent a complete model of human disease. For example, tumor relapse would be especially problematic to study as the usual life span in the majority of mice does not exceed two years. Aside from these underlying basic issues, there have been issues associated with the testing of natural products within these models. Further clarity on the fundamental mechanisms of tumor progression and metastasis and new drug targets will be unveiled as mouse models advance. Until then, we will continue to rely on current disease models and choose such based on disease state and therapeutic targets.

7. Breast cancer signaling pathways

Each of the identified breast cancer subtypes and gene expression patterns are dependent on different oncogenic pathways [105, 182]. The maintenance and differentiation of normal breast tissue is controlled by many signaling pathways and involves cytokines and chemokines, growth factors, steroid hormones, integrins, adhesion molecules and their respective receptors [183]. The regulation of such by single or combined components of the tumor microenvironment (such as fibroblasts, macrophages / lymphocytes, endothelial cells, vessels and proteins of the extracellular matrix (ECM) and stroma) have been implicated in various ways in the promotion, growth invasion and metastasis of breast cancer [184]. Cross talk or communication between the cancer cells and the factors within the tumor environment, including secretion factors from the tumor itself, can modify expression and signaling [184]. Of the several pathways indicated to play a role in cancer and CSC self-renewal, Notch, Wnt/Beta(β)-catenin, and Hedgehog (Hh) have been identified in human mammary cancer [124, 185, 186]. Additionally, evidence has mounted to strengthen the link between nuclear factor kappa-B (NF-κB), stem cells and breast cancer as elegantly reviewed in a recent paper by Shostak and Chariot (2011) [187].

7.1. Notch pathway

Four Notch proteins, namely Notch-1 to Notch-4, are expressed as transmembrane receptors in a variety of stem/progenitor cells [188, 189]. The binding of specific surface-bound ligands are responsible for triggering cleavage events at the Notch proteins by ADAM (A Disintegrin and metalloproteinase domain-containing protein) protease family and γ-secretase [188-191] causing the intracellular domain of Notch to be released and translocate to the nucleus. Once in the nucleus, downstream target genes (including c-Myc, cyclin D1,p21, NF-κB) are activated [190, 192-197]. Known for their ability to modulate the development of various organs and control cell proliferation [198], the notch activated genes and pathways have been reported to drive tumor control through the expansion of CSCs [198-202]. This associated role in self-renewal function of malignant breast cancers CSCs [198], combined with the fact that Notch inhibitors can kill breast cancer cells *in vitro* and *in vivo*, may partially explain why Notch expression and activation has been associated with a poor prognosis in mammary carcinomas [203-205]. In fact, research findings in breast cancer have presented compelling reasons to target Notch as a therapeutic target in solid tumors. In addition to its ability to regulate survival and proliferation in bulk cancer cells [205] and CSCs [206-209], notch plays a pro-angiogenic role in tumor endothelial cells [210, 211]. Farnie *et al* reported that activated Notch-1, Notch-4, and Notch target Her-1 expression in ductal carcinoma mammospheres *in situ* samples, but not from normal breast tissue [206, 212, 213]. Inhibition of Notch with a gamma-secretase inhibitor (GSI) or a neutralizing Notch-4 antibody has been reported to reduce the ability of ductal carcinoma in situ-derived cells to form mammospheres [207, 214]. Such results suggest that Notch inhibition may have significant therapeutic effects in primary lesions, may be able to preferentially target breast CSCs (responsible for reoccurrence and metastatic disease) and counteract angiogenesis [213]. Cross talk with the NF-κB pathway and Notch1 have been reported in a variety of cell interactions [192, 215-219], including the stimulation of NF-κB promoters[217] and the expression of several NF-κB subunits [192, 215-220].

7.2. Wnt/β-catenin pathway

The canonical (Wnt/β-catenin) pathway, including Wnt-1, -3A and -8 is likely the best characterized and traditionally defines Wnt signaling, however other pathways have been described including a non-canonical (planar cell polarity) pathway (including Wnt-5A, - 11) and the Wnt/Ca2+ pathway (protein kinase A pathway) [221-224]. Although it has been more than 25 years since the discovery of the Wnt gene, its structure remains unknown and signaling pathways are not well defined, especially those independent of β-catenin. Perhaps this challenge can be somewhat explained by the recent discovery that differences in cell signaling outcomes may be attributable to precise pairings of Wnt ligands with analogous cellular receptors [225]. For example, if we consider that the mammalian genome codes for 19 Wnt proteins and 10 Fzd receptors, there are potentially 190 Wnt/Fzd pairing combinations [226]. Although all of these ligand/receptor pairings have not been unveiled, we already know that the Wnt/β-catenin pathway has been established for its ability to alter cell proliferation, migration, apoptosis, differentiation and stem cell self-renewal [224, 227-230]. The essential mediator of the canonical pathway is β-catenin, and its two known distinct functions are based on cell specific locations. Accumulation of β-catenin within the cytoplasm leads to activation of Wnt target genes such as c-Jun, c-Myc, fibronectin and cyclin D1 [186, 231-236]. Prior to nuclear translocation, β-catenin operates in the membrane to maintain cell–cell adhesion via cooperation with the epithelial cell–cell adhesion protein E-cadherin [223]. The Wnt signaling pathway is activated via the binding of ligands to transmembrane receptors encoded by the Frizzled (Fzd) gene family and in conjunction with co-receptors, such as low-density lipoprotein receptors (protein 5 and 6) [237] This Wnt-Fzd interaction results in dephosphorylation, accompanied by decreased levels of degradation and causes the accumulation of β-catenin in the nucleus [231]. In the absence of Wnt signaling, β-catenin is quickly degraded in the cytoplasm. Without Wnt signaling, phosphorylation of adenomatous polyposis coli (APC) [238] via a cytoplasmic destruction complex results in ubiquitination of β-catenin which is then prone to proteasomal degradation [231]. Additionally, nuclear levels of β-catenin are lessened by their interaction with APC and Axin, both known for their function in transporting β-catenin back to the cytoplasm. In the nucleus, transcriptional corepressors interact with DNA-binding T-cell factor/lymphoid-enhancer factor (Tcf/Lef) proteins, such as Groucho/TLE, and are enabled to block target-gene expression when β-catenin is held at low levels. [239-242]. Wnt binding to the Fzd or low-density lipoprotein receptor protein-membrane receptors results in the accumulation and stabilization of translocated (from cytoplasm to nucleus) β-catenin [237]. Inhibition of such interactions has been noted by secreted Fzd-related proteins, Dickkopfs, and Wnt inhibitory factor-1 (WIF-1) [243, 244].

Since the initial observation that Wnt overexpression results in malignant transformation of mouse mammary tissue [245], aberrant regulation of the Wnt signaling pathway has emerged as a prevalent theme and continues to develop as a fundamental mechanism in broad cancer biology [246]. While Wnt pathway mutations (genetic and epigenetic) are rare in mammary carcinoma, overactive Wnt signaling has been noted in the majority of breast cancers, including rare classes (i.e.: triple -ve type) via several potential mechanisms [145, 233, 247-256]. Several studies to date have indicated that the expression of both Wnt receptors and their ligands are characteristic of breast cancer and furthermore certain receptors and ligands may be breast cancer type specific. In 2004, Bafico *et al.* reported autocrine Wnt signaling in a panel of breast cancer cell lines, including MDA-MB-231, which were identified by the presence of unstabilized β-catenin and then subsequently reduced upon expression or by the addition of the soluble Wnt inhibitors sFRP1 or DKK1 [257]. The expression of the Wnt receptor FZD7 is characteristic of certain rare types of breast cancer [258]. Additionally, the knockdown of FZD7 in cell lines representative of triple -ve breast cancer reduced the expression of Wnt target genes, inhibited tumorigenesis *in vitro* and greatly retarded the capacity of the MDA-MD-231 cell line to form tumors in mice [246, 259]. With respect to Wnt ligands, secreted frizzled related protein (sFRP)-1, an effective competitor and binding site with FZD receptors for Wnt ligands, has been shown to be ectopically expressed in the MDA-MB-231 cell line [260]. This same study showed that the sFRP1 expressing cells struggled to form tumors upon inoculation into the mammary fat pads of mice and their propensity to metastasize to lung was greatly impaired [260].

Specific to the maintenance of CSCs, Wnt/β-catenin signaling is implicated in many cancers [223, 224, 261-268], including breast cancer [269]. For example, radiation resistance of mouse mammary stem/progenitor cells has been correlated with overexpression of β-catenin in the stem cell survival pathway [266]. Additionally, overexpression of Wnt/β-catenin signaling was reported to promote expansion of the hepatic progenitor cell population in animal studies [267] and the elimination of β-catenin abrogates chemoresistant cell populations endowed with progenitor-like features [57]. Of great interest is the link between Wnt/β-catenin and PI3K (phosphoinositide 3 kinase) /Akt (protein kinase B) pathway as established by several studies. Korkaya *et al.* demonstrated that PI3K/Akt pathway is important in regulating the mammary stem/progenitor cells by promoting β-catenin downstream events through phosphorylation of GSK3β [60, 189]. Other studies have revealed the ability of activated Akt, such as phospho-Akt Ser473 to phosphorylate Ser9 on GSK3β, thereby decreasing the activity of GSK3β, and potentially stabilizing β-catenin [270-272].

In summary, the proof of concept for inhibiting Wnt signaling in cancer is in place. Furthermore there is an increasing amount of evidence to support a role for Wnt signaling in breast cancer; thus, a target has been created for future studies. Specific to breast cancer, the emphasis on target development ranges from antagonizing Wnt ligand secretion or binding to promote β-catenin degradation to specifically blocking β-catenin-mediated transcriptional activity [222]. Nonetheless, as noted several times throughout this chapter, the cooperation of Wnt pathway with other signaling pathways in cancer is an important consideration. Aside from the challenge of determining the most efficacious way to inhibit Wnt related factors, possible safety concerns should be considered; another compelling reason to explore specific targets in the Wnt pathways for all breast cancer sub-types.

7.3. Hh pathway

A crucial mediator of normal tissue development, with recent indications as a regulator of tumor-related vascular formation and function [273], the Hh signaling pathway in cancer is activated by ligand independent mutations in the pathway or through Hh overexpression (ligand-dependent) [189, 274, 275]. In the absence of Hh ligands, (Sonic Hh, Desert Hh and Indian Hh), their transmembrane receptor Patched (Ptch) associates with and blocks the G-protein-coupled phosphoprotein receptor Smoothened (Smo) and is only released when secreted Hh ligands bind to Ptch [189, 276, 277]. This binding triggers the dissociation of glioma-associated (Gli) family of zinc finger transcription factors. The three Gli proteins found in vertebrates include Gli1 and Gli2 (thought to activate Hh target genes) and Gli3 (known to act primarily as a repressor) which lead to the transcription of an assortment of genes including cyclin D, cyclin E, myc and elements of EGF pathway effectors through complex interactions with Costal2 (Cos2), Fused (Fu) and Suppressor of Fu (SuFu) [276-278]. Somatic mutations which activate Hh pathway have been implicated in a variety of human malignancies[278] including basal cell carcinomas, pancreatic cancer, medulloblastomas, leukemia, gastrointestinal, lung, ovarian, breast and prostate cancers [274, 275, 279]. Both *in vitro* and mouse model systems have demonstrated that the Hh signaling pathway plays a crucial role in regulating self-renewal of normal and malignant human mammary stem cells [51, 189]. Hh pathway inhibition has been shown to result in tumor growth inhibition mediated through the stromal microenvironment; as demonstrated in a xenograft model using a tumor and stromal cell co-injection procedure, and consistent with a paracrine signaling mechanism [280]. Although data describing the genetic alteration and the modulation of the expression pattern of Hh pathway components in mammary gland are limited, possible indications for the Hh pathway in development and maintenance of mammary cancer have been proposed [281]. However, a more significant role of Hh signaling has been revealed in prostate cancer studies, demonstrating that autocrine Hh signaling by tumor cells is a requirement for proliferation, viability and invasive behavior [282]. Additionally, the association of accelerated prostate cancer growth and progression with increased Hh signaling has been reported [283]. The Hh signaling pathway has been demonstrated as a critical pathway involved in stem cell self-renewal [276] including the essential role of Hh-Gli signaling in controlling the self-renewal behavior of human glioma CSCs and tumorigenicity [189, 284]. Known for its central role in the control of proliferation and differentiation of both embryonic stem cells and adult stem cells, aberrant activation of Hh signaling could be involved in the generation of CSCs and the development of cancer [278, 285]. In this regard, the development of Hh inhibitors may be a solution in the treatment of human cancers, including prevention of tumor progression. Essential similarities have been noted between Wnt and Hh signaling pathways [286] and their key roles in the physiological and pathological development of both embryonic and stem cells [278] [278]gives rise to the fact that crosstalk exists between the two. Signaling for both are activated by G-protein-coupled receptors [287, 288] and prevents phosphorylation-dependent proteolysis of key effectors (*Cubitus interruptus* or β-catenin) responsible for the conversion of a DNA-binding protein from a repressor to an activator of transcription [278, 289]. Considering the progression model of many cancers, specifically metastasis to bone, it is interesting to note that Wnt signaling has been reported to be downstream of Hh signaling, participating in bone development [278, 290]. Further proof proposing that Wnt signaling is downstream of Hh includes the ability of activated Gli1 to stimulate the transcription of Wnt ligands [276, 278]. It has been noted that molecules involved in Wnt signaling (i.e: GSK-3β) also play a regulatory role in Hh signaling [278, 286]. Furthermore, canonical Wnt/β-catenin signaling is required for the pathological response to oncogenic Hh signaling [278, 291].

7.4. NFκB Pathway

Along with their hallmark roles in cell survival, proliferation, inflammation and immunity, the NF-κB family of transcription factors are often constitutively expressed in breast cancer tumors [292]. Early studies on NF-κB pathway determined its key role in mammary epithelial proliferation, architecture and branching during early post-natal development [293, 294]. However, independent of its effects on mammary development, evidence exists to suggest that NF-κB regulates breast tumor progression [293, 294]. Constitutive activation of NF-κB in several breast tumor cell lines has been shown to profoundly affect the initiation and progression of breast cancer [295]. NF-κB is also required for the induction and maintenance of the EMT a process that critically controls breast cancer progression [296, 297]. Additionally, it is evident that NF-κB mostly acts in specific breast cancer sub-types, namely estrogen receptor (ER)-ve and ErbB2+ve tumors [298, 299] and has been implicated in stem cell expansion in breast cancer studies [187].

Activation of NF-κB results in the constant nuclear localization of proteins including p50, p52, p65, cRel and RelB which subsequently up-regulate anti-apoptotic proteins causing an imbalance between normal cell growth and apoptotic cell death [300]. NF-κB-activation occurs mainly through two well characterized pathways, namely the canonical (classical) and the non-canonical (alternative). Both pathways systematically work in a similar fashion in that they are reliant on signal-induced phosphorylation and degradation of an inhibitory molecule to release and transport nuclear NF-κB proteins. However, they differ in the types of trigger signals, activated kinases, inhibitory molecules and NF-κB proteins utilized in each system. In addition to each of these aforementioned pathways, other NF-κB activating pathways exist and have been indicated in the initiation and progression of breast cancer, however we will not discuss these fully in this chapter other than in the context that they appear in the described and relevant research experiments.

Specifically, the canonical pathway involves translocation of a p50/p65 heterodimer to prompt the expression of genes intricated in cell proliferation as well as their survival, inflammatory properties and role in innate immunity [292]. This process occurs through a transforming growth factor beta activated kinase-1 (TAK1)-dependent pathway and is normally dependent on members of pro-inflammatory cytokines such as tumor necrosis factor-alpha (TNFα) or IL-1β and other pro-inflammatory cytokines to degrade the inhibitor (IκBα) by the NF-κB essential modulator ((NEMO)/IκB kinase (IKK))γ-containing IKK complex [292]. In 2004, Biswas *et al.* published results regarding the activation of NF-κB in human breast tumors and in carcinoma cell lines indicating that the canonical pathway contributes to tumor development [298]. The resulting highlight of this experiment gave rise to activated NF-κB as a therapeutic target for distinctive subclasses of ER-ve breast cancers [298]. Specifically, the (NEMO)-binding domain (NBD) peptide (a selective inhibitor of IKK) blocked heregulin-mediated activation of NF-κB and cell proliferation while inducing apoptosis on proliferating cells substantiating the hypothesis that certain breast cancer cells rely on NF-κB for aberrant cell proliferation and simultaneously avoid apoptosis [298]. More recently, Connelly *et al.* [2011] showed, via genetic approaches, that the canonical NF-κB-activating pathway is inhibited in defined frames during polyoma middle T oncogene (PyVT) tumorigenesis and that interruption of this pathway in the mammary epithelium increases the latency of tumors and decreases tumor burden [301].

The non-canonical pathway, considered to be critical in adaptive immunity, is similar to the canonical cascade as it also relies on an IKKα heterodimer, but not on NEMO/IKKγ [302]. Prior to nuclear shuttling of 52/RelB dimers, the inhibitory molecule p100 is partially degraded through an NF-κB-inducing kinase (NIK)-dependent pathway [292]. Early studies revealed the enhanced expression of the NF-κB protein p52 in breast cancer samples giving rise to the involvement of the non-canonical pathway [303],[304]. The NF-κB protein RelB is increased in ERα-ve breast cancer cells and is required for the maintenance of mesenchymal ERα-ve breast cancer cells partially through the transcriptional induction of BCL2 [305]. Furthermore, RelB/p52 complexes have since been implicated in mammary carcinogenesis. For example, mouse mammary tumors induced by 7,12-dimethylbenz(a)anthracene treatment have been shown to increase RelB/p52 activity and the inhibition of RelB in breast cancer cells repressed cyclin D1 and c-Myc levels and growth in soft agar [306]. Perhaps the most conclusive proof of non-canonical NF-κB-activating pathway involvement occurred in studies employing a novel transgenic mouse model to consider the role of involved mediators (downstream of p100/p52] in both mammary development and tumorigenesis [307]. The results of this study indicated an increase in p100/p52 expression in tumors from mice expressing PyVT in the mammary gland, [307] with no change of nuclear p65 detected; an indication that the observation was limited to a deregulated non-canonical NF-κB-activating pathway [307].

7.4.1. NF-κB and breast cancer stem cell renewal

Recently, studies have strengthened the association between stem cells, breast cancer and NF-κB. Such have been captured in a review by Shostak and Chariot highlighting experiments to date complemented by a compelling rationale for targeting NF-κB and other developmental pathways involved in the self-renewal of normal stem cells [187]. The involvement of NF-κB in various signaling cascades has proven critical in several studies involving breast cancer stem cell expansion.

Cao *et al.* [2007] showed that IKKα is both a regulator of mammary epithelial proliferation and a contributor to ErbB2-induced oncogenesis [308]. Specifically, breast cancer cells from IKKα (AA/AA) knock-in mice (whereby IKKα activation is disrupted) crossed with the Her2 murine breast cancer model, exhibited diminished self-renewal capacity and resulted in the inability to establish secondary tumors [308]. Breast cancers that generate primary, as opposed to secondary mammospheres such as seen in mice used in these experiments, suggests that IKKα is likewise required for the self-renewal of tumor-initiating cells from the Her2 breast cancer model [187]. Additionally, mutated IKKα slowed tumor development following exposure to 7,12-dimethylbenzaanthracene or the MMTV-c-neu (ErbB2/Her2) transgene; however there was no effect on MMTV-v-Ha-ras-induced cancer despite the fact that both of these oncogenes rely on cyclin D1 [308]. In this same series of studies, carcinoma cells from another mouse model (IKKα(AA/AA)/MMTV-c-neu) underwent premature senescence when cultured under conditions used for propagation of mammary gland stem cells. Altogether, these mouse models of breast cancer show that IKKα seems to act as a central protein in the activation of NF-κB during breast cancer stem cell self-renewal [308]. Therefore, the researchers concluded that IKKα may represent a novel and specific target for treatment of ErbB2+ve breast cancer.

While NF-κB appears to be activated in luminal progenitor cells during differentiation of mammary colony-forming cells [309], the mammary stem-like basally located cells are devoid of NF-κB activity [309, 310]. Taken together, these studies suggest that only the canonical NF-κB pathway is active in normal luminal progenitor cells before transformation and is required for the formation of mammary luminal-type epithelial neoplasias [309]; a reminder of the importance of understanding the cellular etiology underpinning breast tumor heterogeneity [310].

Another interesting role for NF-κB signaling involves the link between inflammation and cancer. While the mechanism linking inflammation and cancer has yet to be explained, we do know that the inflammatory cytokine, interleukin(IL)-6 is up-regulated in epithelial cancers, including breast cancer [311]. We also know that NF-κB regulates the expression of anti-apoptotic genes and activates different pro-inflammatory cytokines and chemokines, including IL-6 [312, 313]. Further clarity on the interactions of NF-κB signaling, inflammation and cancer has been gained through a study showing that the temporary activation of Src oncoprotein mediates an epigenetic event whereby immortalized breast cells are stably transformed to a cell lines that represent self-renewing mammospheres containing cancer stem cells [313]. The inflammatory response triggered by the activation of Src and further downstream signaling which inhibits IL-6 expression is mediated by NF-κB [313]. It has been shown that the transformation of cells utilized within this experiment occurs via a positive feedback loop whereby IL-6 mediated STAT3 transcription factor stimulation activates NF-κB [313]. These authors have demonstrated that Src activation triggers a rapid inflammatory response mediated by NF-κB that is critical for cellular transformation. While this study defines Src's role as an oncogenic kinase promoting the expansion of breast cancer stem cells, it also demonstrated the critical involvement of NF-κB in the process [313].

It is known that the onset of progestin-driven breast cancer is affected by the deletion of IKKα in mammary-gland epithelial cells [314]. Such studies are relevant in breast cancers as they consider the importance of associated risk factors between hormone replacement therapy (i.e.: progesterones or synthetic derivatives) and the increased risk of incident of fatal breast cancer [314]. The expression of both receptor activator of NF-κB (RANK) and RANK ligand (RANKL) have been observed in primary breast cancers in humans and breast cancer cell lines [315]. Studies to date indicate that the RANKL/ RANK system is mediated in part by IKK-α–NF-κB signaling and controls the incidence and onset of progestin-driven breast cancer; more specifically a loss of RANK expression significantly impairs the self-renewal capacity of cancer stem cells [314, 316]. Thus, because of the link between the RANKL/RANK system and progestin-driven epithelial carcinogenesis, RANKL inhibition could be considered as a novel approach to the prevention and/or treatment of breast cancer [314].

More recently, a model of Her2-dependent tumorigenesis indicated that breast cancer stem cell renewal is regulated by epithelial NF-κB through a reduction in the expression of key embryonic stem cell regulators, namely Sox2 and Nanog [317]. Specifically, NF-κB was required for both proliferation and colony formation of Her2-derived murine mammary tumor cell lines [317]. Additionally, the rate of initiation of Her2 tumors was governed by NF-κB [317].

7.5. Summarizing pathway interruptions/targets

In many human breast cancers, all three developmental pathways (Wnt, Notch and Hh) appear to be deregulated and control the self-renewal of normal stem cells from a molecular perspective [186]. Additionally, the involvement of NF-κB has emerged as another involved pathway in breast cancer based on what we know about Her2, a membrane bound receptor tyrosine kinase. Her 2 is overexpressed in 30% of breast cancers and critically controls the cancer stem-cell population [318]. Since Her2 activates NF-κB through the canonical pathway [319] [27],

http://dx.doi.org/10.5772/55794

the hypothesis exists that the NF-κB pathway may be involved in the biology of breast cancer stem cells. It is also obvious that these interrupted pathways, and likely others unknown at this time, are responsible for certain stages of cancer progression or cancer cell aggression. If so, then we are in agreement with others who have noted that the development and identification of selective inhibitors of specific signaling pathways is an attractive approach for the prevention of tumor progression and/or treatment of cancers [278]. However, we have also mentioned several examples of cross-talk between the components of different cell signaling pathways. This concept then introduces the task of targeting multiple pathways in an effort to prevent progression and metastasis of cancers. Alternatively, and based on the premise that certain pathways operate downstream of others, it would be more reasonable to focus on inhibitors of overarching pathways, such as NF-κB. In summary, such oncogenic pathway signatures are fundamental in natural product testing. Therapeutic approaches involving natural products may provide a link between pathway deregulation and therapeutic sensitivity indicating an opportunity for the development of target compound(s).

8. Prevention and treatment of breast cancer with natural products: Past successes and promising future treatments

Currently, hormones and cytotoxic drugs remain the standard treatment for metastatic breast cancers. Development of a therapeutic approach for treating tumors, tumor reoccurrence and metastatic tumors is crucial for reducing mortality in cancer patients [6]. There is an urgent need to explore agents that will be effective in preventing and treating metastasis of breast cancer. For centuries, nature has provided us with a rich source of compounds for various disease treatments. Such naturally-derived molecules have been utilized in formal drug discovery platforms of the pharmaceutical industry. Greater than 60% of new chemical entries at the National Cancer Institute from 1981-2002 were either natural products or were derived from natural products [320]. Such naturally-occurring sources can be defined by their origin and include biotic (i.e.: forests, plants, animals, birds and marine organisms) and abiotic (i.e.: land, water, air and minerals such as gold, iron, copper, and silver) components [321]. Within these categories, plants have proven to be a rich source of lead compounds (i.e: alkaloids, morphine, cocaine) or the basis for synthetic drugs (i.e: anesthetics from cocaine) [320, 321]. The complexity and variation of plant structures indicates that their evolution has naturally completed the screening process and that the creation of potent compounds makes them more likely to survive. Plants offer the advantage of abundance, and even with such clinical successes as paclitaxel (Taxol) from the yew tree, and the antimalarial agent artemisinin from *Artemisia annua*, the vast majority have not been studied [320]. Due to promising bioactivity and diversity, the plant environment offers a potential source of natural products. A vast number of studies in the discipline of epidemiology have confirmed an association between fruit and vegetable consumption and the reduced risk of several cancers resulting in an increased interest in the role of naturally occurring dietary compounds in the efficacy of cancer chemoprevention [322]. Thus, the exploration of plant-based molecules as anti-cancer drugs is appropriate.

The history of Tamoxifen and its derivatives in the successful treatment of estrogen receptor (ER)+ve breast cancers are well documented. In the past Tamoxifen was successful in reducing breast cancer mortality rate in hormone receptor+ve breast cancer patients by up to a third and thus was the stronghold of endocrine treatment [323]. Clinical trials have indicated that aromatase inhibitors (AI) have improved efficacy compared with Tamoxifen for the treatment of post-menopausal hormone receptor+ve patients [324-327]. Additionally, the response rate for third generation AIs as first-line agents range from 30%–50% in ER+ve advanced breast cancer. [323]. Leading to these discoveries, and in an effort to capitalize on the advantages of both anti-aromatase and anti-estrogenic activity, many natural products have been tested for their ability to prevent and treat breast cancer, *in vivo* and *in vitro*. Table 4 summarizes plant based compounds that have been indicated for their potential as a prevention or treatment in breast cancer. This list is not exhaustive; however it does capture the extracts studied to date according to activity in cell lines and animal models and represents the most common types of breast cancer. In addition to those listed within Table 4, soy-based extracts, curcumin and piperine have been studied and we will discuss these in detail as the most promising plant based targets in the prevention, treatment and progression of breast cancer.

9. Promising plant based targets in the prevention, treatment and progression of breast cancer

9.1. Summarizing the individual and combined effects of the soy isoflavones, genistein and diadzein, on mammary tumor development, metastases and invasive breast cancer cells *in vivo* and *in vitro*

Genistein, daidzein and glycitein are the main isoflavones present in soybean and soy-based foods [341] [342]. Out of these, genistein is the mostly studied and dominant isoflavone of soy against breast cancer and has progressed to phase II clinical trials [343]. Soy isoflavones acting upon breast cancer cells *in vitro* and *in vivo* have been studied extensively with varying results and the clinical implications specific to breast cancer have been discussed. Soy isoflavones are structurally similar to female androgen estrogen, and thus they are also known as phytoestrogens [344] and may possibly be competing with the physiological estrogens. Genistein and daidazine (but not glycietein) possesses the ability to transactivate the estrogen receptors.

Utilizing cell based assays on MCF-7 human breast cancer cells, estrogenic agonist actions of soy isoflavones have been studied by Matsumura and co-workers whereby genistein and daidzein exert estrogen response in MCF-7 cells [345] via ER with higher affinity to ERβ1. Similarly, in hepatoma cells transfected with ER, genistein and daidazine bind to both ERα and ERβ but with more affinity to ERβ. Genistein is more potent compared to daidazine [346]. However, these phytoestrogens are 400-600 times less potent compared to 17-β estradiol [347].

In vitro, genestein is capable of identifying cells that specifically carry BRCA1 mutation and strongly inhibits the growth of BRCA1 mutant cells compared to cells expressing the wild-type BRCA1 protein [348]. The resistance shown by cells expressing wild type BRCA1 protein has been attributed to increased AKT and decreased p21 (WFA1/CIP1) protein levels [349].

http://dx.doi.org/10.5772/55794

Natural Product; Active Ingredient	Effect	Ref.
White button mushrooms (*Agaricus bisporous*); Conjugated linoleic acid and its derivatives	Decreased both tumor cell proliferation and tumor weight with no effect on rate of apoptosis in MCF-7aro cells and nude mice injected with MCF-7aro cells.	[324]
Taxus brevifolia (Pacific Yew) and other Taxus derivatives; Paclitaxel	Promotes tubulin polymerization and stabilization of microtubules against depolymerization.	[328] [329]
Dysoxylum binectariferum; Flavopiridol	Inhibition of MMP-2 and MMP-9 secretion of in MDA-MB-435 (parental) and 435.eB (stable transfectants) breast cancer cells.	[330]
Green Tea; *Epigallocatechin gallate*	Suppresses receptor (ERα) MBA-MB-231 breast cancer cell growth *in vitro* and *in vivo* in combination with curcumin.	[331]
Bloodroot *(Sanguinaria Canadensis);* Sanguinarine	Induced apoptosis through mediation of ROS production in MDA-MB-231 breast carcinoma cells, decrease in mitochondrial membrane potential, release of cytochrome c, activation of casp-3, and casp-9 and down regulation of Bcl-2.	[332]
Garcinia hanburyi. (Gamboge tree); Gambogic acid	Upregulation of p53 and down regulation of Bcl-2 resulting in apoptosis in MCF-7 cancer cells.	[333]
Ganoderma lucidum; Ganoderic acids	Inhibits AP-1 and NF-κB activity; inhibition of u-PA secretion from MDA-MB-231 cells.	[334]
Ginger; Acetoxychavicolacetate	Decreased cell viability in MCF-7 and MDA-MB-231 cells via casp-3-dependent increase in apoptosis.	[335]
Grapes, fruits, and root extracts of the weed Polygonum cuspidatum); Resveratrol	Suppresses NF-κB activation and cell proliferation in MCF-7 cells, reduced expression of Cox-2 and MMP-9 (with a reduced NF-κB activation).	[336]
Garcinia indica (kokum); Garcinol	Induced apoptosis in MCF-7 and MDA-MB-231 cells via caspase activation and down-regulation of NF-κB regulated genes.	[337]
Plumbago europaea (Plumbago); Plumbagin	Induced apoptosis with concomitant inactivation of Bcl-2 and the DNA binding activity of NF-κB in MCF-7aro breast cancer cells.	[338]
Rotenone; Deguelin	Arrests cells at the S phase resulting in anti-proliferative effect in MDA-MB-231 cancer cells.	[339]
Silymarin; Silibinin	Reduced PMA-induced invasion of MCF-7 cells through specific inhibition of AP-1-dependent MMP-9 expression.	[340]

Table 4. Plant Based Natural Products indicated in Breast Cancer

Cyclooxygenase-2 (COX-2) expression, which is associated breast cancer risk [350], can also be inhibited by soy isoflavones [351]. Thus, it seems that soy isoflavones are capable of curtailing breast cancer risk factors.

The influences of soy isoflavones on cell growth, cell cycle and apoptosis are all relevant to their effectiveness as chemopreventive agents for breast cancer. A number of studies have indicated the potential of genistein to inhibit proliferation of breast cancer cells in culture by causing cell cycle arrest and/or apoptosis. Genistein induces G2/M cell cycle arrest [352-354]. This effect was seen both in hormone sensitive and hormone independent cells [352]. According to Li *et al*. [2008] G2/M cell cycle arrest occurs, via stable activation of ERK1/2 pathway [354].

Demarcation on the relative importance of cell adhesion, invasion and migration for primary tumor growth verses metastatic tumour growth is not clear. However, motility, migration and adhesion are more connected to metastasis which is undoubtedly the most life-threatening aspect of breast cancer. Thus, it is crucial to identify the effects of soy isoflavones on disease metastasis.

Microarray analysis of genistein treated HCC1395 cells, a cell line derived from an early stage primary breast cancer, has indicated up-regulation of genes that inhibit invasion and down-regulation of genes that promote invasion [355]. Genistein enhances the adhesion of breast cancer cells [356, 357]. This may possibly be one method utilized by genistein to reduce metastasis.

A study by Vantyghem *et al* (2005) describes the ability of dietary genistein to affect metastasis in a post–surgical model in mice [358]. This test model mimics the clinical situation where primary tumors are surgically removed and therapeutic strategies are applied to prevent the growth of any cancer cells seeded to other locations prior to surgery. In this study, primary tumours were established by injecting human breast carcinoma cells, MDA-MB-435/HAL, into the mammary fat pad of nude mice. After 5 weeks, tumours were surgically removed and mice were maintained with a soy free diet or genistein supplemented diet. At the end of 5 weeks, a 10 fold reduction in percent lung metastasis in mice fed on a genistein supplemented diet was seen. In another study, as described by Zhang *et al.*, genistein has shown its ability to reduce the number and volume of osteolytic bone metastases in Balb/c(nu/nu) mice injected with MDA-MB-231 human breast cancer cells [359]. As there are clear indications of the ability of this compound to inhibit breast cancer metastasis, as described in the various animal studies, it would be useful to identify the associated molecular mechanisms. Although there are no conclusive findings, a number of different mechanisms have been suggested.

In studies focused on determining related mechanisms, scientists have given more attention to molecules that are overtly expressed in malignant breast tumours. For example, much attention has been invested into the actions of focal adhesion kinase (FAK), a tyrosine protein kinase. As described previously, cell motility is an integral part of metastasis and it is justifiable to investigate the components directly involve in cell motility. FAK has been designated as a regulator of cell migration and invasion [360]. Since over expression of FAK in human tumors occurs, it has been proposed as a potential therapeutic target [361]. Increased expression of FAK expression in invasive breast carcinomas is associated with an aggressive phenotype [362]. In a transgenic model of breast cancer, mammary epithelial specific disruption of FAK blocks transition of premalignant hyperplasias to carcinomas (and their subsequent metastasis) indicating direct involvement in mammary tumor progression [363]. Further, attenuation of FAK function dramatically increased apoptosis in breast cancer cells [364]. Disruption of FAK signaling by expressing the N-terminal domain FAK in human breast carcinoma cells has led to rounding, detachment and apoptosis [365]. To gain insight into the influence of genistein and daidazine in this important pathway in breast cancer, *in vitro* and *in vivo* studies have been conducted. According to an *in vitro* study, the soy isoflavones genistein, daidzein and 17β estradiol increased the number of focal adhesions and FAK activity in ERα +ve (T47D cells) as well as in ERα -ve (MDA-MB-231) breast cancer cells indicating possible involvement of novel signaling pathways and independent of estrogen receptors. Authors of this study suggested a progressive role (to metastasis) for soy isoflavones in the activation of multiple FAK regulated signaling pathways relevant to breast cancer [366], however the mechanism was not investigated. The studies of Mitra and co-workers may possibly explain the mechanism of FAK in breast cancer metastasis [367]. According to this study, reduced FAK activity or expression blocked 4T1 breast cancer cell invasion through matrigel and the blocking was associated with a 2-3 fold reduction in the expression of urokinase plasminogen activator (uPA) [367]. uPA is a serine protease that cleaves extracellulaer matrix and stimulate plasminogen to plasmin. Cancer cells are known to digest the ECM via substances like uPA and matrix metalloproteases (MMPs) as a means of invading surrounding tissue. This idea is supported by the fact that breast cancer patients with higher level of MMP-9 in tissue is associated with lymph node metastasis; thus, MMP-9 levels in serum, tumour tissue and urine are used as prognostic markers [368]. Furthermore, a study on the role of membrane-type 1 matrix metalloproteinase (MT1-MMP) *in vitro* and in SCID mice reports that the down regulation of mammary cancer cell MT1-MMP has no effect on primary tumour growth and lymph node metastasis, but reduces the occurrence of lung metastasis [369]. Interestingly, uPA secretion from mammary carcinoma cells can be influenced by genistein. This property of genistein has been shown *in vitro* and *in vivo* and the implication on tumour angiogenesis has been studied using F3II mammary carcinoma cells in culture as well as in a syngeneic mouse model. Accordingly, non-cytotoxic concentrations of genistein (0.1-50μM) significantly reduced motility in F3II mammary carcinoma cells and inhibited the secretion of uPA from cell monolayers. Once F3II cells were implanted in syngeneic mice receiving a treatment of genistein (10mg/kg/day), anti antiangiogenic effects were evident [357].

These studies indicate the effectiveness of genistein to inhibit angiogenesis and metastasis by inhibiting proteolytic substances such as uPA. In this respect, our attempt to further explore the value of soy isoflavones in modulating metastasis enabled us to review some important findings. Studies by Shao *et al*, [1998] reported that genistein inhibited the invasion of MCF-7 and MDA-MB-231 cells *in vitro* and the inhibition was characterized by down regulation of MMP-9 (matrix mettaloproteinase-9) and up regulation of TIMP-1 (tissue inhibitor of mettaloproteinase-1) [370]. The same effects were seen in nude mouse xenografts of MCF-7 and MDA-MB-231 cells [371]. Furthermore, in MDA-MB-231 xenografts, genistein inhibited tumour growth, stimulated apoptosis, regulated p21 WAF1/CIP1 expression, inhibited angiogenesis with reduced vessel density and decreased the levels of vascular endothelial growth factor and transforming growth factor β1 [370]. Further studies by the same authors reported that genistein inhibits both constitutive and epidermal growth factor stimulated invasion in ER- human breast carcinoma cells as characterized by up regulation of TIMP-1 as well as other trypsin inhibitors like protease nexin-II (PN-II) and alpha 1-antitrypsin (alpha 1-AT) [371]. Kousidou *et al* [2005], examining normal mammary cells (MCF-12A), low invasive (ER+ve) MCF-7 cells and high invasive MDA-MB-231 (ER-ve) cells (in parallel) showed differences in the effect of genistein on highly invasive and low invasive cells. Accordingly, all cell types expressed genes of MMP-2, MMP-9, membrane-type matrix metalloproteinase (MT-1, MT-2, MT-3), MMP and TIMP-1, -2 and -3. However, once genistein was added, down regulation of all MMP genes in highly invasive cells and down regulation of many genes in low invasive MCF-7 cells was observed [372].

Based on the above findings, genistein has a role in reducing metastasis and this appears to arise from its ability to suppress uPA and MMPs thereby invading barriers with no direct effect on the capacity of cell mobility. According to the literature, expression of uPA and MMPs is regulated by NFk-B [373] [307]. Therefore it would be worthwhile to review any association between genistein and the NF-kB pathway.

9.1.1. Genistein may act via inhibition of the NF-κB pathway

The possible connection between NF-κB and breast cancer has been extensively studied [374]. Using a doxycycline-inducible new mouse model to inhibit NF-κB activity, specifically within the mammary epithelium at the time of tumor development, Connelly *et al* (2011) indicated the active contribution of NF-κB in mammary tumor progression [301]. In this model, inhibition of NF-κB activity showed an increase in tumor latency and a decrease in tumor burden [301]. Specifically, soy isoflavones inhibited the tumors by suppressing the NF-κB pathway. Furthermore genistein potentiates the activity of a number of NF-κB mediated chemotherapeutic agents by increasing apoptosis in various cancer cells, including MDA-MB-231 breast cancer cells [375]. In the same cell line, genistein induces G2/M cell cycle arrest via stable activation of ERK1/2 pathway [354],[376]. Furthermore, the MDA-MB-231 cell line has the ability to selectively block NF-κB transactivation of IL-6, a cytokine that is known for estrogen independent tumorigenesis activity [377]. Inhibition of proteosome activity by genistein in MCF-7 breast cancer cells has also been associated with NF-κB inhibition [378]. This property of genistein is particularly important for ER deficient breast cancer as constitutive NF-κB and Mitogen- and Stress- Activated Protein Kinase-1 (MAPK) /MSK activity are linked with aggressiveness and the metastasis.

It is clear that almost all of the studies that show beneficial effects of soy isoflavones utilized genistein. However, within the natural products of soy and soy food not only genistein, but daidzein and glycitein are present. A recent study testing genistein, daidazine and glycitein separately has indicated interesting results. According to this study, only genistein induced apoptosis in MCF-7 breast carcinoma cells whereas daidzein caused a slight cell-stimulating effect in the absence of E2; thus, the authors pointed toward the possible risk of breast cancer in postmenopausal women who take soy supplements [379]. This statement is important as a number of soy supplements available in the market contain high levels of daidzein [380, 381].

An animal study using nude mice and MDA-MB-435 breast cancer cells reported the individual and combined soy isoflavones exerting differential effects on metastatic cancer progression

[382]. As described in this study, daidazine increased mammary tumour growth by 38% while genistein decrease tumor growth by 33%. Moreover, the combined isoflavones increased metastasis to all the organs examined, although no effect on primary tumour growth was noted. These results have led authors to include the consumption of soy foods as a cause of increased breast cancer metastasis. Also, a number of studies by Ju *et al* [383-385] have cited enhanced growth effects of soy components in ER+ve breast cancers. However, with these studies conducted in immune compromised mice, the relevance of these findings have been criticized [386], especially as pre-treatment with genistein has shown to been protective against mammary tumors [387]. More recently, the antiproliferative activity of both genistein and quercetin has been indicated in the prevention and treatment of HER2-overexpressing breast cancer via inhibition of NFκB signaling [388]. In this study, these specific phytoestrogens inhibited proliferation in MCF-7 cell lines accompanied by an increase in intrinsic apoptotic indicators, induction of the extrinsic apoptosis pathway (up-regulating p53), a reduction in the phosphorylation level of IκBα, and negated the nuclear translocation and subsequent phosphorylation of nuclear p65 [388].

9.1.2. Sources of soy

Soybeans can be considered as the richest source of isoflavones in the human diet [389, 390], and are available in fermented and non-fermented forms. Fresh green soy beans, whole dry soybeans, whole-fat soy flour, soy milk and soymilk products such as tofu, okara and yuba are non-fermented while soy sauce, temphe, miso and natto are fermented products [391]. Additionally, products such as soy dairy substitutes, soy cheese, soy yogurt, and soy burgers seem to be popular in Western countries. The isoflavone content in various soy-based food products greatly differ. Other than soy food products, soy supplemented (categorized as a class of complementary medicine) nutraceuticals are widely consumed by Western communities. The quality and standard of these supplements are questionable. For instance, a survey carried out in the Eastern Washington Region of U.S.A. tested 13 products (7 tablet and 6 capsule formulations) by HPLC and showed that only 4 of the 13 products contained the minimum of 90% isoflavone content claimed on the label and variations in composition over time were noted [392]. Interestingly, a recent review shows that overall, most commercially available nutraceuticals are poor in quality [393].

9.1.3. Clinical studies

Although there have been a large number of studies carried out to evaluate a possible soy-breast cancer link, evidence is inconclusive. The two main theories tested involve the effect of soy isoflavone consumption in risk of breast cancer incidence and its effect on recurrence. The largest population based cohort study, including 5,042 female breast cancer survivors, shows that soy food consumption is significantly associated with decreased risk of death and recurrence [394]. Another cohort of 1,954 female breast cancer survivors, who consumed soy isoflavones at the levels comparable to the Asian population, while undergoing tamoxifen therapy showed a reduction in the risk of cancer recurrence and no interference in the efficacy of tamoxifen [395]. Further studies have indicated that soy intake prior to cancer diagnosis is unrelated to disease-free breast cancer survival and that the association between soy protein intake and breast cancer survival does not differ according to the presence of other risk factors such as ER/PR status, tumor stage, age at diagnosis, body mass index (BMI), waist to hip ratio (WHR), or stage of menopause [396]. No variations were noted in the soy-survival association of indicated polymorphisms in ERα and ERβ indicating that soyfoods do not have an adverse effect on breast cancer survival. A recent meta-analysis by Dong and Qin (4 studies of breast cancer recurrence and 14 studies of breast cancer incidence) revealed that the consumption of soy isoflavone is inversely associated with risk of breast cancer incidence [397]. However, the protective effect is only observed among studies conducted in Asian populations, unlike those reported in Western populations [397]. One of the previous meta-analysis studies by Wu *et al* [2008] show a similar trend. Accordingly, in Asian populations a higher intake of soy isoflavones, as compared with lower intake, is associated with 29% reduction in the risk of developing breast cancer [398]. Hence, the consumption of soy food at levels similar to those consumed by Asian populations may have protective effects. However, there is evidence in the literature to show possible adverse effects of soy due to its known stimulatory effect on the premenopausal female breast as indicated by increased secretion of breast fluid, the appearance of hyperplastic epithelial cells and elevated levels of plasma estradiol [399]. Some animal studies support the idea of related disadvantages of consuming soy isoflavones. In overiectomized athymic nude mice, physiological concentrations of dietary genistein stimulates the growth of estrogen dependent MCF-7 tumors in a dose dependent manner [383, 400]. Furthermore, the same test model showed that dietary genistein reverses the inhibitory effect of tamoxifen on the growth of MCF-7 tumors [384].

9.2. The role of curcumin and piperine in breast cancer prevention and its effects on normal human breast stem cell renewal and signaling

Curcumin is a plant derived polyphenol which gives rise to the yellow colour in the spice, tumeric. This pigment is obtained from the plant *Curcuma longa* and has been noted to have power against cancer. In their review of the mechanisms of cell cycle regulation by curcumin, Gaurisankar and Das have named it as a multiple edged sword [401] because of its ability to regulate the cell cycle as well as apoptosis. Distorted cell cycle regulation and programmed cell death/apoptosis are characteristic features of cancer and curcumin has been shown to target both mechanisms. The ability of curcumin to inhibit telomerase activity [402] and to disrupt mitotic spindle structure causing [403] micronucleation in MCF-7 breast carcinoma cells has been reported. Also, curcumin is known to induce anti-proliferative activity via the decreased expression of cyclin D1 and CDK-4 in MCF-7 breast carcinoma cells [404] and can induce apoptosis through p53 dependent Bax induction [405]. Curcumin is able to disrupt breast tumor growth, but also to inhibit metastasis.

As with genestein, curcumin has been shown to mediate its anti-cancer effects via regulation of the NF-κB signaling pathway. In the nude mouse model, curcumin suppresses the paclitaxel-induced NF-κB pathway resulting in the inhibition of lung metastasis of human breast cancer [406]. The modification of NF-kB signaling eventually leads to pro-apoptotic events and perhaps inhibition of ECM breakdown. Curcumin induced apoptosis in MDA-MB-231 cells

http://dx.doi.org/10.5772/55794

in vitro is associated with IkB and p65 phosphorylation and hence reduced activation of NFkB [407]. This leads to reduced expression on MMPs, diminished invasion through a reconstituted basement membrane and a lower number of metastases in immunodeficient mice injected with tumor cells via intra cardiac route [407]. The high level of of MMP-3 expression noted in MDA-MB-231 invasive breast carcinoma cells is not evident on MCF-7 non-invasive breast cancer cells, implicating its importance in invasion and metastasis. The possibility of using the major forms of curcuminoids, curcumin, demethoxycurcumin, and bisdemethoxycurcumin (all of which are found in turmeric powder) as MMP-3 inhibitors to modulate MMP-3 expression has been suggested [408]. According to Chiu and Su (2009), curcumin inhibits proliferation by increasing the Bax to Bcl-2 ratio while inhibiting the migration via decreasing NF-kB p65 expression in breast cancer MDA-MB-231 cells [409]. Utilizing microarray gene expression analysis on MDA-MB-231 breast cancer cells, Bachmeier *et al.* demonstrated the ability of curcumin to downregulate inflammatory cytokines CXCL-1 and -2 via suppression of NF-κB translocation. Moreover, silencing CXCL-1 and -2 resulted in a downregulation of several metastasis promoting genes [410].

Interestingly, curcumin can interfere with estrogen-mimicking pesticides such as endosulfane, DDT and chlordane [411].

9.2.1. Sources of curcumin

Curcumin is generally considered to be the most active component and the principal curcuminoid found in tumeric [411]. The spice tumeric is commonly used in curries and contains 2-8% of this active ingredient [412], however a supplement form is also available.

9.2.2. Clinical trials

Little data is available on the pharmacokinetics and metabolism of curcumin in humans. Dose-limiting toxicity is not reported and high oral doses of curcumin (up to 12g/day) have been tested [220, 413, 414]. In a phase one clinical trial involving individuals with non-invasive cancer and pre-cancerous conditions, oral dosing of 4g, 6g and 8g of curcumin yielded peak serum concentrations of 0.51 +/- 0.11microM, 0.63 +/- 0.06 microM, and 1.77 +/- 1.87 microM, respectively. Peak serum concentrations of curcumin are seen 1-2 hours after oral intake and this gradually declines within 12 hours [220]. In another phase I clinical trial involving 15 patients with advanced colorectal cancer, 3.6g of curcumin daily for up to 4 months was well-tolerated [413]. Another study examined the pharmacokinetics of 450mg-3600mg curcumin (daily for 1 week) in twelve patients with hepatic metastatic disease from primary colorectal adenocarcinomas. Using a high-performance liquid chromatography assay, low nanomolar levels of the parent compound and its glucuronide and sulphate conjugates were found in the peripheral or portal circulation; despite its absence in liver tissue, trace levels of products of its metabolites were detected [415]

Due to the poor bioavailability of curcumin systemically, high priority has been given to study its potential against colorectal cancers. A very recent publication on a phase IIa clinical trial involving men and women 40 years of age or over and smokers that carry 8 or more colorectal aberrant crypt foci (ACF) indicates that oral dosing of curcumin (4g per day for 30 days) significantly reduces colorectal ACF, a biomarker of colon carcinogenesis. [416] The reported anti-carcinogenic effect of curcumin is not associated with increased levels of curcumin in local tissue but increased levels of conjugate concentrations in suggesting that curcumin may mediate its effects by cuccumin conjugates delivered systemically. The same study showed that the presence of curcumin conjugates in plasma and tissue prior to treatment (believed to be originated from the normal diet of the studied population) were accompanied by a steady increase of curcumin conjugates following the month-long daily dosing [416]. A study examining the pharmacokinetics of curcumin at the concentrations of 10g and 12g in twelve healthy volunteers indicates comparable results. Accordingly, a single dose of orally administered curcumin resulted in the detection of conjugates, glucuronides and sulfates in plasma in all subjects while free curcumin was evident in only one subject [414]. Even though curcumin conjugates and other breakdown products have not been assessed for their anticarcinogenic properties [416], these findings shed some light on the potential of curcumin as a treatment of all cancers, including those of colorectal origin. This may offer a likely explanation of how continuous exposure to small quantities of curcumin via normal diets protects Asian women from breast cancer.

A phase I dose escalation trial of combined effects of docetaxel and curcumin in patients with advanced and metastatic breast cancer was published very recently. This study involved 14 patients and demonstrated the feasibility, safety and tolerability of a combination of curcumin with a standard dose of docetaxel which warrants further investigation and progression to a Phase II clinical trial [417]. Similarly, the curcumin inhibiting effects of chemotherapy induced apoptosis in models of human breast cancer have been identified [418].

9.2.3. Curcumins' ability to destroy cancer stem cells

The properties of CSC's are connected with major signaling pathways. The signaling pathways active in mammary stem cells are shown to be Wnt/β catenin, Hh and Notch [60],[51],[185],[206],[269].

A recent study by Karkarala *et al.* has demonstrated the potent inhibitory effect of curcumin and piperine on Wnt/β-catenin signaling in primary human breast epithelial cells [419]. In this study, inhibition of Wnt signaling pathway was shown to affect breast stem cell renewal by inhibiting the mammosphere formation. According to the authors, curcumin and piperine (separately and in combination) inhibited breast stem cell self-renewal; however toxicity to differentiated cells was not reported. The plasma concentration of curcumin in people taking high oral doses has been shown to be very low due to many reasons such as metabolism of the compound in the intestine and the liver, as reviewed by Burgos-Moron *et al.* [420].

The lack of bioavailability of curcumin was known as a potential disadvantage for years and various strategies have been investigated to overcome the problem. One such strategy has been the use of piperine in combination of curcumin. Accordingly, concomitant administration of piperine and curcumin tends to increase the bioavailability (up to 2000%) compared to administration of curcumin alone in an experimental group of people [421]. This finding could well be a possibility as piperine has been shown to inhibit P-glycoproteins and CYP3A4 expressed in enterocytes where the bioavailability of many orally ingested compounds are determined [422]. Alternatively, increasing the solubility of curcumin by heat as means of increasing the bio availability has been suggested [423]. This method is easily achievable and a well-cooked curry with tumeric and piperine could be a tasty way of obtaining the goodness of these natural compounds.

Based on the ability of curcumin and piperine to inhibit CSC's as described above, curcumin has great potential as a possible therapeutic agent against breast cancer. The majority of the breast cancer patients have tumors that respond to the naturally occurring hormone, estrogen. Therefore, most of the currently available drugs known to be effective against breast cancer can prevent the action of estrogen and are thus referred to as selective estrogen receptor modulators (SERM). Unfortunately, there is a cohort of patients whose tumours do not express estrogen receptor. SERMs are of no use for this group with ER -ve breast cancers. The potential of curcumin and piperine to suppress the self-renewal of stem cells could prove beneficial in ER +ve as well as ER -ve breast cancer patients.

10. Summary

Considering the existence of CSC's in breast cancer, and the inability of current therapeutic approaches to destroy such, we propose targeting CSC's as a tool to investigate the effect of natural dietary compounds. Specifically, we suggest isolates of soy and turmeric, and their effects on breast cancer tumors and metastasis reoccurrence in breast cancer. Similar to other developmental agents aimed at cancer signaling pathways, the optimal dosing, dosing regimens and adverse effects will have to be refined. However, these prospects are notably different than conventional therapeutics in several ways and such should be contemplated upon exploring such molecules. For example, consider the complex cross-talk of both inter- and intra-cell signaling pathways and how feedback mechanism effects may eliminate inhibitors via the actions of a single pathway. Figure 2 summarizes targeted areas of interruption via the major pathways involved in stem cell renewal as well as those pathways that may be responsible for downstream signaling to these major pathways. Additionally, if CSC's are primary targets, then metastasis incidence and/or cancer free survival may be a more appropriate efficacy endpoint in clinical trials than tumor volume. Perhaps then it would be more strategic in breast cancer to design preclinical trials based on incorporating combination regimens at the early stages of drug development while targeting multiple pathways and focusing on appropriate endpoints; all to avoid missing potentially important therapeutic benefits. While plant based derivatives, such as those considered in this chapter hold promise in breast cancer treatment and management, their development should be pursued systematically, guided by sound scientific principles.

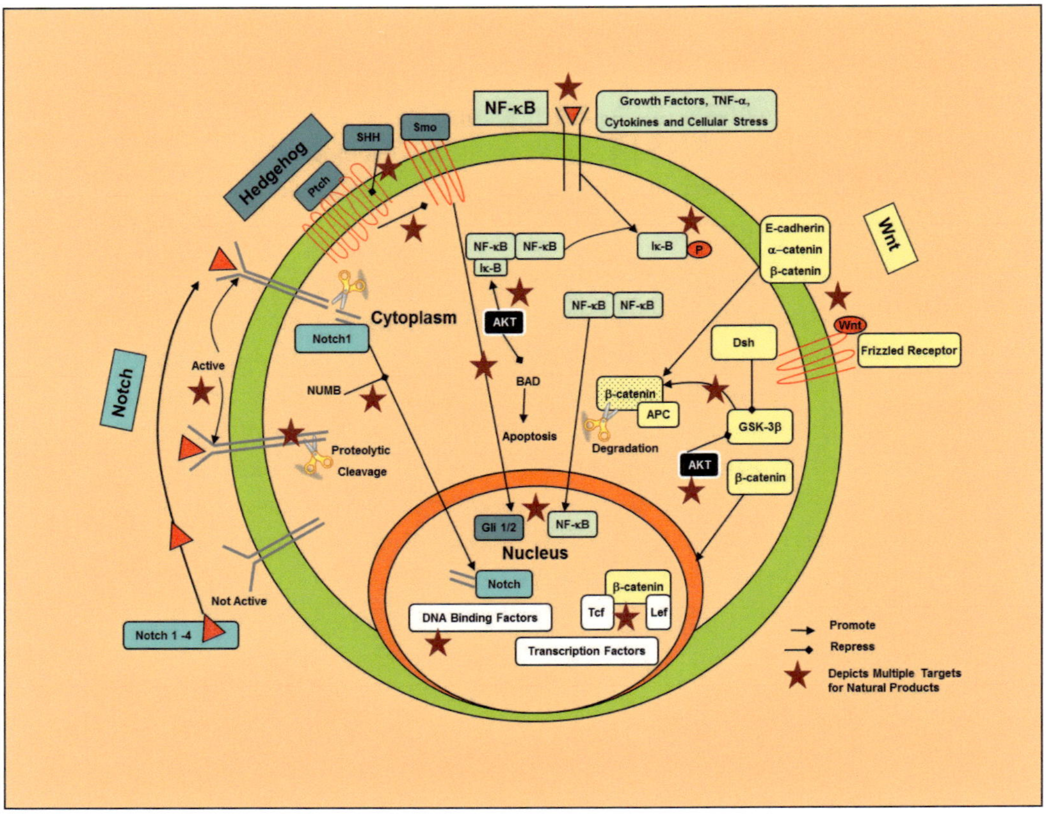

Figure 2. (Tobin, GA, 2012) An Overview of the Major Signaling Networks Involved in Breast Cancer and CSC Self-renewal, including Notch, NFκB, Wnt and Hh. Symbols and acronyms have been discussed previously, with the exception of P = phosphorylation, BAD = Bcl-2-associated death promoter, and SHH = Sonic Hh. Also, NUMB references the Protein numb homolog that in humans is encoded by the NUMB gene.

Acknowledgements

We would like to acknowledge funding and support from: 1. Canadian Institutes for Health Research (CIHR). 2. Innovation PEI and the Department of Innovation and Advanced Learning, PEI, Canada. 3. Canadian Breast Cancer Foundation (CBCF). 4. Beatrice Hunter Cancer Research Institute, Halifax, Nova Scotia, Canada. 5. Department of Biomedical Sciences, Atlantic Veterinary College, UPEI, PEI, Canada. 6. National Research Council (NRC) Institute for Nutrisciences and Health, Charlottetown, PEI, Canada. We are grateful for funds from the Thunder Cove Breast Cancer Award to cover publication costs related to this chapter. We would like to recognize the involvement of Mr. Mike Thomas (mikethomasgraphicdesign.com) in finalizing Figure 1. Last, but certainly not least, we would like to thank Drs. Robert Hurta and Shelia Drover for their comments and suggestions.

http://dx.doi.org/10.5772/55794

Author details

Gailene Tobin[1], Ruwani Kalupahana[2] and Marianna Kulka[1,3*]

*Address all correspondence to: Marianna.Kulka@nrc-cnrc.gc.ca

1 Department of Biomedical Sciences. University of Prince Edward Island, Charlottetown, PE, Canada

2 Department of Veterinary Public Health and Pharmacology, Faculty of Veterinary Medicine and Animal Science, University of Peradeniya, Peradeniya, Sri Lanka

3 Security and Disruptive Technologies, Technologies de Sécurité et de Rupture, National Institute of Nanotechnology, National Research Council Canada, Conseil national de Recherches, Edmonton, AB, Canada

References

[1] Coughlin SS, Ekwueme DU. Breast cancer as a global health concern. Cancer Epidemiol. 2009 Nov;33(5):315-8. PubMed PMID: 19896917.

[2] Canadian Cancer Statistics. 2012. Available at: http://www.cancer.ca/en/cancer-information/cancer-101/cancer-statistics-at-a-glance/?region=on

[3] McClure C. Prince Edward Island Cancer Trends: 1980 - 2009. 2012 August. Document Publishing Center, Charlottetown, Prince Edward Island.

[4] National Cancer Institute. SEER. Cancer Survival Statistics. 2009.

[5] Weigelt B, Peterse JL, van 't Veer LJ. Breast cancer metastasis: markers and models. Nat Rev Cancer. 2005 Aug;5(8):591-602. PubMed PMID: 16056258.

[6] Zhu S, Lee DA, Li S. IL-12 and IL-27 sequential gene therapy via intramuscular electroporation delivery for eliminating distal aggressive tumors. J Immunol. 2010 Mar 1;184(5):2348-54. PubMed PMID: 20139275.

[7] Hanahan D, Weinberg RA. The hallmarks of cancer. Cell. 2000 Jan 7;100(1):57-70. PubMed PMID: 10647931.

[8] Pecorino L. Molecular Biology of Cancer. Mechanisms, Targets and Therapeutics. 2008 (Second Edition).

[9] Merck Manual. Professiional Edition. Ch. 253, Breast Cancer. Website: http://www.merckmanuals.com/professional/gynecology_and_obstetrics/breast_disorders/breast_cancer.html

[10] Porter RS, Justin L. Breast Cancer Merck Manual Professional Editional. 2010;Ch. 253.

[11] Vernig B. Ductal carcinoma in situ of the breast: a systematic review of incidence, treatment and outcomes. Journal of the National Cancer Institute. 2010;102(3):170-8.

[12] Sobin LH Wittekind GM. TNM Classification of Malignant Tumors. 2009;7th ed:310 pages.

[13] Giuliano AE, Hunt KK, Ballman KV, Beitsch PD, Whitworth PW, Blumencranz PW, et al. Axillary dissection vs no axillary dissection in women with invasive breast cancer and sentinel node metastasis: a randomized clinical trial. JAMA. 2011 Feb 9;305(6):569-75. PubMed PMID: 21304082.

[14] Marrazzo A, Taormina P, Gebbiab V, David M, Riili I, Lo Gerfo D, et al. Is sentinel lymph node biopsy more accurate than axillary dissection for staging nodal involvement in breast cancer patients? Chir Ital. 2007 Sep-Oct;59(5):693-9. PubMed PMID: 18019642.

[15] Perou CM, Borresen-Dale AL. Systems biology and genomics of breast cancer. Cold Spring Harbor perspectives in biology. 2011 Feb;3(2). PubMed PMID: 21047916.

[16] Perou CM, Jeffrey SS, van de Rijn M, Rees CA, Eisen MB, Ross DT, et al. Distinctive gene expression patterns in human mammary epithelial cells and breast cancers. Proc Natl Acad Sci U S A. 1999 Aug 3;96(16):9212-7. PubMed PMID: 10430922.

[17] Perou CM, Parker JS, Prat A, Ellis MJ, Bernard PS. Clinical implementation of the intrinsic subtypes of breast cancer. Lancet Oncol. 2010 Aug;11(8):718-9; 20-1. PubMed PMID: 20688274.

[18] Perou CM. Molecular stratification of triple-negative breast cancers. The oncologist. 2011;16 Suppl 1:61-70. PubMed PMID: 21278442.

[19] Sotiriou C, Pusztai L. Gene-expression signatures in breast cancer. N Engl J Med. 2009 Feb 19;360(8):790-800. PubMed PMID: 19228622.

[20] Prat A, Perou CM. Deconstructing the molecular portraits of breast cancer. Mol Oncol. 2011 Feb;5(1):5-23. PubMed PMID: 21147047.

[21] Ross JS. Multigene classifiers, prognostic factors, and predictors of breast cancer clinical outcome. Adv Anat Pathol. 2009 Jul;16(4):204-15. PubMed PMID: 19546609.

[22] Herschkowitz JI, He X, Fan C, Perou CM. The functional loss of the retinoblastoma tumour suppressor is a common event in basal-like and luminal B breast carcinomas. Breast Cancer Res. 2008;10(5):R75. PubMed PMID: 18782450.

[23] Perou CM, Sorlie T, Eisen MB, van de Rijn M, Jeffrey SS, Rees CA, et al. Molecular portraits of human breast tumours. Nature. 2000 Aug 17;406(6797):747-52. PubMed PMID: 10963602.

[24] Perou CM. Molecular stratification of triple-negative breast cancers. The Oncologist. 2010;15 Suppl 5:39-48. PubMed PMID: 21138954.

[25] Peppercorn J, Perou CM, Carey LA. Molecular subtypes in breast cancer evaluation and management: divide and conquer. Cancer Invest. 2008 Feb;26(1):1-10. PubMed PMID: 18181038.

[26] Hu X, Stern HM, Ge L, O'Brien C, Haydu L, Honchell CD, et al. Genetic alterations and oncogenic pathways associated with breast cancer subtypes. Mol Cancer Res. 2009 Apr;7(4):511-22. PubMed PMID: 19372580.

[27] Bild AH, Parker JS, Gustafson AM, Acharya CR, Hoadley KA, Anders C, et al. An integration of complementary strategies for gene-expression analysis to reveal novel therapeutic opportunities for breast cancer. Breast Cancer Res. 2009;11(4):R55. PubMed PMID: 19638211.

[28] Hugh J, Hanson J, Cheang MC, Nielsen TO, Perou CM, Dumontet C, et al. Breast cancer subtypes and response to docetaxel in node-positive breast cancer: use of an immunohistochemical definition in the BCIRG 001 trial. J Clin Oncol. 2009 Mar 10;27(8): 1168-76. PubMed PMID: 19204205.

[29] Kwan ML, Kushi LH, Weltzien E, Maring B, Kutner SE, Fulton RS, et al. Epidemiology of breast cancer subtypes in two prospective cohort studies of breast cancer survivors. Breast Cancer Res. 2009;11(3):R31. PubMed PMID: 19463150.

[30] Myal Y, Leygue E, Blanchard AA. Claudin 1 in breast tumorigenesis: revelation of a possible novel "claudin high" subset of breast cancers. J Biomed Biotechnol. 2010;2010:956897. PubMed PMID: 20490282.

[31] Vargo-Gogola T, Rosen JM. Modelling breast cancer: one size does not fit all. Nat Rev Cancer. 2007 Sep;7(9):659-72. PubMed PMID: 17721431.

[32] Nicholson RI, Johnston SR. Endocrine therapy--current benefits and limitations. Breast Cancer Res Treat. 2005;93 Suppl 1:S3-10. PubMed PMID: 16247594.

[33] Rakha EA, Elsheikh SE, Aleskandarany MA, Habashi HO, Green AR, Powe DG, et al. Triple-negative breast cancer: distinguishing between basal and nonbasal subtypes. Clin Cancer Res. 2009 Apr 1;15(7):2302-10. PubMed PMID: 19318481.

[34] Herschkowitz JI, Simin K, Weigman VJ, Mikaelian I, Usary J, Hu Z, et al. Identification of conserved gene expression features between murine mammary carcinoma models and human breast tumors. Genome Biol. 2007;8(5):R76. PubMed PMID: 17493263.

[35] MacFarlane R SC, Masoudi H, Chia S. . Molecular changes in the primary breast cancer versus the relapsed/metastatic lesion from a large population based database and tissue microarray series. J Clin Oncol. 2008.;26(15S):1000.

[36] Ravdin PM, Siminoff LA, Davis GJ, Mercer MB, Hewlett J, Gerson N, et al. Computer program to assist in making decisions about adjuvant therapy for women with early breast cancer. J Clin Oncol. 2001 Feb 15;19(4):980-91. PubMed PMID: 11181660.

[37] Olivotto IA, Bajdik CD, Ravdin PM, Speers CH, Coldman AJ, Norris BD, et al. Population-based validation of the prognostic model ADJUVANT! for early breast cancer. J Clin Oncol. 2005 Apr 20;23(12):2716-25. PubMed PMID: 15837986.

[38] Silverstein MJ, Craig PH, Lagios MD, Waisman JK, Lewinsky BS, Colburn WJ, et al. Developing a prognostic index for ductal carcinoma in situ of the breast. Are we there yet? Cancer. 1996 Sep 1;78(5):1138-40. PubMed PMID: 8780555.

[39] Silverstein MJ, Lagios MD, Craig PH, Waisman JR, Lewinsky BS, Colburn WJ, et al. A prognostic index for ductal carcinoma in situ of the breast. Cancer. 1996 Jun 1;77(11):2267-74. PubMed PMID: 8635094.

[40] Dawson SJ, Makretsov N, Blows FM, Driver KE, Provenzano E, Le Quesne J, et al. BCL2 in breast cancer: a favourable prognostic marker across molecular subtypes and independent of adjuvant therapy received. Br J Cancer. Aug 24;103(5):668-75. PubMed PMID: 20664598.

[41] Urruticoechea A, Smith IE, Dowsett M. Proliferation marker Ki-67 in early breast cancer. J Clin Oncol. 2005 Oct 1;23(28):7212-20. PubMed PMID: 16192605.

[42] Hofseth LJ, Raafat AM, Osuch JR, Pathak DR, Slomski CA, Haslam SZ. Hormone replacement therapy with estrogen or estrogen plus medroxyprogesterone acetate is associated with increased epithelial proliferation in the normal postmenopausal breast. J Clin Endocrinol Metab. 1999 Dec;84(12):4559-65. PubMed PMID: 10599719.

[43] Scholzen T, Gerdes J. The Ki-67 protein: from the known and the unknown. J Cell Physiol. 2000 Mar;182(3):311-22. PubMed PMID: 10653597.

[44] Dowsett M, Smith IE, Ebbs SR, Dixon JM, Skene A, A'Hern R, et al. Prognostic value of Ki67 expression after short-term presurgical endocrine therapy for primary breast cancer. J Natl Cancer Inst. 2007 Jan 17;99(2):167-70. PubMed PMID: 17228000.

[45] Ponti D, Costa A, Zaffaroni N, Pratesi G, Petrangolini G, Coradini D, et al. Isolation and *in vitro* propagation of tumorigenic breast cancer cells with stem/progenitor cell properties. Cancer Res. 2005 Jul 1;65(13):5506-11. PubMed PMID: 15994920.

[46] Polyak K. Breast cancer stem cells: a case of mistaken identity? Stem Cell Rev. 2007 Jun;3(2):107-9. PubMed PMID: 17873341.

[47] Polyak K. Breast cancer: origins and evolution. J Clin Invest. 2007 Nov;117(11):3155-63. PubMed PMID: 17975657.

[48] Simpson PT, Reis-Filho JS, Gale T, Lakhani SR. Molecular evolution of breast cancer. J Pathol. 2005 Jan;205(2):248-54. PubMed PMID: 15641021.

[49] Pardal R, Clarke MF, Morrison SJ. Applying the principles of stem-cell biology to cancer. Nat Rev Cancer. 2003 Dec;3(12):895-902. PubMed PMID: 14737120.

[50] Al-Hajj M, Wicha MS, Benito-Hernandez A, Morrison SJ, Clarke MF. Prospective identification of tumorigenic breast cancer cells. Proc Natl Acad Sci U S A. 2003 Apr 1;100(7):3983-8. PubMed PMID: 12629218.

[51] Liu S, Dontu G, Mantle ID, Patel S, Ahn NS, Jackson KW, et al. Hedgehog signaling and Bmi-1 regulate self-renewal of normal and malignant human mammary stem cells. Cancer Res. 2006 Jun 15;66(12):6063-71. PubMed PMID: 16778178.

[52] Ginestier C, Hur MH, Charafe-Jauffret E, Monville F, Dutcher J, Brown M, et al. ALDH1 is a marker of normal and malignant human mammary stem cells and a predictor of poor clinical outcome. Cell stem cell. 2007 Nov;1(5):555-67. PubMed PMID: 18371393.

[53] Charafe-Jauffret E, Ginestier C, Iovino F, Wicinski J, Cervera N, Finetti P, et al. Breast cancer cell lines contain functional cancer stem cells with metastatic capacity and a distinct molecular signature. Cancer Res. 2009 Feb 15;69(4):1302-13. PubMed PMID: 19190339. Pubmed Central PMCID: 2819227.

[54] Mani SA, Guo W, Liao MJ, Eaton EN, Ayyanan A, Zhou AY, et al. The epithelial-mesenchymal transition generates cells with properties of stem cells. Cell. 2008 May 16;133(4):704-15. PubMed PMID: 18485877. Pubmed Central PMCID: 2728032.

[55] Bonnet D, Dick JE. Human acute myeloid leukemia is organized as a hierarchy that originates from a primitive hematopoietic cell. Nat Med. 1997 Jul;3(7):730-7. PubMed PMID: 9212098.

[56] Singh SM, Murphy B, O'Reilly RL. Involvement of gene-diet/drug interaction in DNA methylation and its contribution to complex diseases: from cancer to schizophrenia. Clin Genet. 2003 Dec;64(6):451-60. PubMed PMID: 14986824.

[57] Yang DG, Liu L, Zheng XY. Cyclin-dependent kinase inhibitor p16(INK4a) and telomerase may co-modulate endothelial progenitor cells senescence. Ageing Res Rev. 2008 Apr;7(2):137-46. PubMed PMID: 18343732.

[58] Yang W, Lam P, Kitching R, Kahn HJ, Yee A, Aubin JE, et al. Breast cancer metastasis in a human bone NOD/SCID mouse model. Cancer Biol Ther. 2007 Aug;6(8):1289-94. PubMed PMID: 17704641.

[59] Hambardzumyan D, Squatrito M, Holland EC. Radiation resistance and stem-like cells in brain tumors. Cancer Cell. 2006 Dec;10(6):454-6. PubMed PMID: 17157785.

[60] Korkaya H, Paulson A, Charafe-Jauffret E, Ginestier C, Brown M, Dutcher J, et al. Regulation of mammary stem/progenitor cells by PTEN/Akt/beta-catenin signaling. PLoS Biol. 2009 Jun 2;7(6):e1000121. PubMed PMID: 19492080.

[61] Reya T, Morrison SJ, Clarke MF, Weissman IL. Stem cells, cancer, and cancer stem cells. Nature. 2001 Nov 1;414(6859):105-11. PubMed PMID: 11689955.

[62] Shafee N, Smith CR, Wei S, Kim Y, Mills GB, Hortobagyi GN, et al. Cancer stem cells contribute to cisplatin resistance in Brca1/p53-mediated mouse mammary tumors. Cancer Res. 2008 May 1;68(9):3243-50. PubMed PMID: 18451150.

[63] Zhou BB, Zhang H, Damelin M, Geles KG, Grindley JC, Dirks PB. Tumour-initiating cells: challenges and opportunities for anticancer drug discovery. Nat Rev Drug Discov. 2009 Oct;8(10):806-23. PubMed PMID: 19794444.

[64] Bapat SA. Evolution of cancer stem cells. Semin Cancer Biol. 2007 Jun;17(3):204-13. PubMed PMID: 16787749.

[65] Han JS, Crowe DL. Tumor initiating cancer stem cells from human breast cancer cell lines. Int J Oncol. 2009 May;34(5):1449-53. PubMed PMID: 19360358.

[66] Miller SJ, Lavker RM, Sun TT. Interpreting epithelial cancer biology in the context of stem cells: tumor properties and therapeutic implications. Biochim Biophys Acta. 2005 Sep 25;1756(1):25-52. PubMed PMID: 16139432.

[67] Allred DC, Wu Y, Mao S, Nagtegaal ID, Lee S, Perou CM, et al. Ductal carcinoma in situ and the emergence of diversity during breast cancer evolution. Clin Cancer Res. 2008 Jan 15;14(2):370-8. PubMed PMID: 18223211.

[68] Hu M, Yao J, Carroll DK, Weremowicz S, Chen H, Carrasco D, et al. Regulation of in situ to invasive breast carcinoma transition. Cancer Cell. 2008 May;13(5):394-406. PubMed PMID: 18455123.

[69] Klein CA. Cancer. The metastasis cascade. Science. 2008 Sep 26;321(5897):1785-7. PubMed PMID: 18818347.

[70] Husemann Y, Geigl JB, Schubert F, Musiani P, Meyer M, Burghart E, et al. Systemic spread is an early step in breast cancer. Cancer Cell. 2008 Jan;13(1):58-68. PubMed PMID: 18167340.

[71] Ansieau S, Hinkal G, Thomas C, Bastid J, Puisieux A. Early origin of cancer metastases: dissemination and evolution of premalignant cells. Cell cycle. 2008 Dec;7(23): 3659-63. PubMed PMID: 19029812.

[72] Podsypanina K, Du YC, Jechlinger M, Beverly LJ, Hambardzumyan D, Varmus H. Seeding and propagation of untransformed mouse mammary cells in the lung. Science. 2008 Sep 26;321(5897):1841-4. PubMed PMID: 18755941.

[73] Kim MY, Oskarsson T, Acharyya S, Nguyen DX, Zhang XH, Norton L, et al. Tumor self-seeding by circulating cancer cells. Cell. 2009 Dec 24;139(7):1315-26. PubMed PMID: 20064377.

[74] Carroll J. Breast cancer breakthrough spotlights sequencing impact. Fierce Biotech Research. 2009.

[75] Ahmed M, Lalloo F, Evans DG. Update on genetic predisposition to breast cancer. Expert Rev Anticancer Ther. 2009 Aug;9(8):1103-13. PubMed PMID: 19671030.

[76] Lynch HT, Marcus JN, Rubinstein WS. Stemming the tide of cancer for BRCA1/2 mutation carriers. J Clin Oncol. 2008 Sep 10;26(26):4239-43. PubMed PMID: 18779610.

[77] Thompson ME. BRCA1 16 years later: an overview. 2010 Aug;277(15):3071. PubMed PMID: 20608973.

[78] Walsh T, Casadei S, Coats KH, Swisher E, Stray SM, Higgins J, et al. Spectrum of mutations in BRCA1, BRCA2, CHEK2, and TP53 in families at high risk of breast cancer. Jama. 2006 Mar 22;295(12):1379-88. PubMed PMID: 16551709.

[79] Campeau PM, Foulkes WD, Tischkowitz MD. Hereditary breast cancer: new genetic developments, new therapeutic avenues. Hum Genet. 2008 Aug;124(1):31-42. PubMed PMID: 18575892.

[80] Hashizume T, Fukuda T, Nagaoka T, Tada H, Yamada H, Watanabe K, et al. Cell type dependent endocytic internalization of ErbB2 with an artificial peptide ligand that binds to ErbB2. Cell Biol Int. 2008 Jul;32(7):814-26. PubMed PMID: 18442934.

[81] Kinzler KW, Vogelstein B. Cancer-susceptibility genes. Gatekeepers and caretakers. Nature. 1997 Apr 24;386(6627):761, 3. PubMed PMID: 9126728.

[82] Hall J, Montesano R. DNA alkylation damage: consequences and relevance to tumour production. Mutat Res. 1990 Nov-Dec;233(1-2):247-52. PubMed PMID: 2233806.

[83] Hall JG. Genomic imprinting: review and relevance to human diseases. Am J Hum Genet. 1990 May;46(5):857-73. PubMed PMID: 2187341.

[84] Rosnoblet C, Vischer UM, Gerard RD, Irminger JC, Halban PA, Kruithof EK. Storage of tissue-type plasminogen activator in Weibel-Palade bodies of human endothelial cells. Arterioscler Thromb Vasc Biol. 1999 Jul;19(7):1796-803. PubMed PMID: 10397700.

[85] Miki Y, Swensen J, Shattuck-Eidens D, Futreal PA, Harshman K, Tavtigian S, et al. A strong candidate for the breast and ovarian cancer susceptibility gene BRCA1. Science. 1994 Oct 7;266(5182):66-71. PubMed PMID: 7545954.

[86] Starita LM, Parvin JD. The multiple nuclear functions of BRCA1: transcription, ubiquitination and DNA repair. Curr Opin Cell Biol. 2003 Jun;15(3):345-50. PubMed PMID: 12787778.

[87] Duncan JA, Reeves JR, Cooke TG. BRCA1 and BRCA2 proteins: roles in health and disease. Mol Pathol. 1998 Oct;51(5):237-47. PubMed PMID: 10193517.

[88] Yoshida K, Toge T. [Telomerase activity in gastrointestinal, bladder and breast carcinomas and their clinical applications]. Nihon Rinsho. 2004 Jul;62(7):1368-76. PubMed PMID: 15283158.

[89] Rotman G, Shiloh Y. ATM: from gene to function. Hum Mol Genet. 1998;7(10): 1555-63. PubMed PMID: 9735376.

[90] Thompson D, Antoniou AC, Jenkins M, Marsh A, Chen X, Wayne T, et al. Two ATM variants and breast cancer risk. Hum Mutat. 2005 Jun;25(6):594-5. PubMed PMID: 15880680.

[91] Antoniou AC, Easton DF. Models of genetic susceptibility to breast cancer. Oncogene. 2006 Sep 25;25(43):5898-905. PubMed PMID: 16998504.

[92] Hoekstra MF. Responses to DNA damage and regulation of cell cycle checkpoints by the ATM protein kinase family. Curr Opin Genet Dev. 1997 Apr;7(2):170-5. PubMed PMID: 9115420.

[93] Xu Y, Baltimore D. Dual roles of ATM in the cellular response to radiation and in cell growth control. Genes Dev. 1996 Oct 1;10(19):2401-10. PubMed PMID: 8843193.

[94] Birch JM, Hartley AL, Tricker KJ, Prosser J, Condie A, Kelsey AM, et al. Prevalence and diversity of constitutional mutations in the p53 gene among 21 Li-Fraumeni families. Cancer Res. 1994 Mar 1;54(5):1298-304. PubMed PMID: 8118819.

[95] Li FP, Correa P, Fraumeni JF, Jr. Testing for germ line p53 mutations in cancer families. Cancer Epidemiol Biomarkers Prev. 1991 Nov-Dec;1(1):91-4. PubMed PMID: 1845175.

[96] Malkin D, Li FP, Strong LC, Fraumeni JF, Jr., Nelson CE, Kim DH, et al. Germ line p53 mutations in a familial syndrome of breast cancer, sarcomas, and other neoplasms. Science. 1990 Nov 30;250(4985):1233-8. PubMed PMID: 1978757.

[97] Hirao A, Kong YY, Matsuoka S, Wakeham A, Ruland J, Yoshida H, et al. DNA damage-induced activation of p53 by the checkpoint kinase Chk2. Science. 2000 Mar 10;287(5459):1824-7. PubMed PMID: 10710310.

[98] Lee JM, Lee YC, Yang SY, Shi WL, Lee CJ, Luh SP, et al. Genetic polymorphisms of p53 and GSTP1,but not NAT2,are associated with susceptibility to squamous-cell carcinoma of the esophagus. Int J Cancer. 2000 Sep 20;89(5):458-64. PubMed PMID: 11008209.

[99] Matsuoka S, Huang M, Elledge SJ. Linkage of ATM to cell cycle regulation by the Chk2 protein kinase. Science. 1998 Dec 4;282(5395):1893-7. PubMed PMID: 9836640.

[100] Chu EC, Tarnawski AS. PTEN regulatory functions in tumor suppression and cell biology. Med Sci Monit. 2004 Oct;10(10):RA235-41. PubMed PMID: 15448614.

[101] Steck PA, Pershouse MA, Jasser SA, Yung WK, Lin H, Ligon AH, et al. Identification of a candidate tumour suppressor gene, MMAC1, at chromosome 10q23.3 that is mutated in multiple advanced cancers. Nat Genet. 1997 Apr;15(4):356-62. PubMed PMID: 9090379.

[102] Huntsman DG, Chin SF, Muleris M, Batley SJ, Collins VP, Wiedemann LM, et al. MLL2, the second human homolog of the Drosophila trithorax gene, maps to 19q13.1

and is amplified in solid tumor cell lines. Oncogene. 1999 Dec 23;18(56):7975-84. PubMed PMID: 10637508.

[103] Semb H, Christofori G. The tumor-suppressor function of E-cadherin. Am J Hum Genet. 1998 Dec;63(6):1588-93. PubMed PMID: 9837810.

[104] Wong AS, Gumbiner BM. Adhesion-independent mechanism for suppression of tumor cell invasion by E-cadherin. J Cell Biol. 2003 Jun 23;161(6):1191-203. PubMed PMID: 12810698.

[105] Desmedt C, Haibe-Kains B, Wirapati P, Buyse M, Larsimont D, Bontempi G, et al. Biological processes associated with breast cancer clinical outcome depend on the molecular subtypes. Clin Cancer Res. 2008 Aug 15;14(16):5158-65. PubMed PMID: 18698033.

[106] Lange CA. Challenges to defining a role for progesterone in breast cancer. Steroids. 2008 Oct;73(9-10):914-21. PubMed PMID: 18243264.

[107] Lange CA, Richer JK, Horwitz KB. Hypothesis: Progesterone primes breast cancer cells for cross-talk with proliferative or antiproliferative signals. Mol Endocrinol. 1999 Jun;13(6):829-36. PubMed PMID: 10379882.

[108] Fang H, Tong W, Shi LM, Blair R, Perkins R, Branham W, et al. Structure-activity relationships for a large diverse set of natural, synthetic, and environmental estrogens. Chem Res Toxicol. 2001 Mar;14(3):280-94. PubMed PMID: 11258977.

[109] Lin C-Y, SO. Discovery of estrogen receptor alpha target genes and response elements in breast tumor cells. Genome Biol. 2004 5(9):R66(PMID- 15345050).

[110] Dowsett M, Houghton J, Iden C, Salter J, Farndon J, A'Hern R, et al. Benefit from adjuvant tamoxifen therapy in primary breast cancer patients according oestrogen receptor, progesterone receptor, EGF receptor and HER2 status. Ann Oncol. 2006 May; 17(5):818-26. PubMed PMID: 16497822.

[111] Miller K. Choices in Breast Cancer Treatment. 2008. ISBN-10: 0801886848 ISBN-13: 978-0801886843.

[112] Lupulescu A. Estrogen use and cancer incidence: a review. Cancer Invest. 1995;13(3): 287-95. PubMed PMID: 7743382.

[113] Cummings SR, Duong T, Kenyon E, Cauley JA, Whitehead M, Krueger KA. Serum estradiol level and risk of breast cancer during treatment with raloxifene. Jama. 2002 Jan 9;287(2):216-20. PubMed PMID: 11779264.

[114] Panico S, Pisani P, Muti P, Recchione C, Cavalleri A, Totis A, et al. Diurnal variation of testosterone and estradiol: a source of bias in comparative studies on breast cancer. J Endocrinol Invest. 1990 May;13(5):423-6. PubMed PMID: 2380505.

[115] Tesarik J, Garrigosa L, Mendoza C. Estradiol modulates breast cancer cell apoptosis: a novel nongenomic steroid action relevant to carcinogenesis. Steroids. 1999 Jan-Feb; 64(1-2):22-7. PubMed PMID: 10323669.

[116] Ahmed MI, Lennard TW. Breast cancer: role of neoadjuvant therapy. Int J Surg. 2009 Oct;7(5):416-20. PubMed PMID: 19524705.

[117] Weber BL, Nathanson KL. Low penetrance genes associated with increased risk for breast cancer. Eur J Cancer. 2000 Jun;36(10):1193-9. PubMed PMID: 10882856.

[118] Kurzer MS. Hormonal effects of soy in premenopausal women and men. J Nutr. 2002 Mar;132(3):570S-3S. PubMed PMID: 11880595.

[119] Lasfargues EY OL. Cultivation of human breast carcinomas. J Natl Cancer Inst. 1958; 21:1131-47.

[120] Lacroix M, Leclercq G. Relevance of breast cancer cell lines as models for breast tumours: an update. Breast Cancer Res Treat. 2004 Feb;83(3):249-89. PubMed PMID: 14758095.

[121] Fillmore C, Kuperwasser C. Human breast cancer stem cell markers CD44 and CD24: enriching for cells with functional properties in mice or in man? Breast Cancer Res. 2007;9(3):303. PubMed PMID: 17540049.

[122] Kuperwasser C, Chavarria T, Wu M, Magrane G, Gray JW, Carey L, et al. Reconstruction of functionally normal and malignant human breast tissues in mice. Proc Natl Acad Sci U S A. 2004 Apr 6;101(14):4966-71. PubMed PMID: 15051869.

[123] Radisky DC, Bissell MJ. Cancer. Respect thy neighbor! Science. 2004 Feb 6;303(5659): 775-7. PubMed PMID: 14764858.

[124] Dontu G, Al-Hajj M, Abdallah WM, Clarke MF, Wicha MS. Stem cells in normal breast development and breast cancer. Cell Prolif. 2003 Oct;36 Suppl 1:59-72. PubMed PMID: 14521516.

[125] Rae JM, Ramus SJ, Waltham M, Armes JE, Campbell IG, Clarke R, et al. Common origins of MDA-MB-435 cells from various sources with those shown to have melanoma properties. Clinical & experimental metastasis. 2004;21(6):543-52. PubMed PMID: 15679052.

[126] Rae JM, Creighton CJ, Meck JM, Haddad BR, Johnson MD. MDA-MB-435 cells are derived from M14 melanoma cells--a loss for breast cancer, but a boon for melanoma research. Breast Cancer Res Treat. 2007 Jul;104(1):13-9. PubMed PMID: 17004106.

[127] Ellison G, Klinowska T, Westwood RF, Docter E, French T, Fox JC. Further evidence to support the melanocytic origin of MDA-MB-435. Mol Pathol. 2002 Oct;55(5):294-9. PubMed PMID: 12354931. Pubmed Central PMCID: 1187258.

[128] Christgen M, Lehmann U. MDA-MB-435: the questionable use of a melanoma cell line as a model for human breast cancer is ongoing. Cancer Biol Ther. 2007 Sep;6(9): 1355-7. PubMed PMID: 17786032.

[129] Neve RM, Chin K, Fridlyand J, Yeh J, Baehner FL, Fevr T, et al. A collection of breast cancer cell lines for the study of functionally distinct cancer subtypes. Cancer Cell. 2006 Dec;10(6):515-27. PubMed PMID: 17157791.

[130] Hollestelle A NJ, Smid M, Lam S, Elstrodt F, Wasielewski M, Ng SS, French PJ PJ, Rozendaal MJ, Riaz M, Koopman DG, Ten Hagen TL, de Leeuw BH ZE, Teunisse A, van der Spek PJ, Klijn JG, Dinjens WN, Ethier SP CH, Jochemsen AG, den Bakker MA, Foekens JA, Martens JW, M S. : Distinct gene mutation profi les among luminal-type and basaltype breast cancer cell lines. Breast Cancer Res Treat. 2010; 121:53-64.

[131] Koch M, Hussein F, Woeste A, Grundker C, Frontzek K, Emons G, et al. CD36-mediated activation of endothelial cell apoptosis by an N-terminal recombinant fragment of thrombospondin-2 inhibits breast cancer growth and metastasis *in vivo*. Breast Cancer Res Treat. 2011 Jul;128(2):337-46. PubMed PMID: 20714802. Pubmed Central PMCID: 3291836.

[132] Bachmeier B, Fichtner I, Killian PH, Kronski E, Pfeffer U, Efferth T. Development of resistance towards artesunate in MDA-MB-231 human breast cancer cells. PLoS One. 2011;6(5):e20550. PubMed PMID: 21637790. Pubmed Central PMCID: 3102747.

[133] Holliday DL, Speirs V. Choosing the right cell line for breast cancer research. Breast Cancer Res. 2011;13(4):215. PubMed PMID: 21884641. Pubmed Central PMCID: 3236329.

[134] Eccles SA, Welch DR. Metastasis: recent discoveries and novel treatment strategies. Lancet. 2007 May 19;369(9574):1742-57. PubMed PMID: 17512859.

[135] Vernon AE, Bakewell SJ, Chodosh LA. Deciphering the molecular basis of breast cancer metastasis with mouse models. Rev Endocr Metab Disord. 2007 Sep;8(3):199-213. PubMed PMID: 17657606.

[136] Kim IS, Baek SH. Mouse models for breast cancer metastasis. Biochem Biophys Res Commun. 2010 Apr 9;394(3):443-7. PubMed PMID: 20230796.

[137] Jonkers J, Derksen PW. Modeling metastatic breast cancer in mice. J Mammary Gland Biol Neoplasia. 2007 Sep;12(2-3):191-203. PubMed PMID: 17587153.

[138] Maglione JE, Moghanaki D, Young LJ, Manner CK, Ellies LG, Joseph SO, et al. Transgenic Polyoma middle-T mice model premalignant mammary disease. Cancer Res. 2001 Nov 15;61(22):8298-305. PubMed PMID: 11719463.

[139] Blackburn AC, Jerry DJ. Knockout and transgenic mice of Trp53: what have we learned about p53 in breast cancer? Breast Cancer Res. 2002;4(3):101-11. PubMed PMID: 12052252.

[140] Ye Y, Qiu TH, Kavanaugh C, Green JE. Molecular mechanisms of breast cancer progression: lessons from mouse mammary cancer models and gene expression profiling. Breast Dis. 2004;19:69-82. PubMed PMID: 15687699.

[141] Julien SG, Dube N, Read M, Penney J, Paquet M, Han Y, et al. Protein tyrosine phosphatase 1B deficiency or inhibition delays ErbB2-induced mammary tumorigenesis and protects from lung metastasis. Nat Genet. 2007 Mar;39(3):338-46. PubMed PMID: 17259984.

[142] Maroulakou IG, Oemler W, Naber SP, Tsichlis PN. Akt1 ablation inhibits, whereas Akt2 ablation accelerates, the development of mammary adenocarcinomas in mouse mammary tumor virus (MMTV)-ErbB2/neu and MMTV-polyoma middle T transgenic mice. Cancer Res. 2007 Jan 1;67(1):167-77. PubMed PMID: 17210696.

[143] DeNardo DG, Barreto JB, Andreu P, Vasquez L, Tawfik D, Kolhatkar N, et al. CD4(+) T cells regulate pulmonary metastasis of mammary carcinomas by enhancing protumor properties of macrophages. Cancer Cell. 2009 Aug 4;16(2):91-102. PubMed PMID: 19647220.

[144] Sharpless NE, Depinho RA. The mighty mouse: genetically engineered mouse models in cancer drug development. Nat Rev Drug Discov. 2006 Sep;5(9):741-54. PubMed PMID: 16915232.

[145] Lin SC, Lee KF, Nikitin AY, Hilsenbeck SG, Cardiff RD, Li A, et al. Somatic mutation of p53 leads to estrogen receptor alpha-positive and -negative mouse mammary tumors with high frequency of metastasis. Cancer Res. 2004 May 15;64(10):3525-32. PubMed PMID: 15150107.

[146] Fantozzi A, Christofori G. Mouse models of breast cancer metastasis. Breast Cancer Res. 2006;8(4):212. PubMed PMID: 16887003.

[147] Aslakson CJ, Miller FR. Selective events in the metastatic process defined by analysis of the sequential dissemination of subpopulations of a mouse mammary tumor. Cancer Res. 1992 Mar 15;52(6):1399-405. PubMed PMID: 1540948.

[148] Pulaski BA, Terman DS, Khan S, Muller E, Ostrand-Rosenberg S. Cooperativity of Staphylococcal aureus enterotoxin B superantigen, major histocompatibility complex class II, and CD80 for immunotherapy of advanced spontaneous metastases in a clinically relevant postoperative mouse breast cancer model. Cancer Res. 2000 May 15;60(10):2710-5. PubMed PMID: 10825145.

[149] Pulaski BA, Ostrand-Rosenberg S. Reduction of established spontaneous mammary carcinoma metastases following immunotherapy with major histocompatibility complex class II and B7.1 cell-based tumor vaccines. Cancer Res. 1998 Apr 1;58(7): 1486-93. PubMed PMID: 9537252.

[150] Yang J, Mani SA, Donaher JL, Ramaswamy S, Itzykson RA, Come C, et al. Twist, a master regulator of morphogenesis, plays an essential role in tumor metastasis. Cell. 2004 Jun 25;117(7):927-39. PubMed PMID: 15210113.

[151] Hurst J, Maniar N, Tombarkiewicz J, Lucas F, Roberson C, Steplewski Z, et al. A novel model of a metastatic human breast tumour xenograft line. Br J Cancer. 1993 Aug; 68(2):274-6. PubMed PMID: 8394103.

[152] Fogh J, Giovanella BC. The Nude Mouse in Experimental and Clinical Research. Academic Press; 1982.

[153] Schuler W, Bosma MJ. Nature of the scid defect: a defective VDJ recombinase system. Current topics in microbiology and immunology. 1989;152:55-62. PubMed PMID: 2805798.

[154] Dewan MZ, Terunuma H, Ahmed S, Ohba K, Takada M, Tanaka Y, et al. Natural killer cells in breast cancer cell growth and metastasis in SCID mice. Biomed Pharmacother. 2005 Oct;59 Suppl 2:S375-9. PubMed PMID: 16507413.

[155] Ottewell PD, Coleman RE, Holen I. From genetic abnormality to metastases: murine models of breast cancer and their use in the development of anticancer therapies. Breast Cancer Res Treat. 2006 Mar;96(2):101-13. PubMed PMID: 16319986.

[156] Lu X, Kang Y. Metalloproteinases and osteoblast EGFR signaling in osteolytic bone metastasis of breast cancer. Cell Cycle. 2009 Dec;8(23):3804-5. PubMed PMID: 19934661.

[157] Alonso DF, Farias EF, Urtreger A, Ladeda V, Vidal MC, Bal De Kier Joffe E. Characterization of F3II, a sarcomatoid mammary carcinoma cell line originated from a clonal subpopulation of a mouse adenocarcinoma. Journal of Surgical Oncology. 1996 Aug;62(4):288-97. PubMed PMID: 8691844.

[158] Alonso DF, Farina HG, Skilton G, Gabri MR, De Lorenzo MS, Gomez DE. Reduction of mouse mammary tumor formation and metastasis by lovastatin, an inhibitor of the mevalonate pathway of cholesterol synthesis. Breast Cancer Res Treat. 1998 Jul; 50(1):83-93. PubMed PMID: 9802623.

[159] Simstein R, Burow M, Parker A, Weldon C, Beckman B. Apoptosis, chemoresistance, and breast cancer: insights from the MCF-7 cell model system. Exp Biol Med (Maywood). 2003 Oct;228(9):995-1003. PubMed PMID: 14530507.

[160] Levenson AS, Jordan VC. MCF-7: the first hormone-responsive breast cancer cell line. Cancer Res. 1997 Aug 1;57(15):3071-8. PubMed PMID: 9242427.

[161] Soule HD, Vazguez J, Long A, Albert S, Brennan M. A human cell line from a pleural effusion derived from a breast carcinoma. J Natl Cancer Inst. 1973 Nov;51(5):1409-16. PubMed PMID: 4357757.

[162] Bos PD, Zhang XH, Nadal C, Shu W, Gomis RR, Nguyen DX, et al. Genes that mediate breast cancer metastasis to the brain. Nature. 2009 Jun 18;459(7249):1005-9. PubMed PMID: 19421193.

[163] Minn AJ, Gupta GP, Siegel PM, Bos PD, Shu W, Giri DD, et al. Genes that mediate breast cancer metastasis to lung. Nature. 2005 Jul 28;436(7050):518-24. PubMed PMID: 16049480.

[164] Qi Q, Gu H, Yang Y, Lu N, Zhao J, Liu W, et al. Involvement of matrix metalloproteinase 2 and 9 in gambogic acid induced suppression of MDA-MB-435 human breast carcinoma cell lung metastasis. J Mol Med. 2008 Dec;86(12):1367-77. PubMed PMID: 18777017.

[165] Charafe-Jauffret E, Ginestier C, Birnbaum D. Breast cancer stem cells: tools and models to rely on. BMC Cancer. 2009;9:202. PubMed PMID: 19555472.

[166] Elstrodt F, Hollestelle A, Nagel JH, Gorin M, Wasielewski M, van den Ouweland A, et al. BRCA1 mutation analysis of 41 human breast cancer cell lines reveals three new deleterious mutants. Cancer Res. 2006 Jan 1;66(1):41-5. PubMed PMID: 16397213.

[167] Kuperwasser C, Dessain S, Bierbaum BE, Garnet D, Sperandio K, Gauvin GP, et al. A mouse model of human breast cancer metastasis to human bone. Cancer Res. 2005 Jul 15;65(14):6130-8. PubMed PMID: 16024614.

[168] Sotoca AM, Gelpke MD, Boeren S, Strom A, Gustafsson JA, Murk AJ, et al. Quantitative proteomics and transcriptomics addressing the estrogen receptor subtype-mediated effects in T47D breast cancer cells exposed to the phytoestrogen genistein. Mol Cell Proteomics. 2010 Jan;10(1):M110 002170. PubMed PMID: 20884965.

[169] Baselga J, Norton L, Albanell J, Kim YM, Mendelsohn J. Recombinant humanized anti-HER2 antibody (Herceptin) enhances the antitumor activity of paclitaxel and doxorubicin against HER2/neu overexpressing human breast cancer xenografts. Cancer Res. 1998 Jul 1;58(13):2825-31. PubMed PMID: 9661897.

[170] Sporn JR, Bilgrami SA. Weekly paclitaxel plus Herceptin in metastatic breast cancer patients who relapse after stem-cell transplant. Ann Oncol. 1999 Oct;10(10):1259-60. PubMed PMID: 10586349.

[171] Davis AL, Klitus M, Mintzer DM. Chemotherapy-induced amenorrhea from adjuvant breast cancer treatment: the effect of the addition of taxanes. Clin Breast Cancer. 2005 Dec;6(5):421-4. PubMed PMID: 16381625.

[172] Semenza GL. A new weapon for attacking tumor blood vessels. N Engl J Med. 2008 May 8;358(19):2066-7. PubMed PMID: 18463385.

[173] Pollack A. FDA Rejects Use of Drugs in Breast Cancer. 2010; December 16. Available at: http://www.nytimes.com/2010/12/17/health/policy/17drug.html?_r=0

[174] Hurwitz H, Fehrenbacher L, Novotny W, Cartwright T, Hainsworth J, Heim W, et al. Bevacizumab plus irinotecan, fluorouracil, and leucovorin for metastatic colorectal cancer. N Engl J Med. 2004 Jun 3;350(23):2335-42. PubMed PMID: 15175435.

[175] Mateos MV, Hernandez JM, Hernandez MT, Gutierrez NC, Palomera L, Fuertes M, et al. Bortezomib plus melphalan and prednisone in elderly untreated patients with multiple myeloma: results of a multicenter phase 1/2 study. Blood. 2006 Oct 1;108(7): 2165-72. PubMed PMID: 16772605.

[176] Mitsiades N, Mitsiades CS, Richardson PG, Poulaki V, Tai YT, Chauhan D, et al. The proteasome inhibitor PS-341 potentiates sensitivity of multiple myeloma cells to conventional chemotherapeutic agents: therapeutic applications. Blood. 2003 Mar 15;101(6):2377-80. PubMed PMID: 12424198.

[177] Moreau P, Hulin C, Facon T. Frontline treatment of multiple myeloma in elderly patients. Blood Rev. 2008 Nov;22(6):303-9. PubMed PMID: 18550234.

[178] Yang JC, Haworth L, Sherry RM, Hwu P, Schwartzentruber DJ, Topalian SL, et al. A randomized trial of bevacizumab, an anti-vascular endothelial growth factor antibody, for metastatic renal cancer. N Engl J Med. 2003 Jul 31;349(5):427-34. PubMed PMID: 12890841.

[179] Kaplan RN, Riba RD, Zacharoulis S, Bramley AH, Vincent L, Costa C, et al. VEGFR1-positive haematopoietic bone marrow progenitors initiate the pre-metastatic niche. Nature. 2005 Dec 8;438(7069):820-7. PubMed PMID: 16341007.

[180] Radiloff DR, Rinella ES, Threadgill DW. Modeling cancer patient populations in mice: complex genetic and environmental factors. Drug Discov Today Dis Models. 2008;4(2):83-8. PubMed PMID: 19122874.

[181] Prendergast GC, Jaffee EM. Cancer immunologists and cancer biologists: why we didn't talk then but need to now. Cancer Res. 2007 Apr 15;67(8):3500-4. PubMed PMID: 17413003.

[182] Burstein HJ. The distinctive nature of HER2-positive breast cancers. N Engl J Med. 2005 Oct 20;353(16):1652-4. PubMed PMID: 16236735.

[183] Hansen RK, Bissell MJ. Tissue architecture and breast cancer: the role of extracellular matrix and steroid hormones. Endocr Relat Cancer. 2000 Jun;7(2):95-113. PubMed PMID: 10903527.

[184] Hiscox SG, Julia: Nicholson, L . Therapeutic Resistance to Anti-Hormonal Drugs in Breast Cancer. New Molecular Aspects and their Potential as Targets. 2009:87.

[185] Dontu G, Jackson KW, McNicholas E, Kawamura MJ, Abdallah WM, Wicha MS. Role of Notch signaling in cell-fate determination of human mammary stem/progenitor cells. Breast Cancer Res. 2004;6(6):R605-15. PubMed PMID: 15535842.

[186] Liu S, Dontu G, Wicha MS. Mammary stem cells, self-renewal pathways, and carcinogenesis. Breast Cancer Res. 2005;7(3):86-95. PubMed PMID: 15987436.

[187] Shostak K, Chariot A. NF-kappaB, stem cells and breast cancer: the links get stronger. Breast Cancer Res. 2011;13(4):214. PubMed PMID: 21867572. Pubmed Central PMCID: 3236328.

[188] Mumm JS, Kopan R. Notch signaling: from the outside in. Dev Biol. 2000 Dec 15;228(2):151-65. PubMed PMID: 11112321.

[189] Li Y, Wicha MS, Schwartz SJ, Sun D. Implications of cancer stem cell theory for cancer chemoprevention by natural dietary compounds. The Journal of nutritional biochemistry. 2011 Sep;22(9):799-806. PubMed PMID: 21295962. Pubmed Central PMCID: 3248810.

[190] Borggrefe T, Oswald F. The Notch signaling pathway: transcriptional regulation at Notch target genes. Cell Mol Life Sci. 2009 May;66(10):1631-46. PubMed PMID: 19165418.

[191] Wu JY, Rao Y. Fringe: defining borders by regulating the notch pathway. Curr Opin Neurobiol. 1999 Oct;9(5):537-43. PubMed PMID: 10508746.

[192] Oswald F, Liptay S, Adler G, Schmid RM. NF-kappaB2 is a putative target gene of activated Notch-1 via RBP-Jkappa. Mol Cell Biol. 1998 Apr;18(4):2077-88. PubMed PMID: 9528780.

[193] Palomero T, Lim WK, Odom DT, Sulis ML, Real PJ, Margolin A, et al. NOTCH1 directly regulates c-MYC and activates a feed-forward-loop transcriptional network promoting leukemic cell growth. Proc Natl Acad Sci U S A. 2006 Nov 28;103(48): 18261-6. PubMed PMID: 17114293.

[194] Rangarajan A, Talora C, Okuyama R, Nicolas M, Mammucari C, Oh H, et al. Notch signaling is a direct determinant of keratinocyte growth arrest and entry into differentiation. EMBO J. 2001 Jul 2;20(13):3427-36. PubMed PMID: 11432830.

[195] Ronchini C, Capobianco AJ. Induction of cyclin D1 transcription and CDK2 activity by Notch(ic): implication for cell cycle disruption in transformation by Notch(ic). Mol Cell Biol. 2001 Sep;21(17):5925-34. PubMed PMID: 11486031.

[196] Satoh Y, Matsumura I, Tanaka H, Ezoe S, Sugahara H, Mizuki M, et al. Roles for c-Myc in self-renewal of hematopoietic stem cells. J Biol Chem. 2004 Jun 11;279(24): 24986-93. PubMed PMID: 15067010.

[197] Weng AP, Millholland JM, Yashiro-Ohtani Y, Arcangeli ML, Lau A, Wai C, et al. c-Myc is an important direct target of Notch1 in T-cell acute lymphoblastic leukemia/lymphoma. Genes Dev. 2006 Aug 1;20(15):2096-109. PubMed PMID: 16847353.

[198] Wang Z, Li Y, Banerjee S, Sarkar FH. Emerging role of Notch in stem cells and cancer. Cancer Lett. 2009 Jun 28;279(1):8-12. PubMed PMID: 19022563.

[199] Kakarala M, Wicha MS. Implications of the cancer stem-cell hypothesis for breast cancer prevention and therapy. J Clin Oncol. 2008 Jun 10;26(17):2813-20. PubMed PMID: 18539959.

[200] Peacock CD, Watkins DN. Cancer stem cells and the ontogeny of lung cancer. J Clin Oncol. 2008 Jun 10;26(17):2883-9. PubMed PMID: 18539968.

[201] Scoville DH, Sato T, He XC, Li L. Current view: intestinal stem cells and signaling. Gastroenterology. 2008 Mar;134(3):849-64. PubMed PMID: 18325394.

[202] Wilson A, Radtke F. Multiple functions of Notch signaling in self-renewing organs and cancer. FEBS Lett. 2006 May 22;580(12):2860-8. PubMed PMID: 16574107.

[203] Dickson BC, Mulligan AM, Zhang H, Lockwood G, O'Malley FP, Egan SE, et al. High-level JAG1 mRNA and protein predict poor outcome in breast cancer. Mod Pathol. 2007 Jun;20(6):685-93. PubMed PMID: 17507991.

[204] Reedijk M, Odorcic S, Chang L, Zhang H, Miller N, McCready DR, et al. High-level coexpression of JAG1 and NOTCH1 is observed in human breast cancer and is associated with poor overall survival. Cancer Res. 2005 Sep 15;65(18):8530-7. PubMed PMID: 16166334.

[205] Rizzo P, Miao H, D'Souza G, Osipo C, Song LL, Yun J, et al. Cross-talk between notch and the estrogen receptor in breast cancer suggests novel therapeutic approaches. Cancer Res. 2008 Jul 1;68(13):5226-35. PubMed PMID: 18593923.

[206] Farnie G, Clarke RB. Mammary stem cells and breast cancer-role of Notch signalling. Stem Cell Rev. 2007 Jun;3(2):169-75. PubMed PMID: 17873349.

[207] Farnie G, Clarke RB, Spence K, Pinnock N, Brennan K, Anderson NG, et al. Novel cell culture technique for primary ductal carcinoma in situ: role of Notch and epidermal growth factor receptor signaling pathways. J Natl Cancer Inst. 2007 Apr 18;99(8): 616-27. PubMed PMID: 17440163.

[208] Sansone P, Storci G, Giovannini C, Pandolfi S, Pianetti S, Taffurelli M, et al. p66Shc/Notch-3 interplay controls self-renewal and hypoxia survival in human stem/progenitor cells of the mammary gland expanded *in vitro* as mammospheres. Stem Cells. 2007 Mar;25(3):807-15. PubMed PMID: 17158237.

[209] Sansone P, Storci G, Tavolari S, Guarnieri T, Giovannini C, Taffurelli M, et al. IL-6 triggers malignant features in mammospheres from human ductal breast carcinoma and normal mammary gland. J Clin Invest. 2007 Dec;117(12):3988-4002. PubMed PMID: 18060036.

[210] Noguera-Troise I, Daly C, Papadopoulos NJ, Coetzee S, Boland P, Gale NW, et al. Blockade of Dll4 inhibits tumour growth by promoting non-productive angiogenesis. Novartis Found Symp. 2007;283:106-20; discussion 21-5, 238-41. PubMed PMID: 18300417.

[211] Ridgway J, Zhang G, Wu Y, Stawicki S, Liang WC, Chanthery Y, et al. Inhibition of Dll4 signalling inhibits tumour growth by deregulating angiogenesis. Nature. 2006 Dec 21;444(7122):1083-7. PubMed PMID: 17183323.

[212] Pannuti A, Foreman K, Rizzo P, Osipo C, Golde T, Osborne B, et al. Targeting Notch to target cancer stem cells. Clin Cancer Res. 2010 Jun 15;16(12):3141-52. PubMed PMID: 20530696. Pubmed Central PMCID: 3008160.

[213] Foreman K, Rizzo, P, Osipo C, and Miele, L. . Stem Cells and Cancer: The Cancer Stem Cell Hypothesis; Cancer Drug Discovery and Development 2009:pp 3-14.

[214] Tominaga Y, Wang A, Wang RH, Wang X, Cao L, Deng CX. Genistein inhibits Brca1 mutant tumor growth through activation of DNA damage checkpoints, cell cycle arrest, and mitotic catastrophe. Cell Death Differ. 2007 Mar;14(3):472-9. PubMed PMID: 17024228.

[215] Chen Y, Shu W, Chen W, Wu Q, Liu H, Cui G. Curcumin, both histone deacetylase and p300/CBP-specific inhibitor, represses the activity of nuclear factor kappa B and Notch 1 in Raji cells. Basic Clin Pharmacol Toxicol. 2007 Dec;101(6):427-33. PubMed PMID: 17927689.

[216] Cho OH, Shin HM, Miele L, Golde TE, Fauq A, Minter LM, et al. Notch regulates cytolytic effector function in CD8+ T cells. J Immunol. 2009 Mar 15;182(6):3380-9. PubMed PMID: 19265115.

[217] Jang MS, Miao H, Carlesso N, Shelly L, Zlobin A, Darack N, et al. Notch-1 regulates cell death independently of differentiation in murine erythroleukemia cells through multiple apoptosis and cell cycle pathways. J Cell Physiol. 2004 Jun;199(3):418-33. PubMed PMID: 15095289.

[218] Nickoloff BJ, Qin JZ, Chaturvedi V, Denning MF, Bonish B, Miele L. Jagged-1 mediated activation of notch signaling induces complete maturation of human keratinocytes through NF-kappaB and PPARgamma. Cell Death Differ. 2002 Aug;9(8):842-55. PubMed PMID: 12107827.

[219] Wang Y, Chan SL, Miele L, Yao PJ, Mackes J, Ingram DK, et al. Involvement of Notch signaling in hippocampal synaptic plasticity. Proc Natl Acad Sci U S A. 2004 Jun 22;101(25):9458-62. PubMed PMID: 15190179.

[220] Cheng AL, Hsu CH, Lin JK, Hsu MM, Ho YF, Shen TS, et al. Phase I clinical trial of curcumin, a chemopreventive agent, in patients with high-risk or pre-malignant lesions. Anticancer Res. 2001 Jul-Aug;21(4B):2895-900. PubMed PMID: 11712783.

[221] Milele LT, N. Ivy, PS. The Cancer Stem Cell Hypothesis, Embtyonic Signaling Pathways, and Therapeutic: Targeting an Elusive Concept. 2009.

[222] Prosperi JR, Goss KH. A Wnt-ow of opportunity: targeting the Wnt/beta-catenin pathway in breast cancer. Current drug targets. 2010 Sep;11(9):1074-88. PubMed PMID: 20545611.

[223] Nelson WJ, Nusse R. Convergence of Wnt, beta-catenin, and cadherin pathways. Science. 2004 Mar 5;303(5663):1483-7. PubMed PMID: 15001769.

[224] Akiyama T. Wnt/beta-catenin signaling. Cytokine Growth Factor Rev. 2000 Dec;11(4): 273-82. PubMed PMID: 10959075.

[225] Goss KH, Kahn M. Targeting the Wnt pathway in cancer. New York: Springer; 2011.

[226] van Amerongen R, Mikels A, Nusse R. Alternative wnt signaling is initiated by distinct receptors. Sci Signal. 2008;1(35). PubMed PMID: 18765832.

[227] Polakis P. The many ways of Wnt in cancer. Curr Opin Genet Dev. 2007 Feb;17(1): 45-51. PubMed PMID: 17208432.

[228] Polakis P. Wnt signaling and cancer. Genes Dev. 2000 Aug 1;14(15):1837-51. PubMed PMID: 10921899.

[229] Turashvili G, Bouchal J, Burkadze G, Kolar Z. Wnt signaling pathway in mammary gland development and carcinogenesis. Pathobiology. 2006;73(5):213-23. PubMed PMID: 17314492.

[230] Yamaguchi TP. Genetics of Wnt signaling during early mammalian development. Methods Mol Biol. 2008;468:287-305. PubMed PMID: 19099264.

[231] Clevers H. Wnt/beta-catenin signaling in development and disease. Cell. 2006 Nov 3;127(3):469-80. PubMed PMID: 17081971.

[232] He TC, Sparks AB, Rago C, Hermeking H, Zawel L, da Costa LT, et al. Identification of c-MYC as a target of the APC pathway. Science. 1998 Sep 4;281(5382):1509-12. PubMed PMID: 9727977.

[233] Lin SY, Xia W, Wang JC, Kwong KY, Spohn B, Wen Y, et al. Beta-catenin, a novel prognostic marker for breast cancer: its roles in cyclin D1 expression and cancer progression. Proc Natl Acad Sci U S A. 2000 Apr 11;97(8):4262-6. PubMed PMID: 10759547.

[234] Mann B, Gelos M, Siedow A, Hanski ML, Gratchev A, Ilyas M, et al. Target genes of beta-catenin-T cell-factor/lymphoid-enhancer-factor signaling in human colorectal carcinomas. Proc Natl Acad Sci U S A. 1999 Feb 16;96(4):1603-8. PubMed PMID: 9990071.

[235] Orsulic S, Huber O, Aberle H, Arnold S, Kemler R. E-cadherin binding prevents beta-catenin nuclear localization and beta-catenin/LEF-1-mediated transactivation. J Cell Sci. 1999 Apr;112 (Pt 8):1237-45. PubMed PMID: 10085258.

[236] Tetsu O, McCormick F. Beta-catenin regulates expression of cyclin D1 in colon carcinoma cells. Nature. 1999 Apr 1;398(6726):422-6. PubMed PMID: 10201372.

[237] Finch PW, He X, Kelley MJ, Uren A, Schaudies RP, Popescu NC, et al. Purification and molecular cloning of a secreted, Frizzled-related antagonist of Wnt action. Proc Natl Acad Sci U S A. 1997 Jun 24;94(13):6770-5. PubMed PMID: 9192640.

[238] Barker N, Clevers H. Mining the Wnt pathway for cancer therapeutics. Nat Rev Drug Discov. 2006 Dec;5(12):997-1014. PubMed PMID: 17139285.

[239] Bilic J, Huang YL, Davidson G, Zimmermann T, Cruciat CM, Bienz M, et al. Wnt induces LRP6 signalosomes and promotes dishevelled-dependent LRP6 phosphorylation. Science. 2007 Jun 15;316(5831):1619-22. PubMed PMID: 17569865.

[240] Davidson G, Wu W, Shen J, Bilic J, Fenger U, Stannek P, et al. Casein kinase 1 gamma couples Wnt receptor activation to cytoplasmic signal transduction. Nature. 2005 Dec 8;438(7069):867-72. PubMed PMID: 16341016.

[241] Roose J, Molenaar M, Peterson J, Hurenkamp J, Brantjes H, Moerer P, et al. The Xenopus Wnt effector XTcf-3 interacts with Groucho-related transcriptional repressors. Nature. 1998 Oct 8;395(6702):608-12. PubMed PMID: 9783587.

[242] Zeng X, Tamai K, Doble B, Li S, Huang H, Habas R, et al. A dual-kinase mechanism for Wnt co-receptor phosphorylation and activation. Nature. 2005 Dec 8;438(7069): 873-7. PubMed PMID: 16341017.

[243] Glinka A, Wu W, Delius H, Monaghan AP, Blumenstock C, Niehrs C. Dickkopf-1 is a member of a new family of secreted proteins and functions in head induction. Nature. 1998 Jan 22;391(6665):357-62. PubMed PMID: 9450748.

[244] Hsieh JC. Specificity of WNT-receptor interactions. Front Biosci. 2004 May 1;9:1333-8. PubMed PMID: 14977548.

[245] Nusse R, van Ooyen A, Cox D, Fung YK, Varmus H. Mode of proviral activation of a putative mammary oncogene (int-1) on mouse chromosome 15. Nature. 1984 Jan 12-18;307(5947):131-6. PubMed PMID: 6318122.

[246] Polakis P. Drugging Wnt signalling in cancer. EMBO J. 2012 Jun 13;31(12):2737-46. PubMed PMID: 22617421. Pubmed Central PMCID: 3380214.

[247] Howe EN, Cochrane DR, Cittelly DM, Richer JK. miR-200c Targets a NF-kappaB Up-Regulated TrkB/NTF3 Autocrine Signaling Loop to Enhance Anoikis Sensitivity in Triple Negative Breast Cancer. PLoS One. 2012;7(11):e49987. PubMed PMID: 23185507. Pubmed Central PMCID: 3503774.

[248] Lacroix-Triki M, Geyer FC, Lambros MB, Savage K, Ellis IO, Lee AH, et al. beta-catenin/Wnt signalling pathway in fibromatosis, metaplastic carcinomas and phyllodes tumours of the breast. Mod Pathol. 2010 Nov;23(11):1438-48. PubMed PMID: 20693983.

[249] Lin X, Zhang X, Wang Q, Li J, Zhang P, Zhao M, et al. Perifosine downregulates MDR1 gene expression and reverses multidrug-resistant phenotype by inhibiting

PI3K/Akt/NF-kappaB signaling pathway in a human breast cancer cell line. Neoplasma. 2012;59(3):248-56. PubMed PMID: 22329846.

[250] Lu W, Lin C, King TD, Chen H, Reynolds RC, Li Y. Silibinin inhibits Wnt/beta-catenin signaling by suppressing Wnt co-receptor LRP6 expression in human prostate and breast cancer cells. Cellular signalling. 2012 Dec;24(12):2291-6. PubMed PMID: 22820499. Pubmed Central PMCID: 3466371.

[251] Wu Y, Ginther C, Kim J, Mosher N, Chung S, Slamon D, et al. Expression of Wnt3 Activates Wnt/beta-Catenin Pathway and Promotes EMT-like Phenotype in Trastuzumab-Resistant HER2-Overexpressing Breast Cancer Cells. Mol Cancer Res. 2012 Nov 27. PubMed PMID: 23071104.

[252] Howe LR, Brown AM. Wnt signaling and breast cancer. Cancer Biol Ther. 2004 Jan; 3(1):36-41. PubMed PMID: 14739782.

[253] Khramtsov AI, Khramtsova GF, Tretiakova M, Huo D, Olopade OI, Goss KH. Wnt/beta-catenin pathway activation is enriched in basal-like breast cancers and predicts poor outcome. The American journal of pathology. 2010 Jun;176(6):2911-20. PubMed PMID: 20395444. Pubmed Central PMCID: 2877852.

[254] Milovanovic T, Planutis K, Nguyen A, Marsh JL, Lin F, Hope C, et al. Expression of Wnt genes and frizzled 1 and 2 receptors in normal breast epithelium and infiltrating breast carcinoma. Int J Oncol. 2004 Nov;25(5):1337-42. PubMed PMID: 15492823.

[255] Nguyen A, Rosner A, Milovanovic T, Hope C, Planutis K, Saha B, et al. Wnt pathway component LEF1 mediates tumor cell invasion and is expressed in human and murine breast cancers lacking ErbB2 (her-2/neu) overexpression. Int J Oncol. 2005 Oct; 27(4):949-56. PubMed PMID: 16142310.

[256] Xu W, Lin H, Zhang Y, Chen X, Hua B, Hou W, et al. Compound Kushen Injection suppresses human breast cancer stem-like cells by down-regulating the canonical Wnt/beta-catenin pathway. Journal of experimental & clinical cancer research : CR. 2011;30:103. PubMed PMID: 22032476. Pubmed Central PMCID: 3219673.

[257] Bafico A, Liu G, Goldin L, Harris V, Aaronson SA. An autocrine mechanism for constitutive Wnt pathway activation in human cancer cells. Cancer Cell. 2004 Nov;6(5): 497-506. PubMed PMID: 15542433.

[258] Sorlie T, Tibshirani R, Parker J, Hastie T, Marron JS, Nobel A, et al. Repeated observation of breast tumor subtypes in independent gene expression data sets. Proc Natl Acad Sci U S A. 2003 Jul 8;100(14):8418-23. PubMed PMID: 12829800.

[259] Yang L, Wu X, Wang Y, Zhang K, Wu J, Yuan YC, et al. FZD7 has a critical role in cell proliferation in triple negative breast cancer. Oncogene. 2011 Oct 27;30(43):4437-46. PubMed PMID: 21532620.

[260] Matsuda Y, Schlange T, Oakeley EJ, Boulay A, Hynes NE. WNT signaling enhances breast cancer cell motility and blockade of the WNT pathway by sFRP1 suppresses

MDA-MB-231 xenograft growth. Breast Cancer Res. 2009;11(3):R32. PubMed PMID: 19473496. Pubmed Central PMCID: 2716500.

[261] Chien AJ, Moore EC, Lonsdorf AS, Kulikauskas RM, Rothberg BG, Berger AJ, et al. Activated Wnt/beta-catenin signaling in melanoma is associated with decreased proliferation in patient tumors and a murine melanoma model. Proc Natl Acad Sci U S A. 2009 Jan 27;106(4):1193-8. PubMed PMID: 19144919.

[262] Kawaguchi H. Regulation of osteoarthritis development by Wnt-beta-catenin signaling through the endochondral ossification process. J Bone Miner Res. 2009 Jan;24(1): 8-11. PubMed PMID: 19016582.

[263] Khan NI, Bradstock KF, Bendall LJ. Activation of Wnt/beta-catenin pathway mediates growth and survival in B-cell progenitor acute lymphoblastic leukaemia. Br J Haematol. 2007 Aug;138(3):338-48. PubMed PMID: 17614820.

[264] Schulenburg A, Cech P, Herbacek I, Marian B, Wrba F, Valent P, et al. CD44-positive colorectal adenoma cells express the potential stem cell markers musashi antigen (msi1) and ephrin B2 receptor (EphB2). J Pathol. 2007 Oct;213(2):152-60. PubMed PMID: 17708598.

[265] Teng Y, Wang X, Wang Y, Ma D. Wnt/beta-catenin signaling regulates cancer stem cells in lung cancer A549 cells. Biochem Biophys Res Commun. 2010 Feb 12;392(3): 373-9. PubMed PMID: 20074550.

[266] Woodward WA, Chen MS, Behbod F, Alfaro MP, Buchholz TA, Rosen JM. WNT/beta-catenin mediates radiation resistance of mouse mammary progenitor cells. Proc Natl Acad Sci U S A. 2007 Jan 9;104(2):618-23. PubMed PMID: 17202265.

[267] Yang W, Yan HX, Chen L, Liu Q, He YQ, Yu LX, et al. Wnt/beta-catenin signaling contributes to activation of normal and tumorigenic liver progenitor cells. Cancer Res. 2008 Jun 1;68(11):4287-95. PubMed PMID: 18519688.

[268] Ysebaert L, Chicanne G, Demur C, De Toni F, Prade-Houdellier N, Ruidavets JB, et al. Expression of beta-catenin by acute myeloid leukemia cells predicts enhanced clonogenic capacities and poor prognosis. Leukemia. 2006 Jul;20(7):1211-6. PubMed PMID: 16688229.

[269] Li Y, Welm B, Podsypanina K, Huang S, Chamorro M, Zhang X, et al. Evidence that transgenes encoding components of the Wnt signaling pathway preferentially induce mammary cancers from progenitor cells. Proc Natl Acad Sci U S A. 2003 Dec 23;100(26):15853-8. PubMed PMID: 14668450.

[270] Cohen P, Frame S. The renaissance of GSK3. Nat Rev Mol Cell Biol. 2001 Oct;2(10): 769-76. PubMed PMID: 11584304.

[271] Pap M, Cooper GM. Role of translation initiation factor 2B in control of cell survival by the phosphatidylinositol 3-kinase/Akt/glycogen synthase kinase 3beta signaling pathway. Mol Cell Biol. 2002 Jan;22(2):578-86. PubMed PMID: 11756553.

[272] Yost C, Torres M, Miller JR, Huang E, Kimelman D, Moon RT. The axis-inducing activity, stability, and subcellular distribution of beta-catenin is regulated in Xenopus embryos by glycogen synthase kinase 3. Genes Dev. 1996 Jun 15;10(12):1443-54. PubMed PMID: 8666229.

[273] Geng L, Cuneo KC, Cooper MK, Wang H, Sekhar K, Fu A, et al. Hedgehog signaling in the murine melanoma microenvironment. Angiogenesis. 2007;10(4):259-67. PubMed PMID: 17762973.

[274] Chari NS, McDonnell TJ. The sonic hedgehog signaling network in development and neoplasia. Adv Anat Pathol. 2007 Sep;14(5):344-52. PubMed PMID: 17717435.

[275] Evangelista M, Tian H, de Sauvage FJ. The hedgehog signaling pathway in cancer. Clin Cancer Res. 2006 Oct 15;12(20 Pt 1):5924-8. PubMed PMID: 17062662.

[276] Cohen MM, Jr. The hedgehog signaling network. Am J Med Genet A. 2003 Nov 15;123A(1):5-28. PubMed PMID: 14556242.

[277] Lewis MT, Veltmaat JM. Next stop, the twilight zone: hedgehog network regulation of mammary gland development. J Mammary Gland Biol Neoplasia. 2004 Apr;9(2): 165-81. PubMed PMID: 15300011.

[278] Sarkar FH, Li Y, Wang Z, Kong D. The role of nutraceuticals in the regulation of Wnt and Hedgehog signaling in cancer. Cancer metastasis reviews. 2010 Sep;29(3):383-94. PubMed PMID: 20711635. Pubmed Central PMCID: 2974632.

[279] Yang L, Xie G, Fan Q, Xie J. Activation of the hedgehog-signaling pathway in human cancer and the clinical implications. Oncogene. 2010 Jan 28;29(4):469-81. PubMed PMID: 19935712.

[280] Yauch RL, Gould SE, Scales SJ, Tang T, Tian H, Ahn CP, et al. A paracrine requirement for hedgehog signalling in cancer. Nature. 2008 Sep 18;455(7211):406-10. PubMed PMID: 18754008.

[281] Kasper M, Jaks V, Fiaschi M, Toftgard R. Hedgehog signalling in breast cancer. Carcinogenesis. 2009 Jun;30(6):903-11. PubMed PMID: 19237605.

[282] Anton Aparicio LM, Garcia Campelo R, Cassinello Espinosa J, Valladares Ayerbes M, Reboredo Lopez M, Diaz Prado S, et al. Prostate cancer and Hedgehog signalling pathway. Clin Transl Oncol. 2007 Jul;9(7):420-8. PubMed PMID: 17652055.

[283] Vezina CM, Bushman AW. Hedgehog signaling in prostate growth and benign prostate hyperplasia. Curr Urol Rep. 2007 Jul;8(4):275-80. PubMed PMID: 18519011.

[284] Clement V, Sanchez P, de Tribolet N, Radovanovic I, Ruiz i Altaba A. HEDGEHOG-GLI1 signaling regulates human glioma growth, cancer stem cell self-renewal, and tumorigenicity. Curr Biol. 2007 Jan 23;17(2):165-72. PubMed PMID: 17196391.

[285] Medina V, Calvo MB, Diaz-Prado S, Espada J. Hedgehog signalling as a target in cancer stem cells. Clin Transl Oncol. 2009 Apr;11(4):199-207. PubMed PMID: 19380296.

[286] Kalderon D. Similarities between the Hedgehog and Wnt signaling pathways. Trends Cell Biol. 2002 Nov;12(11):523-31. PubMed PMID: 12446114.

[287] Huelsken J, Birchmeier W. New aspects of Wnt signaling pathways in higher vertebrates. Curr Opin Genet Dev. 2001 Oct;11(5):547-53. PubMed PMID: 11532397.

[288] Ingham PW, McMahon AP. Hedgehog signaling in animal development: paradigms and principles. Genes Dev. 2001 Dec 1;15(23):3059-87. PubMed PMID: 11731473.

[289] Price MA, Kalderon D. Proteolysis of the Hedgehog signaling effector Cubitus interruptus requires phosphorylation by Glycogen Synthase Kinase 3 and Casein Kinase 1. Cell. 2002 Mar 22;108(6):823-35. PubMed PMID: 11955435.

[290] Day TF, Yang Y. Wnt and hedgehog signaling pathways in bone development. J Bone Joint Surg Am. 2008 Feb;90 Suppl 1:19-24. PubMed PMID: 18292352.

[291] Yang SH, Andl T, Grachtchouk V, Wang A, Liu J, Syu LJ, et al. Pathological responses to oncogenic Hedgehog signaling in skin are dependent on canonical Wnt/beta3-catenin signaling. Nat Genet. 2008 Sep;40(9):1130-5. PubMed PMID: 19165927.

[292] Hayden MS, Ghosh S. Shared principles in NF-kappaB signaling. Cell. 2008 Feb 8;132(3):344-62. PubMed PMID: 18267068.

[293] Brantley DM, Chen CL, Muraoka RS, Bushdid PB, Bradberry JL, Kittrell F, et al. Nuclear factor-kappaB (NF-kappaB) regulates proliferation and branching in mouse mammary epithelium. Molecular biology of the cell. 2001 May;12(5):1445-55. PubMed PMID: 11359934. Pubmed Central PMCID: 34596.

[294] Cao Y, Bonizzi G, Seagroves TN, Greten FR, Johnson R, Schmidt EV, et al. IKKalpha provides an essential link between RANK signaling and cyclin D1 expression during mammary gland development. Cell. 2001 Dec 14;107(6):763-75. PubMed PMID: 11747812.

[295] Sovak MA, Bellas RE, Kim DW, Zanieski GJ, Rogers AE, Traish AM, et al. Aberrant nuclear factor-kappaB/Rel expression and the pathogenesis of breast cancer. J Clin Invest. 1997 Dec 15;100(12):2952-60. PubMed PMID: 9399940.

[296] Huber MA, Azoitei N, Baumann B, Grunert S, Sommer A, Pehamberger H, et al. NF-kappaB is essential for epithelial-mesenchymal transition and metastasis in a model of breast cancer progression. J Clin Invest. 2004 Aug;114(4):569-81. PubMed PMID: 15314694. Pubmed Central PMCID: 503772.

[297] Chua HL, Bhat-Nakshatri P, Clare SE, Morimiya A, Badve S, Nakshatri H. NF-kappaB represses E-cadherin expression and enhances epithelial to mesenchymal transition of mammary epithelial cells: potential involvement of ZEB-1 and ZEB-2. Oncogene. 2007 Feb 1;26(5):711-24. PubMed PMID: 16862183.

[298] Biswas DK, Shi Q, Baily S, Strickland I, Ghosh S, Pardee AB, et al. NF-kappa B activation in human breast cancer specimens and its role in cell proliferation and apopto-

sis. Proc Natl Acad Sci U S A. 2004 Jul 6;101(27):10137-42. PubMed PMID: 15220474. Pubmed Central PMCID: 454178.

[299] Nakshatri H, Bhat-Nakshatri P, Martin DA, Goulet RJ, Jr., Sledge GW, Jr. Constitutive activation of NF-kappaB during progression of breast cancer to hormone-independent growth. Mol Cell Biol. 1997 Jul;17(7):3629-39. PubMed PMID: 9199297. Pubmed Central PMCID: 232215.

[300] Karin M, Lin A. NF-kappaB at the crossroads of life and death. Nature immunology. 2002 Mar;3(3):221-7. PubMed PMID: 11875461.

[301] Connelly L, Barham W, Onishko HM, Sherrill T, Chodosh LA, Blackwell TS, et al. Inhibition of NF-kappa B activity in mammary epithelium increases tumor latency and decreases tumor burden. Oncogene. 2011 Mar 24;30(12):1402-12. PubMed PMID: 21076466.

[302] Oeckinghaus A, Hayden MS, Ghosh S. Crosstalk in NF-kappaB signaling pathways. Nature immunology. 2011 Aug;12(8):695-708. PubMed PMID: 21772278.

[303] Dejardin E, Bonizzi G, Bellahcene A, Castronovo V, Merville MP, Bours V. Highly-expressed p100/p52 (NFKB2) sequesters other NF-kappa B-related proteins in the cytoplasm of human breast cancer cells. Oncogene. 1995 Nov 2;11(9):1835-41. PubMed PMID: 7478612.

[304] Cogswell PC, Guttridge DC, Funkhouser WK, Baldwin AS, Jr. Selective activation of NF-kappa B subunits in human breast cancer: potential roles for NF-kappa B2/p52 and for Bcl-3. Oncogene. 2000 Feb 24;19(9):1123-31. PubMed PMID: 10713699.

[305] Wang X, Belguise K, Kersual N, Kirsch KH, Mineva ND, Galtier F, et al. Oestrogen signalling inhibits invasive phenotype by repressing RelB and its target BCL2. Nature cell biology. 2007 Apr;9(4):470-8. PubMed PMID: 17369819. Pubmed Central PMCID: 2394707.

[306] Demicco EG, Kavanagh KT, Romieu-Mourez R, Wang X, Shin SR, Landesman-Bollag E, et al. RelB/p52 NF-kappaB complexes rescue an early delay in mammary gland development in transgenic mice with targeted superrepressor IkappaB-alpha expression and promote carcinogenesis of the mammary gland. Mol Cell Biol. 2005 Nov; 25(22):10136-47. PubMed PMID: 16260626. Pubmed Central PMCID: 1280249.

[307] Connelly L, Robinson-Benion C, Chont M, Saint-Jean L, Li H, Polosukhin VV, et al. A transgenic model reveals important roles for the NF-kappa B alternative pathway (p100/p52) in mammary development and links to tumorigenesis. J Biol Chem. 2007 Mar 30;282(13):10028-35. PubMed PMID: 17261585.

[308] Cao Y, Luo JL, Karin M. IkappaB kinase alpha kinase activity is required for self-renewal of ErbB2/Her2-transformed mammary tumor-initiating cells. Proc Natl Acad Sci U S A. 2007 Oct 2;104(40):15852-7. PubMed PMID: 17890319. Pubmed Central PMCID: 2000410.

[309] Pratt MA, Tibbo E, Robertson SJ, Jansson D, Hurst K, Perez-Iratxeta C, et al. The canonical NF-kappaB pathway is required for formation of luminal mammary neoplasias and is activated in the mammary progenitor population. Oncogene. 2009 Jul 30;28(30):2710-22. PubMed PMID: 19483731.

[310] Visvader JE. Keeping abreast of the mammary epithelial hierarchy and breast tumorigenesis. Genes Dev. 2009 Nov 15;23(22):2563-77. PubMed PMID: 19933147. Pubmed Central PMCID: 2779757.

[311] Sasser AK, Sullivan NJ, Studebaker AW, Hendey LF, Axel AE, Hall BM. Interleukin-6 is a potent growth factor for ER-alpha-positive human breast cancer. FASEB journal : official publication of the Federation of American Societies for Experimental Biology. 2007 Nov;21(13):3763-70. PubMed PMID: 17586727.

[312] Naugler WE, Karin M. NF-kappaB and cancer-identifying targets and mechanisms. Curr Opin Genet Dev. 2008 Feb;18(1):19-26. PubMed PMID: 18440219. Pubmed Central PMCID: 2587362.

[313] Iliopoulos D, Hirsch HA, Struhl K. An epigenetic switch involving NF-kappaB, Lin28, Let-7 MicroRNA, and IL6 links inflammation to cell transformation. Cell. 2009 Nov 13;139(4):693-706. PubMed PMID: 19878981. Pubmed Central PMCID: 2783826.

[314] Schramek D, Leibbrandt A, Sigl V, Kenner L, Pospisilik JA, Lee HJ, et al. Osteoclast differentiation factor RANKL controls development of progestin-driven mammary cancer. Nature. 2010 Nov 4;468(7320):98-102. PubMed PMID: 20881962. Pubmed Central PMCID: 3084017.

[315] Jones DH, Nakashima T, Sanchez OH, Kozieradzki I, Komarova SV, Sarosi I, et al. Regulation of cancer cell migration and bone metastasis by RANKL. Nature. 2006 Mar 30;440(7084):692-6. PubMed PMID: 16572175.

[316] Gonzalez-Suarez E, Jacob AP, Jones J, Miller R, Roudier-Meyer MP, Erwert R, et al. RANK ligand mediates progestin-induced mammary epithelial proliferation and carcinogenesis. Nature. 2010 Nov 4;468(7320):103-7. PubMed PMID: 20881963.

[317] Liu M, Sakamaki T, Casimiro MC, Willmarth NE, Quong AA, Ju X, et al. The canonical NF-kappaB pathway governs mammary tumorigenesis in transgenic mice and tumor stem cell expansion. Cancer Res. 2010 Dec 15;70(24):10464-73. PubMed PMID: 21159656. Pubmed Central PMCID: 3010731.

[318] Korkaya H, Paulson A, Iovino F, Wicha MS. HER2 regulates the mammary stem/progenitor cell population driving tumorigenesis and invasion. Oncogene. 2008 Oct 16;27(47):6120-30. PubMed PMID: 18591932. Pubmed Central PMCID: 2602947.

[319] Merkhofer EC, Cogswell P, Baldwin AS. Her2 activates NF-kappaB and induces invasion through the canonical pathway involving IKKalpha. Oncogene. 2010 Feb 25;29(8):1238-48. PubMed PMID: 19946332. Pubmed Central PMCID: 2829103.

[320] Cragg GM, Newman DJ, Yang SS. Natural product extracts of plant and marine origin having antileukemia potential. The NCI experience. Journal of natural products. 2006 Mar;69(3):488-98. PubMed PMID: 16562862.

[321] Miller GT, and S. Spoolman. Living in the Environment: Principles, Connections, and Solutions. Brooks-Cole, Belmont, CA. 2011.

[322] Li Y, Wicha MS, Schwartz SJ, Sun D. Implications of cancer stem cell theory for cancer chemoprevention by natural dietary compounds. J Nutr Biochem. Sep;22(9): 799-806. PubMed PMID: 21295962.

[323] Anderson H, Hills M, Zabaglo L, A'Hern R, Leary AF, Haynes BP, et al. Relationship between estrogen receptor, progesterone receptor, HER-2 and Ki67 expression and efficacy of aromatase inhibitors in advanced breast cancer. Ann Oncol. 2011 Feb 1. PubMed PMID: 21285137.

[324] Chen S, Oh SR, Phung S, Hur G, Ye JJ, Kwok SL, et al. Anti-aromatase activity of phytochemicals in white button mushrooms (Agaricus bisporus). Cancer Res. 2006 Dec 15;66(24):12026-34. PubMed PMID: 17178902.

[325] Ellis MJ, Coop A, Singh B, Mauriac L, Llombert-Cussac A, Janicke F, et al. Letrozole is more effective neoadjuvant endocrine therapy than tamoxifen for ErbB-1- and/or ErbB-2-positive, estrogen receptor-positive primary breast cancer: evidence from a phase III randomized trial. J Clin Oncol. 2001 Sep 15;19(18):3808-16. PubMed PMID: 11559718.

[326] Goss PE, Ingle JN, Martino S, Robert NJ, Muss HB, Piccart MJ, et al. A randomized trial of letrozole in postmenopausal women after five years of tamoxifen therapy for early-stage breast cancer. N Engl J Med. 2003 Nov 6;349(19):1793-802. PubMed PMID: 14551341.

[327] Winer EP, Hudis C, Burstein HJ, Chlebowski RT, Ingle JN, Edge SB, et al. American Society of Clinical Oncology technology assessment on the use of aromatase inhibitors as adjuvant therapy for women with hormone receptor-positive breast cancer: status report 2002. J Clin Oncol. 2002 Aug 1;20(15):3317-27. PubMed PMID: 12149306.

[328] Ahmad A, Ali S, Wang Z, Ali AS, Sethi S, Sakr WA, et al. 3, 3'-diindolylmethane enhances taxotere-induced growth inhibition of breast cancer cells through down-regulation of FoxM1. Int J Cancer. 2011 Dec 10. PubMed PMID: 21154750.

[329] Manfredi JJ, Horwitz SB. Taxol: an antimitotic agent with a new mechanism of action. Pharmacol Ther. 1984;25(1):83-125. PubMed PMID: 6149569.

[330] Li Y, Bhuiyan M, Alhasan S, Senderowicz AM, Sarkar FH. Induction of apoptosis and inhibition of c-erbB-2 in breast cancer cells by flavopiridol. Clin Cancer Res. 2000 Jan; 6(1):223-9. PubMed PMID: 10656453.

[331] Somers-Edgar TJ, Scandlyn MJ, Stuart EC, Le Nedelec MJ, Valentine SP, Rosengren RJ. The combination of epigallocatechin gallate and curcumin suppresses ER alpha-

breast cancer cell growth *in vitro* and *in vivo*. Int J Cancer. 2008 May 1;122(9):1966-71. PubMed PMID: 18098290.

[332] Choi WY, Kim GY, Lee WH, Choi YH. Sanguinarine, a benzophenanthridine alkaloid, induces apoptosis in MDA-MB-231 human breast carcinoma cells through a reactive oxygen species-mediated mitochondrial pathway. Chemotherapy. 2008;54(4): 279-87. PubMed PMID: 18667818.

[333] Gu H, Rao S, Zhao J, Wang J, Mu R, Rong J, et al. Gambogic acid reduced bcl-2 expression via p53 in human breast MCF-7 cancer cells. J Cancer Res Clin Oncol. 2009 Dec;135(12):1777-82. PubMed PMID: 19582475.

[334] Jiang J, Grieb B, Thyagarajan A, Sliva D. Ganoderic acids suppress growth and invasive behavior of breast cancer cells by modulating AP-1 and NF-kappaB signaling. International journal of molecular medicine. 2008 May;21(5):577-84. PubMed PMID: 18425349.

[335] Campbell CT, Prince M, Landry GM, Kha V, Kleiner HE. Pro-apoptotic effects of 1'-acetoxychavicol acetate in human breast carcinoma cells. Toxicol Lett. 2007 Sep 28;173(3):151-60. PubMed PMID: 17766064.

[336] Banerjee S, Bueso-Ramos C, Aggarwal BB. Suppression of 7,12-dimethylbenz(a)anthracene-induced mammary carcinogenesis in rats by resveratrol: role of nuclear factor-kappaB, cyclooxygenase 2, and matrix metalloprotease 9. Cancer Res. 2002 Sep 1;62(17):4945-54. PubMed PMID: 12208745.

[337] Ahmad A, Wang Z, Ali R, Maitah MY, Kong D, Banerjee S, et al. Apoptosis-inducing effect of garcinol is mediated by NF-kappaB signaling in breast cancer cells. J Cell Biochem. 2010 Apr 15;109(6):1134-41. PubMed PMID: 20108249.

[338] Ahmad A, Banerjee S, Wang Z, Kong D, Sarkar FH. Plumbagin-induced apoptosis of human breast cancer cells is mediated by inactivation of NF-kappaB and Bcl-2. J Cell Biochem. 2008 Dec 15;105(6):1461-71. PubMed PMID: 18980240.

[339] Murillo G, Peng X, Torres KE, Mehta RG. Deguelin inhibits growth of breast cancer cells by modulating the expression of key members of the Wnt signaling pathway. Cancer Prev Res (Phila). 2009 Nov;2(11):942-50. PubMed PMID: 19861542.

[340] Lee SO, Jeong YJ, Im HG, Kim CH, Chang YC, Lee IS. Silibinin suppresses PMA-induced MMP-9 expression by blocking the AP-1 activation via MAPK signaling pathways in MCF-7 human breast carcinoma cells. Biochem Biophys Res Commun. 2007 Mar 2;354(1):165-71. PubMed PMID: 17214970.

[341] Cornwell T, Cohick W, Raskin I. Dietary phytoestrogens and health. Phytochemistry. 2004 Apr;65(8):995-1016. PubMed PMID: 15110680.

[342] Murphy PA, Song T, Buseman G, Barua K, Beecher GR, Trainer D, et al. Isoflavones in retail and institutional soy foods. J Agric Food Chem. 1999 Jul;47(7):2697-704. PubMed PMID: 10552547.

[343] Amin AR, Kucuk O, Khuri FR, Shin DM. Perspectives for cancer prevention with natural compounds. J Clin Oncol. 2009 Jun 1;27(16):2712-25. PubMed PMID: 19414669.

[344] Sirtori CR, Arnoldi A, Johnson SK. Phytoestrogens: end of a tale? Ann Med. 2005;37(6):423-38. PubMed PMID: 16203615.

[345] Matsumura A, Ghosh A, Pope GS, Darbre PD. Comparative study of oestrogenic properties of eight phytoestrogens in MCF7 human breast cancer cells. The Journal of steroid biochemistry and molecular biology. 2005 Apr;94(5):431-43. PubMed PMID: 15876408.

[346] Casanova M, You L, Gaido KW, Archibeque-Engle S, Janszen DB, Heck HA. Developmental effects of dietary phytoestrogens in Sprague-Dawley rats and interactions of genistein and daidzein with rat estrogen receptors alpha and beta *in vitro*. Toxicological sciences: an official journal of the Society of Toxicology. 1999 Oct;51(2):236-44. PubMed PMID: 10543025.

[347] Chrzan BG, Bradford PG. Phytoestrogens activate estrogen receptor beta1 and estrogenic responses in human breast and bone cancer cell lines. Mol Nutr Food Res. 2007 Feb;51(2):171-7. PubMed PMID: 17266178.

[348] Privat M, Aubel C, Arnould S, Communal Y, Ferrara M, Bignon YJ. Breast cancer cell response to genistein is conditioned by BRCA1 mutations. Biochem Biophys Res Commun. 2009 Feb 13;379(3):785-9. PubMed PMID: 19126406.

[349] Privat M, Aubel C, Arnould S, Communal Y, Ferrara M, Bignon YJ. AKT and p21 WAF1/CIP1 as potential genistein targets in BRCA1-mutant human breast cancer cell lines. Anticancer Res. 2010 Jun;30(6):2049-54. PubMed PMID: 20651350.

[350] Subbaramaiah K, Norton L, Gerald W, Dannenberg AJ. Cyclooxygenase-2 is overexpressed in HER-2/neu-positive breast cancer: evidence for involvement of AP-1 and PEA3. J Biol Chem. 2002 May 24;277(21):18649-57. PubMed PMID: 11901151.

[351] Lau TY, Leung LK. Soya isoflavones suppress phorbol 12-myristate 13-acetate-induced COX-2 expression in MCF-7 cells. Br J Nutr. 2006 Jul;96(1):169-76. PubMed PMID: 16870006.

[352] Cappelletti V, Fioravanti L, Miodini P, Di Fronzo G. Genistein blocks breast cancer cells in the G(2)M phase of the cell cycle. J Cell Biochem. 2000 Sep 14;79(4):594-600. PubMed PMID: 10996850.

[353] Choi YH, Zhang L, Lee WH, Park KY. Genistein-induced G2/M arrest is associated with the inhibition of cyclin B1 and the induction of p21 in human breast carcinoma cells. Int J Oncol. 1998 Aug;13(2):391-6. PubMed PMID: 9664138.

[354] Li Z, Li J, Mo B, Hu C, Liu H, Qi H, et al. Genistein induces G2/M cell cycle arrest via stable activation of ERK1/2 pathway in MDA-MB-231 breast cancer cells. Cell Biol Toxicol. 2008 Oct;24(5):401-9. PubMed PMID: 18224451.

[355] Lee WY, Huang SC, Tzeng CC, Chang TL, Hsu KF. Alterations of metastasis-related genes identified using an oligonucleotide microarray of genistein-treated HCC1395 breast cancer cells. Nutr Cancer. 2007;58(2):239-46. PubMed PMID: 17640171.

[356] Bergan R, Kyle E, Nguyen P, Trepel J, Ingui C, Neckers L. Genistein-stimulated adherence of prostate cancer cells is associated with the binding of focal adhesion kinase to beta-1-integrin. Clinical & experimental metastasis. 1996 Sep;14(4):389-98. PubMed PMID: 8878413.

[357] Farina HG, Pomies M, Alonso DF, Gomez DE. Antitumor and antiangiogenic activity of soy isoflavone genistein in mouse models of melanoma and breast cancer. Oncology reports. 2006 Oct;16(4):885-91. PubMed PMID: 16969510.

[358] Vantyghem SA, Wilson SM, Postenka CO, Al-Katib W, Tuck AB, Chambers AF. Dietary genistein reduces metastasis in a postsurgical orthotopic breast cancer model. Cancer Res. 2005 Apr 15;65(8):3396-403. PubMed PMID: 15833874.

[359] Zhang Y, Zhu G, Gu S, Chen X, Hu H, Weng S. Genistein inhibits osteolytic bone metastasis and enhances bone mineral in nude mice. Environmental Toxicology and Pharmacology. 2010; 30:37-44.

[360] Hauck CR, Hsia DA, Schlaepfer DD. The focal adhesion kinase--a regulator of cell migration and invasion. IUBMB Life. 2002 Feb;53(2):115-9. PubMed PMID: 12049193.

[361] McLean GW, Carragher NO, Avizienyte E, Evans J, Brunton VG, Frame MC. The role of focal-adhesion kinase in cancer - a new therapeutic opportunity. Nat Rev Cancer. 2005 Jul;5(7):505-15. PubMed PMID: 16069815.

[362] Lark AL, Livasy CA, Dressler L, Moore DT, Millikan RC, Geradts J, et al. High focal adhesion kinase expression in invasive breast carcinomas is associated with an aggressive phenotype. Mod Pathol. 2005 Oct;18(10):1289-94. PubMed PMID: 15861214.

[363] Lahlou H, Sanguin-Gendreau V, Zuo D, Cardiff RD, McLean GW, Frame MC, et al. Mammary epithelial-specific disruption of the focal adhesion kinase blocks mammary tumor progression. Proc Natl Acad Sci USA. 2007 Dec 18;104(51):20302-7. PubMed PMID: 18056629.

[364] Xu LH, Yang X, Bradham CA, Brenner DA, Baldwin AS, Jr., Craven RJ, et al. The focal adhesion kinase suppresses transformation-associated, anchorage-independent apoptosis in human breast cancer cells. Involvement of death receptor-related signaling pathways. J Biol Chem. 2000 Sep 29;275(39):30597-604. PubMed PMID: 10899173.

[365] Beviglia L, Golubovskaya V, Xu L, Yang X, Craven RJ, Cance WG. Focal adhesion kinase N-terminus in breast carcinoma cells induces rounding, detachment and apoptosis. The Biochemical journal. 2003 Jul 1;373(Pt 1):201-10. PubMed PMID: 12659633.

[366] Azios NGaD, S. Role of phytoestrogens modulating focal adhesions and focal adhesion kinase (FAK) activity in breast cancer cells. Li J, Li SA, Llombart-Bosch, A, editor. NY: Springer-Verlag; 2005.

[367] Mitra SK, Lim ST, Chi A, Schlaepfer DD. Intrinsic focal adhesion kinase activity controls orthotopic breast carcinoma metastasis via the regulation of urokinase plasminogen activator expression in a syngeneic tumor model. Oncogene. 2006 Jul 27;25(32):4429-40. PubMed PMID: 16547501.

[368] Wu ZS, Wu Q, Yang JH, Wang HQ, Ding XD, Yang F, et al. Prognostic significance of MMP-9 and TIMP-1 serum and tissue expression in breast cancer. Int J Cancer. 2008 May 1;122(9):2050-6. PubMed PMID: 18172859.

[369] Perentes JY, Kirkpatrick ND, Nagano S, Smith EY, Shaver CM, Sgroi D, et al. Cancer cell associated MT1-MMP promotes blood vessel invasion and distant metastasis in triple-negative mammary tumors. Cancer Res. 2011 May 13. PubMed PMID: 21571860.

[370] Shao ZM, Wu J, Shen ZZ, Barsky SH. Genistein exerts multiple suppressive effects on human breast carcinoma cells. Cancer Res. 1998 Nov 1;58(21):4851-7. PubMed PMID: 9809990.

[371] Shao ZM, Wu J, Shen ZZ, Barsky SH. Genistein inhibits both constitutive and EGF-stimulated invasion in ER-negative human breast carcinoma cell lines. Anticancer Res. 1998 May-Jun;18(3A):1435-9. PubMed PMID: 9673352.

[372] Kousidou OC, Mitropoulou TN, Roussidis AE, Kletsas D, Theocharis AD, Karamanos NK. Genistein suppresses the invasive potential of human breast cancer cells through transcriptional regulation of metalloproteinases and their tissue inhibitors. Int J Oncol. 2005 Apr;26(4):1101-9. PubMed PMID: 15754008.

[373] Silva D. Signaling pathways responsible for cancer cell invasion as targets for cancer therapy. Current cancer drug targets. 2004;Jun 4(4):327-36.

[374] Cao Y, Karin M. NF-kappaB in mammary gland development and breast cancer. J Mammary Gland Biol Neoplasia. 2003 Apr;8(2):215-23. PubMed PMID: 14635796.

[375] Li Y, Ahmed F, Ali S, Philip PA, Kucuk O, Sarkar FH. Inactivation of nuclear factor kappaB by soy isoflavone genistein contributes to increased apoptosis induced by chemotherapeutic agents in human cancer cells. Cancer Res. 2005 Aug 1;65(15): 6934-42. PubMed PMID: 16061678.

[376] Li Z, Li J, Mo B, Hu C, Liu H, Qi H, et al. Genistein induces cell apoptosis in MDA-MB-231 breast cancer cells via the mitogen-activated protein kinase pathway. Toxicol *In Vitro*. 2008 Oct;22(7):1749-53. PubMed PMID: 18761399.

[377] Vanden Berghe W, Dijsselbloem N, Vermeulen L, Ndlovu MN, Boone E, Haegeman G. Attenuation of mitogen- and stress-activated protein kinase-1-driven nuclear fac-

tor-kappaB gene expression by soy isoflavones does not require estrogenic activity. Cancer Res. 2006 May 1;66(9):4852-62. PubMed PMID: 16651441.

[378] Kazi A, Daniel KG, Smith DM, Kumar NB, Dou QP. Inhibition of the proteasome activity, a novel mechanism associated with the tumor cell apoptosis-inducing ability of genistein. Biochemical pharmacology. 2003 Sep 15;66(6):965-76. PubMed PMID: 12963483.

[379] Sakamoto T, Horiguchi H, Oguma E, Kayama F. Effects of diverse dietary phytoestrogens on cell growth, cell cycle and apoptosis in estrogen-receptor-positive breast cancer cells. The Journal of nutritional biochemistry. 2010 Sep;21(9):856-64. PubMed PMID: 19800779.

[380] Clarke DB, Bailey V, Lloyd AS. Determination of phytoestrogens in dietary supplements by LC-MS/MS. Food Addit Contam Part A Chem Anal Control Expo Risk Assess. 2008 May;25(5):534-47. PubMed PMID: 18478479.

[381] Khaodhiar L, Ricciotti HA, Li L, Pan W, Schickel M, Zhou J, et al. Daidzein-rich isoflavone aglycones are potentially effective in reducing hot flashes in menopausal women. Menopause. 2008 Jan-Feb;15(1):125-32. PubMed PMID: 18257146.

[382] Martinez-Montemayor MM, Otero-Franqui E, Martinez J, De La Mota-Peynado A, Cubano LA, Dharmawardhane S. Individual and combined soy isoflavones exert differential effects on metastatic cancer progression. Clinical & experimental metastasis. 2010 Oct;27(7):465-80. PubMed PMID: 20517637.

[383] Ju YH, Allred CD, Allred KF, Karko KL, Doerge DR, Helferich WG. Physiological concentrations of dietary genistein dose-dependently stimulate growth of estrogen-dependent human breast cancer (MCF-7) tumors implanted in athymic nude mice. J Nutr. 2001 Nov;131(11):2957-62. PubMed PMID: 11694625.

[384] Ju YH, Doerge DR, Allred KF, Allred CD, Helferich WG. Dietary genistein negates the inhibitory effect of tamoxifen on growth of estrogen-dependent human breast cancer (MCF-7) cells implanted in athymic mice. Cancer Res. 2002 May 1;62(9): 2474-7. PubMed PMID: 11980635.

[385] Ju YH, Fultz J, Allred KF, Doerge DR, Helferich WG. Effects of dietary daidzein and its metabolite, equol, at physiological concentrations on the growth of estrogen-dependent human breast cancer (MCF-7) tumors implanted in ovariectomized athymic mice. Carcinogenesis. 2006 Apr;27(4):856-63. PubMed PMID: 16399773.

[386] Messina MJ, Wood CE. Soy isoflavones, estrogen therapy, and breast cancer risk: analysis and commentary. Nutr J. 2008;7:17. PubMed PMID: 18522734.

[387] Guo TL, Chi RP, Hernandez DM, Auttachoat W, Zheng JF. Decreased 7,12-dimethylbenz[a]anthracene-induced carcinogenesis coincides with the induction of antitumor immunities in adult female B6C3F1 mice pretreated with genistein. Carcinogenesis. 2007 Dec;28(12):2560-6. PubMed PMID: 17916904.

[388] Seo HS, Choi HS, Choi HS, Choi YK, Um JY, Choi I, et al. Phytoestrogens induce apoptosis via extrinsic pathway, inhibiting nuclear factor-kappaB signaling in HER2-overexpressing breast cancer cells. Anticancer Res. 2011 Oct;31(10):3301-13. PubMed PMID: 21965740.

[389] Fletcher RJ. Food sources of phyto-oestrogens and their precursors in Europe. Br J Nutr. 2003 Jun;89 Suppl 1:S39-43. PubMed PMID: 12725655.

[390] Munro IC, Harwood M, Hlywka JJ, Stephen AM, Doull J, Flamm WG, et al. Soy isoflavones: a safety review. Nutr Rev. 2003 Jan;61(1):1-33. PubMed PMID: 12638461.

[391] Golbitz P. Traditional soyfoods: processing and products. J Nutr. 1995 Mar;125(3 Suppl):570S-2S. PubMed PMID: 7884535.

[392] Chua R, Anderson K, Chen J, Hu M. Quality, labeling accuracy, and cost comparison of purified soy isoflavonoid products. J Altern Complement Med. 2004 Dec;10(6): 1053-60. PubMed PMID: 15674001.

[393] Lockwood GB. The quality of commercially available nutraceutical supplements and food sources. J Pharm Pharmacol. 2011 Jan;63(1):3-10. PubMed PMID: 21155809.

[394] Shu XO, Zheng Y, Cai H, Gu K, Chen Z, Zheng W, et al. Soy food intake and breast cancer survival. Jama. 2009 Dec 9;302(22):2437-43. PubMed PMID: 19996398.

[395] Guha N, Kwan ML, Quesenberry CP, Jr., Weltzien EK, Castillo AL, Caan BJ. Soy isoflavones and risk of cancer recurrence in a cohort of breast cancer survivors: the Life After Cancer Epidemiology study. Breast Cancer Res Treat. 2009 Nov;118(2):395-405. PubMed PMID: 19221874.

[396] Boyapati SM, Shu XO, Ruan ZX, Dai Q, Cai Q, Gao YT, et al. Soyfood intake and breast cancer survival: a followup of the Shanghai Breast Cancer Study. Breast Cancer Res Treat. 2005 Jul;92(1):11-7. PubMed PMID: 15980986.

[397] Dong JY, Qin LQ. Soy isoflavones consumption and risk of breast cancer incidence or recurrence: a meta-analysis of prospective studies. Breast Cancer Res Treat. 2011 Jan; 125(2):315-23. PubMed PMID: 21113655.

[398] Wu AH, Yu MC, Tseng CC, Pike MC. Epidemiology of soy exposures and breast cancer risk. Br J Cancer. 2008 Jan 15;98(1):9-14. PubMed PMID: 18182974.

[399] Petrakis NL, Barnes S, King EB, Lowenstein J, Wiencke J, Lee MM, et al. Stimulatory influence of soy protein isolate on breast secretion in pre- and postmenopausal women. Cancer Epidemiol Biomarkers Prev. 1996 Oct;5(10):785-94. PubMed PMID: 8896889.

[400] Allred CD, Ju YH, Allred KF, Chang J, Helferich WG. Dietary genistin stimulates growth of estrogen-dependent breast cancer tumors similar to that observed with genistein. Carcinogenesis. 2001 Oct;22(10):1667-73. PubMed PMID: 11577007.

[401] Sa G, Das T. Anti cancer effects of curcumin: cycle of life and death. Cell Div. 2008;3:14. PubMed PMID: 18834508.

[402] Ramachandran C, Fonseca HB, Jhabvala P, Escalon EA, Melnick SJ. Curcumin inhibits telomerase activity through human telomerase reverse transcritpase in MCF-7 breast cancer cell line. Cancer Lett. 2002 Oct 8;184(1):1-6. PubMed PMID: 12104041.

[403] Holy JM. Curcumin disrupts mitotic spindle structure and induces micronucleation in MCF-7 breast cancer cells. Mutat Res. 2002 Jun 27;518(1):71-84. PubMed PMID: 12063069.

[404] Liu Q, Loo WT, Sze SC, Tong Y. Curcumin inhibits cell proliferation of MDA-MB-231 and BT-483 breast cancer cells mediated by down-regulation of NFkappaB, cyclinD and MMP-1 transcription. Phytomedicine : international journal of phytotherapy and phytopharmacology. 2009 Oct;16(10):916-22. PubMed PMID: 19524420.

[405] Choudhuri T, Pal S, Agwarwal ML, Das T, Sa G. Curcumin induces apoptosis in human breast cancer cells through p53-dependent Bax induction. FEBS Lett. 2002 Feb 13;512(1-3):334-40. PubMed PMID: 11852106.

[406] Aggarwal BB, Shishodia S, Takada Y, Banerjee S, Newman RA, Bueso-Ramos CE, et al. Curcumin suppresses the paclitaxel-induced nuclear factor-kappaB pathway in breast cancer cells and inhibits lung metastasis of human breast cancer in nude mice. Clin Cancer Res. 2005 Oct 15;11(20):7490-8. PubMed PMID: 16243823.

[407] Bachmeier B, Nerlich AG, Iancu CM, Cilli M, Schleicher E, Vene R, et al. The chemopreventive polyphenol Curcumin prevents hematogenous breast cancer metastases in immunodeficient mice. Cellular physiology and biochemistry : international journal of experimental cellular physiology, biochemistry, and pharmacology. 2007;19(1-4):137-52. PubMed PMID: 17310108.

[408] Boonrao M, Yodkeeree S, Ampasavate C, Anuchapreeda S, Limtrakul P. The inhibitory effect of turmeric curcuminoids on matrix metalloproteinase-3 secretion in human invasive breast carcinoma cells. Arch Pharm Res. 2010 Jul;33(7):989-98. PubMed PMID: 20661707.

[409] Chiu TL, Su CC. Curcumin inhibits proliferation and migration by increasing the Bax to Bcl-2 ratio and decreasing NF-kappaBp65 expression in breast cancer MDA-MB-231 cells. International journal of molecular medicine. 2009 Apr;23(4):469-75. PubMed PMID: 19288022.

[410] Bachmeier BE, Mohrenz IV, Mirisola V, Schleicher E, Romeo F, Hohneke C, et al. Curcumin downregulates the inflammatory cytokines CXCL1 and -2 in breast cancer cells via NFkappaB. Carcinogenesis. 2008 Apr;29(4):779-89. PubMed PMID: 17999991.

[411] Verma SP, Salamone E, Goldin B. Curcumin and genistein, plant natural products, show synergistic inhibitory effects on the growth of human breast cancer MCF-7 cells 68 Natural Product Discovery – From the Field, to the Lab Bench, to the Medicine

Cabinet induced by estrogenic pesticides. Biochem Biophys Res Commun. 1997 Apr 28;233(3):692-6. PubMed PMID: 9168916.

[412] Sharma RA, Gescher AJ, Steward WP. Curcumin: the story so far. Eur J Cancer. 2005 Sep;41(13):1955-68. PubMed PMID: 16081279.

[413] Sharma RA, Euden SA, Platton SL, Cooke DN, Shafayat A, Hewitt HR, et al. Phase I clinical trial of oral curcumin: biomarkers of systemic activity and compliance. Clin Cancer Res. 2004 Oct 15;10(20):6847-54. PubMed PMID: 15501961.

[414] Vareed SK, Kakarala M, Ruffin MT, Crowell JA, Normolle DP, Djuric Z, et al. Pharmacokinetics of curcumin conjugate metabolites in healthy human subjects. Cancer Epidemiol Biomarkers Prev. 2008 Jun;17(6):1411-7. PubMed PMID: 18559556.

[415] Garcea G, Jones DJ, Singh R, Dennison AR, Farmer PB, Sharma RA, et al. Detection of curcumin and its metabolites in hepatic tissue and portal blood of patients following oral administration. Br J Cancer. 2004 Mar 8;90(5):1011-5. PubMed PMID: 14997198.

[416] Carroll RE, Benya RV, Turgeon DK, Vareed S, Neuman M, Rodriguez L, et al. Phase IIa clinical trial of curcumin for the prevention of colorectal neoplasia. Cancer Prev Res (Phila). 2011 Mar;4(3):354-64. PubMed PMID: 21372035.

[417] Bayet-Robert M, Kwiatkowski F, Leheurteur M, Gachon F, Planchat E, Abrial C, et al. Phase I dose escalation trial of docetaxel plus curcumin in patients with advanced and metastatic breast cancer. Cancer Biol Ther. Jan;9(1):8-14. PubMed PMID: 19901561.

[418] Somasundaram S, Edmund NA, Moore DT, Small GW, Shi YY, Orlowski RZ. Dietary curcumin inhibits chemotherapy-induced apoptosis in models of human breast cancer. Cancer Res. 2002 Jul 1;62(13):3868-75. PubMed PMID: 12097302.

[419] Kakarala M, Brenner DE, Korkaya H, Cheng C, Tazi K, Ginestier C, et al. Targeting breast stem cells with the cancer preventive compounds curcumin and piperine. Breast Cancer Res Treat. 2010 Aug;122(3):777-85. PubMed PMID: 19898931.

[420] Burgos-Moron E, Calderon-Montano JM, Salvador J, Robles A, Lopez-Lazaro M. The dark side of curcumin. Int J Cancer. 2010 Apr 1;126(7):1771-5. PubMed PMID: 19830693.

[421] Shoba G, Joy D, Joseph T, Majeed M, Rajendran R, Srinivas PS. Influence of piperine on the pharmacokinetics of curcumin in animals and human volunteers. Planta Med. 1998 May;64(4):353-6. PubMed PMID: 9619120.

[422] Bhardwaj RK, Glaeser H, Becquemont L, Klotz U, Gupta SK, Fromm MF. Piperine, a major constituent of black pepper, inhibits human P-glycoprotein and CYP3A4. J Pharmacol Exp Ther. 2002 Aug;302(2):645-50. PubMed PMID: 12130727.

[423] Kurien BT, Scofield RH. Oral administration of heat-solubilized curcumin for potentially increasing curcumin bioavailability in experimental animals. Int J Cancer. 2009 Oct 15;125(8):1992-3. PubMed PMID: 19618459.